HANDBOOK OF CRITICAL CARE NURSING

Springhouse Corporation
Springhouse, Pennsylvania

Staff

Senior Publisher, Trade and Textbooks
Minnie B. Rose, RN, BSN, MEd

Art Director
John Hubbard

Senior Editors
Diane Labus, David Moreau

Editors
Janice Fisher, Kathy Goldberg, Marguerite Kelly

Acquisitions Editor
Patricia Fischer, RN, BSN

Associate Acquisitions Editors
Louise Quinn, Betsy Snyder

Clinical Consultant
Susan Galea, RN, MSN

Copy Editors
Diane Armento, Janet Hodgson, Suzanne Kozischek, Pamela Wingrod

Design
Stephanie Peters (senior associate art director), Elaine Ezrow, Donald G. Knauss, Mary Ludwicki

Manufacturing
Debbie Meiris, T.A. Landis, Andreas Hess

Editorial Assistants
Stephanie Franchetti, Jeanne Napier

Printed in the United States of America. For information, write Springhouse Corporation,

1111 Bethlehem Pike, P.O. Box 908, Springhouse, PA 19477-0908.

HCCN-010196

ℛ A member of the Reed Elsevier plc group

Library of Congress Cataloging-in-Publication Data

Handbook of critical care nursing.
    p. cm.
  Includes bibliographical references and index.
  1. Intensive care nursing—Handbooks, manuals, etc.
  I. Springhouse Corporation.
  [DNLM: 1. Critical care—methods—handbooks. 2. Critical care—nurses' instruction. WY 49 H235 1996]
RT120.I5H362 1996
610.73'61—dc20
DNLM/DLC   95-41588
ISBN 0-87434-774-2 (alk. paper)   CIP

Contents

Contributors

Esam Al-Khasib, RN, MSN
Clinical Nurse Specialist
Amal Cancer Center
Amman, Jordan
(Immunosuppression)

Ruthie Bach, RN, MSN, CNS, CCRN, CEN
Director Case Management
Doctors Hospital
Groves, Texas
(Abdominal trauma, Bowel disorders, Pancreatitis, Thoracic trauma)

Tracy Banks, RN, BS, CCRN
Senior Clinical Nurse
Bone Marrow Transplant Unit
The Johns Hopkins Oncology Center
Baltimore, Maryland
(Disseminated intravascular coagulation)

Ellie Franges, RN, MSN, CNRN, CCRN
Neuroscience Coordinator
Sacred Heart Hospital
Allentown, Pennsylvania
(Cerebral aneurysm, Head trauma)

Susan Breda Galea, RN, MSN, CCRN
Critical Care Nurse, Surgical Intensive Care Unit
Hospital of the University of Pennsylvania
Philadelphia, Pennsylvania
(Angina, Burns)

Cynthia Hermey, RN, MN, CCRN, CS
Critical Care Nurse Manager
Oconee Memorial Hospital
Seneca, South Carolina
(Pneumonia)

Joyce Johnson, RN, PhD, CCRN
Assistant Professor
Georgia State University
Atlanta, Georgia
(Documentation)

Martha Merritt Kennedy, BSN, RN, CCRN
Critical Care Instructor
The Johns Hopkins Oncology Center
Baltimore, Maryland
(Aspiration, Gastrointestinal hemorrhage, Hepatic failure, Pulmonary embolism)

Sharon Kumm, RN, MN, CCRN
Clinical Instructor
University of Kansas Medical Center, School of Nursing
Kansas City, Kansas
(Near drowning)

Sheila Lawton, RN, MSN
Education Specialist
Bergen Mercy Medical Center
Omaha, Nebraska
(Asthma)

Tamara Luedtke, RN, BSN, CCRN
Nurse Manager, Critical Care Unit
Hendrick Medical Center
Abilene, Texas
(Adult respiratory distress syndrome)

Dawna Martich, RN, MSN
Director, Clinical/Educational Program Development
Idea Exchange
Pittsburgh, Pennsylvania
(Cerebrovascular accident, Hypertensive crisis, Peripheral vascular disease, Renal failure, Renal trauma, Respiratory failure, Spinal cord injury, Nursing Diagnoses appendix)

Carrie McCoy, RN, MSN, CEN
Associate Professor of Nursing
Northern Kentucky University
Highland Heights, Kentucky
(Toxic ingestion)

Leanna Miller, RN, MN, CCRN, CEN
Critical Care Nurse Specialist
Children's Hospital Medical Center of
Central Georgia
Macon, Georgia
(Diabetes insipidus, Diabetic ketoacidosis, Hypoglycemia, HHNS, Organ transplantation, SIADH, Shock)

Chris Nicolai, RN, CS, MS, CNP
Certified Nurse Practitioner
Critical Care Department
Sioux Valley Hospital
Sioux Falls, South Dakota
(Aortic aneurysm)

Barbara B. Ott, RN, PhD, CCRN
Assistant Professor
Villanova University
Villanova, Pennsylvania
(Ethical decision making)

Brenda Kay Shelton, RN, MS, CCRN, OCN
Critical Care Clinical Nurse Specialist
The Johns Hopkins Oncology Center
Baltimore, Maryland
(Acquired immunodeficiency syndrome, Immunosuppression)

Mary Stahl, RN, MSN, CCRN
Cardiovascular Clinical Nurse Specialist
Mid America Heart Institute of St.
Luke's Hospital
Kansas City, Missouri
(Arrhythmias, Myocardial conduction defects)

Johanna K. Stiesmeyer, RN, MS, CCRN
Cardiovascular Education Specialist
Camino Healthcare
Mountain View, California
(Angina)

Patricia L. Vaska, RN, MSN, CNP, CCRN
Cardiovascular Surgery Nurse Practitioner
Clinical Nurse Specialist
Sioux Valley Hospital
Sioux Falls, South Dakota
(Cardiomyopathy, Congestive heart failure, Pericarditis, Valvular heart disease)

Sharon Walker, RN, MSN, CCRN, CNRN
Clinical Nurse Specialist - ICU/CCU
Lovelace Health Systems
Albuquerque, New Mexico
(Brain tumors, Encephalopathy, Seizures)

Joni Walton, RN, RRT, MSN
Critical Care Clinical Nurse Specialist
Saint Luke's Hospital of Kansas City
Kansas City, Missouri
(Cardiac trauma, Pneumothorax)

Sandra K. Williams, RN, MSN, CNN, ACLS
Nurse Manager
Lenoir Memorial Hospital
Kinston, North Carolina
(Electrolyte imbalances)

Reviewers

Susan C. Baltrus, RN,C, MSN
Instructor of Nursing Science
Central Maine Medical Center, School
of Nursing
Lewiston, Maine

Zara R. Brenner, RN, CS, MS
Assistant Professor of Nursing
SUNY-Brockport
Clinical Nurse Specialist, Surgery
The Genesee Hospital
Rochester, New York

Renee Cantwell, RN, MSN, CPHQ
Clinical Quality Management Specialist
VA Medical Center
Philadelphia, Pennsylvania

Lois M. Catts, RN, MS, CCRN
Critical Care Clinical Nurse Specialist
St. Elizabeth Medical Center
Yakima, Washington

**Ellie Z. Franges, RN, MSN, CNRN,
CCRN**
Neuroscience Coordinator
Sacred Heart Hospital
Allentown, Pennsylvania

Sara T. Fry, RN, PhD, FAAN
Henry R. Luce Professor of Nursing
Ethics
Boston College School of Nursing
Chestnut Hill, Massachusetts

Debra R. Hanna, RN, MSN, CNRN
Assistant Director of Nursing, Acute
Care
Bergen Pines County Hospital
Paramus, New Jersey

Cynthia Hermey, RN, MN, CCRN, CS
Critical Care Nurse Manager
Oconee Memorial Hospital
Seneca, South Carolina

Nancy Holloway, RN, MSN
Critical Care Educator
Orinda, California

**Marguerite McMillan Jackson,
RN, MS, CIC, FAAN**
Administrative Director, Epidemiology
Unit
University of California San Diego Medical Center
San Diego, California

**Sharon Lehmann, RN, MS, CCRN,
CNSN**
CV/Interventional Radiology Nurse Clinician
University of Minnesota Hospital
Minneapolis, Minnesota

Carrie A. McCoy, RN, MSN, CEN
Associate Professor of Nursing
Northern Kentucky University
Highland Heights, Kentucky

Teresa A. Palmer, RN, MSN, CNP
Adult Nurse Practitioner
Assistant Professor, Clinical Nursing
Acute Care Nurse Practitioner Track
University of Medicine and Dentistry
Newark, New Jersey

George Saunderlin, RN, BSN, CGRN
Staff Nurse, Endoscopy Suite
Medical College of Virginia Hospitals
Richmond, Virginia

Cathy Sellergren, RN, MSN, CCRN
Pulmonary Case Manager
Hinsdale Hospital
Hinsdale, Illinois

Julie A. Shinn, RN, MA, CCRN, FAAN
Cardiovascular Clinical Specialist
Stanford University Medical Center
Stanford, California

Leslie Ann Siconolfi, RN, MSN,
CCRN
Case Manager, Liver & Renal Trans-
plant Services
University of Pittsburgh Medical Center
Pittsburgh, Pennsylvania

Patricia Smith-Regojo, RN, BSN
Care Coordinator
Franciscan Health System
St. Agnes Medical Center
Philadelphia, Pennsylvania

Linda Stahl, RN, MSN, CCRN
Assistant Professor of Nursing
Mesa State College
Department of Nursing and Allied
Health
Grand Junction, Colorado

Jeanne M. Urban, RN, MSN
Clinical Nurse Specialist
Cardiothoracic Surgery, Ltd.
St. Louis, Missouri

Steven A. Weinman, RN, CEN
Emergency Department Clinical Educa-
tor
Truman Medical Center
Kansas City, Missouri

Foreword

Health care continues to be ever-changing, both from a scientific and an economic perspective. Nurses have witnessed a steady increase in the number of beds needed in intensive care units and other critical care settings due to the rise in patient acuity levels over the past decade. Critical care nurses must therefore keep pace with the latest technological advances and nursing interventions to meet the demands of acutely ill patients, many of whom have multiple, complex medical problems.

Handbook of Critical Care Nursing, an excellent resource for bedside nurses and advanced practitioners, presents the pathophysiology, medical treatments, and nursing care of patient-focused diagnoses most commonly encountered by critical care nurses. Arranged alphabetically, the diagnoses follow a carefully plotted format to ensure quick access to vital facts. Hundreds of tables, flowcharts, and illustrations accompany the entries, providing succinct descriptions and accurate visual renderings of essential information.

Each entry begins with a brief introduction to the disorder. *Pathophysiology* then presents in-depth explanations of underlying causes. *Clinical assessment* provides essential information about history taking and physical findings. *Diagnosis* covers common diagnostic findings, along with normal and abnormal laboratory test results for comparative analysis. *Treatment and care* offers a thorough discussion of standard and state-of-the-art medical treatments and related nursing care. Finally, each entry concludes with *Prognosis* and relevant *Discharge planning* guidelines. Key nursing interventions and potential complications are highlighted throughout, making this handy reference practical to use at the patient's bedside.

Appendices offer quick-reference charts on emergency drugs, laboratory values, therapeutic and toxic drug levels, normal hemodynamic variables, and nursing diagnoses relevant to critical care. *Selected references* provide further suggestions for review, and the detailed *Index* lets you find essential information fast.

Each topic in *Handbook of Critical Care Nursing* has been carefully reviewed by experts to ensure accuracy, currentness, and clarity. Contributors have included significant information about ongoing research that will undoubtedly impact the future care of patients with critical care disorders. *Handbook of Critical Care Nursing* is a succinctly written, up-to-date quick reference that will benefit the bedside critical care nurse for years to come.

Susan J. Quaal, RN,PhD,CVS,CCRN
Cardiovascular Clinical Specialist
Department of Veterans Affairs Medical Center
Associate Clinical Professor
University of Utah Health Sciences
Salt Lake City, Utah

Issues in
Critical Care
Nursing

Documentation in critical care

In intensive care units (ICUs), the acuity of illness and often rapid changes in patient status and treatment regimens make clear and accurate communication a major priority. Because patient care is so intensive and time-consuming, nurses also should try to be as concise as possible when documenting, allowing more time for hands-on care. And because many specialized health care personnel contribute to the care of the critically ill patient, any written communication about the patient's status should be easily interpreted and readily accessible to enhance collaborative care.

Legal implications of documentation

Documentation typically is a major concern in any legal claim involving nursing malpractice. Lack of documentation about a specific observation or action suggests that the observation or action was never performed, and improper documentation of the observation or action lends credence to the malpractice claim. To avoid the legal pitfalls of documentation, make sure that all procedures, actions, and observations are recorded clearly and thoroughly (see *General principles of documentation*).

Patient care guidelines and outcome standards

Standards of nursing care are structural guidelines for planning and delivery of expected patient care. They are designed to direct nursing practice and to protect the public. Standards represent agreed-upon strategies for management that fall within the range of acceptable practice as based on the most current research and literature and established by experts in health care.

Standards have been outlined by various national and specialty nursing organizations and state boards of nursing to ensure quality patient care in all patient settings, including ICUs. Most health care facilities use

General principles of documentation

The following principles are the cornerstone of proper documentation. Use them as a guide to help avoid a lawsuit. Additionally, always follow unit and institutional documentation protocols to conform with established norms.

Ensure accuracy
• Record the patient's name and identification number and the full date on each page of the patient's chart.
• Record the entries in consecutive order as close as possible to the time care was given or an observation was noted.
• Do not skip lines between entries.
• When charting an observation, limit the description to only pertinent or supporting facts.
• Avoid labeling the patient's behaviors; use the patient's own words to describe reported symptoms.
• Do not erase or obliterate a mistake; instead, draw a thin line through the erroneous information to keep the original information intact. Include your initials.

Strive for brevity and clarity
• Do not duplicate in your narrative data that is recorded on another form (graphic sheet, checklist).
• Use concise phrases and standard abbreviations.
• Avoid using vague or inflammatory phrases, such as "appears to be" or "somehow this happened."
• Omit statements of blame.

Ensure comprehensiveness, but stick to the facts
• Record your interpretations of abnormal data and the actions taken to address these concerns.
• Use patient-sensitive language without subjective terminology.
• Use objective observations with data to support analyses.
• Document the time the health care providers were notified or paged, and document when the call was returned.

standards developed by the Joint Commission for Accreditation of Healthcare Organizations (JCAHO) as their basis for health care practice, because these are the standards by which the facility will be judged for accreditation.

In addition, nurses in many health care facilities are involved in outcome or case management systems that rely on critical pathways to outline the course of a hospital stay for specific patient populations. A critical pathway is a detailed treatment regimen that includes all of the basic elements of care to be provided for a specific patient population to achieve desired outcomes. The pathways contain required services needed from all disciplines involved in the patient's care and map the care to be provided each day, from admission through discharge. When a patient's course of progress does not follow the designed map, the variance and its cause are identified and a plan is designed to restore the patient to the pathway (or to place the patient on a different pathway if indicated).

The advantages of outcome management for critical care nurses using critical pathways include:

• clearly stated expectations related to the progress of a patient and the multidisciplinary care needed to meet those expectations

• interdisciplinary collaboration

• proactive nature of nursing care that is designed to promote the smooth progression of the patient through the ICU stay

• improved consistency and continuity of care.

Disadvantages of using critical pathways include:

• lack of individualization inherent in these paths, which are based on the normal progression of a typical patient (many ICU patients do not progress normally because of their complex problems, which might require a combination of paths)

• possible suppression of creativity in caregivers who rely on pathways and become less sensitive to patient responses that might require a deviation from the path to meet the desired outcome.

Nursing documentation

Regardless of which standards are used in the ICU, quality patient care must be provided and documented. JCAHO standards clearly speak to the need to assess actions and document improvement, as well as the need to communicate relevant information. Documentation is a key element in monitoring and evaluating the quality of patient care and identifying variances from an expected path of progress. Standards guide nursing care and documentation, whereas documentation provides the mechanism for evaluation and refinement of standards and critical pathways.

Plans of care

The JCAHO standards of nursing care, which focus on documenting evidence of planning and evaluation of quality patient care, dictate that critical care nurses have a written plan of care for each patient. In critical care units, as in other patient care settings, these plans of care may guide the oral and written communication of patient care. The most common format for care planning in the ICU is the standardized plan of care.

Standardized plans of care are based on established nursing care standards and techniques that address common, expected patient problems. Typically organized by nursing diagnoses or patient problems, these plans include an overall patient goal (often expressed in terms of outcome criteria) as well as independent and interdependent nursing interventions for achieving the goal. The nurse uses the outcome criteria to evaluate the plan's effectiveness and to revise the plan as needed.

Advantages to using standardized plans of care include:
• ability of nurses to care for many types of patients because plans are standardized
• time saved by nurses preparing a plan of care
• consistently high level of the plans of care and documentation by nurses
• greater depth of care by nurses using these detailed plans.

Disadvantages include:
• limitations of plans for use in complex cases, such as ICU patients with problems that change frequently and involve a multitude of contributing factors
• the inclusion of obvious, simple interventions.

Variations in documentation

Narrative documentation is still the most common form of nursing documentation in patient care. A freeform type of reporting, narrative documentation varies in length and content, depending on the nurse and patient situation.

Various types of narrative charting have been developed over the years. The most common types are outlined below:

• Charting by exception: Charting in which only the deviations from normal data are documented and a checklist is used to record assessment of normal findings and routine activities.

• SOAPIE(R) charting: A form of narrative charting that allows the nurse to discuss Subjective and Objective data, an Assessment of the data, a Plan of action, the Implementation of the plan, the Evaluation of the plan, and in some cases Revision of the plan.

• Focus charting: A more abbreviated form of narrative charting in which notes are centered around a specific patient problem or focus. Nurses write a narrative of Data, Action, and Response related to a specific focus. Routine nursing activities are entered on a checklist.

• ICU flowsheets: Used by many critical care nurses, they are designed to include a record of all or most of the data collected on a patient during a 24-hour period; they also allow space to document, via a checklist or short narrative, the nursing care provided to the patient.

• Computerized documentation: Currently being used in some units to record all patient data (often with the exception of the medication record). In other units, the computer is used to document only portions of patient data; a checklist, flowsheet, or narrative nursing note sheet is used to record other information.

Computer programs are often designed or modified to fit the ICU's patient population. Computerized programs for nurses' notes vary from facility to facility. Some allow for standardized narratives, while other programs allow for freeform typed notes or a combination of standardized and freeform narratives. Some programs even incorporate the nursing process, allowing the nurse to identify whether the information relates to assessment, planning, implementation, or evaluation. Computers may be centralized at the nursing station or located at each patient's bedside. Several computers on the unit allow for accessibility of the same or different aspects of a chart by multiple persons at the same time.

Documentation is an important element in monitoring and evaluating the quality of patient care. Whatever the form of documentation used, it should provide an accurate picture of safe, quality nursing care.

Essential elements for ethical decision making

Critical care nurses often encounter situations that require the understanding of ethical principles and the ability to use and apply ethical decision making skills (see *Ethical principles and nursing interventions,* pages 8 and 9). To be most beneficial, nurses must respond to issues concerning fragmentation of care, increased use of medical technology, withdrawal of life support, and allocation of scarce resources.

Open the lines of communication
The first thing a nurse needs to do when faced with what appears to be an ethical problem is to ensure that all the facts are communicated by all of the people involved, including the patient, the family, the physician, and the nurse. The critical care nurse is the one who typically reassesses the patient's and family's understanding and perception of what has been said and what has been heard.

Supporting end-of-life decisions
Several ethical issues in the care of the critically ill seem to demand more attention than others. One of the most difficult issues is the extended use of sophisticated medical technologies. Sometimes, especially in critical care settings, the use of life-prolonging technologies seems to add to the suffering of the patient. It is then that the patient's goals and values must dictate proper

Ethical principles and nursing interventions

The following ethical principles and related nursing interventions help guide nursing practice in the critical care setting.

Principle	Description*	Nursing Interventions
Autonomy	Upholding the right of the patient to choose his or her own actions. Actions are chosen intentionally, with understanding, and without outside controlling influences.	• Listen carefully to what the patient says. • Encourage ongoing dialogue between the patient and physicians. • Encourage ongoing dialogue between the patient and family. • Support the patient's stated values. • Encourage the patient to enact a living will or durable power of attorney to ensure that wishes for the future are known. • Ensure adequate process of informed consent. • Facilitate the patient's choices. • Advocate for the patient.
Nonmaleficence	Inflicting no evil or harm on another individual. Negligence is an act of nonmaleficence.	• Do nothing to harm the patient. —Do not put the patient at risk of harm. —Remove anything that may harm the patient. • Keep up-to-date in the nursing field to prevent harm from the application of outdated information. • Maintain a high level of competence in nursing skills. • Think critically throughout the nursing process. • Know who to contact (even during the night) if the patient's wishes are not being honored or if good care is not being provided.
Beneficence	Promoting the welfare of others as well as preventing or removing harm. Involves careful analysis of the benefits and burdens of treatments.	• Provide expert nursing care. • Encourage others to provide expert nursing and medical care. • Carefully analyze benefits and burdens to the patient without reverting to physician or nurse paternalistic actions.

Ethical principles and nursing interventions (continued)

Principle	Description*	Nursing Interventions
Beneficence (continued)		• Provide information to help the patient weigh the benefits and burdens of treatment options. • Deliver nursing care in a manner that benefits the patient, not necessarily the staff or the institution. • Help the patient become adequately informed to make sound decisions. • Create ethical patient care policies that enable the nurse to provide good care. • Contribute to a good working environment that is interdisciplinary and patient-centered. • Participate in nursing research. • Contribute to the nursing literature. • Mentor less experienced nurses.
Justice	Ensuring that all people are treated equally and that all similarly situated persons receive their fair share.	• Distribute nursing care fairly on the basis of need. • Maintain equitable allocation of beds in the ICU. • Ensure that the allocation of organs for transplant is equitable. • Ensure that the assignment of nurses to patients is fair and based on the needs of patients. • Create ethical patient care policies that foster the equitable distribution of all scarce resources.

*Definitions of ethical principles are based on those discussed in Beauchamp, T.L., and Childress, J.F. (1994). *Principles of Biomedical Ethics*, New York: Oxford University Press.

medical and nursing interventions. Careful consideration of the patient's and family's goals and values and of the process of obtaining informed consent is essential.

Supporting the patient and family through difficult end-of-life decisions is a vital role of the critical care nurse. Equally difficult is the withdrawal of these life-sustaining technologies from patients who are terminally ill with irreversible conditions. It is difficult, yet ethically sound practice, to either withhold or withdraw life-sustaining treatments from patients who have expressed their wishes not to have these treatments. It also is ethically permissible to withhold or withdraw treatments that are futile.

Many times, it is appropriate to employ a treatment, such as mechanical ventilation, for a time-limited run to see if the patient will improve. If mechanical ventilation is not beneficial, it is ethically legitimate to withdraw the ventilator. The appropriate use of life-sustaining technologies depends on critical ethical analysis. This analysis tells us that there is no moral difference between withdrawing and withholding treatments.

Providing quality care

Fragmentation of care can be a major problem in the critical care unit. The American Association of Critical-Care Nurses encourages a collaborative practice model of patient care, identifying collaboration as a pivotal component of quality critical care. Nurses, physicians, and other health care providers can improve the care of critically ill patients and reduce overall stress with genuine collaborative practice and shared decision making.

The critical care nurse usually is an excellent patient advocate. However, being an advocate is not always without some risk. Institutional politics sometimes requires the successful patient advocate to be understanding and sophisticated while being calm, courteous, and persistent.

Another issue that is sometimes ethically disturbing in critical care is the allocation of scarce nursing resources. As the acuity level rises in critical care units, the problem of allocating nursing resources justly becomes difficult. Each unit should have policies that direct the allocation of beds and adequate numbers of nurses in critical care. The allocation of beds in the critical care unit is sometimes very difficult when more patients need to be admitted than there are beds available.

The challenge to give good care also is threatened if an insufficient number of nurses is available to give needed care. The critical care nurse's ability to prioritize and triage is of utmost importance in these decisions. The fair allocation of critical care resources should consider those with the greatest need and the highest probability of a positive outcome. Nurses cannot allow the financial bottom line to jeopardize patient care, but they can be full partners in holding costs down while demanding adequate staffing from administrators.

The larger question surrounding the value that society places on the benefits of critical care and the consequent costs of that care will be decided by public policy. It is hoped that critical care nurses will continue to add their perspectives to this policy debate and decision-making process.

Every institution that houses a critical care unit should have a hospital-based multidisciplinary patient care ethics committee. This committee should be made available to all patients, patients' families, physicians, nurses, and others (including relatives, social workers, residents, and clergy) who raise concerns about ethical decision making surrounding patient care. The policy and procedure manual in the critical care unit should describe the necessary procedure for a nurse to bring an issue before the committee. It is sometimes beneficial to ask the committee to present inservice education programs specific to the needs of those working in critical care.

Advocating the patient's wishes

The Patient Self-Determination Act encourages patients to put into writing all of their wishes concerning treatments at the end of life. End-of-life decisions may be documented in advance directive documents. The patient may choose to enact a living will or a durable power of attorney for health care. However, it is not mandatory that a patient complete such documents. Laws about advance directives vary from state to state, and it is important to know the laws in your own state. The role of the nurse should include giving the necessary information to enable the patient to make his or her own choices.

Because advance directives provide valuable guidance to the health care team, these documents should be placed in the patient's medical record. It is crucial to remember that, even though a patient has completed a living will or a durable power of attorney for health care, the document can be changed by the patient at any time. A verbal statement by the patient is all that is necessary. It would be wise for a nurse or a physician to have the patient state his wishes to more than one person.

Preserving the moral nursing code

The nurse has professional obligations to the patient and to society reflective of the dignity of individuals and the importance of a just society. The nurse's obligations to the patient must be integrated with an active participation in the moral dialogue regarding patient care. This dialogue is enhanced by effective communication skills and a profound sensitivity to patient needs. General moral rules for professional-patient relationships may help guide the nurse's actions.

The American Nurses Association's Code for Nurses also offers some guidance. The code gives guidance for professional relationships and the responsibilities of practicing nursing. The preamble of The Code for Nurses states that "since clients themselves are the primary decision makers in matters concerning their own health, treatment, and well-being, the goal of nursing actions is to support and enhance the client's responsibility and self-determination to the greatest extent possible" (ANA Code for Nurses, 1985).

Nurses have a moral commitment to uphold the statements in the code. Clinical judgments must be based on an understanding of moral principles. Society places its trust in nurses and therefore demands ethical practice from every nurse.

Care of Patients with Body System Dysfunctions

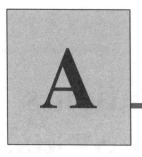

Abdominal trauma

Commonly a part of combined multisystem-multiorgan trauma, abdominal trauma also can occur as a singular injury. Most of those who are injured are under age 50, and half are involved in motor vehicle accidents. Injuries involving abdominal trauma are responsible for 13% to 15% of all trauma deaths in the United States.

Morbidity and mortality for patients with abdominal trauma are directly affected by early diagnosis and prompt treatment. Early detection may prove challenging, because about one third of patients with abdominal injuries show no outward signs of trauma, and some patients develop delayed organ rupture or hemorrhage hours or days after the initial traumatic event. Undetected abdominal injuries may lead to death from hemorrhage, shock, and sepsis.

Pathophysiology

Abdominal trauma can be classified as blunt or penetrating. Both types of injuries may be associated with extensive damage to the abdominal organs, possibly resulting in massive blood loss. Generally, blunt trauma causes greater injury to solid organs (liver, spleen, pancreas, and kidneys), whereas penetrating trauma causes

greater injury to hollow organs (stomach, small intestine, large intestine, and urinary bladder).

Trauma to solid organs typically results in bleeding from lacerations or fractures; trauma to hollow organs results in rupture and release of organ contents into the abdominal cavity, which causes inflammation and infection. Regardless of whether the trauma is blunt or penetrating, the greater the speed or force behind the injury, the greater the degree of trauma sustained.

Blunt trauma

Blunt trauma involves the crushing, shearing, bursting, tearing, or compression of abdominal organs (especially the spleen, liver, pancreas, and intestines) and possibly secondary perforation from fracture fragments. Most commonly caused by motor vehicle accidents or falls, blunt abdominal trauma also may result from injuries sustained during assaults with blunt objects.

Blunt abdominal trauma carries a higher mortality than penetrating trauma because patients can have severe internal damage with little external evidence of injury, resulting in delayed detection and treatment.

Penetrating trauma

Penetrating trauma most often is caused by gunshot or stab wounds. Impalement by various objects also may cause this type of injury. The appearance of entrance and exit wounds does not determine the extent of internal injury. For example, bullets may fragment and change direction once inside the body.

Clinical assessment

All trauma patients admitted to the critical care unit should be suspected of having abdominal trauma. Because changes in the patient's condition may occur rapidly, baseline data and astute assessment skills are essential for timely detection and treatment (see *Abdominal examination techniques,* page 16, for a review of assessment techniques).

Abdominal examination techniques

Assessment of the abdomen involves inspection, auscultation, percussion, and palpation—in that order. Remember to always perform auscultation before percussion or palpation because those maneuvers may alter the frequency of bowel sounds. Additionally, always percuss and palpate painful or tender areas last.

Inspection	Auscultation
Look for: • obvious signs of trauma (examine the back as well) • masses • pulsations • asymmetry • discoloration • abdominal distention.	Listen for: • decreased or absent bowel sounds (may be caused by an irritant, such as blood or intestinal contents outside the bowel) • hyperactive bowel sounds (may be the result of irritants inside the bowel). Special tips: • Listen 3 to 5 minutes to confirm absence. • Listen for bowel sounds in the chest cavity. • Listen for bruits over the abdominal aorta, renal arteries, and femoral arteries (if heard, defer percussion and palpation).
Percussion	**Palpation**
• Useful for identification of air, fluid, and organ size. • Dullness indicates fluid and solid organs. • Tympany indicates air or air-filled organs.	• Palpate close to surface, then deep. • Note rebound pain (may be present with inflammation of the peritoneum). • Note any guarding. • Rectal examination may reveal blood; anterior tenderness may be present with peritoneal irritation.

History

Many patients with abdominal trauma have no obvious signs of injury; consequently, serial abdominal assessments aid in early detection of hidden injuries. During the initial history, the nurse should attempt to ascertain the following:

• the mechanism of injury, including:
 —if a fall, the height and point of impact
 —if a motor vehicle accident, the patient's placement in the car, use of a seat belt, speed and type of impact, any internal damage to the vehicle
 —if a gunshot wound, the caliber of gun and range of fire
 —if a stab wound, the length and type of object, sex of the attacker (males are more likely to stab upward, whereas females tend to stab downward)
• the location and quality of pain
• history of abdominal surgeries
• presence of nausea and vomiting.

 The nurse should be particularly alert to the possibility of abdominal injury in patients with associated spinal, thoracic, or pelvic injuries. Acceleration-deceleration injuries may produce spinal fractures and great vessel disruption, as well as abdominal injuries that may not be apparent for hours to days. Seat-belt restraints may produce pelvic disruption in addition to intraperitoneal or retroperitoneal injuries.

Physical findings

Signs and symptoms of abdominal trauma depend on the specific organs injured (see *Organ injuries and characteristic findings,* pages 18 and 19). Generally, signs and symptoms associated with abdominal trauma include obvious injury to the abdomen, hemodynamic instability, pain, nausea and vomiting, abdominal distention, and decreased or absent bowel sounds. Other findings may include:
• hypovolemic shock (evidenced by agitation, hypotension, tachycardia, decreased urine output, and cool, clammy skin; capillary refill may be delayed)
• increased intra-abdominal pressure
• Cullen's sign (bluish umbilicus suggesting intra-abdominal bleeding)

 The nurse also should observe for coexisting injuries in the trauma patient. Head injuries may result in increased intracranial pressure manifested by decreased

Organ injuries and characteristic findings

Specific organ injuries associated with abdominal trauma as well as their characteristic signs and symptoms are outlined below.

Organ	Characteristic Findings
Diaphragm	• Bowel sounds in chest • Decreased breath sounds • Chest pain
Esophagus	• Pain that radiates to the neck, chest, or shoulders • Possible diffuse abdominal pain • Dysphagia
Stomach	• Blood in nasogastric aspirate or hematemesis • Epigastric pain and tenderness • Signs of peritonitis due to release of acidic gastric contents • Guarding • Decreased or absent bowel sounds • Shock
Duodenum	• Fever • Jaundice • Vomiting • Pain • Peritoneal signs
Pancreas	• Positive Grey Turner's sign (ecchymosis in the flank area, suggesting retroperitoneal bleeding) • Ileus • Epigastric pain radiating to the back or pain in the left upper quadrant • Nausea and vomiting • Positive Kehr's sign (pain in the left shoulder secondary to diaphragmatic irritation by blood)
Spleen	• Left upper quadrant pain radiating to the left shoulder • Shock • Positive Kehr's sign • Positive Ballance's sign (fixed dullness to percussion in the left flank and dullness in the right flank that disappears with a change in position) • Peritoneal irritation • Rigidity
Liver	• Tenderness of right upper quadrant with guarding • Peritoneal irritation

Organ injuries and characteristic findings *(continued)*

Organ	Characteristic Findings
Liver *(continued)*	• Right shoulder pain when lying flat or in Trendelenburg's position • Positive Kehr's sign • Positive Ballance's sign
Small intestine	• Ileus • Peritoneal irritation • Abdominal pain and tenderness • Guarding • Decreased or absent bowel sounds
Colon	• Possible rectal bleeding • Peritoneal irritation due to perforation • Signs of obstruction

level of consciousness, headache, vomiting, visual dysfunction, and motor-sensory disturbances. Thoracic injuries may include pneumothorax, cardiac contusions, cardiac tamponade, and cardiac rupture. Orthopedic injuries also may be present, so X-rays (especially of the cervical spine) should be obtained. With lower left rib fractures, suspect a spleen injury; lower right rib fractures, a liver injury.

Diagnosis

Diagnosing abdominal trauma may be difficult, especially if the patient manifests no outward signs of injury. Because many signs and symptoms of abdominal trauma are nonspecific, certain diagnostic tests are performed to aid in accurate diagnosis (see *Identifying abdominal trauma,* page 20).

Treatment and care

The primary goals of treatment for the patient with abdominal trauma are to maintain hemodynamic stability, maintain organ function, and prevent major complications (see *Major complications of abdominal trauma,* page 21).

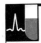

DIAGNOSTIC TESTS

Identifying abdominal trauma

The following diagnostic tests may be ordered to help diagnose abdominal trauma.

Complete blood count (CBC)

An increase in the white blood cell (WBC) count will be noted early as a result of the neuroendocrine stress response. An extreme elevation later may indicate peritoneal inflammation. Hemoglobin (Hb) and hematocrit (HCT) levels will be reduced with hemorrhage. Normal WBC values are 4.5 to 11.5 × 10^3 cells/mm^3. Normal Hb values are 13.5 to 17.5 g/dl for males, 12 to 16 g/dl for females. HCT normally is 41% to 53% for males, 36% to 46% for females.

Amylase level

An elevated serum amylase level may occur with injuries to the duodenum or pancreas. There are numerous sources of amylase, so an increase is not solely an indicator of pancreatic injury. Also, pancreatic injury may be present without a significant rise in serum amylase. Normal values are 25 to 125 U/liter.

Bilirubin level

Increased bilirubin levels may be present in duodenal or liver injuries. Normal direct bilirubin values are 0 to 0.02 mg/dl.

Lipase level

An increase in the lipase level may occur with pancreatic injury. Normal values are 10 to 150 U/liter.

Chest X-ray

This test may reveal lower rib fractures, which carry a high risk of liver or spleen injuries. Abdominal contents in the chest cavity indicate a diaphragmatic tear. Free air within the abdomen also may be identified, indicating perforation of abdominal organs. Right diaphragm elevation may be seen in liver injuries.

Abdominal X-ray

This examination is used to detect free air or the presence of foreign bodies.

Diagnostic peritoneal lavage (DPL)

DPL involves the infusion of warmed saline and the withdrawal and examination of peritoneal fluid for blood, bile, bacteria, or fecal matter. Many clinicians prefer DPL over computed tomography, believing that DPL is more accurate; also, it can be performed rapidly and is less expensive. However, retroperitoneal injuries of the kidneys, duodenum, and colon are not as readily identified with DPL.

Computed tomography (CT scan)

This test may reveal bleeding, organ contusion, laceration, or rupture. Unstable patients may not be candidates for CT because of the time required to perform the examination (typically 30 to 45 minutes).

Fluid and electrolyte homeostasis

Fluid and electrolyte homeostasis is necessary to maintain hemodynamic stability in the trauma patient. Fluid shifts to the bowel wall or irritated peritoneum may de-

Major complications of abdominal trauma

Serious, sometimes fatal complications can follow abdominal trauma. Prevention and early identification of these complications are essential to ensure the best chance for recovery. Other possible complications include hemorrhage, stress ulcers, fistula formation, and alteration of body image.

Complication	Possible Causes
Ileus	Peritonitis, shock, sepsis, manipulation of bowel during surgery
Peritonitis	Contamination by bowel contents or penetrating injuries
Post-traumatic acute cholecystitis	Shock, sepsis, respiratory failure, acute renal failure, total parenteral nutrition, multiple transfusions, high-dose narcotics
Traumatic pancreatitis	Direct trauma to pancreas, vascular compromise
Abscess formation	Contents of ruptured organs (excellent medium for abscess formation if not adequately drained)
Disruption of wound healing	Healing through secondary closure (in cases of contaminated wounds)
Malabsorption syndrome	Removal of more than 200 cm of bowel (this alters the bacterial flora and absorptive segments)
Bowel ischemia, infarction, or obstruction	Bowel injuries, postoperative developments
Overwhelming postsplenectomy infection	Postoperative development due to loss of antibody formation, bacterial infiltration, and enhanced phagocytosis
Sepsis	Contaminated wounds, rupture of organs, causing release of abdominal contents

crease the vascular volume. Fluid loss from wound and fistula drainage also can lead to volume depletion. Hypovolemic shock is common in abdominal trauma and must be addressed promptly to restore intravascular volume and preserve tissue perfusion. Packed red blood cells

are necessary in many cases to maintain a hemoglobin concentration of 10 g/dl and a hematocrit of 30%.

Important nursing interventions to include in the patient's plan of care are outlined below:
• Monitor the patient closely for possible transfusion reactions and volume overload. If administering large quantities of blood, use a blood warmer to prevent hypothermia and its subsequent complications. Other potential complications of massive blood administration include hyperkalemia, hypocalcemia, metabolic acidosis, and coagulopathies.
• Administer crystalloids, such as lactated Ringer's or normal saline solution, to restore vascular volume.
• Monitor electrolyte values closely. Electrolyte depletion can result from wound drainage. Gastrointestinal fluid loss, which can result from vomiting and gastric suctioning, can lead to decreases in serum sodium, potassium, and chloride levels.

Infection control

The patient with abdominal trauma is at risk for wound infections, peritonitis, and sepsis. Broad-spectrum antibiotics may be initiated immediately upon admission, particularly in patients with penetrating wounds or ruptured organs. Appropriate nursing interventions are as follows:
• Monitor for signs of infection, including increasing white blood cell count, fever, and signs of redness, warmth, edema, purulent drainage, or localized pain at the incision or wound site.
• Ensure that the patient's tetanus records are current. Administer tetanus toxoid if necessary.
• Use aseptic technique when changing dressings as well as when handling invasive lines. Some wounds are left open to heal by secondary intention; this may be necessary with significant bowel edema or with contaminated wounds. If the patient has multiple wounds, dress each separately to prevent cross-contamination.
• Occasionally, dehiscence of an incision may occur. In this case, apply a warm, moist saline dressing to the area of dehiscence and prepare the patient for surgery.

• Drains may be used to prevent the formation of an abscess. Be sure to guard against drain leakage, which will affect the patient's skin integrity.

Maintenance of cardiac and respiratory function

The abdominal trauma patient must be monitored closely for signs of cardiac or respiratory compromise; these systems may be affected by coexisting injuries, and many complications can occur. All trauma patients require supplemental oxygen, at least initially, to enhance oxygen supply and meet the organ and tissue oxygen demands. The degree of injury dictates the aggressiveness of oxygen support therapy. Coexisting injuries may necessitate the use of mechanical ventilation for adequate oxygenation.

Specific nursing interventions include the following:
• Administer oxygen, as ordered.
• Initiate pain-control measures to enhance the patient's respiratory status and to prevent shallow respirations and excessive splinting. Respiratory hygiene measures, such as turning, coughing, and deep breathing, are important to prevent secondary complications and are more effective if pain is controlled.
• Monitor for fluid overload, which can occur during aggressive volume replacement. Particularly monitor breath sounds, jugular venous distention, and central venous pressure. Elderly patients and those with preexisting cardiac or renal conditions are at increased risk.

Postoperative course

The decision to perform surgery is based on many factors, including hemodynamic stability, mechanism of injury, wound contamination, and probable organ damage. Some colon injuries may necessitate an ileostomy or a colostomy. Ostomy nurses can be helpful in assisting the patient with ostomy care and psychological adjustment, whether the procedure is permanent or temporary. Many of these patients will require a second trip to the operating room for removal of packing, debridement, or closure of open wounds.

The patient undergoing surgery after abdominal trauma presents a special set of nursing concerns. Specific interventions are as follows:
• Encourage early mobilization to promote peristalsis and help prevent thrombus formation.
• Assess for pain, and monitor the patient's response to analgesics.
• Assist the patient to a position of comfort. An increase in abdominal pain may indicate abscess or fistula formation or delayed viscous rupture.
• Provide emotional support for the patient and family undergoing multiple surgeries.

Prognosis

The outcome for a patient with abdominal trauma depends greatly on prompt identification and treatment of injuries; any delays will increase the patient's morbidity and mortality. Contaminated wounds have a higher morbidity and mortality rate. Other factors that affect the patient's recovery include concomitant injury, extent of organ damage, complications following the injury, preexisting conditions, and age.

Discharge planning

Discharge planning should begin as soon as the patient is stabilized. The following steps should be taken to ensure a smooth discharge:
• Evaluate the patient's support systems.
• Consult social services, if indicated.
• Review the recovery period with the patient and family, including the need for activity, dietary restrictions, and medications.
• Instruct the patient and family on wound care.
• Consult the ostomy nurse, as indicated.
• Ensure that a follow-up appointment has been made.
• Review signs and symptoms of potential complications.
• Discuss the need for a Pneumovax (pneumococcal polysaccharide vaccine) injection, if indicated for the patient who has undergone a splenectomy.

Acquired immunodeficiency syndrome (AIDS)

The severe end disorder of an acquired immune deficit caused by a retroviral infection, AIDS causes abnormalities in cellular immunity that commonly result in opportunistic infections and lymphoreticular cancers. The causative agent of AIDS is human immunodeficiency virus (HIV), which remains active within the afflicted patient's body tissues, blood, or secretions. However, as in other infectious diseases, exposure to the virus may or may not result in transmission to other individuals.

HIV is transmitted primarily through contact with infected blood, semen, and vaginal secretions, as well as through infected breast milk. Infected blood may cross directly from one individual to another through the use of shared needles (common with I.V. drug users), during sexual encounters, during blood transfusions, through placental blood sharing between mother and fetus, or through open-wound contact with infected blood. Blood donor screening has reduced the incidence of HIV in recipients of blood products; however, patients receiving multiple transfusions and administration of multidonor blood products, such as cryoprecipitate, carry a greater risk of contracting the disease via transfusion.

Pathophysiology

HIV is a retrovirus known for its ability to incorporate itself into the normal cell's ribonucleic acid (RNA), causing replication of viral, not normal, cells. HIV cells are impermeable to normal immune surveillance mechanisms because of a protein-coating envelope.

Clinical manifestations of HIV disease are caused by replacement of normal cell deoxyribonucleic acid by HIV, destroying normal T4 helper cells or cells with a CD4 molecule (monocytes). T4 helper cells are primarily responsible for immune surveillance and recognition of mutant (neoplastic), opportunistic, and viral microorganisms. Destruction of these cells leads to cancers and viral or opportunistic infections. Monocytes and macrophages also are infected by this virus, predisposing exposed individuals to infection with encapsulated or intracellular organisms (such as *Mycobacterium intracellulare tubercle* and *Streptococcus*). HIV's effects on monocytes and macrophages lead to tissue infection and liberation of inflammatory mediators, such as tumor necrosis factor. The wasting syndrome associated with AIDS, which is characterized by anorexia, cachexia, and muscle atrophy, may be related to these mediators.

Helper T-cells and monocytes assist in production of immunoglobulin, allograft rejection, and delayed type hypersensitivity. In HIV-infected cells, immunoglobulins may be produced in excessive quantity, but they are ineffective, leading to hyperallergy and an inability to recognize and destroy invading pathogens.

Within 3 to 6 weeks after viral exposure, an infected person may present with transient flu or mononucleosis symptoms. Within 8 to 12 weeks after exposure, 95% of those affected have seroconversion as evidenced by the presence of serum HIV antibodies. Once positive for HIV antibodies, about 35% of individuals exhibit more severe illness within 5 to 6 years and the full clinical spectrum within 8 to 9 years.

Clinical assessment

Primary responsibilities of a critical care nurse are to recognize the signs and symptoms of AIDS and the patients at risk for it. The patient interview and physical assessment provide a basis for diagnostic testing and for monitoring response to therapy. In those with known HIV disease, clinical findings are more sensitive an indicator of improvement or worsening of the disease than diagnostic tests.

History

During the assessment, the nurse should determine the patient's history for risks of exposure.

The nurse also should inquire about manifestation of AIDS-related complications described on the following pages.

Physical findings

The signs and symptoms of HIV infection vary with the specific clinical presentation of the disease. The Centers for Disease Control (CDC) has outlined a classification of AIDS based on cross-referencing the number of affected CD4 cells against a list of common clinical presentations (see *CDC case definitions for AIDS,* pages 28 and 29). Within this grid, the severity of clinical symptoms and refractoriness of the disorders to treatment increase as the CD4 count decreases.

The four major categories of HIV infection symptomatology are acute retroviral infection, neurologic disease, opportunistic infection, and specific cancers. Other clinical complications included in the case definition for AIDS are idiopathic and thrombotic thrombocytopenia purpura, cervical dysplasia or carcinoma in situ, and oral hairy leukoplakia. Although commonly refractory to therapy, these syndromes are treated in the traditional manner.

Individuals at risk for HIV infection and AIDS require frequent total body assessment and patient education regarding reportable symptoms (see *Assessment of AIDS patients,* page 30). Individuals at risk for HIV disease and their significant others should be alert for the most classic symptoms heralding HIV disease, including Kaposi's sarcoma lesions, swollen lymph glands, upper respiratory symptoms, intractable diarrhea, and fevers.

Diagnosis

Diagnosis of HIV infection commonly is made by serum laboratory tests for the presence of HIV or antibodies to the virus (see *Confirming HIV infection*, pages 31 and 32).

CDC case definitions for AIDS

In 1993, the CDC revised its classification system for HIV infection and expanded its surveillance case definition for AIDS. The new classification groups HIV-infected patients according to three ranges of CD4 + T-cell counts and three clinical categories, which include three new AIDS-indicator conditions. The following chart shows the nine mutually exclusive subgroups.

CD4 + T-cell Categories	Clinical Categories		
	A Asymptomatic, acute (primary) HIV, or PGL	B Symptomatic, but not A or C conditions	C AIDS-indicator conditions
≥500/µl	A1	B1	C1
200 to 499/µl	A2	B2	C2
<200/µl AIDS-indicator cell count	A3	B3	C3

CD4 + T-cell categories
These CD4 + T-cell ranges are considered positive markers for HIV infection:
• Category 1: 500 or more cells/µl of blood
• Category 2: 200 to 499 cells/µl of blood
• Category 3: less than 200 cells/µl of blood

Disease categories
The CDC defines three related disease categories as follows:
• Category A: Patients without symptoms, with persistent generalized lymphadenopathy (PGL), or with acute primary HIV infection. Conditions in categories B and C must not have occurred.
• Category B: HIV-infected patients with symptoms or diseases not included in category C, such as bacillary angiomatosis, oropharyngeal or persistent vulvovaginal candidiasis, fever or diarrhea lasting over 1 month, idiopathic thrombocytopenic purpura, pelvic inflammatory disease (particularly if complicated by tubo-ovarian abscess), and peripheral neuropathy.
• Category C: HIV-infected patients with disorders defined by the CDC as AIDS-indicator conditions.

AIDS-indicator conditions
The CDC recognizes the following AIDS-indicator conditions:
• Candidiasis of the bronchi, trachea, or lungs
• Candidiasis of the esophagus
• Cervical cancer, invasive
• Coccidioidomycosis, disseminated or extrapulmonary
• Cryptococcosis, extrapulmonary
• Cryptosporidiosis, chronic intestinal (persisting over 1 month)
• Cytomegalovirus (CMV) disease affecting organs other than the liver, spleen, or lymph nodes
• CMV retinitis with vision loss
• Encephalopathy related to HIV

CDC case definitions for AIDS (continued)

- Herpes simplex, involving chronic ulcers (persisting over 1 month) or herpetic bronchitis, pneumonitis, or esophagitis
- Histoplasmosis, disseminated or extrapulmonary
- Isosporiasis, chronic intestinal (persisting over 1 month)
- Kaposi's sarcoma
- Lymphoma, Burkitt's (or its equivalent)
- Lymphoma, immunoblastic (or its equivalent)
- Lymphoma of the brain, primary

- *Mycobacterium avium* complex or *M. kansasii,* disseminated or extrapulmonary
- *M. tuberculosis* at any site (pulmonary or extrapulmonary)
- *Mycobacterium,* any other species, disseminated or extrapulmonary
- *Pneumocystis carinii* pneumonia
- Pneumonia, recurrent
- Progressive multifocal leukoencephalopathy
- *Salmonella* septicemia, recurrent
- Toxoplasmosis of the brain
- Wasting syndrome caused by HIV.

Treatment and care

Current therapies offer no hope of reversal or cure. The overall goal of all interventions in the acutely ill AIDS patient is to restore and maintain immunologic function at baseline levels. Acute management of HIV-related complications focuses on:
- implementing or maintaining treatment with anti-retroviral agents, the only therapy that halts disease progression
- preventing opportunistic infections
- managing opportunistic infections, cancer, and HIV-related clinical syndromes.

Antiretroviral therapy

Treatment of HIV-positive patients with no accompanying opportunistic infections and those with neurologic disease or some cancers includes the administration of a specific anti-HIV agent, such as zidovudine (azidothymidine [AZT] or Retrovir), zalcitabine (dideoxycytidine [ddC] or Hivid), or dideoxyinosine (ddi). These agents delay or slow RNA transcription of HIV, slowing disease progression for years in some individuals. Transmission from mother to fetus also has been reduced since the implementation of antiretroviral therapy

Assessment of AIDS patients

Patients with AIDS are at risk for various clinical syndromes during their illness. Many of these syndromes precipitate or cause multisystem symptoms. A comprehensive nursing assessment is required to detect early signs and symptoms of emergence or exacerbation of these disorders.

Neurologic system
- Altered cognitive level
- Muscle weakness
- Unequal pupils
- Altered vision
- Peripheral neuropathies

Respiratory system
- Tachypnea and dyspnea
- Crackles, wheezes, and gurgles
- Decreased oxygen saturation
- Cyanosis
- Cough
- Abnormal sputum specimens

Cardiovascular system
- Abnormal heart sounds (gallops, murmurs)
- Elevated jugular venous pulsations
- Altered pulses (weak and thready, full and bounding, unequal)

Gastrointestinal system
- Oral candidiasis and stomatitis (ulcers, redness, soreness)
- Oral hairy leukoplakia
- Xerostomia
- Nausea and vomiting
- Diarrhea
- Abdominal pain
- Abdominal distention
- Enlarged liver
- Enlarged spleen

Genitourinary system
- Dysuria
- Cloudy urine
- Hemorrhagic cystitis

Hematologic and immune systems
- Coagulopathies (bruising, petechiae, bloody secretions, bleeding from orifices, bleeding around catheters)
- Fever
- Pallor

Integumentary system
- Edema
- Kaposi's sarcoma lesions
- Lymphadenopathy

to pregnant HIV-positive women. Antiretroviral therapy is given to patients who meet the following criteria:
- asymptomatic HIV positive with CD4 <200/μl
- symptomatic HIV positive with any CD4 count
- neurologic manifestations of disease
- Kaposi's sarcoma lesions.

The nurse is responsible for monitoring for common adverse effects of antiretroviral therapy; specific nursing measures are included below:
- Administer bone marrow stimulants (erythropoietin-stimulating factors, granulocyte colony-stimulating factor), as ordered.

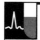

DIAGNOSTIC TESTS

Confirming HIV infection

Diagnosis of HIV infection involves assessing for the presence of antibodies to the disease or actual viral proteins indicating exposure. After diagnosis, lymphocyte counts are followed to monitor progression of disease or response to treatment. Commonly used diagnostic tests are described below.

Diagnostic Test	Methodology
Enzyme-linked im-munosorbent assay (ELISA) *Normal test findings:* immunofluorescence of viral antibody particles	• Used by blood banks to detect infected blood products • Rapid, easy clinical test to perform • False-positive rate of approximately 5% • Inaccurate reflection of HIV status for infants born to HIV-positive mothers
Western blot test *Normal test findings:* absence of HIV core proteins gp 160/120, gp 41, p24	• All positive ELISA test results are followed by this test because of ELISA's false-positive rate • Detects antibodies specific to viral proteins • Positive test result is indicated by testing positive to two of the three HIV components: gp 160/120, gp 41, p24 • Considered 99.5% positive when accompanied by a positive ELISA • Inaccurate reflection of HIV status for infants born to HIV-positive mothers
HIV culture *Normal test findings:* absence of lympho-cyte clumping	• Performed on specific patient tissue when other tests are inconclusive • Clumping of T4 lymphocytes is considered characteristic of HIV infection
Polymerase chain re-action *Normal test findings:* no viral deoxyribo-nucleic acid (DNA) particles noted	• Used only by sophisticated laboratories to test for HIV DNA • Can be positive as much as 2 weeks after exposure to HIV
Absolute T4 helper lymphocyte count *Normal test findings:* helper T count is 600 to 1,200 cells/mm^3 or >12% of total white blood cell count	• Most helpful in predicting patient symptoms and clinical problems • Probably predictive of worsening disease • Below 500 cells/mm^3, immune compromise begins • Below 200 cells/mm^3, opportunistic infections (*Pneumocystis carinii* pneumonia, toxoplasmo-sis) occur

(continued)

Confirming HIV infection (continued)

Diagnostic Test	Methodology
p24 antigen test *Normal test findings:* no p24 core protein detected	• Measures level of viral core protein p24

• Implement infection prevention precautions for the immunocompromised host (no fresh flowers, limiting venipunctures).
• Provide incremental care and frequent rest periods to reduce fatigue or oxygen consumption in those with anemia.
• Administer blood products as ordered.
• Monitor hematologic blood tests routinely.
• Administer antiretroviral agents as close to "around the clock" as possible.
• Follow hazardous material precautions when administering antiretroviral agents.
• Administer ddC with buffered solution on an empty stomach.
• Teach patients and families to be cautious of hand or foot injury due to decreased peripheral sensation.
• Monitor for abdominal pain, nausea, vomiting, and intolerance to fatty foods, which signal pancreatitis.

Prevention of opportunistic infections

Most infections occurring in AIDS patients are from normal environmental flora, which cannot be removed or prevented. Consequently, limited alterations in the barrier defenses are the best tactic for prevention. In the critical care environment, judicious use of invasive lines or planning for routine line changes prevents potential life-threatening infection. Because the infection precedes actual symptoms in infection with contagious illness such as respiratory syncytial virus (RSV) and coxsackievirus, patients are at considerable risk of life-threatening infection if visitors are not properly screened for recent exposure to viral illness.

Food should be monitored carefully to avoid uncooked meats and possible food poisoning. Preventive measures are listed below:

• Implement infection precautions for the immunocompromised patient.

• Limit and screen visitors to monitor for exposure to communicable diseases.

• Avoid the patient's exposure to standing water (such as humidifiers).

• Keep the patient away from areas where ceiling work is being performed and away from sources of direct air blowing, because many structures and air systems encourage growth of fungi.

• Monitor the patient's white blood cell and lymphocyte counts to determine the need for prophylaxis.

• Administer prophylactic antibiotics as indicated (special self-protection precautions and ventilation are required for aerosolized pentamidine).

Treatment of complications of opportunistic infections

In AIDS patients, treatment of opportunistic infections encompasses all types of antimicrobial therapy. Antimicrobial therapy is directed toward the suspected pathogens based on clinical presentation, previous infections, and T4 helper count. The most common infections are the indicator disorders in the CDC definition of AIDS (see *CDC case definitions for AIDS,* pages 28 and 29).

Nursing assessment of body systems for the most common opportunistic infections includes:

• neurologic symptoms: toxoplasmosis, cryptococcosis

• visual problems: cytomegalovirus (CMV)

• pulmonary symptoms: *Pneumocystis carinii* pneumonia, CMV

• sore mouth or throat: candida, streptococcus

• difficulty swallowing: *Candida esophagitis*

• nausea, vomiting, diarrhea: *Cryptosporidium,* CMV, *Salmonella, Isospora*

• dysuria, cloudy urine, urinary frequency: *Streptococcus*.

Cancer treatment

The medical treatment of Kaposi's sarcoma has included local radiation treatments as well as systemic chemotherapy, with only moderate success. Anti-HIV agents, such as zidovudine, have been shown to slow or halt the spread of Kaposi's sarcoma and therefore are the treatment of choice. Symptomatic relief of Kaposi's sarcoma lesions producing serious complications, such as bowel or airway obstruction, have included surgery, brachytherapy (focused beam radiation), and photodynamic therapy. Other agents with limited efficacy against this tumor include vincristine, vinblastine, etoposide, adriamycin, and interferon.

Nursing interventions for patients receiving treatment for Kaposi's sarcoma follow:

• Monitor the number and size of lesions.

• Assess new onset of abdominal pain, nausea and vomiting, or dyspnea, which may signal internal Kaposi's sarcoma lesions.

• Provide skin care with emollients or antimicrobial ointments to areas receiving local radiation treatment.

• Become familiar with the adverse effects of chemotherapy agents given, and prevent symptoms when possible (for example, give an antiemetic prior to adriamycin administration).

The AIDS-related lymphomas have proven resistant to conventional treatment, but usual and investigational chemotherapeutic agents have been used. All lymphoma therapies produce profound bone marrow aplasia and gastrointestinal symptoms, which must be differentiated from symptoms of opportunistic infections. Nursing care includes the following:

• Monitor temperature every 4 hours.

• Administer antimicrobial agents as ordered.

• Monitor cultures of body fluids.

• Monitor blood counts (red blood cells, white blood cells, platelets) daily, and administer replacement blood products as ordered.

• Place the patient on bleeding precautions.
• Provide antiemetics and antidiarrheals as ordered.

AIDS-related neurologic disease may encompass a broad range of mild to severe symptoms that can include short-term memory deficits, peripheral or autonomic neuropathies, confusion, and paranoia. More than half of all AIDS patients manifest neurologic symptoms at some time during their illness. Nursing care includes the following:

• Assess the patient's orientation at least every shift.
• Promote orientation by using a clock and calendar and opening the curtains.
• Implement safety measures, such as maintaining a low bed position, keeping all bedrails up, and providing a room near the nurses' station.
• Administer sedatives, as ordered, for confusion and aggressive behavior.

Restoration of immunologic function

Although antiretroviral agents halt infection of additional normal cells with the virus, they do not restore function of damaged cells. At present, therapies, such as interleukin-2 (aldesleukin), used to accomplish this objective are considered experimental but promising.

Patients with HIV infection are advised to examine their lifestyle and make modifications to enhance health and tissue regeneration and reduce the risk of acquiring infections. In the critical care environment, proper nutrition and rest may improve the health status of these patients. Specific nursing interventions are included below:

• Encourage balanced nutrition with extra protein to enhance body repair.
• Offer and administer vitamin supplements as indicated.
• Monitor the patient's weight for signs and symptoms of malnutrition.
• Calculate caloric needs and intake, and consult a dietitian to supplement and fulfill requirements.
• Use noninvasive monitoring devices that reduce disruption of rest to gather vital signs.

• Develop a progressive activity and exercise regimen similar to that for the patient recovering from critical illness or being weaned from mechanical ventilation.
• Use occupational or physical therapy as indicated.
• Assist the patient in using relaxation techniques or guided imagery.
• Offer clergy services as desired by the patient.

Prognosis

Once a disease known to result in death in a matter of months, AIDS is now met with feelings of despair yet hope for years of quality life, given currently available treatment. Despite measurable success with antiretroviral therapy, overall survival has not significantly improved. In fact, once the clinical criteria for AIDS have been met, about 80% of patients die within 3 years.

Discharge planning

Discharge planning for patients with AIDS requires the nurse to have extensive knowledge of the clinical manifestations of the disease, routine medications, required laboratory tests, and home care resources. Most patients have a permanent indwelling venous access device inserted as the disease progresses into one of the major syndromes, because I.V. medications and blood transfusions frequently are implemented.

The neurologic manifestations of the disease and multiple I.V. medications or blood samples often require skilled nursing care or constant supervision in the home. The disabilities may necessitate purchase or rental of hospital beds, oxygen therapy, and mobility devices. Arrangements for the purchase of medications are essential for successful outpatient therapy. The necessary antibiotics often are expensive and may not be covered by insurers if self-administered. This consideration may drive the decision to have the patient return to the clinic for frequent visits and medication administration. Multiple medications also predispose patients to overlapping adverse effects and to idiosyncratic reactions.

Adult respiratory distress syndrome (ARDS)

A severe form of respiratory failure resulting from diffuse pulmonary injury, ARDS is characterized by a pattern of pathophysiological changes and clinical manifestations that include diffuse alveolar-capillary wall injury, increased alveolar-capillary permeability, noncardiogenic pulmonary edema, atelectasis, and hyaline membrane formation. The clinical manifestations of ARDS can be divided into four stages: Stage I (the initial insult), Stage II (the latent period, with circulatory stability but developing respiratory distress), Stage III (acute respiratory failure), and Stage IV (terminal hypoxia and hypercarbia).

Pathophysiology

Various clinical conditions can lead to the development of ARDS. These causes may be pulmonary (direct) or systemic (indirect). However, the common factor in all conditions appears to be hypoperfusion of the lung parenchyma (see *Precipitating conditions for the development of ARDS,* page 38).

Although the exact mechanism by which a low perfusion state leads to ARDS is unclear, the injury may lead to activation of the complement cascade (including inflammatory mediators, such as histamine, serotonin, prostacyclin, thromboxanes, kinins, and metabolites of arachidonic acid) and the coagulation cascade. As a result of cascade activation, protein and platelet microaggregates form in the circulation and lodge in the pulmonary capillaries. The platelet microemboli release vasoactive amines causing microvascular constriction; chemotaxic factors activate polymorphonuclear neutrophils (PMNs) within the pulmonary circulation.

Once activated, PMNs release noxious products (hydroxyl ions, hypochlorous acid, superoxide ions, and hydrogen peroxide) that damage the pulmonary endothelium and alveolar epithelium. This injury results

Precipitating conditions for the development of ARDS

Pulmonary, or direct, causes
- Aspiration of gastric contents
- Bacterial or viral pneumonia
- Inhalation of smoke or other toxins
- Pulmonary contusion
- Thoracic trauma
- Oxygen toxicity
- Fat, air, or amniotic emboli
- Near drowning

Systemic, or indirect, causes
- Sepsis and other shock states

- Multisystem trauma
- Disseminated intravascular coagulation
- Pancreatitis
- Uremia
- Drug overdose
- Anaphylaxis
- Idiopathic processes
- Multiple blood transfusions
- Cardiopulmonary bypass surgery
- Pregnancy-induced hypertension

in increased permeability at the alveolar-capillary barrier and subsequent extravasation of fluids into the interstitial space. As perivascular edema increases and capillary perfusion decreases, damage to type II pneumocytes occurs, causing decreased surfactant production. This decrease produces an increase in lung interstitial fibrosis, which often is called lung stiffness.

Pulmonary edema
Damage to the pulmonary endothelium and alveolar epithelium results in increased permeability, allowing the movement of protein-rich fluid into interstitial and alveolar spaces. This shift of fluid leads to pulmonary edema, decreased lung compliance, and impaired oxygen transport.

Decreased lung compliance
As interstitial edema increases, fluid begins to flood the alveoli. Decreased surfactant production leads to increased surface tension and the alveoli become smaller. Distal atelectasis and loss of lung volume occur, further impairing gas exchange. The pulmonary congestion and increasing alveolar surface tension result in loss of lung compliance. As compliance decreases, the volume of gas present in the alveoli at the end of expiration (functional residual capacity) is reduced. The volume

of gas may become so small and the surface tension so great that the alveoli collapse completely and cannot reopen.

Hypoxemia

Alveolar collapse and intra-alveolar edema lead to increased shunting. Intrapulmonary shunting occurs in areas where alveoli are perfused with blood but are not ventilated. The normal amount of shunting is 3% to 5% of the cardiac output. However, in a patient with ARDS, the amount of intrapulmonary shunting may be 25% to 50%. Other areas of the lung may have wasted (dead-space) ventilation, which occurs when the lung is ventilated but not perfused.

The lack of perfusion to alveoli results from vasoconstriction, microembolization, leukocyte and platelet aggregation, and pulmonary capillary compression from the edema. The overall result of shunting and wasted ventilation is a mismatch between ventilation and perfusion, and severe, refractory hypoxemia. The decrease in arterial oxygen content and oxygen transport leads to tissue hypoxia.

Inadequate cellular oxygenation causes anaerobic metabolism and increased production of lactic acid, resulting in further damage to the lungs and other organ systems, especially the kidneys and liver, and increasing pulmonary dysfunction. Eventually, the damaged lung tissue becomes fibrotic and lung compliance further decreases. Fibrin and cellular debris form hyaline membranes, which further impede gas exchange.

Clinical assessment

Early detection and initiation of treatment are key to the successful management of ARDS. Members of the health care team should be alert to its development in susceptible patients. Persons with previously normal lung function who suffer either a pulmonary insult (aspiration, inhalation of toxins, pneumonia) or a systemic insult (septic shock, multiple trauma, disseminated intravascular coagulation) should be monitored closely for the development of ARDS.

History

The patient may present in any one of the four stages of ARDS. Depending on the severity of the presenting symptoms and the degree of respiratory failure, obtaining a history may be difficult. The nurse should try to determine the existence of any predisposing clinical events, especially those that have occurred in the previous 24 to 48 hours.

Physical findings

Physical findings depend on the stage of ARDS (see *Clinical findings associated with ARDS,* page 41). In Stage I, abnormalities in the clinical symptomatology or hemodynamic profile may reflect the underlying injury. The patient typically has tachypnea with little or no respiratory distress, and the lungs are clear to auscultation.

In Stage II, the patient appears to be stable. Hyperventilation persists, and the patient exhibits subclinical respiratory distress. Lung sounds may be diminished.

In Stage III, the patient suffers acute respiratory failure, and the clinical signs of pulmonary edema become evident. Auscultation of lungs reveals crackles and wheezes. Physical assessment findings reflect the degree of hypoxemia. By this stage, widespread damage to the pulmonary capillary membrane has occurred, lung compliance has decreased, and increased intrapulmonary shunting is apparent.

Stage IV is marked by severe respiratory failure. Massive pulmonary edema, atelectasis, and fibrosis occur, and lung compliance is further decreased.

Diagnosis

The diagnosis of ARDS requires the correlation of physical findings, a precipitating clinical event, and abnormal laboratory and radiographic findings. The use of a pulmonary artery catheter to measure pulmonary

Clinical findings associated with ARDS

Signs and symptoms and physical findings associated with ARDS are stage-dependent.

Stage	Signs and Symptoms	Physical Findings
I	Tachypnea, restlessness, anxiety	Lungs clear to auscultation, respiratory rate increased, slight respiratory alkalosis (PCO_2 30 to 40 mm Hg), normal PO_2, blood pressure and pulse within normal limits or specific to underlying injury
II	Tachypnea, restlessness, cough, anxiety, fatigue, sudden hypoxemia	Lungs clear, breath sounds possibly diminished, respiratory rate increased, respiratory alkalosis with slight hypoxemia (PCO_2 25 to 30 mm Hg, PO_2 60 mm Hg)
III	Tachypnea with shortness of breath, dyspnea, confusion or changes in mentation, tachycardia	Crackles and wheezes; increased blood pressure, pulse, and respiratory rate; increased hypoxemia and respiratory alkalosis (PO_2 50 to 60 mm Hg, PCO_2 20 to 30 mm Hg)
IV	Overt respiratory distress, profound shortness of breath and dyspnea, diaphoresis, cyanosis, nasal flaring, somnolence or coma	Signs of decreased cardiac output (decreased blood pressure, increased or decreased heart rate, decreased urine output); use of accessory muscles; intercostal, supraclavicular, suprasternal, and substernal retraction; progressive increase in airway pressure; adventitious breath sounds; hypoxemia ($PO_2 < 50$ mm Hg) and hypercarbia ($PCO_2 > 50$ mm Hg)

artery pressures and filling pressures also is useful, especially in determining whether pulmonary edema is cardiogenic or noncardiogenic (see *Confirming ARDS*, pages 42 and 43, for a quick review of diagnostic tests).

Treatment and care

Treatment of ARDS is mainly supportive. The goals of management are to maintain adequate gas exchange, prevent further lung injury, and prevent failure of non-

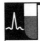

DIAGNOSTIC TESTS

Confirming ARDS

The following tests and laboratory findings will help confirm a diagnosis of ARDS.

Test	Stage I
Arterial blood gas analysis	
Hydrogen ion concentration (7.35 to 7.45)	> 7.45
PO$_2$ (80 to 100 mm Hg)	Normal to slightly low
PCO$_2$ (35 to 45 mm Hg)	Normal to slightly low
Chest X-ray	
	Normal
Hemodynamic parameters	
Pulmonary systolic pressure (15 to 30 mm Hg)	Normal
Pulmonary diastolic pressure (5 to 15 mm Hg)	Normal
Pulmonary capillary wedge pressure (4 to 12 mm Hg)	Normal
Cardiac output (4 to 8 liters/minute)	Normal

pulmonary organs. Meeting these goals requires venti-latory management and hemodynamic, pharmacologic, and nutritional support. The patient should be monitored closely for complications of therapy and tissue hypoxia.

Investigations of experimental therapies aimed at blocking or reducing the effects of the immune-inflammatory response are ongoing. These include the use of prostaglandin E, which inhibits platelet aggregation,

Stage II	Stage III	Stage IV
> 7.50	< 7.35	< 7.20
60 mm Hg; may respond to O_2 administration	50 to 60 mm Hg	< 50 mm Hg; refractory to O_2 administration
25 to 30 mm Hg	20 to 30 mm Hg	> 50 mm Hg
Thickened or blurred margins of bronchi or vessels	"Ground glass" appearance; diffuse, extensive bilateral interstitial and alveolar infiltrates	Consolidation ("white lung")
Normal	Normal to slightly increased	Increased as a result of vasoconstriction
Normal	Normal	Normal to slightly increased
Normal	Normal	Normal
Slightly elevated	> 8 liters/minute	< 4 liters/minute

neutrophil chemotaxis, and macrophage activity; exogenous surfactant, to reduce surface tension in the alveoli; and monoclonal antibodies, which act against adhesion molecules on the white blood cells (WBCs).

The use of extracorporeal membrane oxygenation to oxygenate the blood of the critically ill patient also has been studied. Although the results of its use in neonates were positive, the results with adult patients have been disappointing. Studies so far show no difference in mortality rates and an increase in complications.

Ventilatory management

Patients with moderate to severe ARDS require endotracheal intubation and mechanical ventilation to improve oxygenation and prevent tissue hypoxia. The two major goals of management are to maintain adequate gas exchange and to prevent secondary injury due to the mechanical ventilation.

Oxygen must be given in a concentration sufficient to meet the body's needs. A PO_2 of 60 mm Hg generally is adequate; however, in the patient with ARDS, maintaining adequate oxygenation often requires using concentrations greater than 60%, a level that is toxic to lung tissues and can cause further damage. Conventional ventilatory management of the patient with ARDS includes the use of supraphysiologic tidal volumes (10 to 15 ml/kg), flow rates that establish inspiratory to expiratory (I:E) ratios of less than 1:1, and positive end-expiratory pressure (PEEP).

The use of PEEP can improve gas exchange and allow administration of oxygen at lower levels. PEEP augments decreased lung volumes in the airways and the alveoli and increases the functional residual capacity, thereby decreasing intrapulmonary shunting. When PEEP is being used, the nurse must be alert to two possible complications: reduced cardiac output and barotrauma, such as tension pneumothorax, pneumomediastinum, air emboli, and subcutaneous air. Barotrauma results from overdistension of nondiseased alveoli. Any sudden change in the patient's status can indicate a tension pneumothorax, which is a medical emergency and requires prompt intervention.

PEEP affects cardiac output in two ways. The maintenance of positive pressure may compromise venous return, decreasing preload and potentially reducing cardiac output. Right ventricular afterload also may be increased because the right ventricle now has to pump against increased resistance in the pulmonary circuit. This increased right ventricular afterload can cause a mechanical displacement of the interventricular septum into the left ventricle during systole, causing a decrease in the left ventricular stroke volume. Reduced cardiac output (indicated by direct measurement, decreased blood pressure, and decreased urine output) usually can be corrected by an increase in intravascular volume, careful use of pressor agents, or both (see *Complications of ARDS,* page 46). If the intravascular volume is adequate, inotropic agents (dobutamine, dopamine, and isoproterenol) can be used to improve cardiac output.

Even though mechanical ventilation with PEEP remains the primary treatment for ARDS, several new ventilation techniques are being tried to maximize the benefits of treatment while minimizing the harm. Much literature correlates high peak airway pressures with barotrauma. Pressure-controlled inverse ratio ventilation (PC-IRV) is one technique being used to minimize this risk. This ventilatory mode reverses the conventional I:E ratio, and the mechanical breaths are pressure-limited.

During PC-IRV, prolonged positive pressure is applied during inspiration, creating a less turbulent pattern of flow. Peak airway pressure is decreased, and there is a decrease in the overdistention of the more compliant areas of the lung. Because the inspiration and expiration times are reversed, inspiration occurs before exhalation is complete, and alveolar collapse is avoided. The time for gas exchange is improved, and the surface area for gas exchange increases.

Because this method of ventilation reportedly causes patients to experience the sensation of inability to breathe, the use of neuromuscular blocking agents (pancuronium, atracurium, vecuronium, and mivacurium) in conjunction with sedation has been recommended. When neuromuscular blockade is used, ventilator settings and alarms must be checked frequently, as there is respiratory paralysis. The patient also may experience complications from immobi-

Complications of ARDS

Serious and potentially fatal complications can occur in the patient diagnosed with ARDS. These complications may be the result of the process itself or the result of the treatment. Prevention, early detection, and treatment of these complications are essential for recovery. Common complications are listed below.

Complication	Cause	Assessment Findings
Tension pneumothorax	• Increased intrathoracic pressure due to stiff, noncompliant lungs, high peak airway pressures, or use of positive end-expiratory pressure (PEEP)	• Absent breath sounds on affected side • Asymmetrical chest movement • Increased airway pressures • Falling O_2 saturation
Decreased cardiac output	• Hypoxemia • Decreased venous return due to use of PEEP	• Decreased blood pressure and urine output • Increased pulse rate • Decreased cardiac output (via pulmonary artery catheter)
Cardiac arrhythmias	• Hypoxemia • Electrolyte imbalance related to diuretic therapy	• Irregular cardiac rate and rhythm • Abnormal ECG tracing
Renal failure	• Hypotension • Hypoxia	• Urine output of < 20 ml/hour • Elevated blood urea nitrogen and creatinine levels
Sepsis	• Pneumonia • Underlying infectious process • Immunocompromised condition • Invasive lines	• Tachycardia • Elevated white blood cell count • Decreased clotting factors • Fever progressing to hypothermia • Increased cardiac output during "warm" phase of septic shock

lization, such as foot drop, skin breakdown, and corneal abrasions. Sedation must be used to decrease the patient's anxiety, because paralytic agents do not provide sedative effects.

Another new management technique called permissive hypercapnia is being used to minimize the risk of barotrauma. This ventilatory method limits peak inspiratory pressure to 30 to 40 cm/H_2O and uses synchronized intermittent mandatory ventilation (SIMV) and low tidal volumes (4 to 7 ml/kg). The $PaCO_2$ is allowed to rise to greater than 40 mm Hg. Although CO_2 removal is compromised, there is no treatment of subsequent changes in blood hydrogen oxygen concentration. There is clear evidence that barotrauma is reduced with this method of ventilation, but further study is required to determine the overall efficacy of the technique.

When the patient is receiving mechanical ventilation, the following nursing interventions should be incorporated into the plan of care:
• Auscultate breath sounds at least every 2 hours, or more frequently if the patient's condition indicates.
• Monitor oxygen saturation continuously via pulse oximetry.
• Evaluate arterial blood gas (ABG) studies for degree of hypoxemia and acid-base balance.
• Observe for changes in respiratory rate or pattern (such as asymmetrical chest movement).
• Suction only when indicated, especially if the patient is on PEEP.
• Position the patient to facilitate gas exchange (monitor arterial oxygen saturation while repositioning to determine best positions).
• Pace the patient's activities to tolerance levels. Even routine activities such as turning the patient can cause drastic decreases in PO_2, secondary to the lack of reserve and amount of shunting present.
• Observe for changes in level of consciousness, increased restlessness, or agitation.
• Observe for signs of reduced cardiac output (tachycardia, hypotension, decreased urine output) every hour.

Hemodynamic support
Management of fluid therapy in the patient with ARDS is critical. Intravascular volume must be carefully con-

trolled because of the tendency of protein and fluid to leak into the lung parenchyma. The goal of hemodynamic monitoring is to keep the patient as dry as possible, preventing further pulmonary edema, while maintaining adequate circulation and perfusion.

There is continued debate as to the use of crystalloid versus colloid fluid therapy. Recent research indicates that the increased permeability of the pulmonary vasculature allows colloids to move easily into the pulmonary interstitium, causing increased pulmonary edema. Therefore, crystalloid fluid therapy remains the most common means of support.

The following nursing interventions should be incorporated into the plan of care for the patient receiving hemodynamic monitoring:
• Monitor intake and output hourly.
• Weigh the patient daily.
• Monitor hemodynamic parameters (pulmonary arterial pressures, pulmonary capillary wedge pressure, cardiac output, central venous pressure, pulmonary vascular resistance, systemic vascular resistance) every 2 to 4 hours or more often, if necessary.

Pharmacologic intervention

Presently, most pharmacologic interventions for patients with ARDS are supportive. Drug therapies include antibiotics, bronchodilators, and sedative or paralytic agents. Antibiotics are used to treat infections. Bronchodilators are used to help reverse airway obstruction due to bronchoconstriction. Sedatives and neuromuscular blockers may be necessary to reduce discomfort, decrease anxiety, and decrease oxygen consumption. Paralytic agents are used to reduce skeletal muscle activity, thereby reducing oxygen consumption and decreasing metabolic acidosis. The nurse must always use sedation if a neuromuscular blocker is ordered. Diuretics may be administered in an attempt to decrease interstitial edema.

The use of corticosteroids is controversial, although it is believed by some to reduce pulmonary edema and stabilize pulmonary membranes by stabilizing lyso-somes. A number of risks are associated with corti-costeroid therapy, including sodium retention and potassium loss, muscle wasting, delayed healing, and increased susceptibility to infections. If indicated, vaso-active or inotropic therapy (or both) may be used to treat abnormalities of cardiac output, pulmonary vascu-lar resistance, and systemic vascular resistance.

Nursing interventions to be incorporated in the plan of care include:

• Administer medications as ordered and monitor their effects (such as urine output after administration of di-uretics, hemodynamic parameters).

• Administer neuromuscular blocking agents to elimi-nate skeletal muscle activity if metabolic acidosis oc-curs.

• Monitor the level of paralysis with a nerve stimulator in the patient receiving neuromuscular blockers.

• Administer sedatives as ordered.

Nutritional support

Because the patient with ARDS is in a hypermetabolic state, early, aggressive nutritional support is necessary. If nutritional needs are not met, the patient will remain in a catabolic state, which contributes to further meta-bolic and infectious complications. Malnutrition also slows the weaning process. Because nutritional support can contribute to volume overload and increased CO_2 production, the patient should be monitored closely. Nutrition may be provided by enteral or parenteral means, although the enteral route is preferred whenever possible.

The following nursing interventions should be an-ticipated:

• Monitor the rate of enteral and parenteral infusions closely; use of an infusion pump is recommended.

• Monitor electrolyte, glucose, blood urea nitrogen, and creatinine levels.

• Check gastric residuals every 4 hours or as ordered if the patient is receiving enteral feedings.

Prevention and treatment of additional complications

Prevention, early detection, and treatment of further complications or systemic insults are essential. Routine monitoring of the WBC count and collection of sputum cultures can aid in early identification of infection. Strict aseptic technique must be observed when suctioning the patient or caring for any invasive lines. The patient should be observed closely for any signs of a stress ulcer or other GI bleeding. Antacids, H_2 blockers, and sucralfate may be prescribed to avoid such complications.

Other potential complications include:
• fever (which may result from any of the complications that follow)
• nosocomial pneumonia
• abdominal abscess—especially after abdominal surgery
• sinusitis
• line sepsis
• systemic candidiasis
• drug fever
• renal failure
• liver failure
• multiple organ dysfunction syndrome.

Prognosis

Although the mortality rate for ARDS is 40% to 60%, the final patient outcome is difficult to predict. Many factors, including the etiology, involvement of other organ systems, and amount and duration of required ventilatory support, seem to influence the course. Patients may make a full recovery, with lung volumes and ABG levels returning to normal. Other possible outcomes include:
• the development of mild fibrosis followed by healing and recovery
• initial healing, followed by the development of severe fibrosis and death
• rapid progression to fibrosis and death.

Discharge planning

Ideally, discharge planning should begin as soon as the patient enters the health care system. Education should be geared to the patient's condition, with emphasis on explaining therapies, such as ventilator support. The family should be included in the teaching process and given frequent updates on the patient's condition.

When discharge planning is initiated, the following elements should be included:
• the need for social services, if indicated
• evaluation of the patient's home care abilities, including support systems
• review of any activity restrictions
• review of any therapies, such as oxygen administration, to be continued at home
• review of all medications, including dosage, food and drug interactions, and adverse reactions
• discussion of follow-up visit.

Angina

Unstable angina is a transitory syndrome that results from an insufficient supply of oxygenated blood to the myocardium. This type of angina characteristically strikes in an unpredictable pattern: the patient cannot anticipate when the symptoms will appear, how long they will last, or the degree of severity. It may develop in patients regardless of known or unknown coronary artery disease (CAD). Unstable angina also can occur after a patient has sustained a myocardial infarction (MI), percutaneous transluminal coronary angioplasty (PTCA), or coronary artery bypass grafting (CABG). The patient with this pathology is at significant risk for MI and sudden cardiac death.

Unstable angina may be the first sign of CAD or may signal an acceleration of disease in a patient with an established history of stable CAD. Often the appearance of unstable angina signals the potential for MI, which some patients may experience within days to several weeks after the initial presentation of unstable angina.

Pathophysiology

The pathophysiologic basis of unstable angina is attributed to a significant reduction of the luminal diameter of one or more coronary arteries. The reduced luminal diameter significantly limits the flow of oxygenated blood and nutrients to the myocardial tissue supplied by the artery.

The pathological mechanism that contributes to the unpredictable nature of unstable angina and results in the signs and symptoms experienced by the patient is most commonly related to the disruptive cracking and fissuring of plaque. The clot that subsequently develops increasingly diminishes the flow of oxygenated blood to the myocardium. Other factors also may increase myocardial oxygen demand or decrease myocardial oxygen consumption, resulting in anginal complaints. For further discussion, see *Factors affecting myocardial oxygen consumption*, page 53.

Plaque formation begins when endothelial cells become injured; circulating monocytes and lymphocytes adhere to the endothelial surface and release growth factors and inflammatory mediators. Lipids begin to accumulate in the injured area, and a fatty streak begins to form in the intimal layer. Platelets from the circulation migrate into this area and release growth factors. Concomitantly, smooth muscle cells migrate from the medial layer of the coronary arterial wall, release growth factors, and proliferate in the intima.

The plaque lesion continues to grow. Injury to the endothelial cells also results in diminished vasodilator response, and chemicals such as prostaglandin and angiotensin II exert vasoconstrictive effects that further narrow the luminal diameter. The plaque associated with unstable angina can rupture over time, creating fissures. Platelets, thrombin, fibrinogen, and fibrin migrate into the fissures, adhere to the surface, and form clots over a period of days to weeks in 70% to 90% of

Factors affecting myocardial oxygen consumption

The following table lists various factors that can increase myocardial oxygen demand or decrease myocardial oxygen supply, both of which should be avoided with unstable angina.

Factors increasing myocardial oxygen demand
- Emotional upset
- Excitement
- Stress
- Congestive heart failure
- Exercise
- Hyperthyroidism
- Papillary muscle rupture
- Polycythemia
- Pulmonary hypertension

- Ventricular aneurysm
- Ventricular septal defect

Factors decreasing myocardial oxygen supply
- Clot formation caused by the cracking of the coronary artery plaque
- Cold weather
- Anemia
- Cocaine intoxication

patients with unstable angina. The clot can cause partial or total occlusion of the flow in the artery.

Coronary artery plaque most commonly occurs in the bifurcations and branches of any of the coronary arteries. However, when a lesion in the proximal left anterior descending (LAD) artery causes a significant obstruction to the blood supply of the critical mass of left ventricular tissue, the patient is at serious risk for experiencing hemodynamic demise and death. Unstable angina caused by a plaque in the proximal LAD coronary artery has been termed Wellens' syndrome or critical proximal LAD stenosis. Early recognition and prompt management of this syndrome can preserve the integrity of this tissue and avert a potentially fatal event. For additional information, see *Identifying Wellens' syndrome*, page 54.

When coronary artery flow is significantly reduced, myocardial oxygenation needs are not met. The myocardial cells become ischemic and revert to anaerobic metabolism, an ineffective method of obtaining energy. Because the ischemia is transient, the myocardial cells do not die; the internal integrity of the cell and its intracellular components remains intact.

Identifying Wellens' syndrome

The main indicators of Wellens' syndrome are listed below.

• Electrocardiographic findings: These findings either are seen upon admission to the critical care unit or develop within 24 hours.

—T-wave inversion that initially starts and deepens in V_{2-3} and progresses to include leads V_{1-6}, 1, and aVL.

—ST segments that are either isoelectric or slightly elevated.

—R-wave progression, which indicates a viable anterior wall without necrosis.

• Cardiac enzyme profile: Total creatine phosphokinase (CPK) and CPK-MB (CPK with isoenzymes) normal or slightly elevated.

• Clinical symptoms: New onset of unstable anginal pattern within 1 week of admission.

The electrocardiographic sign of T-wave inversion in the precordial leads may or may not be initially present but most often will evolve. Although the ischemic process may accelerate and cause deepening T-wave inversion, acceleration of the ischemic state is not always accompanied by the clinical symptoms that the patient initially experienced. The patient may be totally asymptomatic, for reasons that are presently unknown. If the escalating ischemia is allowed to progress to total occlusion, the patient will experience extensive anterior-lateral myocardial damage.

The patient with Wellens' syndrome undergoes the same testing procedures as any patient with unstable angina, and treatment is guided by the results of the diagnostic procedures.

Clinical assessment

Clinical assessment is crucial in collecting the data needed to recognize unstable angina. Clinical assessment should include exploring the patient's history, performing a detailed evaluation of physical findings, and obtaining and reviewing the results of diagnostic studies.

History

A patient can present with one of three scenarios: rest angina, new onset angina, or increasing angina. *Rest angina* is defined by the Canadian Cardiovascular Society Classification (CCSC) as "angina occurring at rest and usually prolonged > 20 minutes occurring within a week of presentation." *New onset angina* is described as "angina of at least CCSC III severity with onset within 2 months of initial presentation." *Increasing angina* demonstrates a pattern of angina that lasts and is more severe; the patient's CCSC classification has increased over the last 2 months. For a discussion of the classifications of severity, see *Determining the severity of angina,* page 56.

Pertinent information to obtain includes:
• age
• presence of risk factors: hypercholesterolemia, hypertension, diabetes, smoking history, Type A or B behavior, stress, sedentary lifestyle, diet high in fats (especially saturated fats)
• patient history of CAD or other cardiac disease including MI and subsequent associated complications
• family history of CAD
• duration of condition and associated symptoms
• change in symptoms from previous pattern
• presence of precipitating factors
• medications that relieve the symptoms.

Physical findings

The signs and symptoms of unstable angina are similar to those of MI. The key indicator that distinguishes unstable angina from MI is that the symptoms are transient and typically last no longer than 30 minutes. The patient may exhibit the following:
• unpredictable burning or vice-like chest pressure located behind the sternum or epigastric area; may radiate to jaw, neck, left arm, or back and last between 5 and 30 minutes; most typically occurs at rest and is not related to emotion or stress; usually more severe and of longer duration than other forms of angina
• shortness of breath: can be isolated, unexplained, new-onset, or dyspnea that is worsening
• nausea and vomiting
• diaphoresis and cool, clammy skin
• anxiety
• bradycardia or tachycardia
• cardiac arrhythmias: ventricular ectopy such as premature ventricular contractions, ventricular tachycardia
• elevated respiratory rate, pulmonary congestion
• hypotension or hypertension

ASSESSMENT TIP
Determining the severity of angina

When assessing a patient suspected of having angina, the nurse must identify the degree of activity that causes symptoms. A helpful guide is the classification system developed by the Canadian Cardiovascular Society.

Class I: Ordinary activity does not cause angina. Angina occurs with strenuous, rapid, or prolonged exertion at work or recreation.

Class II: Slight limitation of ordinary activity. Angina occurs on walking or climbing stairs rapidly, walking uphill, walking or stair climbing after meals; or in cold, in wind, or under emotional distress; or only during the few hours after awakening; or walking more than two blocks on the level and climbing more than one flight of ordinary stairs at a normal pace and in normal condition.

Class III: Marked limitation of ordinary physical activity. Angina occurs on walking one or two blocks on the level and climbing one flight of stairs in normal conditions and at a normal pace.

Class IV: Inability to carry on any physical activity without discomfort; anginal symptoms may be present at rest.

Source: Canadian Cardiovascular Society Classification System for Grading Angina Pectoris, U.S. Department of Health & Human Services, 1994, page 10.

• S$_4$ heart sounds.

Atypical signs and symptoms may include absence of pain or pressure in chest, isolated discomfort in elbows or fingers, jaw or tooth pain, and transient sore throat.

Diagnosis

There are three goals in diagnosis: to determine the existence and degree of unstable angina in the patient with elusive and nonspecific symptoms; to differentiate unstable angina from MI or other diseases that may mimic cardiac symptoms, such as hiatal hernia or pulmonary embolism; and to determine the level of treatment necessary. Key diagnostic tests include cardiac enzyme studies, 12-lead electrocardiogram (ECG), and coronary angiography. A detailed description of these tests can be found in *Confirming unstable angina,* page 57, and *Potential ECG changes with unstable angina,* page 58.

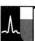

DIAGNOSTIC TESTS
Confirming unstable angina

The following diagnostic tests will provide information on the status of the patient's coronary arteries, hemodynamic parameters, and laboratory findings that may indicate myocardial ischemia and confirm the presence of unstable angina.

Intervention and Description

Cardiac enzyme studies
• Provide information on the presence of total creatine phosphokinase (CPK) and CPK-MB (CPK with isoenzymes) in the systemic circulation. These values indicate if myocardial damage has occurred.

• Unstable angina patients who have not sustained myocardial injury should have total CPK and CPK-MB levels in the normal range.
• The usual routine for obtaining cardiac enzyme studies is to draw blood levels every 12 hours for 36 hours.

Cardiac catheterization
• Provides a hemodynamic profile and assessment of the presence of plaque in the coronary arterial system.
• A catheter is inserted into the femoral artery and guided under fluoroscopy in a retrograde fashion

through the aorta to the openings of the coronary arteries. Contrast medium (dye) is injected into the arteries and will identify perfusion defects and extent of blood flow restriction.
• The procedure guides treatment choices.

Coronary angiography—digital subtraction
• Diagnostic tool that produces high resolution images of cardiovascular structures and is used to evaluate coronary artery flow, myocardial perfusion, and left ventricular func-

tion. Extraneous structures such as bone or soft tissue are eliminated from the image.
• The procedure is the same as for cardiac catheterization, except the dye used is more dilute and less harmful to the patient.

Coronary ultrasound
• Diagnostic tool that provides visualization of the lumen of the coronary arterial wall, plaque characteristics, and blood flow.
• High-frequency sound waves directed to the coronary artery will reflect back to the transducer at fre-

quencies corresponding to the velocity of blood flow through the vessel—the higher the velocity, the higher the frequency.
• Images produced may be hazy secondary to the noninvasive nature of the study and the potential for obstruction from underlying structures.

Exercise ECG or stress tests allow for evaluation of chest pain during physical stress, and thallium imaging can diagnose patency of coronary arteries and evaluate antianginal therapy. Diagnostic tests also may include those described in "Myocardial Infarction," page 424.

Potential ECG changes with unstable angina

Myocardial ischemia has four main indicators, each with a slightly different clinical significance. Note the significance of these patterns as they relate to progressive myocardial ischemia with the potential to lead to myocardial infarction (MI).

Indicator	Electrical Pattern	Significance
T-wave inversion		In ischemic tissue, the repolarization process is delayed; thus, the tissue stays in a negatively charged state longer. Instead of the normal upright appearance of the T wave, the resultant electrical pattern seen, often the classic indicator of ischemia, is a narrow and symmetrical inversion of the T wave in association with an isoelectric ST segment.
ST-segment depression and T-wave depression		If the ischemia is severe but transient, as seen in unstable angina, ST-segment depression with an inverted T wave will be present. This pattern represents ischemia to one or two layers of the ventricular myocardium and is transient in unstable angina.
Hyperacute upright T waves		This pattern represents transmural ischemia to a regionalized section of the ventricular myocardium. It often is the precursor to an MI pattern, which proceeds rapidly after the appearance of hyperacute upright T waves.
ST-segment elevation		This pattern represents transient ischemia to a transmural portion of the ventricular myocardium caused by total occlusion. The lack of collateral circulation contributes to this situation.

Treatment and care

Treatment and care is guided by collection of data derived from the patient's history, physical examination, and 12-lead ECG. Medical and nursing management focus on identifying an escalation in the ischemic process, preserving the integrity of the viable myocardial tissue, providing pharmacologic management and evaluating its effectiveness, and preparing the patient for invasive diagnostic and revascularization procedures.

Preserving the integrity of the myocardium

Efforts should be directed at increasing myocardial perfusion and decreasing myocardial oxygen demand to preserve the integrity of the myocardium. The workload of the already compromised heart must be decreased in order to mitigate any demands. The health care team must frequently reevaluate the patient's status to recognize any deterioration or escalation of the ischemic process early on.

The following nursing interventions necessary to increase oxygen supply and decrease myocardial demand should be incorporated into the plan of care:

• Provide supplemental oxygen.
• Maintain intravenous access.
• Administer antianginal agent as prescribed.
• Administer medications for pain or pressure symptoms as prescribed.
• Advise patient to report return of anginal symptoms.
• Monitor cardiac enzymes for indication or trend of myocardial injury pattern.
• Administer anxiolytics as necessary to decrease factors that would increase myocardial oxygen demand.
• Provide optimal rest periods to reduce or prevent any increased myocardial oxygen demand. Maintain on bed rest (except for bathroom privileges).
• Monitor the patient placed on the intra-aortic balloon pump according to hospital policy.
• Assess the patient every 2 hours and as needed for signs of heart failure and pulmonary congestion.

Nursing interventions aimed at identifying escalation of ischemic process and intervening early on include the following:
• Provide continuous cardiac monitoring.
• Monitor pulse oximetry.
• Report signs of escalating ischemia or MI to the physician immediately.
• Administer antianginal medications as ordered.
• Prepare for cardiac catheterization if needed.

Pharmacologic intervention and evaluation

Pharmacologic management is aimed at decreasing the workload of the heart, subsequently decreasing myocardial oxygen demand, and increasing oxygen supply, depending on the class of antianginal agent used. Specific information regarding pharmacologic management can be found in *Pharmacologic management of unstable angina,* pages 61 and 62.

The following nursing interventions for administering and evaluating antianginal agents should be incorporated into the plan of care:
• Assess efficiency of pharmacologic management.
• Determine whether the patient is symptom-free.
• Report symptoms that are not relieved, and adjust pharmacologic therapy as instructed by the physician.
• Evaluate for adverse reactions to the prescribed antianginal drug, such as hypotension with nitrates.
• Monitor fluid volume status and hemodynamic parameters.
• Observe for symptoms of breathing difficulty, such as bronchoconstriction with beta-adrenergic blockers.
• Provide appropriate education to the patient and family regarding the medications administered.
• Administer heparin as prescribed, and monitor for bleeding.

Invasive diagnostic and revascularization procedures

Many diagnostic and revascularization procedures can be used for a patient with unstable angina. The revascu-

MAJOR DRUGS

Pharmacologic management of unstable angina

Pharmacologic treatment for unstable angina is individualized for the patient and may include aspirin, nitrates, beta blockers, calcium channel blockers, morphine sulfate, heparin, or thrombolytic therapy. For a listing of thrombolytic therapy, see page 440 in "Myocardial Infarction."

Drug and Dosage	Mechanism of Action	Major Adverse Reactions
Aspirin (75 to 324 mg P.O. daily)	• Inhibits platelet aggregation and thromboxane A$_2$ formation. • Can play a significant role in limiting the incidence of fatal infarction.	• GI bleeding • Prolonged clotting time
Beta blockers *Atenolol* (5 mg I.V. loading dose followed by 5 mg I.V. after 5 min. Initiate 50 to 100 mg P.O. daily 1 to 2 hrs after second I.V. dose) *Tenormin (atenolol)* (25 to 50 mg P.O. four times/day) *Propranolol* (0.5 to 1 mg I.V. followed by 40 to 80 mg P.O. every 6 to 8 hrs starting 1 to 2 hrs after initial I.V. dose)	• Reduce myocardial oxygen demand and contribute to pain control. • Decrease the contractility of the heart, resulting in reduced workload. • Decrease heart rate, resulting in reduced oxygen demand.	• Bronchospasm • High-grade atrioventricular (AV) block • Hypotension • Prolonged PR interval • Fluid retention and congestive heart failure • Shock
Calcium channel blockers *Norvasc (amlodipine)* (2.5 to 5 mg P.O. four times/day) *Verapamil* (180 to 240 mg P.O. four times/day) *Diltiazem* (240 mg P.O. four times/day) *Procardia (nifedipine)* (30 mg P.O. four times/day)	• Decrease myocardial oxygen demand by arteriolar constriction with subsequent decreased systemic vascular resistance. • Dilate coronary arteries, resulting in increased myocardial oxygen supply.	• Hypotension • Arrhythmias, such as AV blocks • Pulmonary edema • Left ventricular failure

(continued)

Pharmacologic management of unstable angina *(continued)*

Drug and Dosage	Mechanism of Action	Major Adverse Reactions
Heparin (Bolus of 80 units/kg I.V.; initial bolus may vary depending on physician's preference. I.V. rate of 1,000 units/hr; adjust to keep activated partial thromboplastin time between 1.5 and 2.5 times control)	• I.V. administration may play a significant role in reducing the evolution of the disease into an infarctional state; may help control pain.	• Bleeding disorders • Thrombocytopenia • Hemorrhagic stroke
Nitroglycerin (Begin at 5 to 10 mcg/min I.V. infusion. Titrate to control symptoms while maintaining acceptable blood pressure; titration not to exceed 75 to 200 mcg/min. Oral: 0.4 mg under the tongue every 5 to 10 min up to three times)	• Improved myocardial perfusion as a result of a redistribution of blood flow from the dilation of coronary arteries and collateral network. Results in increased oxygen supply, decreased myocardial oxygen demand, and decreased preload and afterload. • Plays a role in the prevention of coronary artery spasm and reduces the affinity of platelets to aggregate.	• Hypotension • Decreased cardiac output with the decreased preload • Cardiovascular collapse • Severe headache
Morphine sulfate (2 to 5 mg repeated every 5 to 30 min. Titrate for relief of symptoms and to act as sedation; dose does not typically exceed 10 mg/hr)	• Decreases myocardial oxygen requirements by increasing venous capacitance, reducing systemic vascular resistance, and decreasing preload. • Provides pain control.	• Decreased mentation • Hypotension • Respiratory depression

larization procedures available include cardiac catheterization (which should be done within 48 hours of admission), PTCA, angioplasty, directional coronary atherectomy, use of the rotoblade, and CABG. A detailed description of these procedures can be found in

Revascularization procedures, pages 64 and 65. It is important for the patient and family to receive information from the health care team regarding the procedure, risks, and potential complications of these procedures.

The following nursing interventions should be incorporated into the plan of care:

• Obtain current renal function tests if dye is to be used in the procedure; ensure that the patient does not have any allergies to dye.

• Explain invasive diagnostic and revascularization procedures to the patient and family.

• Ensure that the patient has signed a permit for the procedures.

• Institute hospital monitoring protocol postprocedure.

• Monitor for potential complications following the procedure, including potential risk of coronary artery occlusion, aortic dissection, MI, hemorrhage, tamponade, thromboemboli, and infection.

Preventing complications

The unstable nature of the disease and the degree of arterial blockage can cause a variety of complications. Assessment and detection of complications is crucial to preserve the integrity of the myocardial tissue. Complications associated with unstable angina include MI, pump failure leading to decreased cardiac output, pulmonary edema, life-threatening arrhythmias, ventricular arrhythmias, high-grade atrioventricular blocks, and junctional or idioventricular escape rhythms resulting in decreased cardiac output, hypoxia, and impaired perfusion and death.

Prognosis

Over 570,000 patients are admitted to the hospital with unstable angina each year, with mortality rates reported to be as high as 60%. The patient with unstable angina must modify his or her lifestyle (stop smoking, adopt an appropriate diet, maintain a balance between rest and exercise) to improve the prognosis.

Revascularization procedures

Many types of revascularization techniques are used to improve coronary artery circulation. Diagnostic procedures, such as cardiac catheterization, also are frequently used with thrombolytics as revascularization procedures. Some of the most common procedures are described below.

Procedure	Description and Application
Percutaneous coronary artery angioplasty	• Revascularization device that includes a balloon inflated over the site of the plaque in order to increase intraluminal diameter • Requires the injection of dye to visualize effect of inflation
Directional coronary atherectomy	• Revascularization device using a catheter equipped with a cutting edge and a balloon. The cutting edge is positioned over the site of the plaque, the balloon is inflated, and the plaque is shaved off. Plaque remnants are captured and extracted from the vessel
Mechanical rotational atherectomy	• Revascularization device; a high-speed drill or burr is located on the end of a catheter that is powered by an air compressor to create rotational speeds of 190,000 rpm, which is highly effective in cutting calcified plaque located in a tortuous area
Transluminal extraction— endarterectomy device	• Revascularization device; the end of a catheter is fitted with 2 stainless steel blades in a hollow chamber and 2 adjoining windows • A vacuum, catheter drive units, and battery pack also comprise this device • Highly effective in plaque with associated thrombus • Only device that evacuates plaque particles and thrombus
Angioplasty, laser	• An experimental procedure that uses laser beams instead of thrombolytics to vaporize coronary obstructions • A laser catheter is inserted into the diseased artery and rapid bursts of laser are switched on and off for a predetermined time. Between bursts the catheter is rotated and advanced until the vessel is completely opened
Coronary artery stent placement	• Metal devices that are placed into a coronary artery to maximize luminal diameter and maintain patency of the vessel so that blood flow can be maintained • Especially useful for patients with bleeding disorders, which would prohibit the use of anticoagulation therapy, and tortuous vessels, where a large thrombus may exist

Revascularization procedures *(continued)*	
Procedure	**Description and Application**
Coronary artery bypass surgery	• Surgical insertion of the saphenous vein or the internal mammary artery to bypass blockages in one or more coronary arteries

Discharge planning

The overall goal of discharge planning is to prepare the patient to resume normal life activities at the highest possible level. Discharge planning should focus on the following:

• Develop a support structure to alter or decrease the effects of the patient's risks for heart disease (smoking cessation, relaxation, diet control).

• Consult social services or home care as needed.

• Educate the patient on the discharge medication regimen.

• Review the signs and symptoms of angina and of MI. Teach the patient to stop all activity and sit down if any of these are experienced. Usually the physician will order the patient to take nitroglycerin under the tongue and repeat 2 additional times at 5-minute intervals. If symptoms persist, the patient should know how to access emergency aid.

• If appropriate, refer for cardiac rehabilitation.

• Discuss when sexual activity can be resumed. Usually the suggested time period is between 2 and 4 weeks postdischarge, but this should be individualized.

Aortic aneurysm

An aortic aneurysm is the dilation and enlargement of a portion of the aorta in which the diameter increases to more than 50% its normal size. This life-threatening disorder presents a particular challenge to emergency personnel and critical care nurses, who should be familiar with the etiology, salient clinical manifestations, diagnosis, and required treatment because of the high mortality associated with unrecognized cases.

Rare before the fifth decade of life, aortic aneurysms are the tenth-leading cause of death in men over age 55. Those with coronary artery disease, peripheral vascular disease, or femoral or popliteal aneurysms are at highest risk. About 75% of all cases involve the abdominal aorta; the remaining 25%, the thoracic aorta.

Classification of aortic aneurysms

Aortic aneurysms are classified according to their morphology or location (see *Classification of aortic aneurysms,* pages 67 and 68). Morphologically, aneurysms may be either fusiform or saccular. A fusiform aneurysm affects the entire aortic circumference and is cylindrical; a saccular aneurysm involves the outpouching of only a portion of the aortic wall. Fusiform aneurysms are more common, although saccular aneurysms are more prone to rupture. An aortic aneurysm may be located in the thoracic, thoracoabdominal, or abdominal segment of the aorta. The thoracic aorta may be further subdivided into the ascending, transverse arch, and descending thoracic segments. Abdominal aortic aneurysms are almost exclusively fusiform.

Besides traditional, or true, aortic aneurysms, two other aortic disorders—pseudoaneurysms and aortic dissections—are possible. A pseudoaneurysm, or false aneurysm, is a contained aortic rupture in which blood escapes into the space between the aortic wall and the periaortic sheath. A sac develops around this hematoma and is confined to the periaortic area. Thus, the wall of a false aneurysm is not the original aortic wall but rather a mass of connective tissue and structures surrounding the extravasated blood. A communication or channel between the aorta and the sac allows blood to flow in and out of the area; it may be felt as a pulsatile mass.

An aortic dissection (formerly called a dissecting aneurysm) occurs when the intimal layer of the aorta tears and blood surges through, forming a hematoma

Classification of aortic aneurysms

Aortic aneurysms commonly are classified according to morphology or location. Four morphologic types are shown below.

Fusiform: A true aneurysm in which the entire arterial wall is dilated and the aneurysm is circumferential.

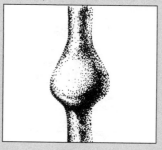

Pseudoaneurysm: A false aneurysm in which a ruptured vessel is confined by surrounding tissue that allows blood to flow in and out.

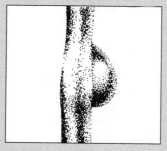

Saccular: A true aneurysm in which a distinct portion of the arterial wall balloons outward.

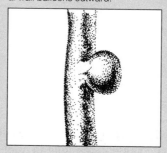

Aortic dissection: A false aneurysm in which a tear in the intimal layer of the aorta results in the formation of a hematoma between the intimal and medial layers, splitting the aorta lengthwise. Aortic dissections commonly are subclassified according to the location of the intimal tear and the extent of the hematoma, as illustrated below.

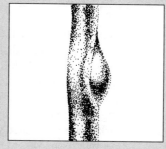

(continued)

Classification of aortic aneurysms *(continued)*

Aneurysms classified by location are shown below. Shading indicates areas that may be affected by dissection.

Type I: Dissection originates at the ascending aorta and extends distally through the aortic arch and down the descending aorta.

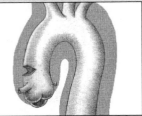

Type III: Dissection originates at or near the left subclavian artery and extends distally down the descending aorta.

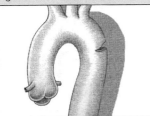

Type II: Dissection is contained in the ascending aorta.

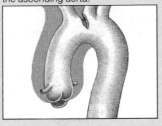

between the intimal and medial layers. Sometimes the blood can form a distal entry site, resulting in a false channel or double-lumen aorta. Dissections commonly are classified according to their point of origin and extent of hematoma formation; most occur in the ascending aorta. Systemic hypertension is the most common risk factor associated with this condition, although connective tissue disorders, such as Marfan's and Ehlers-Danlos syndromes, also are implicated.

Pathophysiology

Aneurysms arise as a result of a defect in the middle layer of the arterial wall. Once the elastic fibers and

Risk factors for aortic aneurysm development

- Advanced age
- Atherosclerosis
- Chronic obstructive pulmonary disease
- Cystic medial necrosis
- Diabetes mellitus

- Hypertension
- Infection
- Inflammatory disorders
- Smoking
- Trauma

collagen in that layer have been damaged, stretching and segmental dilation occur. The medial layer loses some of its elasticity, and fragmentation takes place. Smooth muscle cells are lost, and medial thinning can occur. The thinned wall may contain calcium deposits and atherosclerotic plaque, making the wall brittle.

Once an aneurysm begins to develop, lateral pressure increases, the lumen widens, and blood flow slows. Over time, mechanical stressors contribute to elongation of the aneurysm, causing the aorta to become bowed and tortuous. Hemodynamic forces also may play a role, causing pulsatile stresses on the weakened wall and pressing on the vasa vasorum, the blood vessels that supply nutrients to the arterial wall. Any aneurysm may predispose the patient to the further complications of thrombosis, distal embolization, or rupture.

The exact cause of aneurysms continues to be debated. Recent studies support a diffuse enlargement of all arteries (generalized dilating diathesis). Other studies suggest a hereditary component, in which certain individuals exhibit genetic susceptibility to the disease. There may be increased activity of certain enzymes, such as collagenase and elastase, in the vessel wall. These proteolytic enzymes can destroy the collagen and elastin and cause degeneration of the aortic wall. Most researchers believe that multiple factors contribute to the degenerative structural changes that lead to aortic aneurysm (see *Risk factors for aortic aneurysm development,* page 69).

Clinical assessment

Most aortic aneurysms are diagnosed in the course of testing for other conditions. Usually, a patient who presents to the emergency room has symptoms of an imminent aneurysm rupture, or the rupture has already occurred.

History

When eliciting information about the patient's history, inquire about any family history of aneurysms, such as Ehlers-Danlos or Marfan's syndromes, as well as any contributing factors, such as smoking, hypertension, heart disease, carotid disease, or other aneurysms.

Patients with aortic aneurysms may have multiple aneurysms involving the iliac, femoral, and popliteal arteries. A history of bilateral popliteal aneurysms is considered a marker, because about 33% of patients have concomitant aortic aneurysms. History of inguinal hernias also has been associated with increased incidence of aortic aneurysms.

Physical findings

Signs and symptoms of aortic aneurysm depend on the location and size of the dilation (see *Signs and symptoms of aortic aneurysm,* page 71). Usually, symptoms result from rupture, expansion, embolization, thrombosis, or pressure from the mass on adjacent structures.

The physical examination may provide clues to the presence of aneurysms. Thoracic aneurysm may produce an inequality of pulse and blood pressure in the arms. These aneurysms also may involve the aortic valve and produce an aortic insufficiency murmur. In acute cases of thoracic aneurysm expansion, the patient may present with severe hypertension, acute neurologic signs, and a new murmur of aortic insufficiency. Physical examination also may reveal a right sternoclavicular lift, jugular venous distention, or tracheal deviation.

Aortic aneurysms in the abdominal region should be palpable if the patient is not too obese and does not have ascites and the dilation is at least 5 cm in size. The exam-

Signs and symptoms of aortic aneurysm

The signs and symptoms of aortic aneurysm usually are related to its location and its expansion or encroachment on adjacent structures.

Thoracic aneurysm

• Chest pain that usually is substernal and can radiate to the neck, back, abdomen, or shoulders
• Sharp, tearing pain between the scapula (may indicate impending rupture)
• Hoarseness and coughing (if aneurysm is pressing on laryngeal nerve) or difficulty swallowing (due to esophageal compression)
• Difficulty breathing or hemoptysis (with rupture into tracheobronchial tree); hematemesis (with rupture into esophagus)
• Back pain due to spinal compression
• Regurgitation due to involvement of the aortic valve (if aneurysm involves ascending aorta)
• Obstruction of the coronary arteries, leading to ischemia or infarction (if aneurysm is near sinus of Valsalva)

• Venous congestion with swelling and bluish discoloration of the upper arms and head (if aneurysm is near superior vena cava); jugular venous distention may be noted

Abdominal aneurysm

• Excruciating back pain
• Abdominal pain and tenderness associated with peritoneal irritation
• Pain that radiates to the groin or legs
• Urge to defecate
• Urologic disorders, such as renal colic-type pain, gross hematuria, pulsating urination, testicular or flank pain
• "Blue toe syndrome" (livedo reticularis and bilateral cyanotic toes with palpable pedal pulses)
• Hip pain caused by pressure of the mass on the psoas muscle

ination will reveal a pulsatile mass located in the umbilical region of the abdomen, slightly to the left of midline. Bruits may be heard over the abdomen or femoral arteries.

Ruptures may be contained in surrounding extravascular space, tamponading the bleeding and preventing extravasation. Frank rupture, a vascular catastrophe, includes physical findings of cardiovascular collapse (hypotension, tachycardia, pallor, oliguria, and diaphoresis). Rupture can rapidly lead to death by exsanguination. Mottling of the abdomen and lower extremities, with weakening or loss of pulses, may be present.

Diagnosis

The diagnosis of aortic aneurysm is made through various imaging modalities (see *Imaging methods for diagnosing*

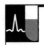

Imaging methods for diagnosing aortic aneurysms

The most useful imaging method for diagnosing aneurysms depends on the location of the lesions. Each modality has advantages and limitations.

Ultrasound
Ultrasound is the simplest and least expensive method for diagnosing and measuring abdominal aortic aneurysms, although it cannot be used to assess thoracic aneurysms. Ultrasound results are reported as two numbers (such as 3.5 × 3.8), indicating the transverse and anterior-posterior diameters of the aneurysm. The larger of the diameters is taken as the size.

Transesophageal echocardiogram (TEE)
TEE allows for visualization of the thoracic aorta and combined use of color Doppler flow to give information on blood flow.

X-ray
Plain films may provide information about the aneurysm; 55% to 85% of aortic walls contain a fine rim of calcium that can be visualized. Widening of the mediastinum suggests thoracic aneurysm.

Computed tomography (CT scan)
CT defines the size and extent in both directions better than ultrasound and visualizes the retroperitoneum, making it possible to identify an unsuspected rupture or other complications.

Magnetic resonance imaging (MRI)
MRI is a more recent advance in imaging than CT, but its role in the diagnosis of aortic aneurysm is not yet fully defined. It provides accurate measurement of aneurysm size and identifies involvement of the renal and iliac artery.

Aortography
Aortography is not as accurate in measuring aneurysm size as CT or MRI, because a thrombus will reduce the lumen size of the artery. However, it can aid in distinguishing the patency of visceral vessels and often is performed in patients who have associated renovascular hypertension or symptoms of mesenteric or peripheral vascular involvement.

aortic aneurysms, page 72). No specific laboratory tests are available to assist in the diagnosis of aneurysms, although leakage of blood may be indicated by leukocytosis and a drop in the hemoglobin and hematocrit.

Treatment and care
The approach to treatment of an aortic aneurysm depends on its size and location and the patient's presentation. The best scenario is when the aortic aneurysm is repaired as an elective surgery. In this instance, coexist-

ing conditions can be assessed and therapy optimized before surgery.

Because thoracic and thoracoabdominal aneurysms pose a greater risk of rupture than abdominal aneurysms, an aggressive surgical approach usually is employed. Small abdominal aortic aneurysms, which are less than 5 cm, may be followed by serial sonography testing every 3 to 6 months. Once the size reaches 5 cm, surgery is advocated.

Initial emergency treatment

Patients with suspected aortic rupture or impending rupture are managed in a critical care setting or taken immediately to surgery. Nursing management is of utmost importance, and time is of the essence (see *Key nursing interventions for patients with aortic aneurysm,* page 74). Interventions include nursing surveillance, drug therapy, general supportive measures, and preparation for surgery.

Blood pressure should be followed with an indwelling arterial cannula with continuous ECG monitoring. A Swan-Ganz pulmonary arterial catheter may be inserted to monitor heart filling pressures. Urine output should be monitored hourly and maintained above 30 ml/hour. If the patient has an acute rupture, urgent blood transfusions are needed. Sedation and pain relief are a priority to prevent agitation and increased blood pressure. Measures should be taken to lower an elevated blood pressure immediately. The drug most widely used is sodium nitroprusside. A beta-adrenergic blocking drug also may be used to slow the heart rate. Propranolol or esmolol commonly is used to reduce the heart rate and pulse pressure, leading to reduced pressure on the aortic wall.

Nursing measures to incorporate into the plan of care are as follows:

• Insert large-bore intravenous catheters for potential rapid fluid resuscitation.

• Assess pain location and intensity. Increased intensity suggests rapid enlargement or imminent rupture.

Key nursing interventions for patients with aortic aneurysm

Care of the patient with aortic aneurysm involves assessment and interventions to ensure tissue perfusion to all extremities and all end organs.

MAINTAIN ADEQUATE TISSUE PERFUSION

Maintain systemic cardiac perfusion	Optimize fluid balance	Maintain cardiac output
• Monitor kidney perfusion by checking urine output and blood urea nitrogen and creatinine levels. • Assess skin temperature and color and Doppler pulses; prevent the development of pressure sores. • Assess nasogastric output, bowel sounds, and stools. • Assess level of consciousness and motor strength. • Monitor the ECG and assess ST segments, chest pain, and creatine phosphokinase isoenzyme levels.	• Assess for fluid excess by monitoring fluid resuscitation and I.V. therapy. —Administer diuretics as ordered. —Monitor cardiac output, wedge pressure, and central venous pressure. • Monitor for fluid deficits by assessing for fluid shifts, third-space loss, insensible loss, and osmotic diuresis; replace lost fluids. • Analyze parameters of weight trends (intake and output, drainage tube amount, hemoglobin [Hb] and hematocrit [HCT], hemodynamic profile). • Administer blood products and I.V. fluids as ordered.	• Assess for hypotension. —Check for evidence of hemorrhage. —Administer I.V. fluids and dopamine as ordered. —Monitor Hb and HCT. • Assess for hypertension. —Check for underlying causes (hypothermia, pain, anxiety). —Administer vasodilators and titrate to desired response. —Administer pain medication to reduce anxiety. • Monitor cardiac function by assessing hemodynamic parameters and aortic valve murmurs.

• Assess for signs and symptoms of rupture, such as hypotension, pallor, cool and clammy skin, and altered mentation.
• Assess the ECG for rate, arrhythmias, and ST segment changes.
• Anticipate the need to administer nitroprusside if the patient is hypertensive, or dopamine if hypotensive.
• Anticipate adequate volume replacement with blood and other products to block the effects of cross-clamping and decrease declamping hypotension during surgery.
• Palpate peripheral pulses; check for pulse deficits.
• Administer medications for pain and agitation as ordered, such as morphine and Valium (diazepam).

Surgical treatment
Surgery of aortic aneurysms may be an emergency procedure in cases of rupture or impending rupture or an elective procedure in stable conditions. Indications for surgery include:
• aneurysm that is progressively increasing in size or greater than 5 cm
• impending rupture
• symptoms of aneurysmal-induced interruptions in circulation, causing cerebral ischemia (loss of consciousness, transient ischemic attacks) or coronary ischemia
• uncontrolled pain
• aortic valve insufficiency.

Postoperative nursing care
Nursing care is similar to that for cardiac surgical patients and focuses on surveillance and prevention of complications (see *Serious complications following aortic aneurysm repair,* page 76). Most patients present to the critical care unit with invasive monitoring lines and ventilator support. Chest tubes may be in place if surgery involved the thoracic aorta.

Postoperative hypertension is common, due to aortic denervation, stimulation of renin-angiotensin system, neural reflexes, and hypothermia during surgery. Nitroprusside or nitroglycerin may be infused and

Serious complications following aortic aneurysm repair

Most complications following aneurysm repair stem from the abrupt cessation of blood flow through the aorta or embolization during surgery, leading to end-organ ischemia and subsequent organ dysfunction.

Complication	Cause
Myocardial dysfunction	Left ventricular failure, arrhythmia, myocardial infarction
Renal failure/acute tubular necrosis	Embolization, contrast dye, ischemia
GI complications	Ileus, pancreatitis, ischemia of left colon
Paralysis	Ischemia to spinal cord
Ischemia to lower extremities (trash foot)	Atheromatous debris
Hemorrhage	Injury to iliac or lumbar veins, coagulopathies, spleen damage

titrated by the nurse to maintain normotension. Pulmonary hygiene requires meticulous attention and involves suctioning, postural drainage, and deep-breathing exercises.

Nursing interventions are as follows:

• Provide continuous ECG monitoring.

• Assess urine output with a Foley catheter to ensure adequate renal perfusion.

• Maintain nasogastric tube patency to decompress the stomach.

• Assist with serial Doppler examination of all extremities to evaluate adequacy of the vascular repair and presence of any embolization.

• Assess for signs of poor arterial perfusion: pain, paresthesia, pallor, pulselessness, paralysis, and poikilothermia (coldness).

Prognosis

The prognosis for patients with aortic aneurysm is grim if surgical repair is not done. The 1- and 3-year survival rates with untreated thoracic aneurysms are 58% and 26%, respectively. The aneurysm will continue to enlarge until rupture and death result. Furthermore, the prognosis is better if the aneurysm is repaired on an elective, nonemergency basis.

If the aneurysm is repaired with Dacron or another type of synthetic graft, fistula development and graft infection are possible. Graft infection is a serious but rare complication that most often occurs after 2 years. Aortoenteric fistula, another rare development, can occur years after surgery. The patient presents with massive GI bleeding, and emergency surgery is required.

Discharge planning

With shortened lengths of postoperative hospital stay, it is imperative to assess the patient's home situation before discharge, ideally at the time of admission. Depending on the patient's self-care ability and social support system, it may be necessary to arrange home visits by public health nurses or nursing case management during the initial period to assess wound healing and overall status.

Discharge instructions should include information on:
• restricting activity and allowing time for rest
• the need for showers or sponge baths initially and avoiding use of lotions or powder at the incision site
• continuing pulmonary hygiene procedures at home
• adhering to a low-fat, low-cholesterol diet if the patient has atherosclerosis
• notifying the physician about any increased abdominal or incision pain, difficulty breathing, signs of infection (fever or draining, reddening, or swelling at the incision site), numbness, coolness, or a change in circulation to hands or feet
• the need to control blood pressure and stop smoking.

Arrhythmias

Arrhythmias are variations in the normal pattern of electrical stimulation of the heart. Lethal arrhythmias, such as ventricular tachycardia and ventricular fibrillation, are a major cause of sudden cardiac death, claiming the lives of over 300,000 people annually in the United States. Arrhythmias can be classified by the region of the heart in which they originate (see *Identifying and treating arrhythmias,* pages 80 to 89).

Pathophysiology

Arrhythmias typically originate from ectopic beats, failure of myocardial tissue to initiate or conduct a beat, escape beats and rhythms, or reentry mechanisms.

Ectopic beats

Ectopic beats can originate in the atria, atrioventricular (AV) junction, or ventricular tissue. Although all of these tissues are capable of automaticity (ability of a cardiac cell to initiate an electrical stimulus), the sinus node has the fastest rate of spontaneous discharge and normally initiates myocardial depolarization. Infrequent ectopic beats occur in the normal heart as a result of transient increases in catecholamine levels, as with exercise. More frequent ectopic beats may result from increased pressure or strain on the atria or ventricles, as occurs with cardiomyopathy, congestive heart failure, and hypertension.

Frequent ectopic beats also are common with electrolyte imbalance, as this disrupts the pattern of myocardial depolarization and repolarization, which depends on the flow of ions across the cell membrane. Ischemia also disrupts the function of the cell membrane by inhibiting transfer of metabolic byproducts out of the cell and by inhibiting normal metabolic functions as a result of the unavailability of oxygen.

Failure to initiate or conduct an impulse

Failure of the sinus node to initiate an impulse at the appropriate time may result in sinus pause or sinus arrest. This may be caused by ischemia at the sinus node, vagal stimulation, or toxicity of various drugs, such as digoxin. Failure of myocardial tissue to conduct an impulse may result in a myocardial block and can be caused by ischemia, myocardial infarction (MI), degenerative changes in the heart's conduction system, or toxicity of various drugs that suppress ectopic beats in those tissues. Sinus exit block results when the atrial tissue surrounding the sinus node fails to respond to or conduct the impulse. Toxic levels of quinidine or procainamide hydrochloride also may produce such a block. (See "Myocardial Conduction Defects," page 409, for a complete discussion of heart blocks.)

Escape beats and rhythms

Escape beats and rhythms occur with suppression or dysfunction of higher intrinsic pacemaker tissues. Thus, a junctional escape rhythm may result when the sinus node is suppressed by vagal stimulation or various medications, such as beta blockers. Following sinus arrest, if the AV junction or a site in the ventricle reaches threshold (the point where the cell can depolarize spontaneously) before the sinus node resumes function, a junctional escape or ventricular escape beat will occur. An idioventricular rhythm will occur if the sinus node and AV junction cease functioning, which may occur with a large MI.

Reentry

The underlying mechanism for most tachycardias, reentry occurs when cardiac conduction along two parallel pathways proceeds in an abnormal fashion, resulting in a blocked impulse and retrograde conduction (see *Reentry mechanisms,* page 90). Micro-reentry, the mechanism underlying paroxysmal atrial tachycardia and ventricular tachycardia, occurs when the reentry circuit is formed by two neighboring cardiac cells.

(Text continues on page 88.)

Identifying and treating arrhythmias

The following chart highlights the characteristics, causes and underlying mechanisms, and treatments of arrhythmias commonly seen by critical care nurses.

Rhythm/Arrhythmia	Characteristics
Sinus rhythm 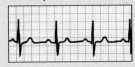	• Regular • P waves normal • Atrial and ventricular (AV) rates 60 to 100/minute • PR interval normal (0.12 to 0.20 second) • QRS complex normal (0.04 to 0.10 second)
Sinus bradycardia 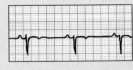	• Regular • P waves normal • AV rates < 60/minute • PR interval normal • QRS complex normal
Sinus tachycardia 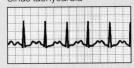	• Regular • P waves normal • AV rates > 100/minute • PR interval normal • QRS complex normal
Sinus arrhythmia 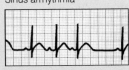	• Irregular • P waves normal • AV rates normal • PR interval normal • QRS complex normal
Sinus pause/arrest 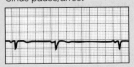	• Irregular • P waves normal, none in pause • AV rates depend on underlying rhythm • PR interval normal • QRS complex normal, none in pause • Pause < 2 sinus cycles; arrest > 2

Causes/Underlying Mechanisms	Treatment
• Normal function	• None
• Impulse originates in sinus node more slowly than usual • Vagal stimulation, beta blockers, calcium channel blockers, ischemia, myocardial infarction (MI)	• Treat only if symptomatic. • Atropine increases sinus rate, resulting in relief of symptoms. • Consider pacemaker if condition persists.
• Impulse originates in sinus node more quickly than usual • Exercise, stress, pain, fever, strong emotion, hypovolemia, MI	• Treat underlying cause.
• Rate increases with inspiration to accommodate increased venous return to right heart, decreases with expiration as return decreases	• None.
• Temporary failure of sinus node to initiate a stimulus, resulting in one or more "dropped" P-QRS • If rare and short, may be normal; antiarrhythmic medications	• Observe patient. • Consider cause, length of pause, and frequency. • If > 3 seconds, report. • If frequent or long, may require pacemaker.

(continued)

Identifying and treating arrhythmias *(continued)*

Rhythm/Arrhythmia	Characteristics
ATRIAL ARRHYTHMIAS	

Rhythm/Arrhythmia	Characteristics
Premature atrial complex (PAC) 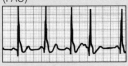	• Irregular • P waves present; premature P waves may differ in shape and may be hidden in preceding T wave • AV rates depend on underlying rhythm • PR interval may be normal, short, or prolonged • QRS complex normal
Nonconducted PAC 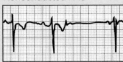	• Irregular • P waves present; premature P waves may differ in shape and may be hidden in preceding T wave • Rate depends on underlying rhythm, A>V rate • No PR interval • No QRS complex
Paroxysmal atrial tachycardia (PAT) 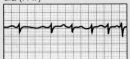	• Regular during tachycardia • P waves present, but during tachycardia may be difficult or impossible to see • Rate 140 to 270/minute during tachycardia • PR interval during tachycardia normal, short, or prolonged • QRS complex usually normal
PAT with block 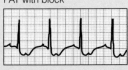	• Regular or irregular • P waves present, regular, and more frequent than QRS complexes • Atrial rate 140 to 270, A>V rate • PR interval constant for conducted beats (normal, short, or long) • QRS complex usually normal
Atrial fibrillation (A-fib) 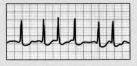	• Irregular • No P waves; atrial activity is coarse or fine fibrillatory waves • Atrial rate 375 to 600/minute; ventricular rate 30 to > 200/minute • No PR interval • QRS complex usually normal

Causes/Underlying Mechanisms	Treatment
• Ectopic site within atrium initiates beat before next sinus beat • May be normal if infrequent; frequent PACs due to atrial strain (in congestive heart failure [CHF]), ischemia, or mechanical irritation (cannulation for heart-lung bypass)	• Consider treating if > 6/minute, as this may indicate irritability that may lead to atrial fibrillation or atrial flutter. • Administer type 1A antiarrhythmics (quinidine, procainamide).
• PAC (as above) reaches AV node before it has repolarized, so impulse is not conducted to ventricles • May be normal if infrequent, or caused by atrial strain, ischemia, or mechanical irritation	• Treatment is same as for PAC above. • If frequent, ventricular rate will be low; assess patient for signs of decreased cardiac output.
• Reentry focus within the atria • May be due to digoxin toxicity	• Have patient cough forcefully or bear down (vagal maneuver). • Physician may perform carotid sinus massage. • Administer type 1A antiarrhythmics (quinidine, procainamide).
• Reentry focus within the atria • Almost always due to digoxin toxicity	• Evaluate for and treat digoxin toxicity. • If not caused by digoxin toxicity, treat with type 1A antiarrhythmics.
• Multiple foci in atria simultaneously initiate impulses with only a small area of tissue responding to each; atria do not contract in a coordinated fashion, but rather quiver • Mechanical irritation, atrial strain (from CHF or chronic obstructive pulmonary disease [COPD])	• Quinidine, procainamide, or amiodarone may suppress the ectopic foci. • Digoxin increases chance of remaining in sinus rhythm in the event of conversion. • I.V. verapamil or diltiazem hydrochloride will control a fast ventricular rate. • Pacing cardioversion or synchronized electrical cardioversion may be needed. • Some patients with enlarged atria will remain in A-fib.

(continued)

Identifying and treating arrhythmias *(continued)*

Rhythm/Arrhythmia	Characteristics

ATRIAL ARRHYTHMIAS *(continued)*

Atrial flutter (A-flutter) 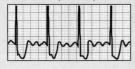	• Regular or irregular • No P waves; atrial activity is regular flutter waves ("sawtooth" baseline); no PR interval • Atrial rate 275 to 350/minute; ventricular rate depends on ratio of conduction • No PR interval • QRS complex may be distorted by flutter waves
Wandering atrial pacemaker 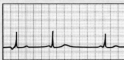	• Regular or slightly irregular • P waves differ in shape (at least 3 shapes seen) • Atrial and ventricular rates 60 to 100/minute • PR interval varies • QRS complex normal
Multifocal atrial tachycardia 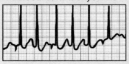	• Irregular • P waves differ in shape (at least 3 shapes seen) • AV rates > 100/minute • PR interval varies • QRS complex usually normal
Supraventricular tachycardia (SVT) 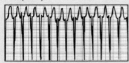	• Regular • P waves present but may be hidden • AV rates > 100/minute • PR interval constant; may be normal, short, or long • QRS complex usually normal; if QRS wide, see criteria for wide complex (page 92)

JUNCTIONAL RHYTHMS AND ARRHYTHMIAS

Premature junctional complex (PJC) 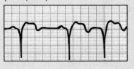	• Irregular • P waves inverted in Lead II, seen before or after QRS, or occur during QRS and so are hidden • Rates depend on underlying rhythm • PR interval < 0.12 second if P waves before QRS complex; otherwise not measured for PJC • QRS complex normal

Causes/Underlying Mechanisms	Treatment
• Reentry focus within the atria • Mechanical irritation, atrial strain	• Vagal maneuvers may slow ventricular rate so flutter waves are visible. • I.V. verapamil or diltiazem will control fast ventricular rate. • Quinidine, procainamide, or digoxin may alter reentry pathway. • Synchronized electrical cardioversion needed.
• Slowing of sinus node from vagal stimulation allows other atrial sites to reach threshold and initiate a beat.	• No treatment needed.
• Multiple ectopic foci in atria initiate beats at a rapid rate • Severe stretch on the atria due to advanced, generally end-stage COPD	• Rhythm is not treated; rather, treat the underlying COPD.
• May be sinus tachycardia, PAT, rapid A-flutter, or junctional tachycardia; "SVT" is used generically until further evidence allows more accurate rhythm identification	• Try vagal maneuvers to slow or convert rhythm. • I.V. adenosine or procainamide may convert rhythm. • Synchronized electrical cardioversion may be needed.
• Early P-QRS disrupts sinus timetable, with a small pause or recovery period following PJC • Ectopic site within AV junction initiates beat before the sinus beat, conduction to atria is retrograde • If infrequent, may be normal • May be due to ischemia or catecholamines	• PJCs are not treated. • If frequent, evaluate for underlying cause.

(continued)

Identifying and treating arrhythmias *(continued)*

Rhythm/Arrhythmia	Characteristics

JUNCTIONAL RHYTHMS AND ARRHYTHMIAS (continued)

Junctional rhythm

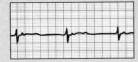

- Regular
- P waves inverted in Lead II, seen before or after QRS, or occur during QRS and so are hidden
- AV rates 40 to 60/minute
- PR interval < 0.12 second if P wave before QRS complex; otherwise not measured
- QRS complex normal

Accelerated junctional rhythm

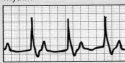

- Regular
- P waves inverted in Lead II, seen before or after QRS complex, or occur during QRS and so are hidden
- AV rates 60 to 100/minute
- PR interval < 0.12 second if P wave before QRS complex; otherwise not measured
- QRS complex normal

Junctional tachycardia

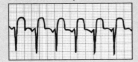

- Regular
- P waves inverted in Lead II, seen before or after QRS complex, or occur during QRS and so are hidden
- AV rates > 100/minute
- PR interval < 0.12 second if P wave before QRS complex; otherwise not measured
- QRS complex normal

VENTRICULAR ARRHYTHMIAS

Premature ventricular complex (PVC)

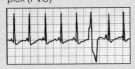

- Irregular
- Usually no P wave before PVC
- Rates depend on underlying rhythm
- PR interval not measured for PVC
- QRS complex wide, generally > 0.16 second

Idioventricular rhythm

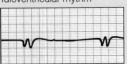

- Regular
- No P waves
- Ventricular rate 10 to 40/minute
- No PR interval
- QRS complex wide, > 0.10 second

Causes/Underlying Mechanisms	Treatment
• Suppression of sinus node allows AV junction to initiate beats at its intrinsic rate • May be due to vagal stimuli, ischemia, or effects of drugs (such as digoxin, beta blockers, or calcium channel blockers)	• Assess patient; this is usually well tolerated. • If symptomatic from rate or loss of AV synchrony, atropine may increase sinus rate and restore sinus rhythm.
• Increased rate of spontaneous depolarization in AV junction • May be due to catecholamine effects or ischemia at AV junction	• No treatment for rhythm. • Assess patient; this is usually well tolerated. • Treat cause.
• Increased rate of spontaneous depolarization in AV junction or reentrant tachycardia involving AV node • May be due to catecholamines or ischemia at AV junction • Reentry pathway may be due to different refractory times among AV nodal tissues	• May respond to type 1A antiarrhythmics (quinidine, procainamide). • Pacing cardioversion or synchronized electrical cardioversion may be needed. • AV nodal reentry may be treated with ablation.
• Ectopic focus in ventricle fires prior to next sinus beat • Electrolyte imbalance (especially hypokalemia), ischemia, MI, catecholamines, cardiomyopathy, abnormal electrical function at border of MI scar	• Consider treating if >6/minute, increasing frequency, occurring in couplets, triplets, or bigeminy. • Treat with antiarrhythmic drugs. • Treat underlying cause.
• Failure of higher pacemakers (sinus node and AV junction); escape rhythm originating in Purkinje fibers • MI, severe hypoxia, severe acidosis	• Begin cardiopulmonary resuscitation (CPR) if pulseless. • Oxygen, atropine, epinephrine may restore higher pacemakers. • Artificial pacemaker may be needed. *(continued)*

Identifying and treating arrhythmias *(continued)*

Rhythm/Arrhythmia	Characteristics
VENTRICULAR ARRHYTHMIAS *(continued)*	
Accelerated idioventricular rhythm 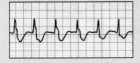	• Regular • No P waves • Ventricular rate 40 to 100/minute • No PR interval • QRS complex wide, > 0.10 second
Ventricular tachycardia (V-tach) 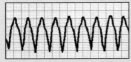	• Regular • P waves present but rarely seen; if seen, are not associated with QRS complex • Ventricular rate > 100/minute • No PR interval • QRS complex wide, > 0.10 second • See criteria for wide complex (page 92)
Ventricular fibrillation (V-fib) 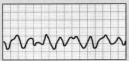	• Irregular • No P waves • No rate • No PR interval • No QRS complex, chaotic electrical activity
Asystole 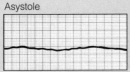	• No rhythm • No P waves • No AV rate • No PR interval • No QRS complex • "Flat line"

Macro-reentry, which occurs in AV nodal reentrant tachycardia and pre-excitation syndromes, involves a larger circuit, generally incorporating the tissue of the AV node as one leg of the reentry circuit (see "Myocardial Conduction Defects," page 409).

Clinical assessment

Differentiation of arrhythmias is crucial to ensure proper treatment; however, the nurse must remember to treat

Causes/Underlying Mechanisms	Treatment
• Suppression of higher pacemakers or increased rate of spontaneous discharge of Purkinje fibers • Vagal or drug suppression of higher pacemakers • Ischemia, MI, myocardial reperfusion	• No treatment unless patient is symptomatic from rate or loss of AV synchrony. • Atropine may restore higher pacemakers.
• Reentry mechanism in ventricles • Ischemia, cardiomyopathy, MI, electrolyte imbalance, abnormal function in tissue bordering MI scar or ventricular aneurysm • Long QT interval (may be induced by type 1A antiarrhythmics)	• Assess patient. • If stable, begin I.V. lidocaine. • If unstable (chest pain, severe dyspnea, hypotension), begin sedation and synchronized cardioversion. • If pulseless, defibrillate and begin CPR.
• Multiple foci in ventricles initiating beats, no coordinated contraction so no cardiac output • Fibrillatory waves may be coarse or fine; coarse are more likely to be converted • MI, severe hypoxia, severe acidosis	• Defibrillate. • Begin CPR. • I.V. epinephrine will increase amplitude of waves and increase chance of successful defibrillation.
• Failure of all pacemakers • MI, severe hypoxia, severe acidosis	• Begin CPR. • I.V. atropine or epinephrine may restore some kind of electrical activity. • Temporary pacemaker may be needed.

the entire patient, not just the rhythm disturbance. For any arrhythmia that might result in hemodynamic compromise, the nurse's primary action is to assess the patient. Once the patient has been stabilized, a complete analysis of the cardiac rhythm can proceed.

History

When a patient presents with a history of symptoms suggestive of arrhythmia or has been treated previously

Reentry mechanisms

Normal conduction along parallel pathways proceeds at equivalent rates. When two impulses meet, each finds the tissue already depolarized by the other impulse, so the conduction of the impulse stops (top). Conduction can progress only to neighboring cells that have not already been depolarized. In reentry tissue, one pathway conducts rapidly, while a parallel pathway conducts slowly, resulting in a blocked impulse (bottom). When the impulse from the fast pathway reaches the previously blocked area, it finds the tissue sufficiently repolarized to conduct the impulse slowly in a backward (retrograde) fashion. When the impulse has conducted retrograde through the slow tissue and reaches the fast pathway, it finds the tissues of the fast pathway repolarized and ready to conduct the impulse again. The result is a circular movement down the fast pathway and up the slow pathway. With each circuit, the impulse also is conducted to adjacent tissues, resulting in repetitive beats at regular intervals—a tachycardia.

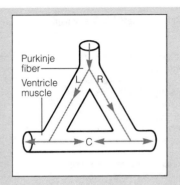

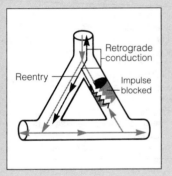

for an arrhythmia, the nurse should ask a few basic questions addressing:
• precipitating factors (exercise, smoking, sleep, emotional stress, exposure to heat or cold, caffeine intake, position changes, recent illnesses)
• any attempts to alleviate symptoms (coughing, rest, medications, taking deep breaths)
• any previous experience of these symptoms (timing and duration of symptoms, what alleviated them)
• sensations of heart rhythm (palpitations, irregular beating, skipped beats, rapid or slow heart rate)

Physical findings

These findings will vary considerably, depending on the arrhythmia and degree of hemodynamic compromise. Circulatory failure along with an absence of pulse and respirations is seen with asystole, ventricular fibrillation, and idioventricular rhythm and sometimes occurs with ventricular tachycardia. Other assessment findings may include:

• hypotension
• irregular, rapid, or slow pulse
• dyspnea, tachypnea
• chest discomfort
• diaphoresis
• change in level of consciousness, vision changes, light-headedness, dizziness, slurred speech, or other neurologic symptoms
• pallor
• jugular cannon A waves
• variation in the timing and intensity of S_1 and S_2 heart sounds.

Diagnosis

A definitive diagnosis or identification of the type of arrhythmia generally is made by careful examination of the electrocardiogram (ECG) rhythm strip. Wide-complex ectopic beats and tachycardias may require examination of additional leads of the 12-lead ECG (see *Differentiating between ectopy and aberrancy,* pages 92 and 93). Given the best diagnostic criteria, there is a 10% inaccuracy in diagnosis of wide-complex tachycardias.

Electrophysiologic testing can provide accurate diagnosis of these tachycardias and can be used to help guide and evaluate treatment. Other diagnostic tests, such as signal-averaged ECG and Holter monitoring, also are important, as are monitoring antiarrhythmic therapeutic drug levels and serum electrolyte levels.

The regularity of rhythm, presence of P waves, atrial and ventricular rates, PR interval, and QRS duration should be evaluated on all rhythm strips. Failure to look

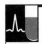

ASSESSMENT TIP

Differentiating between ectopy and aberrancy

Differentiating ectopy from aberrant conduction is among the most difficult of rhythm diagnoses as well as one of the most important due to differences in patient management. Specific criteria for surface ECG differentiation of premature ventricular complexes (PVCs) from aberrant ventricular conduction and ventricular tachycardia (V-tach) from supraventricular tachycardia (SVT) with aberrant conduction have been developed and validated with data from EP studies. The criteria were developed for V1 and V6 leads, but have been validated for MCL1 and MCL6 monitoring. Criteria of QRS duration, morphology, and axis allow 90% accuracy in rhythm diagnosis:

QRS DURATION
• QRS of 0.12 to 0.14 second favors aberrant conduction
• QRS of ≥ 0.16 second favors ventricular origin

QRS MORPHOLOGY
When the wide complex is **mainly positive in V1,** ventricular origin is favored by:
• rabbit ear configuration, with the left peak taller in V1 (see figure 1)

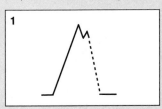

• monophasic complex in V1 (see figure 1) or biphasic complex in V1 (see figure 2)

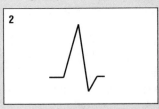

• an S wave deeper than the R wave is tall in V6 (see figure 3)

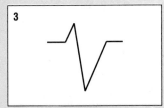

When the wide complex is **mainly positive in V1,** aberrant conduction is favored by:
• triphasic complex in V1 or V6 (see figure 4)

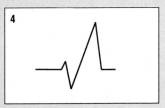

When the wide complex is **mainly negative in V1,** ventricular origin is favored by:
• R wave of ≥ 0.04 second in V1 (see figure 5)

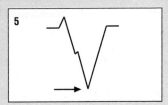

Differentiating between ectopy and aberrancy *(continued)*

• notched or slurred downstroke of S or QS wave in V1 (see figure 5)
• a distance of ≥ 0.07 second from the onset of QRS in V1 to the nadir (most negative point of deflection) indicated by the arrow in figure 5
• any Q wave in V6

QRS AXIS
• axis of -90 to -180 degrees favors V-tach (quick reference tip: QRS complex will be mostly negative in both Lead I and AVF)
• if tachycardia is mostly positive in V1, left axis deviation (> -30 degrees) or right axis deviation (> +120 degrees) favors V-tach

OTHER CRITERIA FAVORING V-TACH
• concordant V leads (QRS mainly positive or mainly negative in all V leads)
• atrioventricular (AV) dissociation (P waves seen through run of tachycardia with no relationship to QRS complexes)
• capture beats (sinus beat occurs during run of tachycardia)
• fusion beats (isolated QRS complex in tachycardia is a fusion of depolarization from sinus node along the normal conduction pathway and depolarization progressing from ventricular focus)

---

at all of these may result in misdiagnosis and inappropriate treatment. This information is compared to the criteria for the different arrhythmias to arrive at a definitive diagnosis (see *Identifying and treating arrhythmias,* pages 80 to 89).

Treatment and care

Treatment must be individualized to the patient's clinical presentation and may involve observation, pharmacologic management, or the use of synchronized electrical cardioversion or unsynchronized electrical defibrillation (specific treatments for each arrhythmia are listed in *Identifying and treating arrhythmias,* pages 80 to 89). Nursing management focuses on maintaining cardiac output, promoting cardiac perfusion, and controlling arrhythmias (see *Key nursing interventions for patients with arrhythmias,* page 94).

Pharmacologic management

Medications are a significant part of the therapeutic management of the patient with arrhythmias. *Antiarrhythmic drugs,* pages 95 and 96, identifies major drug

ESSENTIAL ELEMENTS

Key nursing interventions for patients with arrhythmias

The flowchart below highlights key interventions that nurses typically perform when a patient has an arrhythmia resulting in hemodynamic compromise.

Maintain hemodynamic status		
Maintain cardiac output	**Promote cardiac perfusion**	**Control arrhythmias**
• Have patient lie down. • Remove transdermal nitrates; consider decreasing or stopping I.V. vasodilators. • Elevate the patient's legs, if not contraindicated. (*Note:* Do not place the patient in Trendelenburg's position, which promotes a shift of abdominal viscera toward the thorax and may impede diaphragmatic excursion and cardiac filling.) • Administer I.V. fluids as volume expander (commonly normal saline solution).	• Administer oxygen. • Limit the patient's activity. • Allay anxiety by explaining to patient what is happening.	• Monitor ECG rhythm. • Monitor electrolyte levels and obtain orders to correct imbalances, especially potassium and magnesium. • Administer antiarrhythmics as ordered; observe response. • Be prepared to defibrillate, if needed. • Prepare patient for therapeutic interventions: —placement of an implantable cardioverter defibrillator —ablation —pacemaker placement.

groups and lists indications and nursing considerations for each. Careful monitoring of the cardiac rhythm for a possible proarrhythmic effect is an essential element of nursing care for patients receiving antiarrhythmic agents, particularly when a new drug is initiated or a dose is adjusted.

MAJOR DRUGS

Antiarrhythmic drugs

Antiarrhythmic drugs are categorized according to their effects on the action potential of the cardiac cell. Differences in effectiveness for particular problems or individual patients' tolerance of adverse reactions will affect drug choice.

Drug	Indications	Nursing Considerations
Type 1A: quinidine, procainamide, disopyramide	• Atrial and ventricular arrhythmias • Blocking of accessory bypass pathway conduction	• During first 24 hours, monitor for prolonged QT interval, which indicates risk for torsade de pointes.
Type IB: lidocaine, mexiletine, tocainide, phenytoin	• Ventricular arrhythmias, particularly those that result from cell injury and acute ischemia	• Observe for signs of central nervous system toxicity (slurred speech, tremors, confusion).
Type IC: flecainide, encainide, propafenone	• Life-threatening ventricular arrhythmias	• Observe for prolonged PR and QRS. • A 50% increase in QRS or a QRS of 0.20 second may require discontinuation of drug. • Observe for proarrhythmic effect.
Type II: beta blockers (propranolol, acebutolol, esmolol)	• Catecholamine-induced arrhythmias • Suppression of ectopic pacemakers • Atrioventricular (AV) nodal reentry tachycardias • Esmolol is used for supraventricular tachycardia (SVT), particularly atrial fibrillation (A-fib) and atrial flutter (A-flutter)	• Observe for prolonged PR interval and sinus bradycardia.
Type III: amiodarone, sotalol, bretylium	• Life-threatening ventricular arrhythmias • Amiodarone also is effective for atrial arrhythmias, particularly refractory A-fib or A-flutter	• Monitor for prolonged QT interval. • Sotalol also has beta-blocking effects; watch PR interval. • Amiodarone can cause pulmonary interstitial fibrosis. • Orthostatic hypotension is common with bretylium.

(continued)

Antiarrhythmic drugs *(continued)*

Drug	Indications	Nursing Considerations
Type IV: calcium channel blockers (verapamil, diltiazem)	• SVTs using the sinus or AV nodes as part of the reentry circuit • Ventricular rate control with A-fib or A-flutter	• Contraindicated in patient with A-fib and accessory bypass pathways. • Observe for hypotension.
Adenosine	• SVTs using the AV node, particularly AV nodal reentrant tachycardia	• Administer drug as rapidly as possible and flush afterward (very short half-life). • Markedly decrease dose if given through central line or to patient on dipyridamole.
Digoxin	• Atrial arrhythmias and SVTs involving the AV node	• Signs of digoxin toxicity include GI effects and visual disturbances, such as blurred vision and yellow borders around objects.

Cardiac defibrillation

Some patients with recurrent ventricular tachycardia or fibrillation who cannot be managed adequately with antiarrhythmic drugs benefit by using an implantable cardioverter defibrillator (ICD). This device can detect ventricular tachycardia or fibrillation and deliver a variety of therapies to terminate the arrhythmia, including pacing capabilities to terminate ventricular tachycardia with single, paired, or bursts of rapid-pacing stimuli, and delivery of an electric shock to defibrillate the heart, allowing it to return to a normal rhythm. To defibrillate, the device delivers 25 to 35 joules through patches placed on the epicardial surface, subcutaneous patches, or transvenous lead wires.

Nursing interventions for ICDs include:
• Be familiar with the device's capabilities and if it is turned on or off.
• For a patient who develops ventricular tachycardia or fibrillation, assess the patient; if stable, allow the device to attempt to convert the rhythm.

• Be aware that contact with the patient during a defibrillation attempt will result in a 2-joule shock felt at the skin surface; wear latex or other examination gloves for insulation.

• If the ICD is unsuccessful in converting the rhythm, provide same treatment as for any patient with the same rhythm and clinical picture:

—drug therapy for a stable patient

—synchronized cardioversion for a conscious patient who is unstable

—unsynchronized defibrillation and cardiopulmonary resuscitation (CPR) for an unconscious patient.

• Keep in mind that modifications to external defibrillation procedures may be required if the patient has epicardial or subcutaneous patches as part of the ICD system. Such patches will insulate the heart against external defibrillation, so higher energy levels may be required. Because one patch commonly is placed at the apex of the heart, external paddles may be more effective if placed anterior and posterior, rather than the standard apex and sternum placement.

• Note that, in rare instances, defibrillator devices have responded to other tachycardias, such as a rapid atrial fibrillation. In these cases, the patient may receive numerous inappropriate shocks; wear protective gloves until the device can be deactivated.

Ablation

A popular treatment for supraventricular tachycardias, ablation is accomplished by delivering radiofrequency energy through an ablation catheter tip at the exact part of the endocardial surface involved in the reentry circuit, damaging the tissue so that it can no longer participate in producing tachyarrhythmias. This procedure is technically more difficult for ventricular tachycardia because of the difficulty in isolating the reentry circuit.

Prognosis

Prognosis for patients with non-life-threatening arrhythmias is related to the underlying process that caused the arrhythmia, whereas the prognosis for those with life-threatening arrhythmias depends on both the underlying cardiac problem and the degree to which the arrhythmia can be controlled.

Discharge planning

The following general discharge instructions should be addressed with any arrhythmia patient:

• medications (drug regimen, adverse reactions, food and drug interactions, warnings about not stopping the drug without consulting the physician and not double-dosing to make up for missed doses)

• symptoms to report, such as recurrence of presenting symptoms, near-syncope or syncope, and an increase in frequency or duration of palpitations.

Instructions for patients with recurrent ventricular tachycardia or fibrillation include explanations about:

• activity restrictions (because of the potential for sudden loss of consciousness, these patients commonly are instructed not to drive)

• what to do in an emergency (call 911, lie down)

• the need for family to participate in CPR training.

Additionally, patients discharged with an ICD should be instructed on:

• follow-up appointments for evaluation of ICD

• what to do if the device discharges

• the need to avoid strong electromagnetic fields (may inactivate or activate the device)

• the need to avoid contact sports or activities that may cause impact over the device.

Aspiration

The introduction of a foreign substance into the pulmonary system, aspiration is a commonly diagnosed disorder among critically ill patients. Depending on the type and extent of substance aspirated, patients may suffer either mild lung damage, with minimal inflammation and compromise to respiration and oxygenation, or severe damage, resulting in destruction of alveolar function, pulmonary edema, and respiratory failure.

Aspirated substances commonly are grouped according to their physical properties (liquid or solid, large or particulate, acidic or alkalotic, or infectious or noninfectious). The qualities of the aspirated content have direct clinical implications for both morbidity and care requirements.

Pathophysiology

Aspiration is classified in one of four ways: aspiration of gastric contents, "bland" aspiration, infectious aspiration, and aspiration of solid materials.

Aspiration of gastric contents

This form of aspiration often is associated with patients who have the following conditions:

• autonomic pathology (as with bulbar palsy or vocal cord paralysis)

• depressed cough reflex (as in spinal cord injury, chronic ventilator or tracheostomy tube use, alcohol or narcotic intoxication, or following anesthesia)

• impaired mucociliary action (chronic aspiration that hinders the esophageal ciliary escalator)

• placement of nasogastric (NG) tubes that compromise the gastroesophageal sphincters

• tracheobronchial fistula.

Regardless of the underlying condition, the result is introduction of acidic gastric contents into the pulmonary tree (Mendelson's syndrome). The severity of pulmonary compromise resulting from the aspiration is directly related to the hydrogen ion concentration (pH) and composition of materials. Aspiration of water-soluble contrast media and materials with a pH of less than 2.5 is associated with severe bronchospasm, epithelial damage, and chemical pneumonitis within minutes. Depending on the underlying condition, pulmonary compromise may resolve rapidly with symptomatic treatments or deteriorate into complete respiratory failure with subsequent development of a bacterial superinfection.

"Bland" aspiration

Aspiration of small quantities of moderate pH fluids, which commonly occurs during sleep, is less likely to cause severe problems than the aspiration of large amounts of gastric contents. Pulmonary aspiration of non-acidic materials (water, blood, and bland fluids) causes transient inflammation of the tracheobronchial tree but usually does not result in severe compromise unless the volume of aspirate is large. In most cases, the clinical presentation improves over 24 to 48 hours. If the aspirated materials include lipoid substances (milk or oil-based compounds), acute or chronic pneumonia may result.

Infectious aspiration

Aspiration of infectious materials occurs when pharyngeal or airway secretions colonize and migrate into the lungs. Although gastric contents usually are sterile because of their low pH, aspirated contents can pick up organisms when traversing the oropharynx, especially if the mucociliary escalator is less functional than it should be (as in elderly patients or alcohol abusers) or if the gag reflex is compromised.

The typical patient who presents with this problem has been sick for several days with infectious and proteinaceous material in the alveoli, altered immune access to the damaged areas, and increased pulmonary susceptibility.

Aspiration of solid materials

Aspiration of solid material that becomes trapped at the entrance of the glottis causes airway blockage. The normal response of the individual is to inhale deeply in hope of coughing out the blockage; however, this usually drives the object deeper, causing asphyxia, cyanosis, and disorientation. The blockage must be removed by abdominal thrust or an invasive procedure in order to restore function.

If the aspirated materials are small, the airway itself is unlikely to become blocked. During vomiting, for example, particles of food enter the smaller segments of

Risk factors for pulmonary aspiration

Decreased level of consciousness
- Chronic alcohol or narcotic abuse
- General anesthesia
- Near-drowning
- Neurologic deficits
- Seizure disorders
- Smoke or irritant inhalation

Decreased swallowing ability and mechanical disturbances
- Age extremes (very old or very young)
- Endotracheal intubation
- General anesthesia
- Nasogastric tube placement
- Nasotracheal intubation
- Neurologic impairments (stroke, spinal cord injury)

- Smoke or irritant inhalation

Decreased esophageal sphincter competence
- General anesthesia
- Hiatal hernia
- Increased abdominal pressure

Miscellaneous
- Emergency surgery (insufficient time between meals and abdominal surgery, intubation)
- Increased abdominal pressure (obesity, ascites, pregnancy, delayed gastric emptying)
- Structural abnormalities (fistulas, carcinomas, Zenker's diverticulum)

the lower respiratory tract, carried by liquid GI contents. When this occurs, the resulting inflammatory response may cause areas distal to the blockage to become susceptible to infection and atelectasis.

Clinical assessment

The priority for assessing a patient for pulmonary aspiration is to determine what, if any, risk factors the patient may exhibit (see *Risk factors for pulmonary aspiration*). Chronic alcohol or narcotic abusers and those with hiatal hernia are at risk for chronic aspiration of upper airway secretions because of decreased level of consciousness and diminished esophageal sphincter competence, respectively. Patients with delayed gastric emptying, NG tube placement, or enteral feedings are more prone to aspirate when lying down than when the head of the bed is elevated.

Some patients experience "silent" aspirations, which are subclinical and remain unrecognized until complications ensue (for a list of common clinical manifestations, see *Signs and symptoms of pulmonary aspi-*

Signs and symptoms of pulmonary aspiration

Clinical manifestations may be apparent initially or within a few days after the aspiration event. The most common signs and symptoms are included below.

General manifestations
- Bronchospasm
- Chest pain
- Coughing
- Cyanosis
- Decreased PaO_2 level
- Dyspnea
- Fever
- Hemodynamic instability (hypotension, decreased central venous pressure as a result of fluid shifts)
- Minimal sputum production
- Rales or rhonchi
- Tachycardia

- Vomitus or particulate material in the oropharynx
- Wheezes over affected area

If accompanied by bacterial pneumonia
- Complaints of low-grade fever, malaise, and sputum production
- Foul-smelling sputum (consider anaerobic pneumonia, present for at least 1 week)
- Recurring fever (3 or more days after the initial event)

ration, page 102). Therefore, immediate and thorough assessment of the patient with possible pulmonary aspiration is critical. When possible, the nurse should inspect the oropharynx for the presence of particulate or liquid material to determine the nature of the injury. Intubated patients should have suction material tested for glucose, especially if tube feedings are required. Large aspirations will cause bilateral diffuse alveolar and interstitial infiltrates, although the presentation may be altered depending on the patient's position when the aspiration occurred.

Diagnosis

Evaluation of the patient for physical signs and symptoms of pulmonary aspiration should be the first diagnostic procedure undertaken. Obviously, if the patient aspirates solid material in front of witnesses, the primary diagnosis will not be difficult; in such cases, it is important to evaluate for secondary effects of the event. For some patients who have aspirated without apparent cause, studies to evaluate swallowing mechanics may be appropriate, especially for patients with neurologic injuries.

Primary diagnostic measures include pulmonary auscultation, evaluation of arterial blood gases, chest X-rays, glucose testing of tracheal aspirate, and bacterial culturing of sputum and endotracheal suction materials (see *Diagnosing pulmonary aspiration,* pages 104 and 105). Other diagnostic evaluations include a complete blood count and evaluation for pulmonary shunting.

Treatment and care

Treatment of the patient who has aspirated is largely supportive. Providing adequate ventilation and oxygenation, promoting healing, and preventing complications are key components of therapy.

Preventing complications in a patient who has aspirated involves minimizing the adverse reactions of treatments and preventing further aspirations. This includes monitoring for adverse reactions of oxygen therapy, providing pulmonary hygiene, maintaining fluid balance, decreasing oxygen requirements, and promoting weaning from mechanical support.

Ventilatory support

Ensuring adequate oxygenation and ventilation is a clinical priority, because it will determine the overall patient outcome. This may be accomplished by administering oxygen via nasal cannula, face mask, endotracheal intubation, or mechanical ventilation. Key nursing interventions are included below:

• Administer supplemental oxygen via nasal cannula, face mask, and intermittent positive-pressure breathing treatments. If saturations cannot be maintained with supplemental noninvasive oxygen, consider intubation.

• Evaluate mechanical ventilatory modes for coordination with the patient's respiratory effort. Keep in mind that some patients can tolerate a lower oxygen concentration and saturation because other organ systems are healthy; others may require higher concentrations to

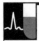

Diagnosing pulmonary aspiration

Early recognition and diagnosis of pulmonary aspiration is necessary to ensure the best possible patient management. The following information is provided to help prioritize diagnostic approaches.

Auscultation

Used to identify or isolate areas of compromise.

• *Bacterial aspiration pneumonia:* Bronchial breath sounds over affected area

• *Chemical aspiration:* Rhonchi and wheezes in affected area

• *Lobar collapse:* Lack of breath sounds over an area where gases have been absorbed distal to a plugged airway

• *Microatelectasis:* End inspiratory rales, improving after coughing, associated with insufficient tidal volume

• *Viral pneumonias:* More diffuse, scattered rales and rhonchi

Chest X-ray

Used to evaluate pulmonary beds for both obvious and subtle signs of aspiration and related complications.

• X-ray findings may vary with patient position during aspiration

-*Decubitus position:* Multiple or all segments of one lung, while other is not affected

-*Prone position:* Anterior segments of the upper and lower lobes, middle lobe, or lingula

-*Supine position:* Superior segments of upper and lower lobes

• *Infected material:* Gravity-dependent pneumonia-like presentation

• *Massive aspiration:* Bilateral diffuse alveolar and interstitial infiltrates

• *New focal opacities:* May be normal if only small amounts of water, blood, or other bland fluid is aspirated, or early in the event

• *Pleural effusion:* Corresponding with affected area

• *Solid material:* Airway obstruction with distal atelectasis, pneumonia

Glucose testing, sputum culture

Performed to evaluate the potential cause of aspiration pneumoniae.

• *Bacterial cultures:* Detect gram-negative bacilli and gram-positive organisms

• *Glucose testing:* Evaluates for presence of food contents in pulmonary aspirate

• *Viral cultures:* Identify respiratory syncytial virus, viral influenzae (less common than bacterial organisms)

Saturation monitoring

About 97% of oxygen is attached to hemoglobin (Hb); this is measured by arterial saturation monitors. The strength of bonds between Hb and oxygen is directly related to blood acid-base balance, body temperature, and 2,3-diphosphoglycerate (DPG) levels.

• *Decreased hydrogen ion concentration (pH), increased temperature, increased $PaCO_2$ level, and increased 2,3-DPG:* Increase dissociation of oxygen from the Hb, enhancing oxygen delivery to the tissues

• *Increased pH, decreased temperature, low $PaCO_2$ level, and decreased 2,3-DPG:* Decrease dissociation of oxygen from the Hb, decreasing oxygen delivery to the tissues

• In aspiration, SaO_2 would be decreased

Diagnosing pulmonary aspiration *(continued)*

Arterial blood gas (ABG) analysis

About 3% of oxygen is dissolved in the plasma; this content is measured by the PaO_2

- *Acidosis:* With decreased ventilation, increased CO_2, increased lactic acid concentration
- *Alkalosis:* With hyperventilation and decreased CO_2
- *Hypoxia:* $O_2 < 80$ torr
- *Aspiration:* PaO_2 levels may be decreased; hyperventilation leading to decreased CO_2 levels may cause an increased pH; ventilation compromise with resultant CO_2 retention may cause decreased pH.

Hemodynamic monitoring

Central venous pressure (CVP) and pulmonary capillary wedge pressure (PCWP) are taken to monitor fluid status and cardiovascular response to pulmonary compromise.

- *Chemical aspiration or massive fluid aspiration:* Increased pulmonary artery pressures due to hypoxia and resulting pulmonary vasoconstriction
- *Decreased CVP and PCWP:* Decreased circulating volume following shifting of fluid from vascular to interstitial or pulmonary tissues
- *Increased CVP and PCWP:* Fluid balance greater than the individual can tolerate, which may be related to altered cardiac function; pressures may also be increased secondary to hypoxic vasoconstriction and pulmonary shunting

handle the additional stressors associated with the aspiration.

• Minimize the percentage of supplemental oxygen (keep under 50% or 60%, if possible) to decrease the risk of complications related to increased alveolar oxygen concentration.

• Use positive end-expiratory pressure to facilitate oxygenation and ventilation, especially to overcome the loss of volume and stretch accompanying supine positioning.

• Promote pulmonary hygiene, including frequent coughing and deep-breathing exercises, incentive spirometry, chest physiotherapy, and gravitational drainage, to mobilize and remove secretions.

• Change the patient's position every 2 to 4 hours to enhance the matching of well-ventilated alveolar units with pulmonary perfusion. If tolerated, move the patient to a chair to promote full diaphragmatic expansion and gravitational perfusion.

• If the disease is unilateral, maintain the healthy lung in a dependent position (this can dramatically increase oxygenation, as ventilation is matched by perfusion). Take care, however, that secretions do not accumulate in that lung and compromise oxygen delivery; position changes are still recommended.

• Monitor the patient's tidal volume by incentive spirometry to measure lung capacity and ventilatory strength.

• Take appropriate measures to decrease metabolic demand, which increases oxygen use. Fever, agitation, anxiety, shivering, increased respiratory demand, sepsis, and overfeeding are only a few of the events that dramatically increase the oxygen and metabolic requirements of a compromised patient. Sedation, relaxation techniques, antipyretics, and coordination of nursing care with rest periods may counteract some of these physical stressors. In severe cases, pharmacologic paralysis with deep sedation may be required to decrease metabolic and oxygen demands.

Tissue oxygenation

Ensuring tissue perfusion and oxygenation requires that the patient have a sufficient oxygen content within the circulating blood and adequate cardiac function to deliver blood to tissues; therefore, interventions to increase oxygen delivery are focused in these areas. Saturation of hemoglobin (Hb) by oxygen is affected by alterable factors. For example, an alkalotic environment makes it harder for oxygenated Hb to dissociate and donate oxygen to tissues; correction of acid-base imbalances facilitates oxygen delivery. Hypothermia decreases oxygen dissociation and tissue delivery and must be corrected to enhance tissue oxygenation. Banked blood contains significant amounts of 2,3-diphosphoglyceric acid, which impairs oxygen dissociation; frequent or rapid transfusions may have oxygenation ramifications. Fortunately, the additional Hb resulting from transfusions facilitates oxygen transport and delivery.

Nursing interventions should focus on returning the patient to a state of pH balance, thereby maximizing oxygen delivery and uptake, as indicated below:

• Manipulate the ventilated patient's tidal volume, respiratory rate, degree of ventilatory support, and paralysis and sedation to decrease or increase CO_2 concentrations as necessary.

• Sedate the unventilated patient who is overbreathing and alkalotic to decrease respirations and CO_2 removal. If oversedation has led to decreased respirations and acidosis, reversal agents, such as naloxone and flumazenil, may be used. If narcotics are necessary for the patient's comfort and care, mechanical ventilation may be indicated.

• Carefully administer sodium bicarbonate to decrease serum acidosis. If serum acidosis is the result of lactic acid accumulation from hypoxic episodes and anaerobic metabolism, administer supplemental oxygen and consider sufficiency of circulating volume to increase perfusion and reverse the acidosis.

Fluid volume replacement

Following aspiration of acidic gastric contents, alveolar-capillary damage results from circulating fluid leaking into interstitial tissues and pulmonary tissues. The end result is hypovolemia and hypotension. Therapy is aimed at replenishing circulating volume, usually with crystalloids, saline solution, or both, without overloading the cardiovascular system or increasing the hydrostatic component of the capillary leak. Appropriate nursing interventions are as follows:

• Maintain central venous pressure (CVP) between 2 and 8 mm H_2O and pulmonary capillary wedge pressure (PCWP) between 4 and 12 mm Hg. The patient with a history of cardiac or pulmonary disease may have higher values, and fluid management must reflect the patient's presentation. Increased PCWP and CVP may correlate with replenishment that is either overzealous or too forceful for the patient's cardiac status.

• Assess for signs and symptoms of pulmonary edema or congestion, including:
—increasing airway pressure
—decreased oxygen saturation and arterial oxygen (PaO_2)
—decreasing urine output (output less than intake) that accompanies fluid repletion
—increased respiratory distress, increased work of breathing, accessory muscle use, dyspnea, air hunger, restlessness, and anxiety
—increasing edema (generalized swelling and pitting edema)
—rales, rhonchi, and wheezing.

Nutritional support

The critically ill patient requires maximal nutrition to promote healing. If enteral feedings via a feeding tube are ordered, minimizing the risks of further aspiration is crucial. Important nursing interventions are included below:

• Confirm placement of the feeding tube via fluoroscopy or X-ray and manipulation. This is especially important when gastric tubes are advanced, because they sometimes curl within the stomach or esophagus.

• Monitor the patient's bowel activity, peristalsis, and residuals to help determine how well feedings are tolerated and to evaluate for increasing abdominal pressure associated with constipation and slowed bowel activity. Use of peristaltic stimulators, such as metoclopramide, may be appropriate to help increase the patient's tolerance of feedings.

• If the patient's hemodynamic status permits, elevate the head of the bed during and after feedings.

• Discontinue tube feedings at least 8 hours before surgery or other procedures requiring anesthesia.

Pharmacologic therapy

If the patient is at risk for continuing aspiration, alkalinization of the gastric contents with histamine blockers, sucralfate, and antacids may be indicated. Because the prognosis for a patient is poorer if the aspirated contents are very acidic, creating an alkaline gastric content will protect the esophageal tissues from constant exposure to acids and the lungs from the disruption resulting from aspiration. However, aspiration of alkalotic gastric juices predisposes the patient to infection, because the decreased acidity of the gastric contents permits bacterial growth.

Prophylactic antibiotic treatment is not recommended unless the patient presents with signs of infectious aspiration; injudicious use of antibiotics may result in bacterial overgrowth or development of resistant bacteria strains. Antibiotic therapy is recommended only after an infection has been confirmed, either by sputum or blood cultures or development of a fever without a second source of infection. The choice of antibiotic therapy is determined by the results of the gram stain, culture, and sensitivity.

Prognosis

Recovery from aspiration is directly related to the nature of the injury. Obviously, the patient who aspirates a large quantity of gastric juices is likely to be in much worse condition than the patient who has a brief choking episode that was resolved with an abdominal thrust. The risk of developing adult respiratory distress syndrome increases with the severity of the gastric aspiration, increasing the morbidity and mortality associated with aspiration.

Discharge planning

Discharge instructions depend on the cause of the aspiration. If the patient had an acute episode of choking on a large piece of food that was quickly removed, instructions should focus on preventing a second occurrence and education regarding the signs and symptoms of pulmonary compromise in the unlikely event that complications develop. However, if the patient requires constant tube feedings on an outpatient basis, both the patient and family should be educated regarding:

• positioning during and after feedings (elevated head of bed or upright Fowler's position)
• checking for residuals before and during feedings (to determine a critical amount of residual that should preclude further feedings)
• signs and symptoms of respiratory distress (increased respiratory rate, shortness of breath, cyanosis, diaphoresis, confusion, disorientation, and anxiety).

Any patient with spinal cord injury or other cause of mechanical disruption of the swallowing process, especially a chronic tracheostomy patient, requires constant observation for complications. Referral to rehabilitation and swallowing clinics or specialists can be of great benefit to the patient and family.

Asthma

A lung disease with reversible components, asthma is characterized by obstructed airflow resulting from inflammation, edema, and contraction of bronchial smooth muscle following exposure to extrinsic or intrinsic stimuli. Status asthmaticus, the acute exacerbation of the disease, occurs when standard therapies are ineffective in controlling the effects of stimuli exposure.

Asthmatic patients typically require intensive care for aggressive treatment and continual monitoring because of limited respiratory reserves, increased susceptibility to respiratory infections, and respiratory failure. Also, lifesaving interventions, such as intubation and mechanical ventilation, can be instituted more readily in this setting.

Pathophysiology

Although asthma can be classified several ways, the most common classification is by etiology (see *Classifying asthma by etiology,* page 111). The common denominator of all classification systems is hyperactivity of the airways.

Classifying asthma by etiology

Etiologic classifications help to identify the cause of asthma, determine treatment options, and prevent future attacks through patient teaching at discharge.

Type of Asthma	Defining Characteristics
Extrinsic (allergic)	• Results when inhaled allergen (pollen, dust, feathers, animal dander) causes IgE release of mediators on surface of bronchial mast cells • Diagnosis is made when signs and symptoms correspond to allergen exposure • Most common in patients age 4 to 40
Intrinsic	• Occurs without release of IgE mediators • Commonly results from viral respiratory infection; may result from exposure to tobacco smoke, perfumes, or cold air • Most common in patients over age 40
Mixed	• Triggered by combination of intrinsic and extrinsic factors (such as allergic reaction and infection) • More common in younger patients
Potentially fatal	• Respiratory failure from asthma • Need for endotracheal intubation • Two or more episodes of status asthmaticus despite use of oral steroids • Two or more instances of pneumothorax or pneumomediastinum resulting from asthma
Aspirin-induced	• Induced within 2 to 3 hours after ingestion of aspirin or another nonsteroidal anti-inflammatory drug
Occupational	• Caused by pulmonary sensitizer in workplace (fumes, odors, vapors, wood products) • Occurs in less than 2% of U.S. population
Exercise-induced	• Results directly from exercise • Possibly related to increased blood release or mediator release due to osmotic changes
Coexistent asthma and chronic obstructive pulmonary disease (COPD)	• Thought to result from significant airway hyper-reactivity that occurs with COPD
Factitious	• Appears to be asthma but really is not • Patient typically mimics asthma symptoms, either consciously or unconsciously

Airway hyperactivity may be related to the antigen-antibody reaction that occurs with sensitivity to an inhaled antigen. Mediators released as a result of this interaction include histamine bradykinins, leukotrienes, and prostaglandins. Histamine promotes airway narrowing, severe bronchial smooth muscle contraction, and increased bronchial wall thickness related to mucosal edema and mucus plugging. Leukotrienes are responsible for the airway inflammatory response and bronchospasm. Circulation of these substances stimulates activation of eosinophils and neutrophils in the blood, leading to epithelial lung cell damage and mucociliary alterations.

In some individuals, bronchoconstriction results from upper airway irritation via vagus nerve stimulation, which encourages mucus production and is responsible for the accompanying cough and hyperventilation. As the ability to remove mucus deteriorates, alveoli collapse and hypoxemia worsens.

As plugging occurs, air becomes trapped behind the occluded smaller airways, resulting in hyperinflation of the lungs. The higher end-expiratory volumes associated with air entrapment decrease lung compliance and increase the work of breathing. The diaphragm flattens as air is trapped behind mucus plugs, decreasing its ability to contract to aid in ventilation. The patient feels an overwhelming need to take in a new breath before the last one is emptied and becomes dyspneic. As the work of breathing increases, the patient resorts to using sternocleidomastoid (accessory) muscles to maintain oxygenation. CO_2 levels are decreased from the hyperventilation; as airflow obstruction continues, alveolar hypoventilation occurs, CO_2 levels increase, and respiratory acidosis ensues.

Hypoxemia combined with pulmonary hyperinflation increases vascular resistance in the pulmonary tree. Hyperinflation increases more negative pressures within the thoracic cavity, increasing afterload on the left side of the heart. As the heart's pumping ability becomes impaired, signs of cardiopulmonary compromise become evident. Arrhythmias, such as tachycardia, can occur as a result of the ventilation-perfusion mismatching.

The hallmark of impending respiratory arrest is overwhelming respiratory failure resulting from fatigue and hypercapnia. The presence of lactic acidosis in status asthmaticus is a poor prognostic sign, usually indicating imminent respiratory failure.

Clinical assessment

In the asthmatic patient, ongoing rapid assessments and early therapeutic measures can significantly increase the survival rate and decrease complications. General assessments include level of alertness, color of skin and mucous membranes, signs of respiratory distress, and general fluid status (important because patients tend to be dehydrated and have secretions that are thick and difficult to remove). Once the patient is stabilized, additional information regarding lifestyle and management therapies can be obtained.

History

The patient experiencing a severe asthma attack will appear breathless and anxious. The nurse must listen carefully to obtain key information that will help in caring for the patient and in preserving respiratory reserves. Information to elicit includes:
• the time the attack began
• precipitating factors or triggers
• initial symptoms and their progression of severity as the patient presents for treatment (such as how the symptoms have limited activities or exercise tolerance)
• medications currently taken
• previous asthma attacks and how they were managed or treated (such as whether the patient was ever intubated as a result of an attack)
• compliance with maintaining current medical therapy.

Physical findings

The asthmatic patient may have the following findings:
• anxiety or restlessness, with trouble talking and breathing simultaneously

• desire to sit upright or at an angle greater than 30 degrees
• dehydration (evidenced by dry, sticky mucous membranes or weight loss)
• pallor or cyanosis
• pulsus paradoxus of 12 mm Hg or greater (late sign indicative of impending respiratory failure)
• tachycardia
• tachypnea with rates above 30 breaths/minute
• wheezing (an unreliable symptom; the severity of attack cannot be gauged by the amount of wheezing).

Diagnosis

Diagnostic tests include those listed in *Diagnosing asthma,* page 115. The complete blood count (CBC) may show evidence of a left shift and eosinophilia, indicating a concurrent infection. Electrolyte studies may be consistent with fluid imbalances.

Treatment and care

The primary goals of management for the patient with status asthmaticus are to optimize gas exchange, tissue oxygenation, and airway clearance and to maintain hydration. Close monitoring is essential in preventing such complications as respiratory failure, congestive heart failure, hypotension, dehydration, and metabolic imbalances.

Pharmacologic treatment

Parenteral and aerosolized bronchodilators and corticosteroids are commonly given to decrease bronchoconstriction, reduce edema of the bronchial airways, and increase pulmonary ventilation (see *Major drugs for treating asthma,* pages 116 to 118). Commonly prescribed bronchodilators include methylxanthines (theophylline and aminophylline) and sympathomimetics (epinephrine, albuterol, metaproterenol, and terbutaline). Albuterol and terbutaline are considered first-line agents because they tend to result in fewer adverse reactions than epinephrine. Corticosteroids (hydrocortisone

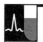

DIAGNOSTIC TESTS

Diagnosing asthma

Diagnostic tests can help clarify and determine exact diagnosis once a thorough physical assessment is completed. Each provides additional information that may be helpful in the treatment of the patient.

Chest X-ray
Valuable in determining infiltrates, atelectasis, or pneumothorax, if present. Should be obtained if auscultated breath sounds are unequal or if patient complains of chest pain.

Complete blood count (CBC)
Can help identify infection as the trigger. White blood cell, neutrophil, and eosinophil counts will be elevated with infection.

Serum electrolyte studies
Serum potassium levels may be low related to the beta-antagonist therapy. If muscle weakness is present, serum magnesium and potassium levels may be low.

Sputum culture
Serious asthma attacks often are precipitated by either a viral or bacterial infection; a sputum culture may identify the offending organism. Sputum samples may appear foamy, clear, or white with mild cases; purulent, thick, and tenacious (green-yellow) with infection.

Arterial blood gas (ABG) studies
Should be used in conjunction with other subjective and objective information. May help in identifying worsening asthma as the $PaCO_2$ and PaO_2 change. Initially, hydrogen ion concentration (pH) is normal, PO_2 is low (40 to 60 mm Hg), and PCO_2 is normal to slightly low. Later, pH is low (acidosis), PO_2 is low, and PCO_2 continues to rise as respiratory decompensation occurs.

Pulse oximetry
Noninvasive measurement of oxygen saturation blood levels and response to therapy in the absence of pending respiratory failure. Normal level is 98% to 100%; goal is 92%.

Peak expiratory flow rate (PEFR)
Nonspecific measure of airway obstruction; it is easier to obtain in patients with severe distress and is helpful in judging bronchospasm severity. Average values: for males, 10 liters/second (600 liters/minute); for females, < 10 liters/second.

Forced expiratory flow (FEF)
Measure of average flow over the middle 50% of the functional residual capacity; non-effort-dependent, and values indicative of obstructive disease can be obtained early and at the bedside. FEF values < 20 liters/minute indicate severe obstruction.

Electrocardiogram (ECG)
Helpful in identifying right axis deviation and tachycardia; may help rule out concurrent cardiac problems.

and methylprednisolone) are prescribed for their anti-inflammatory and immunosuppressive effects. If the asthma results from an infection, antibiotics also are prescribed.

(Text continues on page 118)

MAJOR DRUGS

Major drugs for treating asthma

The cornerstone of therapy of acute asthma exacerbation is early, aggressive treatment aimed at reversing bronchospasm as well as the underlying inflammation. The following table provides usual adult dosages for agents used to manage status asthmaticus.

Drug	Dosage	Adverse Reactions
Bronchodilators: Methylxanthines		
Theophylline	• Dosage should be calculated individually based on body weight • Loading dose: 4.7 mg/kg I.V. for those not currently receiving theophylline; 2.5 mg/kg I.V. generally acceptable for those currently on therapy • Loading dose given over 20 to 30 minutes	• Nausea, vomiting, abdominal cramps • Headache, hyperexcitability • Tachycardia, increased heart rate • Hypersensitivity, twitching, tachypnea, cardiac arrest with rapid I.V. administration
Aminophylline	• Dosing guidelines individualized • Loading dose: 6 mg/kg I.V. for those not currently on theophylline therapy; 2.5 mg/kg I.V. for those currently on theophylline	• Nausea, vomiting, abdominal cramps • Headache, hyperexcitability • Tachycardia, increased heart rate • Hypersensitivity, twitching, tachypnea, cardiac arrest with rapid I.V. administration
Bronchodilators: Sympathomimetics		
Epinephrine Primatene Mist Sus-Phrine	• 0.1 to 1.5 mg S.C. or I.M. • S.C.: may be given at 20-minute to 4-hour intervals; no single dose should exceed 1 mg • Continuous I.V. infusions should start at 1 to 4 μg/minute	• Tachycardia, palpitations, angina, chest pain, ventricular fibrillation • Anxiety, fear, headache, tremor, excitability • Necrosis at injection sites due to vasoconstriction • Metabolic acidosis (possible with prolonged use or overdose) • Bronchial edema or irritation, rebound bronchospasms (may occur with inhalation therapy)

Major drugs for treating asthma *(continued)*

Drug	Dosage	Adverse Reactions
Bronchodilators: Sympathomimetics *(continued)*		
Albuterol Ventolin Proventil	• Nebulizer: 2.5 to 5 mg every 20 minutes for 6 doses • By mouth (P.O.): 2 to 4 mg 3 or 4 times daily • Extended-release tablets: 4 to 8 mg every 12 hours • For elderly patients: initial dose of 2 mg 3 to 4 times daily; may gradually increase to 8 mg daily .	Most adverse reactions are dose-related: • Tachycardia, palpitations, low blood pressure, peripheral vasodilation, angina • Nausea, vomiting, abdominal cramps, hypokalemia • Dilated pupils, hyperactivity
Metaproterenol Alupent Metaprel	• Nebulizer: 2.5 ml of 0.4% or 0.6% solution diluted per nebulizer provides 10 mg or 15 mg respectively; can be repeated every 4 hours • P.O.: 20 mg 3 to 4 times daily	Most adverse reactions are dose-related: • Tachycardia, tremors, palpitations, hypertension • Nausea, vomiting • Cramping in extremities (rare) • Hypersensitivity Note: Concurrent administration with theophylline may increase cardiotoxic effects; concurrent use of other sympathomimetics may have additive effects.
Terbutaline Brethine Brethaire Bricanyl	• Orally inhaled: 400 µg (2 inhalations 1 minute apart) every 4 to 6 hours • P.O.: initially, 2.5 mg 3 to 4 times daily; maintenance dose, 5 mg 3 times daily 6 hours apart while awake	Adverse reactions are dose-related: • Tachycardia, increased blood pressure, arrhythmias, headache, angina • Nausea, vomiting • Seizures (rare), vertigo
Corticosteroids		
Hydrocortisone Cortef Solu-Cortef	• I.V.: initially 100 to 500 mg over 30 seconds and every 2 to 10 hours as needed	• Nausea, vomiting, abdominal distension, delayed healing of peptic ulcers

(continued)

Major drugs for treating asthma *(continued)*

Drug	Dosage	Adverse Reactions
Corticosteroids (continued)		
Hydrocortisone *(continued)*	• High doses should not be continued over 48 to 72 hours	• Decreased glucose tolerance, hyperglycemia, aggravated or precipitated diabetes mellitus, sodium retention, potassium loss • Thrombocytopenia • Restlessness, seizures, increased intracranial pressures with withdrawal of therapy, dry mouth
Methylprednisolone Medrol Solu-Medrol	• I.V.: 10 to 250 mg; may be repeated up to 6 times daily • Dosage range is 10 mg to 1.5 g daily	• Similar to hydrocortisone

The following nursing interventions should be incorporated into the plan of care:

• Administer medications as prescribed. When giving parenterally, administer a loading dose and follow with an I.V. drip (use an infusion control device).

• Monitor continuously for ECG changes, possible arrhythmias, and cardiopulmonary status changes.

• Assess respiratory status for changes indicating improvement or deterioration, such as decreased breath sounds, crackles, or rhonchi.

• If theophylline is used, monitor serum drug levels to ensure therapeutic range.

• If the patient is receiving systemic corticosteroids, observe for complications, such as elevated blood glucose levels and fluid retention.

• Assess for possible adverse reactions.

• Prepare to switch to oral forms and inhalers as the patient's condition improves.

Ventilatory management

Ventilatory management goals are to promote effective gas exchange, tissue oxygenation, airway clearance, and breathing. Measures include oxygen therapy, suctioning, breathing techniques, chest physiotherapy, and, if necessary, endotracheal intubation and mechanical ventilation. Low-flow humidified oxygen is used to treat dyspnea, cyanosis, and hypoxemia. The amount delivered is designed to maintain the PaO_2 between 65 and 85 mm Hg, as determined by ABG studies. Mechanical ventilation is necessary if the patient does not respond to initial ventilatory support and pharmacologic treatment or develops respiratory failure.

The following nursing interventions should be included in the plan of care:

• Administer low-flow humidified oxygen via nasal cannula or Venturi mask at prescribed levels; be prepared to adjust flow rate according to ABG results.

• Continually assess all respiratory parameters, including vital signs, tidal volume, accessory muscle use, cough, and depth and character of respirations.

• Auscultate lungs frequently, noting the degree of wheezing and quality of air movement.

• Obtain serial ABG studies, pulmonary function tests, and chest X-rays, as ordered; monitor for acidosis and atelectasis.

• Continually assess pulse oximeter readings to evaluate oxygen saturation levels; maintain oxygen saturation above 85%.

• Consult the respiratory therapist to initiate aerosol therapy. Monitor response to aerosol therapy, and check peak flows before and after therapy.

• Maintain high Fowler's position; turn every 2 hours.

• Promote relaxation to decrease the work of breathing (pursed-lip breathing, reducing environmental stimulation).

• Allow for rest periods between procedures and treatments.

• Perform chest physiotherapy to mobilize secretions; encourage coughing and deep breathing every 2 to 4 hours.

• Suction as needed to remove sputum and clear the airway.

• Provide supplemental oxygen, temporarily increasing liter flow to minimize hypoxemic effect during procedures.

• Monitor for signs and symptoms of pulmonary infection (fever, elevated white blood cell count, sputum color changes), and administer antibiotics as ordered.

• Assess for signs and symptoms of deteriorating status, including increasing respiratory distress, diminished breath sounds, altered level of consciousness, decreased oxygen saturation, and increased $PaCO_2$.

• Anticipate intubation and mechanical ventilation if the patient fails to maintain adequate oxygenation.

For a patient receiving mechanical ventilation, the following additional nursing interventions should be included in the plan of care:

• Suction as needed to remove secretions and clear the airway, hyperventilating with 100% oxygen before and after the procedure.

• Prevent oxygen toxicity by monitoring and decreasing fraction of inspired oxygen to less than 50%.

• Institute positive end-expiratory pressure (PEEP) if indicated. PEEP holds the alveoli open, thus increasing functional residual capacity, decreasing shunting and hypoxemia; however, it also can decrease cardiac output, increase the risk of oxygen toxicity, and cause fluid overload.

Fluid therapy

Initially, fluid therapy is administered I.V., usually 2,000 to 4,000 ml/day or as ordered. Oral fluids are included once the patient can tolerate them. Careful monitoring is essential because aggressive hydration may lead to fluid overload in patients with compromised cardiovascular status. Patients receiving systemic corticosteroids also require close monitoring because of the increased risk of cushingoid effects.

The following nursing interventions should be incorporated into the plan of care:
• Monitor serial serum electrolyte, hematocrit, and hemoglobin levels for changes.
• Weigh the patient daily.
• Administer I.V. and oral fluid therapy, as ordered.
• Assess the patient's fluid status through hourly intake and output, skin turgor, condition of mucous membranes, sputum characteristics, presence or absence of edema, and urine specific gravity.

Prognosis

Recovery from status asthmaticus largely depends on awareness of allergic triggers, early recognition of respiratory symptoms, and prompt medical treatment. Factors that can affect recovery include previous hospitalizations for asthma attacks, use of oral corticosteroids in the maintenance phase, previous hospitalizations requiring intubation and mechanical ventilation support, patient education, and compliance with self-management.

Discharge planning

Once the acute phase of the illness has been successfully managed, attention must be directed at assisting the patient to manage the condition and recognize potential complications. Discharge instructions should cover:
• identification of personal asthma triggers
• normal lung function, activity level, and dietary management
• correct use of metered-dose inhalers and home nebulizers and peak flow rate monitoring
• medication instructions (dosages, actions, adverse reactions, and potential drug interactions)
• the need to contact a physician or nurse regarding respiratory problems and complications.

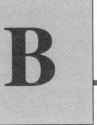

Bowel disorders

Normal bowel function depends on three physiologic conditions: an open lumen, adequate circulation, and adequate innervation. Alterations in one or more of these conditions may result in intestinal ischemia, obstruction, or perforation—all potentially fatal bowel disorders that can occur alone or in combination.

Intestinal ischemia is caused by a disruption in adequate circulation, possibly resulting from obstruction or perforation. Intestinal obstruction results when the bowel lumen has a blockage, which may be mechanical or nonmechanical in origin. Intestinal perforation can result from obstruction, ischemia, or a traumatic injury.

Because the presenting symptoms often are nonspecific and sometimes mimic those of other disorders, bowel disorders require keen assessment skills and a high index of suspicion for correct diagnosis. Delays in diagnosis and treatment can have serious consequences, ranging from mild, reversible dysfunction to sepsis, peritonitis, and death.

Pathophysiology

Each of the bowel disorders described here may occur singly or concurrently; in many cases, disease takes a more progressive course—beginning with ischemia or obstruction and ending in perforation. In all cases, the patient experiences some degree of fluid and electrolyte imbalance due to decreased oxygenation, perfusion, and bowel motility.

Massive fluid losses can result from third-space shifting, impaired reabsorption, or hemorrhage. Third-space shifting may be caused by pressure within the obstructed bowel, which forces fluid to pass from the intestine into the peritoneal cavity. Impaired reabsorption may be due to alterations in normal reabsorptive abilities caused by distention or inadequate intestinal perfusion. Electrolyte imbalances, such as hyponatremia and hypokalemia, typically occur during the early stages of intestinal obstruction. Electrolyte loss also results from increased intestinal secretions, vomiting, nasogastric (NG) suctioning, and diarrhea.

Intestinal ischemia

Intestinal ischemia results from decreased oxygen supply caused by inadequate intestinal perfusion. Acute ischemia can result from arterial or venous occlusion or from nonocclusive causes, such as vasoconstriction of mesenteric vascular beds due to decreased cardiac output from shock or congestive heart failure (CHF).

Other conditions that can lead to intestinal ischemia include embolism or thrombosis; low hematocrit (HCT) level; use of digoxin, cocaine, estrogen, vasopressin, or psychotropic drugs; aneurysms; disseminated intravascular coagulation; vascular surgery; direct trauma with or without perforation; abdominal tumors; intestinal obstructions; vasculitis; sickle-cell crisis; and competitive long-distance running. Regardless of the cause of ischemia, the end result is the same: a progressive degeneration of the intestinal wall that ultimately leads to infarction, overgrowth of toxic bacteria, sepsis, and perforation of the bowel wall if untreated.

Intestinal obstruction

Intestinal obstructions can be mechanical or nonmechanical. Mechanical obstructions affect the lumen of

Examples of mechanical obstructions

An adhesion (A) is a closed obstruction in which two segments of the bowel are joined by fibrous tissue. A volvulus (B) is a strangulated obstruction in which a bowel segment becomes twisted. Intussusception (C), another type of strangulated obstruction, involves the invagination or telescoping of one bowel section into another.

B. Volvulus

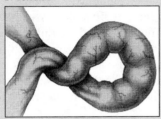

A. Adhesion

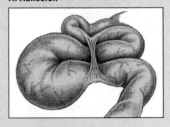

C. Intussusception

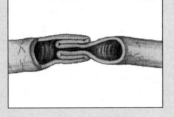

the bowel and account for about 90% of all obstructions. Located mainly in the small intestine, they commonly are classified according to cause: extrinsic (hernias, adhesions, and volvulus), intrinsic (ischemia, inflammation, tumors, and intussusception), and the presence of foreign bodies (fecal and barium impactions). Such obstructions also can be classified as simple (obstruction is in one place, with no impaired blood flow), closed (obstruction is in two places and may impair blood flow), or strangulated (blood flow to part or all of the obstructed segment is occluded). All types of mechanical obstruction can progress to strangulated when blood flow to the bowel area is impaired (see *Examples of mechanical obstructions,* page 124).

Nonmechanical obstructions (also known as functional obstructions, adynamic bowel, or ileus) affect peristalsis and involve neuromuscular dysfunction or ischemia. Causes may be categorized as intra-abdominal or extra-abdominal (see *Causes of intra-abdominal and extra-abdominal obstructions,* page 126).

At some point, mechanical and nonmechanical obstructions cause the passage of bowel contents to cease, resulting in fluid and electrolyte abnormalities. About 7 to 8 liters of extracellular fluid enter the small intestine each day; reabsorption is impaired as these fluids and electrolytes accumulate above the obstruction. Early during the obstruction, water, sodium, and potassium are secreted into the intestinal lumen, causing distention. This leads to hypovolemia and such electrolyte imbalances as hyponatremia and hypokalemia.

Intestinal perforation

Various conditions can cause intestinal perforation, which allows the spillage of intestinal contents and development of peritonitis. Common causes include obstruction, trauma (see "Abdominal Trauma," page 14), diverticulitis, Crohn's disease, appendicitis, diagnostic or therapeutic tests (such as endoscopy or barium enema), and ingestion of bones or fruit pits.

Clinical assessment

A careful clinical assessment is indicated for a patient with suspected intestinal ischemia, obstruction, or perforation. The patient's outcome depends on timely diagnosis and treatment.

History

The nurse should elicit the following information from a patient with suspected intestinal ischemia:
• history of CHF, myocardial infarction
• episodes of atrial fibrillation
• hypotensive episodes secondary to pancreatitis, hemorrhage, or burns
• previous arterial emboli
• history of peripheral vascular disease
• medication use
• abdominal pain after meals that lasts 1 to 2 hours and is associated with nausea, vomiting, and diarrhea

Causes of intra-abdominal and extra-abdominal obstructions

Type	Common Causes
Intra-abdominal	• Inflammation from peritonitis or pancreatitis • Intestinal ischemia • Vasculitis • Diabetic ketoacidosis • Postoperative ileus
Extra-abdominal	• Pneumonia • Pulmonary embolus • Electrolyte abnormalities • Metabolic disturbances • Medications (anticholinergics, opiates, chemotherapeutics, tricyclic antidepressants, digoxin, diuretics)

• history of hypercoagulable states (pregnancy or polycythemia vera)
• history of lupus or sickle cell disease
• previous abdominal surgeries or malignancies.

For a patient with suspected intestinal obstruction, the following information is important:
• previous abdominal surgeries or irradiation
• history of diverticulitis, hernias, gallstones, tumors, pancreatitis, ulcers, inflammatory bowel disease, or previous obstructions
• ingestion of a foreign body
• bowel habits, including last stool and consistency
• medication use
• history of abdominal pain, distention, nausea, and vomiting

For a patient with suspected intestinal perforation, the following information is important:
• history of abdominal trauma or surgery, inflammatory bowel diseases
• recent diagnostic or therapeutic examinations.

Physical findings

Signs and symptoms are similar for patients presenting with bowel disorders and may include:
• crampy abdominal pain (may be intermittent or relieved by vomiting), back pain
• nausea or vomiting
• abdominal distention, rigidity, guarding, or peristaltic waves on inspection
• rebound tenderness or palpable mass
• hyperresonance to percussion
• bowel sounds (normal, absent, hypoactive, or hyperactive, depending on stage of disease)
• diarrhea or constipation
• leukocytosis
• Cullen's sign (bluish umbilicus associated with intestinal bleeding)
• Turner's sign (flank ecchymosis associated with intestinal bleeding)
• fever
• tachycardia
• shallow respirations due to pain
• bloody stool
• hypotension
• increased serum amylase level, metabolic acidosis
• evidence of dehydration
• diaphoresis.

Diagnosis

Diagnostic tests, in conjunction with history and physical assessment findings, contribute to the timely and accurate diagnosis of intestinal disorders (see *Confirming intestinal ischemia, obstruction, and perforation,* page 128, for helpful tests).

Treatment and care

The primary goals of treatment for patients with bowel disorders are restoration of healthy bowel function, maintenance of fluid and electrolyte balance, and the adequate treatment of infection. The patient with intestinal ischemia may require bowel rest. If the patient's

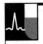

DIAGNOSTIC TESTS

Confirming intestinal ischemia, obstruction, and perforation

Various clinical tests can assist in confirming a diagnosis of intestinal ischemia, obstruction, or perforation. The most common tests are described below.

Abdominal X-rays

An increase in gas and fluid may be noted above the blockage in mechanical obstruction. In nonmechanical obstructions, increased gas and fluid may be seen throughout the intestine. Patients with intestinal ischemia may have normal X-rays; however, some reveal a marked decrease in gas patterns, an isolated distention of the transverse colon, or a distended bowel with a thickened, irregular bowel wall (thumbprinting). In cases of perforation, free air may be seen below the diaphragm.

Selective angiography

This is the primary form of diagnosis for occlusive and nonocclusive forms of intestinal ischemia. Angiography localizes the occlusion and reveals the severity of disease. Intra-arterial infusion of vasodilators directly into the circulation may be accomplished at this time.

Endoscopy or colonoscopy

These examinations allow direct visualization and may be used to diagnose ischemia, infarction, obstruction, and perforation. The nurse will need to administer drugs for conscious sedation and monitor the patient closely. The patient must be on nothing-by-mouth (NPO) status for endoscopy; the bowel must be evacuated for colonoscopy.

Upper and lower GI series

These can pinpoint the location of an obstruction and identify perforations. Barium should not be used in cases of suspected perforation or infarction. Also, use of barium can preclude the use of other diagnostic studies. The patient must be NPO for an upper GI; for a lower GI, the bowel must be evacuated.

Computed tomography (CT scan)

CT may reveal evidence of superior mesenteric artery obstruction. Contrast media often are used. This exam may last up to 60 minutes and requires the patient to lie still.

Complete blood count (CBC)

Leukocytosis, which is common in intestinal ischemia, is evidenced by a white blood cell count of $15,000/mm^3$ with a left shift; however, some elderly and immunosuppressed patients do not manifest significant leukocytosis.

Serum amylase levels

The serum amylase level often is elevated in intestinal ischemia. Normal values are 25 to 125 U/liter.

nothing-by-mouth status is anticipated to last beyond 7 days, total parenteral nutrition should be initiated; the patient may have dry mouth and thirst and will require frequent oral care. The patient experiencing intestinal perforation is usually suffering from concurrent conditions; treatment will consist of surgical correction and antibiotic coverage to prevent peritonitis and sepsis. In all cases, the nurse should promote hemodynamic stability. Volume replacement will be required, and supplemental oxygen may be necessary.

Prevention of complications is important. Short bowel syndrome (characterized by weight loss, diarrhea, steatorrhea, and malnutrition secondary to fluid and electrolyte disturbances and malabsorption) can occur in patients who have had 200 to 300 cm of bowel removed. This significant resection of the small bowel can result in a drastic reduction in absorptive functions. Symptoms and treatment will depend on the length and area of bowel removed. Nutritional therapies range from modified eating habits to enteral feedings or lifelong parenteral therapy.

Fluid and electrolyte balance

Because significant volume loss can occur with bowel disorders, fluid resuscitation is essential to prevent hypovolemia and shock. Blood replacement, to provide hemoglobin (Hb) and increase oxygen carrying capacity, may be required in addition to crystalloids.

The following nursing interventions are appropriate:
• Monitor hemodynamic parameters, including blood pressure, central venous pressure, pulmonary capillary wedge pressure, pulse rate, and cardiac output.
• Monitor Hb and HCT values.
• Assess for fluid overload when administering blood and fluids and in the postoperative patient as fluid moves back into the vascular space.
• Monitor electrolyte levels carefully.
• Monitor intake and output and daily weights.
• Assess for abdominal distention.

Sepsis prevention

Intestinal ischemia can lead to necrosis and infarction, allowing translocation of bacteria into the bloodstream that leads to septicemia. Penetration of the bowel wall leads to spillage of contents and peritonitis, which also leads to septicemia. Broad-spectrum antibiotic coverage may be initiated to prevent infection. Treatment includes administration of dopamine for hypotension and broad-spectrum antibiotics to treat the infection.

The nurse should initiate these interventions:

• Monitor for signs and symptoms of early septic shock, including fever, increased white blood cell count, hypotension, tachycardia, increased cardiac output, decreased systemic vascular resistance, decreased level of consciousness, bounding peripheral pulses, shallow respirations, and warm, flushed, dry skin.

• Obtain blood cultures before giving antibiotics.

• Administer antibiotics as prescribed.

• Use aseptic technique during dressing changes and with drain manipulation.

• Provide early nutritional support to decrease the risk of sepsis.

Pain control

Pain, which can result from distention, inflammation, and tissue damage, usually is treated with intravenous narcotics. An NG tube is used to decompress the stomach and reduce distention. Interventions include:

• If volume depletion occurs, avoid giving I.M. medications because the drugs will be poorly absorbed.

• Maintain proper functioning of the NG tube and suction equipment.

Pharmacologic interventions

Vasodilators may be introduced through an angiographic catheter to control the embolic, thrombotic, and nonocclusive causes of intestinal ischemia. Papaverine, the current standard, produces splanchnic vasodilation and prevents vasoconstriction, thereby restoring blood flow to the affected bowel segment and preventing bowel infarction. Cisapride may be used to stimulate intestinal motility in patients with bowel obstruction and in those with postoperative ileus. Low-dose dopamine and oxygen therapy may be needed to improve oxygenation and tissue perfusion.

Appropriate nursing interventions include the following:

• Monitor for signs of hypotension (common with papaverine use).

• In the case of intestinal ischemia, consult the physician about discontinuation of vasoconstrictors.

• Anticipate the need for dopamine and oxygen therapy.

Invasive measures

Surgical and nonsurgical measures vary with the type of bowel disorder. Treatment of intestinal ischemia may include use of thrombolytics and angioplasty in high-risk operative patients (although limited success has been achieved with this method) and surgery in cases of increasing abdominal tenderness, guarding, fever, and paralytic ileus. Acute superior mesenteric artery embolism may be treated with embolectomy. Vascular bypass grafting also is an option. A laparotomy is performed, and the bowel is assessed for viability. Nonviable areas are resected. In some cases, such as gangrenous bowel, a temporary colostomy or ileostomy may be required. A second laparotomy may be required in 12 to 36 hours for reassessment.

With bowel obstructions, a nonsurgical approach is preferred whenever possible; however, surgery often is necessary. Common indications for surgery include total obstruction, most cases of volvulus, gallstone ileus, strangulation, obstructing hernia, and obstruction that leads to infarction or perforation.

In the case of small bowel obstruction without evidence of strangulation, a double-lumen Miller-Abbott nasointestinal tube may be used to decompress the small bowel, thereby relieving edema and promoting the return of peristalsis. The tube is most useful in small bowel obstructions caused by adhesions.

Volvulus may be treated differently, depending on the location. A cecal volvulus may be treated with colonoscopy. If the location is in the sigmoid colon, a rectal tube may be employed.

Intestinal perforation always warrants surgery. The affected bowel section is removed, and the abdominal cavity is irrigated with copious amounts of antibiotic solution. A colostomy may be necessary.

Prognosis

The prognosis for patients with intestinal ischemia, obstruction, or perforation depends largely on timely diagnosis and treatment. All can eventually lead to peritonitis, sepsis, and death if not adequately treated. Factors associated with an increased mortality rate include advanced age, concurrent illness, malignant obstruction, and strangulation.

Discharge planning

A smooth and timely discharge depends on early planning. The nurse should address:
• the patient's support systems and need for social services, if indicated
• the recovery period, including activity and medications
• nutrition or dietary instruction, including instructions on home enteral or parenteral feedings
• wound care management
• signs and symptoms to report to the physician
• follow-up appointments.

Brain tumors

The second-leading cause of death from intracranial disease (after stroke), brain tumors constitute 10% of all cancers. Such tumors may be classified as primary or metastatic. Primary tumors arise from cells located within the cranium; metastatic tumors originate from structures outside the cranium.

Brain tumors may develop at any age; however, peak incidence is bimodal, occurring from ages 3 to

12 or from ages 50 to 80. Incidence is slightly higher in males than females.

Although the cause of primary brain tumors is unknown, some (epidermoid tumors and craniopharyngiomas) are congenital, and others (von Recklinghausen's disease and tuberous sclerosis) have a hereditary basis. Head injury, nutritional and environmental factors (except radiation), and stress do not cause primary brain tumors.

Metastatic brain tumors originate from migratory tumor cells of the lungs, breast, and gastrointestinal and genitourinary tracts. Primary neoplasms arise from anaplastic transformation of normal brain cells (see *Overview of common brain tumors,* pages 134 to 136).

Pathophysiology

Brain tumors are classified as either malignant or benign. However, space-occupying lesions located within the rigid confines of the skull are often fatal, even if they are histologically benign. Surgically inaccessible yet nonmalignant tumors destroy surrounding tissue and compress vital structures.

The pathophysiology of brain tumors is directly related to the expansion of elements within the cranial vault. The brain has a limited ability to compensate for increases in intracranial volume. Compensatory mechanisms include the shifting of cerebral spinal fluid (CSF) into the spinal subarachnoid space and the displacement of cerebral blood volume, largely by the compression of venules surrounding the tumor. When the limits of these mechanisms are exceeded, increased intracranial pressure (ICP) and neurologic deterioration result.

Compensation for increased intracranial volume depends on the rate of lesion expansion. Although fast-growing lesions result in rapid deterioration, slow-growing tumors may be present for years without manifestations. Pathophysiologic processes related to the expansion of intracranial lesions are cerebral edema, increased ICP, and herniation syndromes.

(Text continues on page 136.)

Overview of common brain tumors

The following table provides an overview of the most common types of intracranial neoplasms, including general characteristics, symptoms, and prognosis.

Tumor	Characteristics	Prognosis
Astrocytoma	• Most common type of glial tumor • Graded according to degree of malignancy	
Grades I and II	• Arises from astrocytes • Benign, invasive, slow-growing tumor • Constitutes 20% of all gliomas • Most common in those age 20 to 40	• Complete removal is difficult because of tumor's invasiveness • Average survival after surgery is 6 to 10 years • Low-grade gliomas may transform to a higher grade and become malignant
Grades III and IV	• Grade III is called anaplastic astrocytoma; Grade IV also is called glioblastoma multiforme and is the most common and lethal of all primary tumors • Highly malignant, vascular, and invasive • Peak occurrence is ages 40 to 60 • Constitutes 20% of all brain tumors • Male:female ratio is 2:1	• Survival after surgery and radiotherapy for Grade III is less than 2 years; for Grade IV, survival is 6 months to 1 year
Oligoden-drocytoma	• Arises from oligodendrocytes • Usually benign and relatively avascular; tends to be encapsulated • Slow-growing tumor commonly graded I to IV • Bimodal occurrence: commonly manifests between ages 6 and 12 or between ages 30 and 40 • Constitutes 5% to 7% of all gliomas • Male:female ratio is 2:1	• Long-term survival is possible with complete removal and radiotherapy • High-grade tumors are associated with less than 5-year survival, even with chemotherapy

Overview of common brain tumors *(continued)*

Tumor	Characteristics	Prognosis
Ependymoma	• Arises from ependymal cells lining the ventricles • More common in children and young adults (average age is 22) • Invasive, variable growth rate, dependent on grade • Constitutes 5% of all gliomas • Male:female ratio is 2:1	• Complete removal is difficult • 50% 1-year mortality without complete removal
Medulloblastoma	• Arises from embryonic cells of the posterior cerebellar vermis • Rapid-growing, highly malignant tumor of childhood (common in ages 4 to 8) • Constitutes 4% of all brain tumors • Male:female ratio is 3:1	• Highly radiosensitive • 60% 5-year survival with surgery, chemotherapy, and radiotherapy
Meningioma	• Arises from arachnoid cells • Benign, slow-growing, encapsulated, and compressive tumor • Peak incidence is ages 50 to 70 • Constitutes 10% of all brain tumors • Female:male ratio is 2:1	• Permanent cure with complete removal • Radiation for residual tumor associated with long-term survival
Pituitary adenoma	• Arises from pituitary cells (chromophobes, basophils, eosinophils) • Slow-growing; involves anterior pituitary • Incidence increases with each decade	• Good prognosis with complete surgical excision • Tumors that extend outside the sella may require radiation and extensive surgery
Acoustic neuroma	• Arises from Schwann cells surrounding the eighth nerve • Slow-growing, benign, encapsulated, and usually unilateral • Most commonly manifests from age 40 to 60 • Constitutes 7% of all brain tumors	• Good prognosis with complete removal using surgery and radiosurgery • May regrow if not completely removed • 30% mortality within 3 to 4 years if not completely removed

(continued)

Overview of common brain tumors *(continued)*

Tumor	Characteristics	Prognosis
Craniopharyngioma	• Congenital tumor arising from the embryonic remnants of tissue located near infundibular stem and pituitary • Bimodal occurrence: childhood and middle age	• Tumor is extremely radiosensitive • Complete removal may be difficult; recurrence is possible if not totally removed
Metastatic lesions	• May be single or multiple • Arise from lung, breast, skin (melanoma), and gastrointestinal and genitourinary tracts • About 25% of all cancer patients have central nervous system metastasis	• May arise months or years after the primary cancer; death usually results from the primary cancer • Treatment is palliative; surgical excision is an option when primary cancer is controlled and may improve the quality of life

Cerebral edema

Cerebral edema is the most important factor in the pathophysiology of tumor growth. If edema is severe enough, sequelae include displacement of normal brain tissue, increased ICP, and herniation syndromes. Two types of edema, vasogenic and cytotoxic, may occur.

Vasogenic edema is vascular in nature. When vessels adjacent to the tumor are compressed, increased capillary pressure and permeability force plasma to leak into the interstitium. Edema forms and primarily affects white matter surrounding the tumor.

The squeezing nature of a tumor also produces cytotoxic edema. As vessels become compressed by tumor growth, local blood flow is diminished. The resultant cellular hypoxia leads to formation of intracellular edema, which results in cell death.

Increased intracranial pressure

As the tumor expands and cerebral edema increases, so does the pressure within the cranial cavity. As the intracranial volume and pressure increase, the surrounding blood vessels become compressed, resulting in decreased cerebral blood flow and perfusion. Inadequate cerebral perfusion leads to cellular hypoxia, anaerobic metabolism, and acidosis.

Herniation syndromes
Infoldings of tough, inelastic dura mater separate the major components of the cranial vault into compartments. Space-occupying intracranial lesions shift or herniate brain tissue from one compartment to another.

Two syndromes common with brain tumors are subfalcial (cingulate) and transtentorial (uncal) herniation. Subfalcial herniation occurs when the cingulate gyrus of a cerebral hemisphere pushes under the falx and displaces the other hemisphere. As a result, cerebral tissue and local blood vessels are compressed, causing ischemia, hypoxia, edema, and increased ICP.

Transtentorial herniation occurs when the uncus of the temporal lobe is forced through the tentorial notch through which the midbrain passes. Midbrain displacement and compression of the oculomotor nerve, posterior cerebral artery, and cerebral peduncle may occur, producing ipsilateral pupillary dilation, ptosis, ipsilateral hemiplegia, decreased level of consciousness (LOC), and respiratory changes. With continued pressure on the brain stem, further deterioration and eventually death occur from respiratory arrest, cardiac arrest, or both.

Clinical assessment
The manifestations of brain tumors are diverse and may be subtle or dramatic. While some patients experience vague symptoms, others have dramatic signs, including seizures, focal deficits, and hydrocephalus. Clinical manifestations of brain tumors are both general and specific. General findings, such as headache, decreased LOC (may present as subtle drowsiness or as confusion, restlessness, stupor, and finally coma), seizures, and papilledema, are more closely related to cerebral edema, increased ICP, and herniation than to direct tu-

mor invasion. Conversely, specific findings often depend on the type and location of the tumor.

History

Because brain tumors can affect mentation, patients with intracranial neoplasms may provide a poor history. If this is the case, someone who knows the patient well should be questioned carefully about the following:
• history of behavior or cognitive changes
• history of seizures (generalized or partial)
• motor or sensory (especially visual) deficits
• manifestations of increased ICP
• endocrine abnormalities
• signs of hydrocephalus.

Physical findings

For specific signs and symptoms related to particular tumor locations, see *Manifestations of brain tumors,* page 139.

Common physical findings include:
• behavioral and cognitive deficits (irritability, emotional lability, lack of initiative, flat affect, deterioration in social skills, difficulty concentrating, forgetfulness, faulty insight, slowed mental processing)
• seizure activity (partial or generalized seizures occur in up to 50% of all brain tumor patients; sudden-onset seizures may herald presence of a neoplasm)
• focal sensory or motor deficits (may include hemiparesis or hemiplegia, possible hyperesthesia, paresthesia, loss of two-point discrimination, astereognosis, and agraphia; these deficits may indicate not only the presence but also the location of a tumor within the motor or sensory cortices; visual deficits are a common initial sign of many tumors)
• hydrocephalus (tumors involving the ventricular system typically obstruct the flow of CSF; manifestations of noncommunicating hydrocephalus include headache, declining mental and physical activity, gait disturbances, and sphincter incontinence)
• increased ICP (head pain, changes in LOC, and vomiting; although variable in nature, headache is an early

Manifestations of brain tumors

The manifestations of brain tumors are related to the anatomic location of the lesion, as outlined below.

Frontal lobe
Frontal lobe syndrome (inappropriate behavior, including impulsiveness, loss of social graces, difficulty concentrating and problem solving, emotional lability, memory impairment, flat affect, and slowed responses), headache, expressive aphasia, seizures (especially focal motor), sphincter incontinence, hemiparesis or hemiplegia, conjugate eye deviation

Parietal lobe
Sensory deficits (hyperesthesia, paraesthesia, loss of two-point discrimination, astereognosis, anosognosia, agraphia, acalculia), sensory focal seizures, headache, receptive aphasia, homonymous hemianopia

Temporal lobe
Complex partial seizures (psychomotor), headache, receptive aphasia with dominant-side involvement, irritability, depression, memory impairment

Occipital lobe
Visual impairment (contralateral homonymous hemianopia, visual agnosia, cortical blindness), visual hallucinations, seizures, headache

Pituitary and hypothalamic areas
Endocrine manifestations (Cushing's syndrome, giantism, acromegaly, hypopituitarism), visual deficits, sleep disturbance, fat and carbohydrate metabolism abnormalities, water balance problems, temperature abnormalities, headache, sexual dysfunction

Ventricular system
Hydrocephalus, headaches, vomiting, signs of increased intracranial pressure, compression of the cerebellum and brain stem (if fourth ventricle is involved), loss of swallow and gag reflexes (with lower cranial nerve involvement)

Brain stem
Cranial nerve dysfunction, vertigo, dizziness, vomiting, motor and sensory deficits, gait disturbances, sudden death (from involvement of cardiorespiratory centers)

Cerebellum
Ataxia, incoordination, falling spells, tremors, cerebellar seizures, brain stem compression, headache, vomiting

symptom in 33% of all brain tumor patients and typically is bifrontal but worse ipsilaterally, worsens when the patient bends over, and may be described as sharp or dull, constant or intermittent, or severe or mild)
• papilledema (hyperemia and edema of the optic disk; occurs in over 70% of brain tumor patients, signals intracranial hypertension, and often is associated with vi-

sual disturbances, such as decreased acuity, diplopia, and visual field deficits)
• cranial nerve deficits (depend on the type and location of brain tumor; see *Common cranial nerve deficits associated with intracranial neoplasms,* pages 141 and 142).
• gait difficulties (incoordination and frequent falls, commonly associated with hydrocephalus and posterior fossa tumors) and speech difficulties (dysarthria, aphasia, and dysphonia are common with tumors involving the cerebellum, dominant cerebral hemisphere, or vagus nerve).

Diagnosis
The diagnosis of intracranial neoplasms is made on the basis of clinical presentation, neurologic examination, and diagnostic procedures (for a list of common diagnostic tests, see *Confirming a brain tumor,* page 143).

Treatment and care
Treatment of a brain tumor depends on its type, size, and location. Common treatments are surgery, radiotherapy, and chemotherapy. For an overview of nursing goals and interventions, see *Key nursing interventions for patients with brain tumors,* page 144.

Surgery
Surgery remains the treatment of choice for most brain tumors. However, inaccessibility or extensive infiltration makes complete resection of some neoplasms impossible. Computed tomography–guided stereotactic surgery may be used to obtain a needle biopsy.

Laser surgery, alone or in combination with conventional methods, can be used to treat some tumors. For example, acoustic neuromas and craniopharyngiomas may be vaporized by directing a narrow laser beam at the neoplasm.

Nursing interventions related to intracranial surgery consist of preoperative education (including fami-

Common cranial nerve deficits associated with intracranial neoplasms

Cranial nerve deficits may result when the tumor arises from the nerve itself, as a result of tumor infiltration, or from compression of the nerve from an expanding intracranial mass. Common cranial nerve deficits associated with brain tumors are outlined in the chart below.

Cranial Nerve	Type of Tumor	Physical Findings
I (olfactory)	Anterior fossa tumors, meningiomas	Unilateral or bilateral anosmia (loss of smell)
II (optic)	Pituitary tumors pressing on optic chiasma, optic nerve astrocytomas, orbital tumors	Visual disturbances, bitemporal hemianopsia (loss of temporal visual fields), papilledema
III (oculomotor)	Meningiomas, osteomas, orbital tumors	Pain, ophthalmoplegia (paralysis of eye muscles), abnormal pupillary response, ptosis
IV (trochlear)	Meningiomas, osteomas, orbital tumors	Ophthalmoplegia, diplopia, pain
V (trigeminal)	Acoustic neuromas involving the fifth nerve, trigeminal neuromas, sinus tumors	Loss of corneal reflex and keratitis, facial pain and loss of sensation
VI (abducens)	Cerebellar tumors involving the fourth ventricle, meningiomas, osteomas, orbital tumors	Strabismus, diplopia, pain, ophthalmoplegia
VII (facial)	Acoustic neuromas involving the seventh nerve, osteomas	Ipsilateral facial paralysis, loss of taste
VIII (vestibulo-cochlear)	Acoustic neuroma, meningioma	Tinnitus, decreased hearing, dizziness and balance deficits
IX (glossopharyngeal)	Acoustic neuromas involving the ninth nerve, posterior fossa tumors, meningiomas	Absent gag reflex, diminished or lost taste, dysphagia

(continued)

Common cranial nerve deficits associated with intracranial neoplasms *(continued)*

Cranial Nerve	Type of Tumor	Physical Findings
X (vagus)	Meningiomas, posterior fossa tumors	Dysphagia, ipsilateral loss of gag reflex and vocal cord paralysis
XI (accessory)	Meningiomas, posterior fossa tumors, spinal cord tumors	Weakness of the sternocleidomastoid and trapezius muscles
XII (hypoglossal)	Meningiomas, angiomas, spinal cord tumors	Ipsilateral paralysis and atrophy of the tongue, dysphagia

ly members) and postoperative evaluation. Appropriate nursing interventions are listed below:

• Inform the patient and family of what to expect following craniotomy, including possible admission to the intensive care unit.

• Explain the purpose of frequent assessment, turning, antiembolic stockings, and early ambulation.

• Provide instructions for the use of an incentive spirometry, and evaluate the patient's understanding.

• Postoperatively, monitor hourly intake and output, vital signs, and neurologic signs for early detection of diabetes insipidus (especially after pituitary surgery), increased ICP, and altered cerebral perfusion.

• Depending on the nature of the surgery, monitor cranial nerve function. Before the patient eats or drinks, always assess the gag and cough reflexes.

• For the patient with decreased LOC, maintain a side-lying position and continually assess airway patency.

• Immediately report any rise in ICP, change in LOC, or other neurological deterioration.

• Treat pain and nausea promptly.

• Foster a supportive atmosphere to ensure the well-being of patient and family.

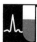

Confirming a brain tumor

The following tests may help with positively diagnosing a brain tumor.

Computed tomography (CT scan)

CT is extremely useful in revealing intracranial lesions. CT technology can scan the brain in successive layers (slices) from 1.5 to 10 mm in thickness, allowing for detection of small lesions. A brain tumor will appear on CT as an area of increased density. Additionally, displacement of intracranial structures (ventricles) and abnormalities in the size, shape, and location of structures are common.

Magnetic resonance imaging (MRI)

Like CT, MRI provides "slice images" of the brain. However, the sharp detail of MRI is superior to CT. MRI is especially effective in detecting deep or small tumors, particularly in areas difficult to visualize, such as the brain stem and basal skull. However, unlike CT, MRI cannot be used for patients with implanted metallic equipment (pacers, aneurysm clips, or orthopedic hardware), because the magnetic field generated can move these objects.

Visual field and funduscopic examination

Because the visual pathways traverse through all lobes of the brain, visual field evaluations are helpful in localizing brain tumors. A funduscopic examination can reveal papilledema, a common finding in brain tumors associated with increased intracranial pressure.

CT-guided stereotactic biopsy

A CT-guided stereotactic biopsy is especially useful for obtaining biopsies from tumors deep in the cerebral hemispheres or basal ganglion.

Other tests

Because up to 30% of metastatic brain tumors arise from the lungs, a chest X-ray may be helpful in determining the nature and source (primary versus metastatic) of an intracranial lesion and in locating primary tumors as well. Electroencephalography may be performed if seizures are part of the presentation. Positron emission tomography scanning is used in a few large centers to study tumor metabolism. Cerebral angiography can help determine the vascularity of the tumor as well as its proximity to surrounding vessels.

Radiotherapy

A mainstay in the treatment of malignant intracranial tumors, radiotherapy can halt tumor growth and induce shrinkage. It most often is employed to increase survival time after surgical excision of the lesion. Tumors most amenable to radiotherapy are medulloblastomas and deep, surgically inaccessible neoplasms. Drawbacks include radiation-induced edema and necrosis, which can exacerbate symptoms. Specific types of ra-

ESSENTIAL ELEMENTS

Key nursing interventions for patients with brain tumors

Important nursing interventions for the patient with a brain tumor are highlighted below.

Achieve optimal neurologic status		
Recognize and treat increased intracranial pressure (ICP)	**Prevent post-treatment complications**	**Provide an optimally supportive environment**
• Monitor for and report: —decreased level of consciousness —pupil changes —motor and sensory deficits —ICP > 15 mm Hg —vital sign changes. • Treat increased ICP by: —administering osmotic diuretics, and analgesics as ordered —maintaining head in a midline position —avoiding impeding jugular venous outflow —minimizing nursing activities that raise ICP.	• Ensure that the patient turns, deep-breathes, and uses an incentive spirometer every 1 to 2 hours. • Apply antiembolic stockings and a sequential compression device. • Get the patient out of bed as soon as possible. • Maintain optimal nutrition and hydration. • Administer steroids as ordered to decrease cerebral edema. • Discontinue Foley catheters and other invasive devices as soon as possible.	• Always identify yourself to the patient and family. • Inform the patient and family of what you are doing before doing it. • Allow for liberal visiting if the patient so desires. • Obtain social service consult if appropriate. • Offer to call the patient's spiritual advisor. • Assume a positive, empathetic approach with the patient and family.

diotherapy include whole-brain radiation, stereotactic radiosurgery (gamma knife, cyclotrons), interstitial brachytherapy, and tumor heating. Stereotactic radiosurgery is used to destroy deep, inaccessible lesions without opening the cranium.

Related nursing interventions include:
• Inform the patient and family of what to expect before, during, and after treatment. Explain that adverse reactions (alopecia, nausea, vomiting, headache, cerebral edema, and brain necrosis) may occur immediately or may be delayed for years.
• After the procedure, provide skin care to the irradiated site; avoid using tape, alcohol, powder, or cream.
• Promptly treat headache, nausea, vomiting, or diarrhea with appropriate medications.

Chemotherapy

Chemotherapy has limited value in treating intracranial neoplasms; it usually is a last option offered to patients who already have had surgery and radiation therapy. Although chemotherapy rarely induces remission, one class of drugs, the nitrosoureas (carmustine BCNU, lomustine CCNU), may be beneficial in improving the quality, not quantity, of life. Most chemotherapy regimens are delivered IV; however, alternative delivery methods include intra-arterial infusion and use of an Ommaya reservoir.

Nursing interventions include:
• Administer antiemetics before and during chemotherapy.
• Monitor for and protect the patient from infection.
• Monitor for respiratory, liver, kidney, and bone marrow dysfunction.
• Monitor intake and output, and maintain optimum hydration.
• Provide emotional support, and prepare the patient for possible hair loss and other discomforts.

Pharmacologic therapy

Three other types of drugs commonly prescribed for patients with brain tumors include corticosteroids, antiepileptic drugs, and analgesics. Corticosteroids provide an effective treatment for the cerebral edema associated with brain tumors. Antiepileptic drugs, such as phenytoin (Dilantin), are prescribed for patients who experience seizures. Analgesics are used to control pain associated with intracranial neoplasms. Mild head pain usually is treated with acetaminophen; more severe pain may be remedied with codeine or morphine.

Preventing complications
The most common complications of brain tumors are cerebral edema, increased ICP, neurological deficits, and seizures. Although the development of cerebral edema cannot be prevented, the administration of dexamethasone (Decadron) decreases cerebral edema and neurologic deficits. Additionally, controlling cerebral edema is one method for preventing increased ICP.

To help prevent complications arising from cerebral edema and increased ICP, the nurse should monitor for signs and symptoms of increased ICP and neurologic deficits, including deteriorating LOC, pupillary changes, motor and sensory deficits, and changes in vital signs (late findings).

Prognosis
The prognosis for patients with malignant brain tumors is poor. Patients treated by surgery alone have an average survival time of about 17 weeks. When radiotherapy is added to the treatment plan, survival time is about 38 weeks. Adding chemotherapy to the regimen does not increase survival time.

The prognosis for patients with benign brain tumors is highly variable. Outcomes depend on several factors, including size and location of the neoplasm at diagnosis, tumor invasiveness, surgical accessibility, amount of destruction of normal tissue, and the patient's age and general state of health.

Discharge planning
Discharge planning begins as soon as the patient is admitted; education is a key element. The nurse should provide discharge instructions that focus on:
• the patient's and family's understanding of the treatment plan, including medication dosages, schedules, and adverse reactions; appointments for follow-up and

further treatment; reportable signs and symptoms; instructions for activity, wound care, and personal hygiene; diet and fluid restrictions; and how to acquire and use assistive devices
• the need for social service, hospice, pastoral counseling, or psychiatric referrals
• local brain tumor support groups, such as the National Brain Tumor Foundation and the American Brain Tumor Association.

Burns

A tissue injury resulting from contact with a thermal, chemical, or electrical source, a burn can cause cellular skin damage and a systemic response that leads to altered body functions. The severity depends on both the injury's size (level of tissue destruction) and its depth.

Burns typically are classified as partial-thickness (first-degree and second-degree) or full-thickness (third-degree and fourth-degree), according to their physical appearance and the tissue layers affected (see *Burn depth classification,* page 148).

Thermal burns, the most common type of burn injuries, may result from exposure to fire, hot liquids, steam, or fireworks. Ionizing radiation exposure, which commonly is categorized as a type of thermal burn, can cause skin injuries similar to those of partial-thickness thermal burns as well as systemic injury.

Chemical burns, which are caused by direct contact with a chemical or by inhalation or ingestion of a caustic material, usually occur in the work or home setting. Injuries resulting from such burns are due to denaturing of protein within the tissues or to cellular dehydration.

Electrical burns produce heat that subsequently causes burn injury. Common causes are lightning bolts, defective or improperly installed electronic devices, and contact with high-power electric lines.

Burn depth classification

Burns may be classified as either partial-thickness or full-thickness, depending on the skin layers involved. The degree of injury increases with the depth of burn, as shown in the chart below.

Type of Burn	Characteristics
Partial-thickness	
First-degree	• Painful superficial injury involving only the epidermis • Pink to red, with no blisters • Grafting unnecessary • Usually heals within 3 to 5 days
Second-degree	*Superficial* • Painful injury involving the epidermis and dermis • Pale to red, with weeping blisters and no eschar • Usually heals in 2 to 3 weeks *Deep* • Painful injury that damages hair follicles and nerves • Cherry-red, with possible blisters and pronounced weeping; may develop eschar • Usually heals in 3 to 6 weeks
Full-thickness	
Third-degree	• Injury extending through entire dermis and possibly into subcutaneous fat; rarely painful because nerves are damaged • Brown, yellow, red, white, gray, or black • Hard and inelastic, with no blisters • Requires treatment, including grafting, to heal
Fourth-degree	• Painless injury that extends through all skin layers, damaging muscle, bone, and nerves • Charred black • Hard and inelastic, with no blisters • Requires treatment, including grafting, to heal

Pathophysiology

Burn injuries produce local and systemic responses as well as changes at the cellular level.

Local response

Localized changes include a loss of the skin as a protective barrier. The transfer of heat denatures cellular protein, inactivates or blocks thermolabile enzymes, and interrupts vascular supply.

Systemic response

Systemically, increased capillary permeability occurs for the first 2 to 3 weeks after injury, with the most severe changes occurring in the first 24 to 36 hours. The increased permeability leads to extravasation of water, electrolytes, albumin, and protein into the interstitial and intracellular compartments, leading to edema. This process begins immediately after a burn injury and can lead to a 60% loss of intravascular volume if the burn injury is greater than 30% of the body surface area (BSA). An increase in the body's metabolic rate leads to further water loss via the respiratory system. Evaporative fluid loss from the wound also occurs.

The body's systemic response to burn injury also includes thrombosis of the vasculature, which causes impaired circulation and can lead to decreased peripheral perfusion and metabolic acidosis. The obstructed blood flow generally is restored within 24 to 48 hours for partial-thickness wounds but may continue for 3 to 4 weeks with full-thickness injuries.

Cellular response

The cellular inflammatory response associated with burn injury includes convergence of neutrophils in the injured area and phagocytosis of bacteria. The release of vasoactive substances, such as histamine, causes increased vascular permeability and further decreases the intravascular volume. Red blood cell (RBC) hemolysis in the injured area and partial destruction at the wound's periphery also occurs. Disseminated intravascular coagulopathy may occur as a result of decreased platelet and fibrinogen levels. Generally, these levels return to normal within 36 to 72 hours after injury.

Body system changes

Cardiac function is affected by the increased capillary permeability and subsequent intravascular hypovolemia. Cardiac output decreases and requires aggressive fluid resuscitation to prevent burn shock. In patients with greater than 50% BSA injury, myocardial depressant factor is released from prolonged constriction of the splanchnic organs, causing a negative inotropic effect. This subsequently leads to a decrease in cardiac output of 30% during the first 30 minutes after injury.

Pulmonary injuries related to burns typically pose the most immediate threat to life. Carbon monoxide poisoning and smoke inhalation injury are common with burns of the head, neck, and chest. Smoke inhalation, a chemical injury, causes immediate loss of bronchial cilia, decreased alveolar surfactant, atelectasis, mucosal edema, hypoxemia, and hypercarbia. If the chest has a circumferential burn, pulmonary function is affected secondary to the restrictive defects of the thorax. Noncardiogenic pulmonary edema also occurs following fluid shifts into the lung parenchyma, further compromising pulmonary function.

The GI tract responds to hypovolemia by causing splanchnic vasoconstriction with a reflex ileus. Gastric dilation, paralytic ileus, abdominal distention, regurgitation, malabsorption, ulcerations, and hyperacidity are common responses to burn injury. Curling's ulcer, a type of duodenal ulcer, commonly develops in patients with severe burn injury.

Renal function is altered by hypovolemia and the release of antidiuretic hormone. Inadequate fluid resuscitation, myoglobin released during muscle destruction, and hemoglobin released during RBC hemolysis can cause acute tubular necrosis.

The immune system responds to burn injury with an immediate depression of the immunoglobulins IgA, IgG, and IgM. In combination with the loss of skin barrier and abnormal neutrophil function, this lowering of host defenses increases the patient's susceptibility to infection and sepsis.

The hormonal stress response to burn injury includes an increased release of catecholamines, cortisol, and glucagon. Blood sugar levels increase in response to increased adrenal hormone levels and decreased insulin effectiveness. Acceleration of metabolic rate results in the need for greatly increased caloric and protein intake in burn patients.

Clinical assessment

A quick but thorough history and physical assessment will provide information that will dictate the level of expertise required and the appropriate first interventions. Assessment includes estimating the extent of burn injury (see *Estimating the extent of burn injuries using the Rule of Nines,* page 152).

History

The health care team needs to quickly determine the extent of injury, associated complications, and trauma. Questions should focus on information that provides important prognostic indicators of severity and mortality, including:
• cause and anatomical location of the burn injury
• time of the injury and extent or duration of exposure
• where the patient was found (risk of smoke inhalation increases if the patient was in an enclosed space)
• possible contaminants and estimated blood loss
• medical history, including current medications, allergies, tetanus immunization history, disabilities, and age (defines the natural thickness of skin and indicates amount of stress the patient can withstand)
• possible associated injuries
• circumstances that may suggest attempted homicide or suicide, child or elder abuse, or domestic violence.

Physical findings

All burn patients must be evaluated for life-threatening injuries that can cause airway, breathing, and circulatory complications. Pulmonary-related findings may include wheezing and air hunger, atelectasis, hoarseness, tachypnea, cough, stridor, abdominal respirations, severely restricted respiratory excursion, a PaO_2 of less than 60 mm Hg, and a $PaCO_2$ of greater than 45 mm Hg.

Estimating the extent of burn injuries using the Rule of Nines

Nurses can quickly gauge the extent of a burn injury in an adult by dividing the total body surface into percentages based on multiples of nine (note that the perineum counts as only 1%).

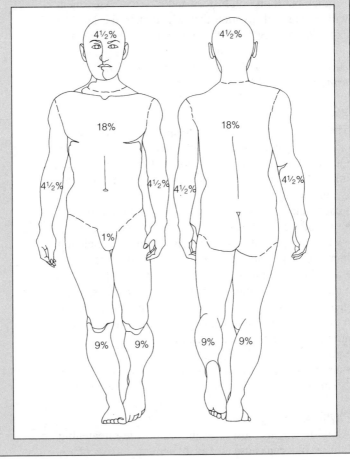

Signs and symptoms of circulatory system injury may include hypotension, tachycardia, decreased peripheral pulses, decreased cardiac output, decreased pulmonary catheter filling pressures, decreased urinary output, increased metabolic rate and increased myocardial oxygen consumption, and hypothermia or hyperthermia.

In addition to the above findings, certain types of burns are associated with specific physical findings, as explained below.

• *Thermal burns:* Depending on the degree of injury, the patient will have signs or symptoms of epidermal, dermal, and subcutaneous involvement.

• *Chemical burns:* Injuries from alkali products are associated with deep burns resulting in more severe damage than that caused by acid products.

• *Electrical burns:* Surface entrance and exit wounds usually represent a small portion of the actual damage. As current passes through the body, immediate damage is done to the heart, lungs, and brain. Bone and fat are more resistant to the current than nerves, muscles, and blood vessels, which tend to be more severely damaged.

Some other general findings and their related etiologies are listed below:

• pain (common and severe in partial-thickness burns; absent in full-thickness burns because of nerve damage)

• singed nasal hair (may be present in face and neck burns; soot in oropharynx suggests pulmonary injury)

• disorientation or combative behavior (may indicate hypoxemia)

• entry and exit wounds (common with electrical burns)

• palpitations (from increased catecholamine release)

• arrhythmia or conduction disturbances (possible with electrical burns)

• headache or changes in level of consciousness (indicate possible neurologic impairment associated with electrical burns, concurrent head injury, hypoxia, or toxic exposure).

Diagnosis

Few tests are required to diagnose a burn. Blood work and laboratory tests are needed to evaluate the patient's response to the burn and body system injury (see *Diagnostic laboratory tests for burn patients,* page 154). Other diagnostic studies, such as fluorescein dye injec-

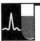

Diagnostic laboratory tests for burn patients

The following tests typically are performed in the evaluation of burn patients. Normal values appear in bold.

Complete blood count

Used to evaluate overall and cellular response to the burn injury in assessing for abnormalities. Decreased red blood cell (RBC) count and increased hemoglobin (Hb) level usually are seen initially; anemia often is seen after the initial stage. **White blood cell count 4 thousand to 11 thousand/μliter; RBC count, 4.3 million to 5.8 million/μliter; Hb level, 13.5 to 17.5 g/dl; hematocrit level, 40% to 52%.**

Serum potassium level

Used to evaluate for elevated potassium levels caused by tissue destruction. **Potassium level 3.5 to 5.3 mmol/liter.**

Clotting studies

Used to assess for thrombocytopenia and for *decreased* fibrinogen and *increased* fibrin split products to detect disseminated intravascular coagulation. **Activated partial thromboplastin time, 25 to 36 seconds; prothrombin time, 10 to 12.5 seconds; platelet levels 11.5% to 14.5%; fibrinogen level, 200 to 400 mg/dl; fibrin degradation products level, < 16 mcg/ml.**

Liver function tests

Used to evaluate specific organ damage, especially if patient has an electrical burn. **Alkaline phosphatase level, 30 to 120 /liter; aspartate aminotransferase level, 8 to 20 /liter; indirect serum bilirubin level, < 1.1 mg/dl; direct serum bilirubin level, < 0.5 mg/dl.**

Blood urea nitrogen (BUN) and serum creatinine levels

Used to assess for renal insufficiency or renal failure exhibited by elevated BUN **(> 10 to 20 mg/dl)** and serum creatinine levels **(> 0.8 to 1.3 mg/dl)**, which are associated with renal insufficiency or renal failure.

Arterial blood gas studies

Used to evaluate for hypoxemia (PO_2 80 mm Hg); carboxyhemoglobin level indicates the degree of smoke and carbon monoxide inhalation **hydrogen ion concentration, 7.35 to 7.45; PO_2, 80 to 100 mm Hg; PCO_2, 35 to 45 mm Hg; HCO_3^-, 22 to 26 mEq/liter; base excess, +2.**

Urine studies

Used to evaluate for myoglobinuria, indicating the breakdown of muscle or hemoglobinuria that indicates the hemolysis of RBCs in burn patients.

tion, electrocardiogram, chest X-ray, and wound culture and sensitivity, help determine burn depth, potential for tissue recovery, and associated injuries. A bronchoscopy may be done for suspected smoke or chemical inhalation to evaluate the extent of injury.

Treatment and care

Primary medical and nursing goals for all burn patients include stabilization of all life-sustaining processes, preservation of body integrity, and prevention of complications (see *Complications associated with major burn injuries,* page 156).

Resuscitative therapy

Initial resuscitative goals are the same for all burn patients, regardless of the burn's etiology. These are outlined below.

• Stop the burning process to decrease the depth and extent of injury. The rescuer at the site often is responsible for this; however, the emergency room or intensive care unit nurse often must clean the injured area thoroughly when a patient has a chemical burn.

• Follow the ABCs of trauma resuscitation. The patient's airway and breathing must be maintained, and evidence of impaired gas exchange and ineffective airway clearance must be identified and corrected. Efforts are made to support cardiovascular and peripheral circulation. Immediate and appropriate fluid resuscitation should also be instituted to prevent burn shock from hypovolemia.

Specific nursing interventions during this stage of treatment are provided below:

• Auscultate breath sounds and assess for signs of laryngeal edema or tracheal obstruction.

• Evaluate for the need for early intubation for facial or neck burns. Assist with intubation, if necessary. Properly maintain endotracheal tube and airway and secure tube with tape.

• Administer humidified oxygen. Adjust the fraction of inspired oxygen (FIO_2) as soon as possible, because carboxyhemoglobin levels generally are reduced within 30 to 60 minutes of receiving 100% FIO_2. (Always use caution when administering oxygen to patients with chronic lung disease.)

• Monitor arterial blood gases and oxygen saturation.

Complications associated with major burn injuries

The list below identifies some of the complications that can occur in the burn patient. The presence of some of these complications, such as acute tubular necrosis and infection, can increase the patient's mortality rate.

• Pulmonary edema
• Decreased pulmonary function
• Hypovolemia
• Increased blood viscosity
• Impaired circulation

• Neurovascular compromise
• Acute tubular necrosis
• Paralytic ileus
• Curling's ulcer
• Infection
• Spinal cord injury
• Neurologic deficits
• Thrombosis
• Contractures
• Scar hypertrophy
• Keloid formation

• Prepare the patient for escharotomy of the chest and neck for deep burns or circumferential injuries, if necessary, to promote lung expansion and decrease pulmonary compromise.

• Provide rapid fluid resuscitation as prescribed (see *Fluid replacement in the burn patient,* page 157). Use a large-bore peripheral catheter or subclavian vein catheter for fluid administration.

• Assess vital signs, temperature, and pulmonary catheter filling pressures every 30 minutes until stable and then as prescribed.

• Monitor for tachycardia, which may indicate intravascular depletion or represent the patient's hypermetabolic state.

• Assess hemodynamic status via laboratory data including hydration level (blood urea nitrogen [BUN]), renal involvement (BUN, serum creatinine), and electrolytes, which may cause hemodynamic instability.

• Insert an indwelling urinary catheter. Monitor for urine output of 1 ml/kg/hour in children, 30 to 50 ml/hour for adults, and 75 to 100 ml/hour for those with electrical burns.

• Administer renal-dose dopamine to promote urine output.

• Assess for bowel signs, because splanchnic constriction is a result of hypovolemia and can lead to ileus.

Fluid replacement in the burn patient

The Parkland formula is used to evaluate fluid replacement needs in the burn patient during the first 24 hours after a burn injury. The formula is:

2 to 4 ml lactated Ringer's solution/kg/% of body surface area burned.

Nursing precautions
• Fluid overresuscitation and underresuscitation must be avoided. Underresuscitation is manifested by signs and symptoms of hypovolemic shock; overresuscitation, by signs and symptoms of congestive heart failure or pulmonary edema.

• Administration of colloids should be avoided in the first 24 hours to avoid potentiating capillary leakage. Controversy exists over administration of hypertonic saline solutions instead of lactated Ringer's solution. The former provides increased sodium chloride in smaller volumes of solution.

Restorative therapy

After the patient is stabilized, continued vigilance is required to maintain homeostasis of fluid, electrolyte, and acid-base balance and the other body systems affected by the burn injury and to prevent complications. The patient also should be evaluated for possible transfer to a burn center, where expert care may be provided.

Meticulous wound care is required, with emphasis on quick identification and treatment of neurovascular compromise and infection. Providing the injured area with an oxygen supply, removing dead material by debridement, and promoting gentle, active range of motion are all key concepts of burn care.

Hydrotherapy, washing of the wound or the entire patient (also referred to as "tubbing" or "tanking"), is useful in removing old dressings and ointments and in assisting with debridement. In addition to debridement, skin grafting may be performed for deep partial-thickness and full-thickness burns to cover an excised wound, protect the wound from contaminants, reduce fluid and heat losses, decrease pain, and lower the metabolic rate. Autografts (which are composed of the patient's own skin), human allografts (from donated or cadaver skin), or xenografts (from another species, such as the pig) may be used during treatment, depending on availability. However, permanent wound closure can be accomplished only with autografts.

Adequate nutrition for increased protein and caloric needs also must be maintained because of the burn patient's hypermetabolic state. Rehabilitative goals are established early to preserve the patient's range of motion and functional ability and to prevent further loss of motion secondary to edema or eschar formation. Throughout recovery, the patient and family are psychologically stressed and require the combined efforts of the entire multidisciplinary team.

Nursing interventions during the restorative phase include the following:

• Assess vital signs, temperature, intake and output, and pulmonary catheter filling pressures, as prescribed.

• Suction the patient every 8 hours and as needed to avoid pooling of pulmonary secretions.

• Use bronchodilators for wheezing, as prescribed.

• Weigh the patient daily.

• Assess Doppler pulses.

• Assess capillary refill in extremities.

• Assess for numbness, tingling, and increased pain in affected extremities.

• Elevate the burned extremity to decrease edema.

• Notify the physician of signs and symptoms of inadequate circulatory perfusion, and prepare the patient for escharotomy or fasciotomy.

• Assess the degree of pain every 2 hours, and evaluate the effectiveness of prescribed analgesics using a quantitative scale. Administer I.V. analgesics because I.M. drugs may not be readily absorbed.

• Administer an analgesic as needed 30 minutes before painful procedures.

• Carefully titrate narcotic doses to provide adequate pain relief. Use patient-controlled analgesia when possible. Teach and encourage the use of relaxation techniques and diversional activities.

• Institute universal precautions and wound and skin precautions to protect the patient. Use reverse isolation to avoid cross-contamination.

• Administer a tetanus prophylaxis.

• Monitor neurovascular status, including pulses, reflexes, paresthesia, color, and temperature of the injured areas.

• Cleanse wounds daily or every 4 hours if needed (see *Wound care for burn patients,* page 160).

• Assist with splinting, positioning, compression therapy, and exercise, as ordered.

• Maintain burned areas in a neutral position. Position neck burns in extension without pillows to prevent contractures. Use 90-degree shoulder abduction and 10-degree elbow flexion in axillae burns to prevent scar band formation. Elevate the head of the bed to decrease edema in facial burns.

• Assess the patient's range of motion and encourage the patient to exercise the burned area if able.

• Inspect the wound frequently for exposed tendons, edema, points of pressure, contracture, banding, or keloid formation so as to treat and reverse the problem.

• Observe wound sites carefully and report signs of infection. Send wound cultures as needed.

• Administer antibiotics as prescribed and evaluate the patient's response.

• Place a nasogastric tube and maintain nothing-by-mouth status, if prescribed, to help prevent paralytic ileus and alleviate the effects from gastric dilatation.

• Administer prophylactic histamine blockers and antacids as ordered to reduce gastrointestinal ulceration.

• Administer appropriate nutrition, when prescribed.

• Assess bowel sounds and institute enteral feedings via a Dobhoff or gastric tube, as prescribed. Maintain the head of the bed at greater than 30 degrees during feedings. Monitor aspirate before and after bolus feedings, and during continuous enteral feedings.

• Use meticulous line and dressing care for parenteral feedings, as the patient is susceptible to infection.

Wound care for burn patients

Wound healing begins immediately after a burn injury, and meticulous care is required to promote optimal healing. The following chart details specific nursing interventions to include in the care of burn patients; these are in addition to the universally applied general principles of using sterile technique and evaluating for signs of infections during all dressing changes.

Superficial (first-degree) burns

• Apply an appropriate dressing, such as a single layer of saline-moistened gauze.
• Instruct the patient to elevate the burned area to prevent swelling and to use an over-the-counter anesthetic spray to manage pain.
• Instruct the patient to perform the above dressing change twice a day, if applicable, and to keep the area clean to prevent infection.
• Teach the patient to report signs and symptoms of infection.
• Tell the patient that complete healing should take place in 3 to 5 days.
• Warn the patient that skin may peel and that scarring should be limited to skin discoloration.

Partial-thickness (second-degree) burns

• Clean and debride the wound with each dressing change. Apply a 1/16" layer of antimicrobial cream, such as silver sulfadiazine, twice a day.
• Cover the clean wound with a sterile dressing to absorb fluid that will leak from the wound.
• Use a wet-to-moist/dry dressing for contaminated wounds to facilitate debridement.
• Minimize edema by elevating the burned area.

• Advise the patient that the wound should heal in 7 to 14 days.
• Inform the patient that deep second-degree burns may convert to full-thickness wounds that will require skin grafting.

Full-thickness (third-degree and fourth-degree) burns

• Clean and debride the wound utilizing topical agents such as silver sulfadiazine if antimicrobial coverage is needed.
• Use enzymatic therapy to prepare wounds for skin grafting.
• Explain to the patient that early excision and grafting help to minimize scarring and decrease infection. Explain that split-thickness skin grafts are meshed to allow for coverage of an area larger than the actual donor site.
• Cover the area of the skin graft with a nonadherent dressing and protect the skin graft from motion and disruption for 72 to 96 hours.
• If an autograft has been performed, care for the donor site by covering it with a synthetic dressing such as Op Site or DuoDerm.
• Treat the donor site with topical antibiotics if the site is infected.
• Explain to the patient that the donor site should heal in 10 to 14 days and that healing of third-degree and fourth-degree burns will take months.

• Provide support and prepare the patient and family for the eventual processes of reconstruction and rehabilitation. Consult psychiatric services.

Prognosis

The prognosis for burn injuries directly correlates with the degree of injury, the development of complications, and the presence of preexisting disease. Psychological adjustment also will affect the patient's ability to accept changes that have occurred. Despite improved fire-safety education, approximately 2 million people are burned each year in the United States, and about 75,000 persons are hospitalized with burn injuries. Although burn care has improved over the last three decades and there has been an increase in the survival rates of large-burn patients, 12,000 die each year from burn injuries and their complications.

Discharge planning

Discharge from the hospital requires not only satisfactory wound healing but also adequate preparation of the patient and examination of the home environment. The following areas should be evaluated:
• presence of competent provider of wound care
• outpatient rehabilitation facilities
• availability of community resources and patient and family support systems.

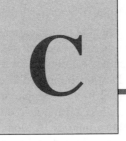

Cardiac trauma

Often dramatic in presentation, cardiac trauma usually is associated with other thoracic injuries and may occur secondary to blunt or penetrating trauma. Thoracic injuries, which include those of the heart, account for 25% of all trauma deaths. Although cardiac trauma can be severe, not all injuries are apparent upon admission to the emergency department or critical care unit, especially when the patient has no external signs of chest-wall damage. Some injuries may not manifest for several hours, and many complications may not be evident for days. Consequently, nurses must maintain a high index of suspicion to identify cardiac injuries and ensuing complications early.

Pathophysiology

Cardiac trauma may occur secondary to blunt or penetrating trauma. Blunt trauma typically results from vehicular accidents or falls. Injuries caused by rapid deceleration involve the heart's striking the anterior chest wall and sternum, resulting in myocardial contusion. Rapid deceleration also may result in shearing forces that tear cardiac structures and cause great-vessel disruption. Falls may cause a rapid increase in intra-abdominal and intrathoracic pressures, which can result

Myocardial contusion

Myocardial contusion may occur during deceleration injuries when the myocardium strikes the sternum. The aorta may be lacerated by shearing forces. The arrows show the forward motion of the aorta and heart that may cause injury. Direct force also may be applied to the sternum, causing injury.

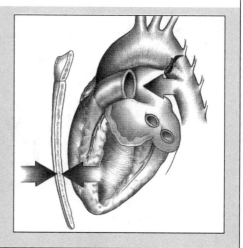

in myocardial rupture, valvular rupture, or both. Crushing and compression forces may result in contusion or rupture, as the heart is compressed between the sternum and vertebral column.

Penetrating trauma to the heart, which carries a high mortality rate and frequently requires immediate thoracotomy and surgical repair, often results from knife or gunshot wounds. Penetrating injuries to the heart result in prehospital death in 60% to 90% of cases, depending on the cause of the injury.

Myocardial contusion
A bruising of the myocardium, myocardial contusion is the most common type of injury sustained from blunt trauma and should be suspected with any blow to the chest. It usually results from a fall or from impact with a steering wheel (see *Myocardial contusion*, page 163). The right ventricle is the most common site of injury because of its location directly behind the sternum.

Cardiac tamponade

This illustration depicts cardiac tamponade resulting from a penetrating injury. Blood fills the pericardial sac, compressing the heart and resulting in decreased cardiac output.

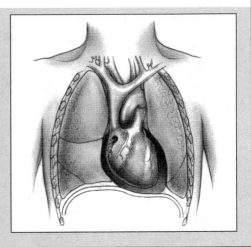

Cardiac tamponade

Cardiac tamponade can result from blunt or, more commonly, penetrating trauma. The pericardial sac is an inelastic membrane surrounding the heart that normally contains 25 ml of fluid. A gradual addition of 50 to 100 ml of blood causes a small rise in intrapericardial pressure. Amounts above this cause a sharp increase in pressure, which leads to compression of the ventricles and decreased ventricular filling. Increased intrapericardial pressure interferes with venous return to the right atrium. Impaired venous return and decreased ventricular filling result in diminished cardiac output, which can be life-threatening (see *Cardiac tamponade,* page 164).

Penetrating injuries can cause a sudden influx of blood into the pericardial sac, whereas blunt injuries to the myocardium usually produce a slower accumulation of fluid. A gradual increase in intrapericardial pressure, as in blunt injury, can be tolerated for longer periods. Therefore, cardiac tamponade may not be evident for several hours following injury.

Other cardiac injuries

Several other, relatively rare cardiac injuries include:
• aortic or mitral valve disruption, which results in signs and symptoms of congestive heart failure (CHF)
• myocardial rupture, which may follow blunt injury and usually is immediately fatal. If the patient survives to the emergency department, emergency thoracotomy and repair are indicated.
• aortic dissection (see "Thoracic Trauma," page 653).
• septal defects, which usually are caused by penetrating trauma. The injuries often are associated with myocardial rupture. However, the septum may be injured when a blow to the chest occurs during an increase in ventricular pressure (late diastole or early systole). These patients may exhibit signs of cardiac failure (due to volume overload and left-to-right shunting) that can occur immediately or days to weeks after the injury.

Clinical assessment

Cardiac injuries initially may be overlooked as other life-threatening injuries are treated. Signs and symptoms of myocardial contusion or tamponade may not be evident for hours. Astute assessment skills are necessary for early detection and prompt treatment.

History

The patient with cardiac injury generally has pain and is apprehensive. During the initial assessment, the nurse should attempt to ascertain the following:
• mechanism of injury
  —motor vehicle accident: how the accident occurred, any internal damage to the car, location of the patient in the car, seat-belt use
  —fall: how far the patient fell, onto what surface, how the patient landed
  —gunshot wound: caliber of gun and range
  —stabbing: size and type of weapon
• previous health history, particularly cardiovascular and pulmonary problems
• presence and nature of pain

• presence of shortness of breath.

The nurse should be especially suspicious of cardiac injury in any patient with the following conditions associated with myocardial contusion or perforation:
• associated head injury
• cervical or thoracic spine injury
• other thoracic injuries (of the lungs, trachea, great vessels, or esophagus)
• upper abdominal injuries
• chest-wall trauma
• fractured ribs.

Physical findings

Signs and symptoms of myocardial contusion include:
• hemodynamic instability
• chest pain that is not relieved by coronary vasodilators
• arrhythmias caused by ventricular irritability
• chest-wall contusion or ecchymosis
• symptoms of CHF and cardiogenic shock
• elevated cardiac enzymes (may or may not be present)
• signs of cardiac tamponade
• pericardial friction rub
• ECG changes including ST and T wave changes that may not be apparent for up to 48 hours after the injury.

Physical findings of cardiac tamponade include:
• hemodynamic instability
• Beck's triad, including hypotension, distended neck veins, and muffled heart sounds. (It is important to note that neck vein distention may not be evident in the hypotensive or volume-depleted patient.)
• tachycardia
• dyspnea
• paradoxical pulse (a 10 mm Hg drop in systolic pressure during inspiration)
• narrowed pulse pressure
• jugular venous distention with an increase in central venous pressure readings
• facial cyanosis
• failure to respond to volume infusion (if hypotensive)

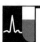

DIAGNOSTIC TESTS
Confirming cardiac trauma

The following diagnostic tests may be helpful in identifying cardiac trauma.

Cardiac enzymes
Specificity in myocardial contusion is uncertain. However, elevations of CPK-MB (creatine phosphokinase with isoenzymes), along with ECG abnormalities, is suggestive of myocardial contusion. Normal CPK is 5 to 200 U/l. Normal MB is less than 3% to 5%.

Cardiac troponin I
This is a sensitive test of myocardial necrosis. It is used in myocardial infarction but has not been widely evaluated in cardiac trauma patients. The normal blood level ranges from 1.5 to 3.1 ng/ml.

Electrocardiogram
Patients with myocardial contusion may show several rhythm disturbances, including premature ventricular contractions, premature atrial contractions, ventricular tachycardia, atrial tachycardia, and ventricular fibrillation, as well as non-specific ST-segment or T-wave changes. Most arrhythmias are apparent within 24 to 48 hours.

Chest X-ray
A chest X-ray may reveal a widened mediastinum in cardiac tamponade. In patients with septal defects, pulmonary engorgement may be present if a left-to-right shunt exists.

Echocardiogram
This noninvasive exam may show cardiac tamponade and valve abnormalities. Patients with myocardial contusion may have abnormalities in ventricular wall movement and decreased ejection fractions. Transesophageal echocardiography also may be safely used for increased visualization of cardiac structures. It may detect aortic disruptions, cardiac tamponade, and atrial and septal defects.

• Kussmaul's sign (distended neck veins during inspiration).

Diagnosis

Diagnosis begins with a high index of suspicion and may be difficult, particularly if there are no external signs of chest trauma. Several diagnostic tests are helpful in identifying cardiac trauma (for a detailed discussion, see *Confirming cardiac trauma,* page 167).

Pericardiocentesis can be a diagnostic tool as well as a treatment in the patient with cardiac tamponade. The patient may initially stabilize with volume infusion. However, a patient who fails to respond may have

Pericardiocentesis

Pericardiocentesis involves the insertion of a large-bore needle into the pericardial sac and the withdrawal of fluid. Preparation for the procedure includes placing the patient in semi-Fowler's position unless contraindicated. Continuous monitoring with 12-lead ECG equipment is necessary to avoid penetration of the myocardium.

The procedure for pericardiocentesis follows:
• Prep the subxiphoid area with an antiseptic solution.
• Assist with administration of local anesthetic.
• Attach a large-bore needle to a 60-ml syringe with a 3-way stopcock.
• Attach one end of an alligator clamp to the hub of the needle and the other end to the V-lead of the ECG monitor.
• Insert the needle just below the xiphoid at a 45-degree angle and direct toward the left shoulder.
• If the needle touches the myocardium, premature ventricular contractions or ST-segment elevation may be observed.

• Aspirate the syringe while advancing the needle. The pericardial sac is entered if blood is aspirated with no ST-segment elevation.
• When blood has been aspirated, attach a clamp to the needle at the level of the skin to prevent further insertion.
    Aspiration of unclotted blood is diagnostic for cardiac tamponade. Pericardial blood does not clot, because it is defibrinated by cardiac motion within the pericardial sac. If the blood does clot rapidly, the needle may have entered the heart. A negative result does not completely rule out tamponade, because a false negative result may occur if the needle becomes obstructed by tissue or clots.

tamponade or hemorrhage and will require immediate treatment. The critical care nurse must be familiar with the signs and symptoms of tamponade because it can develop hours after the patient is admitted. Additionally, because tamponade can be life-threatening, the nurse must be prepared to assist with emergency pericardiocentesis (see *Pericardiocentesis,* page 168).

Treatment and care
Primary goals of treatment for the patient with cardiac trauma are to maintain hemodynamic stability, preserve cardiac function, and prevent major complications (see *Key nursing interventions for patients with cardiac trauma,* page 169).

ESSENTIAL ELEMENTS

Key nursing interventions for patients with cardiac trauma

The following flowchart highlights key interventions that may be performed when a patient is diagnosed with cardiac trauma.

Achieve Optimal Cardiac Status		
Maintain hemodynamic stability	**Preserve cardiac function**	**Prevent major complications**
• Monitor hemodynamic parameters (blood pressure, pulse, central venous pressure, pulmonary capillary wedge pressure, cardiac output) every 1 to 2 hours. • Restore intravascular volume with blood products and fluids as necessary; monitor for transfusion reaction and fluid overload. • Monitor ECG continuously for first 24 to 48 hours for arrhythmias or conduction defects (if patient is hemodynamically stable, ECG monitoring may be discontinued). • Treat decreased cardiac output and ejection fraction with volume or positive inotropes (dopamine, dobutamine, or digitalis), as ordered.	• Administer supplemental oxygen based on oxygen saturation levels. • Prepare patient for emergency pericardiocentesis, surgery, or both, as indicated. • Maintain bed rest and high Fowler's position to decrease myocardial oxygen demand. • Administer analgesia to control pain, which inhibits full chest excursion (predisposing patient to atelectasis), increases cardiac workload, and increases myocardial oxygen consumption. • Promote respiratory hygiene measures, such as turning, coughing, and deep breathing.	• Assess for signs and symptoms of congestive heart failure (shortness of breath, distended neck veins, bilateral rales, edema). • Assess heart sounds for pericardial friction rub. • Monitor for signs of postoperative infection.

Maintaining hemodynamic stability

The most common presentation of patients with cardiac trauma is hemodynamic instability. Penetrating trauma may be associated with massive hemorrhage, leading to acute hypotension and shock. Cardiac tamponade may seriously decrease cardiac output, necessitating immediate treatment. Arrhythmias following myocardial contusion also may affect cardiac output.

Preservation of cardiac and respiratory function

The patient with cardiac trauma must be monitored closely for signs and symptoms of cardiopulmonary compromise. Cardiac trauma often is associated with pulmonary trauma. These patients require supplemental oxygen, with the aggressiveness of oxygen support therapy depending on the degree of injury sustained. Mechanical ventilation may be required for adequate oxygenation. Monitoring of arterial blood gases as well as Qs/Qt (shunt fraction) and compliance is indicated.

Postoperative course

Patients with cardiac trauma may require surgery, particularly to correct septal or valvular defects, as well as penetrating injuries or rupture. Tamponade may be treated surgically if pericardiocentesis is not successful.

In addition to the issues presented above, the following nursing interventions should be incorporated for the patient who has undergone surgery:
• Monitor and assess chest tubes for patency, volume and color of drainage, and presence of air leak.
• Monitor for postoperative infection (increasing white blood cell count; fever; redness, warmth, edema, purulent drainage, or localized pain at the incision site).
• Ensure that the patient's tetanus status is current. Administer a tetanus toxoid injection as indicated.
• Provide emotional support to the patient and family.

In addition, if the injuries are the result of a violent crime, the patient's clothing as well as knives, bullets, or other foreign bodies removed from the patient should be saved for law enforcement officials.

Complications of cardiac trauma

Potentially fatal complications may follow cardiac trauma. Astute assessment skills and prompt intervention are necessary for optimum recovery.

Complication	Possible Causes	Assessment Findings
Congestive heart failure (CHF)	• Septal or valvular damage • Myocardial necrosis	• Shortness of breath • Distended neck veins • Bilateral rales • Peripheral and pulmonary edema • Symptoms sometimes absent for days to weeks after injury
Ventricular aneurysm	• Ligation of coronary artery or suture of ventricular laceration	• Findings of CHF
Cardiac herniation	• May occur through a pericardial incision that reopens postoperatively	• Hemodynamic instability following a pericardial incision
Pneumopericardium (air within the pericardium, creating a tamponade)	• Pleuropericardial defect with pneumothorax • Pericardial defect with bronchial defect (disruption in a main bronchus)	• Signs and symptoms of cardiac tamponade (hypotension, distended neck veins, muffled heart sounds, dyspnea, tachycardia) • Tension pneumothorax
Post-traumatic pericarditis First stage	• Epicardium and pericardium are irritated by blood in the pericardium, causing inflammation and edema secondary to myocardial contusion or disruptions in the pericardium • May develop postoperatively	• Pericarditis with effusion—signs and symptoms of cardiac tamponade • Pericarditis without effusion—pericardial friction rub, fever, chest pain
Post-traumatic pericarditis Second stage	• A serofibrinous effusion develops within the pericardium	• Constrictive pericarditis—signs of right-sided heart failure (peripheral edema, ascites), muffled heart sounds, third heart sound, dyspnea, fever) *(continued)*

Complications of cardiac trauma *(continued)*

Complication	Possible Causes	Assessment Findings
Post-traumatic pericarditis Second stage *(continued)*		• Nonconstrictive pericarditis—chest pain, fever, pericardial friction rub, tachypnea, signs of tamponade • Signs and symptoms sometimes absent for weeks to months

Preventing and treating complications

Patients with cardiac trauma may develop complications days to months after injury and should be monitored during this time. Patients should be aware of signs and symptoms to report to their physician (see *Complications of cardiac trauma,* pages 171 and 172).

Prognosis

The prognosis for a patient with cardiac trauma depends largely upon the extent of cardiac damage and associated injuries. Prompt identification and treatment of injuries is crucial. Careful monitoring is required throughout hospitalization to detect developing complications. Other factors that affect mortality rate include preexisting conditions and age.

Discharge planning

Discharge planning should begin as soon as the patient is stabilized. The following steps should be taken to ensure a smooth discharge:

• Evaluate the patient's support systems.
• Consult social services, if indicated.
• Assess the cause of injury and proceed as appropriate. (For example, if the accident was alcohol-related, the patient may need follow-up for alcohol abuse. If a gunshot wound to a patient who is a minor was gang-related, social services may be able to intervene for

appropriate placement. If an elderly patient has been involved in an automobile accident, appropriateness of the patient driving again may be assessed.)
• Ensure that a follow-up appointment has been made.
• Review signs and symptoms of complications that may occur and the need to report symptoms associated with the complications.

Cardiomyopathy

An idiopathic disorder of myocardial tissue, cardiomyopathy is characterized by structural abnormalities of the myocardium and ventricular changes resulting from reduced myocardial contractility or distensibility. Cardiomyopathy may be classified as dilated, hypertrophic, or restrictive, depending upon the anatomic appearance and physiologic deviations (see *Classifying cardiomyopathy,* page 174).

Pathophysiology

Although the exact cause of cardiomyopathy is unknown, several precipitating conditions have been identified for each type. The most common precipitants of dilated cardiomyopathy are infections, toxins, coronary artery disease, and peripartum causes. Hypertrophic cardiomyopathy frequently is genetic. Connective tissue diseases often are linked with restrictive cardiomyopathy.

Dilated cardiomyopathy

In dilated cardiomyopathy, the heart is flabby, dilated on one or both sides, and globe-shaped. Microscopic evidence of myofibril atrophy with discrete focal zones of cellular necrosis and scar tissue is found. Myocardial biopsy typically demonstrates extensive interstitial and perivascular fibrosis and myocellular hypertrophy.

The initial event is depressed contractility. Reduction of working myofibrils decreases the degree of myofibril shortening and the maximum rate of develop-

Classifying cardiomyopathy

Cardiomyopathy commonly is classified according to cardiac structural changes and the ventricular changes they cause.

Dilated cardiomyopathy is characterized by damaged myocardial muscle fibers and ventricular enlargement, resulting in poor contractility.

Hypertrophic cardiomyopathy is marked by thickening of the interventricular septum that leads to resistance of blood flow from the left atrium and to left ventricular outflow obstruction.

Restrictive cardiomyopathy is characterized by rigid, fibrotic ventricular walls that restrict ventricular filling and result in abnormal diastolic functioning.

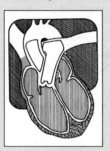
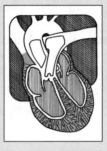
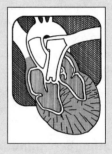

ment of ventricular pressure over time. This produces a large left ventricular end-systolic volume (LVESV) that generates a large left ventricular end-diastolic volume (LVEDV). The chronically increased LVEDV increases the end-diastolic fiber length (preload), resulting in ventricular and atrial dilation.

Initially, the increase in the ventricular chamber size compensates for the loss of contractility via the Frank-Starling mechanism. However, the increase in resting myofibril length requires more time to overcome the increased afterload produced via this mechanism. Consequently, the normal hypertrophic response fails to occur, further increasing ventricular wall tension and dilation. The prognosis is better for patients who develop concomitant hypertrophy, because the heart does not become as dilated.

Hypertrophic cardiomyopathy

In hypertrophic cardiomyopathy, systolic function is vigorous (hyperdynamic), but diastolic function is impaired because of the thick, poorly compliant ventricle. The ventricular septum is affected in about 90% of all patients with this type. Microscopically, the myofibrils are arranged chaotically, which may be responsible for the diastolic stiffness and arrhythmias common in the disorder.

The hypertrophied, stiff ventricular muscle impedes diastolic filling, causing increased left ventricular end-diastolic pressure (LVEDP) and atrial dilation from backward pressure. The most significant consequence of hypertrophic cardiomyopathy is the outflow tract obstruction caused by the septal hypertrophy. A systolic gradient is produced between the body of the left ventricle and the outflow tract beyond the hypertrophic segment. The asymmetrically hypertrophied septum causes the papillary muscle to become misaligned, which pulls the anterior mitral leaflet away from the posterior leaflet during systole, causing inadequate mitral closure and regurgitation.

This systolic anterior motion (SAM) is the hallmark of hypertrophic cardiomyopathy. SAM impedes blood flow from the left ventricle to the aorta, causing left ventricular outflow tract obstruction. Factors that increase inotropy or contractility (such as dopamine) worsen SAM because they increase the pull on the anterior mitral leaflet. The systolic changes are considered dynamic because the magnitude of the pressure gradient and SAM vary during contraction.

Compliance is impaired from loss of myocardial elasticity and increased muscle mass. The result is an elevated LVEDP with decreased diastolic filling time. This diastolic dysfunction coupled with impaired systolic ejection is responsible for most of the symptoms associated with this condition, including dyspnea and inadequate cardiac output.

Restrictive cardiomyopathy

In restrictive cardiomyopathy, systolic function is maintained but diastolic relaxation is markedly impaired by the extremely rigid ventricle. Although both the right and left ventricles are affected, the ventricular chamber size remains unaffected. The ventricles become noncompliant because of a fibrotic endomyocardium or the infiltration of the myocardium by a toxin. The noncompliant ventricle cannot adequately fill, precipitating increased preload and consequently failure of the left and right sides of the heart. Because of inadequate diastolic filling, stroke volume is reduced and symptoms of low cardiac output appear.

Clinical assessment

The onset of disease in patients with dilated or restrictive cardiomyopathy generally is insidious. In the later stages, patients suffering from all types of cardiomyopathy experience frequent exacerbations and hospitalizations. A detailed nursing history and assessment can help identify precipitating factors and may prevent further exacerbations (see *History and clinical findings for patients with cardiomyopathy*, pages 178 and 179).

Dilated cardiomyopathy

Most patients are middle-aged men, whose symptoms may be overlooked until left ventricular failure, the hallmark symptom, occurs. When taking the history, the nurse should evaluate the patient's current condition as compared with the previous 6 to 12 months.

Hypertrophic cardiomyopathy

The clinical presentation of patients is highly variable. Often the presenting symptom is syncope or sudden cardiac death from arrhythmias. The average age of presentation is in the 30s. Many patients are active athletes who are asymptomatic and diagnosed by subtle findings on routine physical examination. Other patients have an insidious onset of symptoms.

Restrictive cardiomyopathy

The patient initially presents with signs of congestive heart failure (CHF) caused by the increased preload and consequent pulmonary edema. Eventually, the inadequate diastolic filling reduces the stroke volume, and signs of inadequate cardiac output appear. Most patients develop biventricular failure.

Diagnosis

Diagnosis of cardiomyopathy is primarily noninvasive. Invasive studies, such as cardiac catheterization, may be performed to rule out ischemia as a cause of the cardiomyopathy as well as to obtain endomyocardial biopsy (see *Diagnosing cardiomyopathy,* pages 180 and 181). Computed tomography (CT) and magnetic resonance imaging (MRI) are gaining importance as tools in the diagnosis of restrictive cardiomyopathy.

Treatment and care

There is no known cure for cardiomyopathy. Specific treatments vary depending on the type of cardiomyopathy. Cardiac transplantation may be considered for end-stage patients.

Dilated cardiomyopathy

Treatment is aimed at relieving symptoms and increasing longevity. Therapy is directed toward reducing afterload, decreasing myocardial oxygen demand, treating life-threatening cardiac arrhythmias, preventing and treating intracardiac thrombus, relieving pulmonary and systemic vascular congestion, and increasing cardiac output.

Because hemodynamic variables may not correlate with the patient's functional capacity, the nurse should monitor for trends in hemodynamic values while continually assessing the patient's overall clinical status. Important nursing interventions are included below (also see *Key nursing interventions for patients with dilated or restrictive cardiomyopathy,* page 182, for overall nursing goals and responsibilities).

History and clinical findings for patients with cardiomyopathy

The following chart compares significant patient history information and clinical findings for each type of cardiomyopathy.

Type of Cardiomyopathy	Significant History Information
Dilated	• Duration of and measures used to relieve symptoms • Medication and alcohol use • Recent pregnancy and previous medical conditions • Physical activity tolerance • Dietary habits • Precipitating factors, including exposure to toxic substances
Hypertrophic	• Precipitating symptoms and measures used to relieve symptoms • Family history of hypertrophic cardiomyopathy or sudden death • Physical response to exercise
Restrictive	• Personal or family history of cancer or autoimmune diseases (especially amyloidosis, scleroderma, or sarcoidosis) • Cancer treatments, especially radiation therapy • History of allergic disorders • Exposure to toxic substances

• Administer unloading agents. Angiotensin-converting enzyme inhibitors help improve the quality of life and increase longevity in patients with severe left ventricular failure and should be used in all patients who have no contraindications to the drugs.

Clinical Findings

- Signs of failure of the left side of the heart (dyspnea, cough, orthopnea, palpitations, hypotension, weakness)
- Signs of failure of the right side of the heart (abdominal pain caused by liver engorgement, generalized aching, lower extremity edema, ascites)
- Cool, clammy extremities
- Peripheral cyanosis
- Jugular vein distention
- Rales
- Pulsatile liver engorgement
- Left precordial heaves (nonsustained)
- Laterally displaced apical impulse
- S_3 or S_4 heart sounds or summation gallop
- Decreased pulse pressure

- Fatigue
- Dyspnea
- Syncope
- Angina (either at rest or with exertion) and chest pain unrelieved by nitrates
- Arrhythmias, especially atrial fibrillation and ventricular tachycardia
- Signs of congestive heart failure (occur during late stages)
- Late systolic murmur (auscultated at the lower, left sternal border and radiating to the axilla, exaggerated by the Valsalva maneuver)
- Abrupt, jerky arterial pulse
- Triple apical impulse (each heartbeat feeling as if it were three movements instead of two)

- Similar to that of dilated cardiomyopathy
- Signs of peripheral congestion (lower extremity edema and liver congestion)

• Administer nitrates, as ordered, to increase the myocardial oxygen supply and relieve anginal symptoms. Although beta-blocking agents and calcium channel blockers decrease the myocardial oxygen demand (MVO_2), they generally are poorly tolerated by the patient with dilated cardiomyopathy. They reduce cardiac

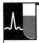

Diagnosing cardiomyopathy

Many tools are useful in diagnosing cardiomyopathy. The most definitive test for confirming the diagnosis is the echocardiogram because it illustrates the anatomic abnormalities that define each type of cardiomyopathy. The chart below shows characteristic findings using each diagnostic tool.

Dilated	Hypertrophic	Restrictive
CHEST X-RAY		
• Enlarged cardiac silhouette • Pulmonary vascular redistribution • Interstitial and alveolar edema • Pleural effusions	• Left atrial enlargement • Left ventricular enlargement • Signs of heart failure in late stages	• Pulmonary vascular redistribution • Interstitial and alveolar edema • Pleural effusions
ELECTROCARDIOGRAM		
• Tachycardia • Atrioventricular (AV) conduction disturbances • Atrial fibrillation (A-fib) • Ventricular ectopy • Left bundle branch block • Pathologic Q-waves (indicate extensive left ventricular fibrosis as opposed to necrosis; new Q-wave mandates evaluation for concurrent myocardial infarction) • Nonspecific ST-T wave abnormalities	• A-fib • Ventricular arrhythmias • Left ventricular hypertrophy • Conduction defects • Left atrial enlargement • Left axis deviation • Pathologic Q-waves • May be normal	• Low voltage • Sinus tachycardia • A-fib • High-grade AV blocks with amyloidosis
ECHOCARDIOGRAM		
• Four-chamber cardiac enlargement • Disproportionate dilatation to hypertrophy • Reduction of ventricular free wall movement • Atrial or ventricular thrombus	• Asymmetric ventricular cavity and septal thickness • Wall motion abnormalities • Systolic anterior motion of the mitral leaflet	• Thick pericardium • Reduced ventricular compliance • Diastolic filling impairment • Atrial and ventricular thrombus

Diagnosing cardiomyopathy (continued)

Dilated	Hypertrophic	Restrictive
RADIONUCLIDE STUDIES (SUCH AS THALLIUM STRESS TEST)		
• Reduced ventricular ejection fraction • Identification of areas of reversible ischemia	• Exercise-induced ischemic defects • Asymmetric septal hypertrophy	• Normal systolic function • Reduced diastolic function • Reduced ejection fraction
CARDIAC CATHETERIZATION		
• Illustration of coronary artery disease • Left ventriculography to directly assess left ventricular function and pressures • Myocardial biopsy (limited role because biopsy is rarely diagnostic and does not alter the therapeutic regimen)	• Pressure gradient within left ventricular outflow tract • Spade-shaped ventricular contour • Increased systolic function • Impaired diastolic compliance	• Endomyocardial biopsy most useful diagnostic tool • Biopsy identifies presence of infiltrates or tumor

contractility and increase LVESV and LVEDV, and they may further deteriorate the patient's condition.

• Administer supplemental oxygen.

• Assess hemodynamic parameters of the patient with an intra-aortic balloon pump. (The pump may benefit the severely compromised patient by increasing coronary blood flow and decreasing afterload.)

• Evaluate electrolyte levels and report abnormal levels. Alterations in potassium and magnesium levels place patients at risk for ventricular arrhythmias.

• Monitor for arrhythmias and administer antiarrhythmic medications. Unfortunately, antiarrhythmic drugs do not prevent death caused by ventricular arrhythmias in these patients. Patients with recurrent ventricular arrhythmias should be referred for electrophysiology studies and possible implantation of an automatic implantable cardioverter defibrillator (AICD).

ESSENTIAL ELEMENTS

Key nursing interventions for patients with dilated or restrictive cardiomyopathy

The following flowchart highlights key interventions that may be performed when a patient is diagnosed with dilated or restrictive cardiomyopathy.

ACHIEVE OPTIMAL CARDIAC FUNCTION

Reduce afterload	Increase myocardial oxygen supply and decrease myocardial oxygen demand	Prevent complications of poor cardiac function
• Administer nitrates (dilated cardiomyopathy only). • Administer angiotensin-converting enzyme inhibitors. • Monitor cardiac index and systemic vascular resistance. • Evaluate effect of dobutamine and nitroprusside infusions. • Assess patient for effects of intra-aortic balloon pump (dilated cardiomyopathy only).	• Administer nitrates (dilated cardiomyopathy only). • Administer beta-adrenergic blockers and calcium channel blockers (restrictive cardiomyopathy only). • Encourage cardiac rehabilitation. • Assist in placement of an intra-aortic balloon pump, and monitor patient for beneficial hemodynamic changes and complications (dilated cardiomyopathy only). • Administer oxygen as needed.	• Observe for and treat arrhythmias. • Monitor serum potassium and magnesium levels. • Refer patient with recurrent ventricular arrhythmias for electrophysiology evaluation (dilated cardiomyopathy only). • Administer anticoagulation for patient with low ejection fraction. • Instruct patient regarding anticoagulation therapy. • Report signs of thromboembolism. • Provide adequate calories and protein with low-sodium diet. • Monitor fluid balance with daily weights, intake and output records, and physical assessment for signs of congestive heart failure.

• Teach the patient receiving warfarin therapy to monitor anticoagulation. Low-dose warfarin may be prescribed for the patient with low ejection fractions. Presence of left atrial or ventricular thrombus may necessitate heparin infusions to prevent stroke and other sequelae of thromboembolism. Antiplatelet drugs, such as Persantine (dipyridamole) or aspirin, may be prescribed for patients who cannot safely take warfarin.

• Provide a salt-restricted diet. It is important to maintain adequate caloric intake without exceeding sodium restriction, to prevent a catabolic state while avoiding factors that can precipitate pulmonary edema.

• Monitor the patient's daily weight and intake and output records. A weight gain of over 2 lb in one week is considered clinically significant.

• Administer digitalis, as ordered. Digitalis can increase cardiac contractility and reduce preload because of more complete ventricular emptying. However, the nurse must use caution when administering any positive inotropic agent, because the MVO_2 can increase and worsen arrhythmias and anginal symptoms.

• Discuss the possibility of permanent pacemaker placement with the patient and family. Dual-chamber pacemakers synchronize atrial and ventricular contraction at a short atrioventricular interval and may subsequently increase the cardiac output.

Hypertrophic cardiomyopathy

The primary goals of medical therapy for the patient with hypertrophic cardiomyopathy are to relieve symptoms and prevent complications. Because many patients are asymptomatic when first diagnosed, they are unaware of the life-threatening ramifications of the disease and require intensive education.

Specific medical treatments are focused on relieving left ventricular outflow tract obstruction, reducing MVO_2, controlling arrhythmia, managing CHF symptoms, and preventing complications. Surgical treatments may include left ventricular septal myotomy and myectomy, pacemaker insertion, and AICD insertion.

Specific nursing interventions for achieving the treatment goals are discussed below (also see *Key nursing interventions for patients with hypertrophic cardiomyopathy,* page 185, for highlights):

• Administer negative inotropic agents, as ordered. Beta-adrenergic blockers prolong diastolic filling time, thus allowing the ventricular chamber size to increase and consequently separating the anterior mitral leaflet from the hypertrophied septum and relieving the outflow tract obstruction. They also reduce the vigor of systolic contraction. Calcium channel blockers reduce systolic function and improve diastolic filling and relaxation, all of which decrease the outflow tract obstruction.

• Avoid the use of positive inotropic agents (digoxin, dopamine, epinephrine), because they worsen the outflow tract obstruction by increasing myocardial contractility and decreasing diastolic filling time.

• Monitor vital signs closely in patients receiving diuretics. Diuretics should be used cautiously because they reduce circulating volume and, subsequently, left ventricular volume, thus exaggerating the outflow tract obstruction. Diuretics should be administered only in combination with beta-adrenergic blockers or calcium channel blockers. Symptoms of severe congestive failure may be an indication for surgical management.

• Provide adequate intravenous volume for surgical patients. A left ventricular septal myotomy and myectomy may be performed. The hypertrophied area is resected at the junction point of the septal-mitral contact. Mitral valve replacement may be performed concomitantly.

• Provide follow-up instructions for patients who receive pacemaker therapy. Conventional ventricular pacing pulls the septum away from the left ventricle during systole, thus reducing the outflow tract obstruction.

• Instruct the patient that nitroglycerin will not relieve angina. Nitrates reduce afterload, resulting in a need for increased cardiac output.

• Instruct the patient that calcium channel blockers and beta blockers are used to prevent angina. These drugs

ESSENTIAL ELEMENTS

Key nursing interventions for patients with hypertrophic cardiomyopathy

The following flowchart highlights key interventions that may be performed when a patient is diagnosed with hypertrophic cardiomyopathy.

PREVENT MORBIDITY AND MORTALITY RELATED TO THE ANATOMIC ABNORMALITY

Relieve left ventricu-lar outflow tract ob-struction	Reduce myocardial oxygen demand	Educate patient about condition and necessary lifestyle changes
• Administer nega-tive inotropic agents as ordered. • Avoid use of posi-tive inotropic agents. • Provide adequate intravenous volume for septal myotomy and myectomy pa-tients. • Instruct patient in rationale and home care for permanent pacemaker place-ment. • Monitor vital signs closely in pa-tient on diuretics.	• Administer beta blockers. • Administer calci-um channel block-ers. • Educate patient that nitrates are in-effective in treating angina. • Advise patient to report any synco-pal episodes. • Monitor for ar-rhythmias.	• Counsel athletic patient regarding danger of strenu-ous activity. • Help athlete to in-corporate alterna-tive activities into lifestyle. • Familiarize patient with American Col-lege of Cardiology guidelines for physi-cal activity. • Maintain adequate circulating blood vol-ume to augment car-diac output during exertion. • Recommend screening and ge-netic counseling for family members. • Encourage partic-ipation in support groups.

treat the angina by reducing heart rate and prolonging diastolic time.

• Advise the patient to report any episode of syncope, a common complication due to arrhythmias and the inability to increase cardiac output during exertion. Lethal arrhythmias are the leading cause of death in young athletic patients with hypertrophic cardiomyopathy; event or Holter monitoring may be indicated in symptomatic patients.

• Administer prophylactic beta-adrenergic blockers, as indicated, to control arrhythmias.

• Administer conventional antiarrhythmic agents in the patient with known arrhythmias; currently, amiodarone is the most promising agent. Because antiarrhythmics have not been demonstrated to prevent sudden death in hypertrophic cardiomyopathy, AICDs may be implanted in some patients.

• Observe the patient who is receiving treatment for CHF for adverse reactions to medications.

• Counsel athletic patients regarding the danger of strenuous activity, and help them to incorporate alternative activities into their lifestyle. Maintain adequate circulating blood volume to augment cardiac output during exertion. Individuals with known hypertrophic cardiomyopathy should follow American College of Cardiology guidelines for athletic activity.

• Counsel and educate patients about lifestyle restrictions. Activities and occupations that require strenuous activity should be avoided. Instruct patients about the course of the disease and the risks of terminating medications even when asymptomatic.

• Discuss familial tendencies and genetic counseling with the patient and family, and recommend screening for family members (especially males). Encourage participation in support groups.

• Instruct the patient about subacute bacterial endocarditis and prophylactic measures. Antibiotic prophylaxis for invasive procedures is mandated.

Restrictive cardiomyopathy

The medical and nursing management is similar to that of dilated cardiomyopathy, with a few exceptions:

• Treatment with beta blockers, calcium channel blockers, or both may improve ventricular filling by increas-

ing diastolic filling time, which decreases the heart rate and reduces contractility.
• Treatment of the underlying cause may include steroids, which can help halt the disease's progress.
• Digitalis and vasodilators are generally ineffective because systolic function is well preserved in these patients (unlike those with dilated cardiomyopathy).
• Patients are particularly prone to intraventricular thrombus formation and therefore require systemic anticoagulation.

Prognosis

Overall the prognosis for patients with cardiomyopathy is dismal, although hypertrophic patients can expect a better long-term outlook if they carefully adhere to medical guidelines. In general, dilated cardiomyopathy has a rapid course of disease progression, with 20% to 50% of patients dying in the first year after diagnosis. The course of hypertrophic cardiomyopathy is variable, but the average patient dies approximately 5 to 10 years after onset of clinical signs and symptoms. In patients who are born with the autosomal dominant trait, the average age of death is 40. The patient with restrictive cardiomyopathy generally has about a 1-year survival rate; however, less than 25% survive when the underlying cause cannot be identified and treated.

Discharge planning

Discharge planning for cardiomyopathy patients requires close medical and nursing follow-up. General guidelines are listed below:
• Consult the community health nurse to monitor the patient's functional status at home and to report signs of physical deterioration.
• Encourage the patient to keep all medical appointments, even when feeling well.
• Advise the patient about the importance of taking all medications as prescribed, and discuss the risk in discontinuing medications against medical advice.

• Instruct the patient discharged on warfarin to carefully monitor the prothrombin time or international ratio with the primary health care provider.

• Provide instructions about a low-sodium diet; recommend adequate nutritional intake to maintain cellular structural integrity and to provide stamina during exacerbations.

• Advise the patient to monitor for fluid and weight gain.

• Discuss the need for lifestyle restrictions, including occupation choices, sports, and physical or strenuous activities.

Cerebral aneurysm

A cerebral aneurysm is a round, saccular dilatation in a cerebral artery that develops as a result of a weakness in the arterial wall, usually at a bifurcation in the arterial system. Subarachnoid hemorrhage, bleeding into the subarachnoid space that can extend into the ventricular system and intraparenchymally, most commonly occurs from a ruptured cerebral aneurysm and accounts for 8% of the strokes seen annually. Although subarachnoid hemorrhage occurs in all age groups, the mean age for aneurysm rupture is 50; nearly 60% of all patients with subarachnoid hemorrhage are female.

Pathophysiology

Cerebral aneurysm results from a weakening in the arterial wall, which eventually dilates into a round, saccular outpouching. The pathogenesis of aneurysm development is unclear and may be multifactorial. One theory holds that aneurysms are congenital and develop secondary to a defect in the arterial wall. Another theory suggests that aneurysms develop as a result of degenerative arterial changes that affect the internal elastic membrane and allow the intima to rupture through the weakened area, such as with atherosclerotic disease. A third theory contends that hypertension or hemodynamic stress may contribute to the development of cerebral aneurysms.

There is no clear-cut explanation of why aneurysms rupture; however, certain conditions may be associated. These include polycystic kidney disease, hypertension, fibromuscular dysplasia, disorders that affect the arterial wall (Ehlers-Danlos and Marfan's syndrome), infections, neoplasms, trauma, and cocaine use.

Most aneurysms are small, measuring less than 1 cm in diameter. However, they can dilate up to 5 cm and present signs and symptoms of increased intracranial pressure (ICP) typical of a space-occupying lesion. They commonly are classified according to size and shape (see *Types of cerebral aneurysms,* page 190). Not all aneurysms rupture; some are found during postmortem examinations.

Aneurysms most frequently are found at bifurcations in the cerebral circulation. About 85% occur in the anterior circulation, which supplies blood to two thirds of the cerebral cortex, usually in the internal carotid and middle cerebral artery (MCA) distribution. In the posterior circulation, which feeds the brain stem and cerebellum, the most common site for aneurysm development is the juncture of the posterior communicating artery and the MCA.

When an aneurysm ruptures, it spreads blood into the subarachnoid space and sometimes into the ventricular system and cerebral tissues. The signs and symptoms that the patient displays are related to the location, degree of ICP, and meningeal irritation caused by the hemorrhage. Neurologic dysfunction often is associated with vasospasm, a narrowing of the arteries that restricts blood flow and contributes to cerebral infarction.

Vasospasm occurs in 40% to 60% of patients with subarachnoid hemorrhage and contributes to the morbidity and mortality associated with cerebral aneurysm. Causes of vasospasm are not clearly understood. One theory describes a neurogenic mechanism that acts on the arterial smooth muscle cell membrane to allow the influx of calcium, which promotes prolonged smooth muscle contraction.

Types of cerebral aneurysms

Aneurysms commonly are classified according to size and shape. The classification becomes very important for the neurosurgeon when evaluating the feasibility of surgical treatment.

Berry (saccular): Small, round aneurysm with a neck; typically less than 2 cm in diameter. The most common type of aneurysm thought to result from a defect in the anatomic development of the vessel wall. If surgically accessible, can be clipped across the neck.
Giant: Aneurysm that is similar to berry but larger (greater than 3 cm in diameter) and acts like a space-occupying lesion. Too large to be clipped but often can be wrapped to reinforce the arterial wall and decrease the risk of bleeding.
Fusiform: Irregular dilatation of the arterial wall, usually resulting from widespread atherosclerotic dis-

ease. Rarely ruptures.
Traumatic: Aneurysm that usually results from arterial stretching but also can be caused by direct injury. Most commonly found in the carotid circulation.
Mycotic: Aneurysm that results from an infection in which septic emboli cause arteritis.
Charcot-Bouchard: Microscopic aneurysm resulting from hypertension that usually is found in the basal ganglia or brain stem.
Dissecting: Aneurysm formed when blood flows between the arterial walls, separating the intima from the muscle layer. Commonly results from arteriosclerotic disease.

Other theories center on the release of spasmogenic substances from the blood clot and direct arterial damage as a result of the aneurysm rupture. A combination of reduction in catecholamines and the release of serotonin during clot lysis creates an environment that promotes vascular contraction. Other blood components that have been identified as possible spasmogens include lysed erythrocytes, oxyhemoglobin, fibrin, and fibrin degradation products.

As with the development of aneurysms, vasospasm probably occurs as a response to a combination of factors, including the release of spasmogenic agents from the blood clot, structural changes in the vessels, and an inflammatory response caused by hemorrhage. Patients who suffer from vasospasm typically present with clinical symptoms that fluctuate with the degree of spasm; these patients are at great risk for permanent neurologic dysfunction or death.

Clinical assessment

Most patients with cerebral aneurysms are asymptomatic until the aneurysm ruptures. A large aneurysm that acts as a space-occupying lesion may become symptomatic before rupture. Such an aneurysm may give subtle signs of increased ICP, including generalized headache, sleepiness, and inability to concentrate. Localized signs, such as hand weakness, correspond to the area of the brain affected by the pressure from the lesion. As long as the signs remain nonspecific and do not impair functioning, patients generally do not seek medical attention.

History

Often the history of the presenting signs leads the nurse to suspect the presence of aneurysmal subarachnoid hemorrhage. The most common presenting sign is the sudden onset of headache. The words "violent" and "explosive" often are used to describe the pain, and many patients speak of "the worst headache of my life." Important history information includes:
- description of the onset of headache
- precipitating factors
- loss of consciousness associated with the headache
- seizure
- nausea or vomiting.

Physical findings

Signs and symptoms associated with subarachnoid hemorrhage are related to meningeal irritation, cerebral dysfunction, and increased ICP. Regardless of the extent of the presenting symptoms, the patient should be considered in serious condition with a guarded prognosis.

Besides a severe headache, other significant findings include:
- nausea and vomiting
- third nerve palsy
- deviations of gaze or loss of visual acuity
- elevated temperature (greater than 100° F)
- seizures (may be focal or generalized)
- photophobia

- nuchal rigidity
- positive Kernig's sign
- positive Brudzinski's sign
- altered level of consciousness
- hemiparesis or hemiplegia
- abnormal posturing.

Aneurysms are graded on the basis of physical assessment findings. The most commonly used grading scale is a modification of the Botterel Scale originally developed in the late 1950s. The Hunt and Hess Scale has become more popular in recent years because it differentiates the unruptured aneurysm from a rupture with minimal symptoms. Grading often is used as a basis for the treatment plan (see *Classification of aneurysmal subarachnoid hemorrhage,* page 193).

Diagnosis

Diagnosis of aneurysmal subarachnoid hemorrhage is based on the history and physical examination findings suggestive of hemorrhage as well as on laboratory studies (see *Confirming aneurysmal subarachnoid hemorrhage,* page 194).

Routine laboratory studies, such as hemoglobin and hematocrit (HCT) levels, serum electrolyte levels, prothrombin time, partial thromboplastin time, and serum osmolarity, should be obtained on admission to provide baseline values, because the routine treatment for vasospasm often precipitates electrolyte abnormalities that are associated with hemodilution.

Treatment and care

Early management of the patient who presents with possible aneurysmal subarachnoid hemorrhage involves stabilization of neurologic status and vital signs so that the necessary diagnostic studies can be performed. Preventing complications from the hemorrhage is key to a successful outcome. The two most common complications of aneurysmal subarachnoid hemorrhage are rebleeding of the aneurysm and vasospasm. Both are associated with high morbidity and

Classification of aneurysmal subarachnoid hemorrhage

The grading of subarachnoid hemorrhage according to clinical symptoms has guided decisions for surgery since the late 1950s. The two most commonly used scales, the Hunt and Hess Scale and the Modified Botterel Scale, are shown below. Note that serious systemic disease and age over 70 generally increase the grading of severity.

Hunt and Hess Scale

Grade	Amount of Bleeding	Clinical Findings
0	No bleeding	Unruptured aneurysm
1	Minimal bleeding	Alertness, slight nuchal rigidity, minimal headache, no focal neurologic signs
2	Mild bleeding	Alertness, nuchal rigidity, mild to severe headache, minimal neurologic deficit (such as third nerve palsy)
3	Moderate bleeding	Drowsiness or confusion, nuchal rigidity, mild focal deficits
4	Moderate to severe bleeding	Stuporousness, mild to severe hemiparesis, nuchal rigidity, possible early decerebration
5	Severe bleeding	Deep coma, decerebrate rigidity, moribund appearance

Modified Botterel Scale

Grade	Description
0	No evidence of rupture or subarachnoid hemorrhage within last 30 days
1	Mild headache, alertness, oriented, no motor or sensory deficits
2	Severe headache, major meningeal findings, mild change in level of consciousness, possible focal deficits
3	Major alteration in level of consciousness, major focal deficit, or both
4	Semicomatose or comatose with or without major lateralizing signs

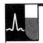

Confirming aneurysmal subarachnoid hemorrhage

The following studies typically are performed to help confirm a diagnosis of aneurysmal subarachnoid hemorrhage.

Lumbar puncture

Usually performed on patients who present with no signs of increased intracranial pressure to identify the presence of blood in the subarachnoid space. Normally, cerebrospinal fluid (CSF) is clear and colorless; with subarachnoid hemorrhage, CSF may be bloody or xanthochromic. Laboratory analysis reveals red blood cells in xanthochromic fluid, increased white blood cell count secondary to meningeal irritation, and increased CSF protein secondary to inflammation from blood in the subarachnoid space.

Computed tomography (CT scan)

Imaging technique of choice for acute patients, CT helps to evaluate the extent of the hemorrhage and the condition of intracranial structures and to determine the presence of hydrocephalus. Presence of an aneurysm may reveal blood in the subarachnoid space, ventricular system, or cerebral tissues as well as hydrocephalus.

Magnetic resonance imaging (MRI) and magnetic resonance angiography (MRA)

Can be performed on the more stable patient. MRI and MRA identify the hemorrhage and may show the source of bleeding.

Cerebral angiography

Shows the intracerebral vasculature and helps identify the location of the aneurysm, the source of hemorrhage, and the presence of vasospasm. Dye is injected into the carotid and vertebral arteries, usually via a femoral puncture, to outline the cerebral vessels and provide information on how the aneurysm fills. If the angiogram does not identify the source bleeding, a second angiogram usually is performed 1 week later to confirm a nonlocalized subarachnoid hemorrhage.

Transcranial Doppler study

Identifies flow velocities in the cerebral circulation via ultrasound over the transtemporal walls, transorbital windows, and foramen magnum. Normal flow velocity is 70 to 80 cm/second. In patients with vasospasm, flow velocities often are greater than 200 cm/second secondary to vessel narrowing.

mortality. Rebleeding most commonly occurs within 7 to 10 days after the initial hemorrhage, possibly as a result of clot lysis. Patients who rebleed face a 50% mortality rate; those who survive the rebleeding usually are left with significant neurologic dysfunction.

Once the diagnosis of cerebral aneurysm has been made, surgical treatment options can be discussed. The decision to proceed with surgery and the timing of the procedure depend on many factors, including the patient's clinical status (grade of subarachnoid hemorrhage),the location and size of the aneurysm, the presence of vasospasm, and the patient's health history.

Early preoperative management

The general goals in the preoperative period are to reduce stress on the patient, limit any stimulus or activity that would increase pressure and contribute to rebleeding, and minimize the discomfort caused by the meningeal irritation from the blood in the subarachnoid space. Continued neurologic assessment is necessary to identify signs of developing vasospasm.

Many patients are restless and agitated because of the headache and altered level of consciousness associated with subarachnoid hemorrhage. Restraints should be avoided whenever possible. However, if hands must be restrained to prevent patients from pulling out tubes, mitts are preferable to wrist restraints. Headache control can be difficult. Because headache can contribute to restlessness and the increase in activity associated with restlessness can contribute to rebleeding, sedation with phenobarbital also may be employed.

Early nursing management includes:
• Keep the patient on bed rest.
• Maintain a dark room with minimal stimulation.
• Administer stool softeners to avoid straining.
• Administer analgesics for headache.
• Evaluate the success of the narcotic analgesic, and institute changes in medication if necessary.
• Administer antiemetics to control nausea.
• Monitor the patient's level of consciousness.
• Assess the size and shape of pupils and their reaction to light.
• Check for motor and sensory function and pronator drift.

- Assess the patient's speech pattern, fluency, and comprehension.
- Perform frequent cranial nerve assessments.
- Assess for any increase in nuchal rigidity or photophobia.
- Assess for seizures.
- Assess for signs of increasing ICP.

Hypertensive, hypervolemic, and hemodilution therapy

The standard of care to prevent vasospasm, this therapy incorporates fluid and drug therapy to maintain arterial patency (by inducing hypertension), to maintain perfusion and prevent cerebral ischemia and infarction (by adding more volume), and to reduce the sludging of red blood cells (RBCs) along the interior of vessels (via hemodilution), thereby improving blood flow and decreasing the risk of vasospasm.

In the preoperative period, therapy must be carefully titrated because extremes of hypertension can contribute to rebleeding from the aneurysm. Postoperatively, therapies can be more aggressive because the potential for rebleeding is reduced. In a younger patient with no history of cardiovascular disease, therapy can be managed by monitoring central venous pressure (CVP). For older patients or those with a history of cardiovascular problems, it is important to have a pulmonary artery catheter in place so that the effect of fluid load on the heart may be evaluated.

The most common fluid therapy combination is a crystalloid (such as $D_5W_{1/2}NS$) and 5% albumin, at a rate sufficient to raise the CVP above 10 mm Hg. If a pulmonary artery catheter is being used, the pulmonary capillary wedge pressure should be maintained between 16 and 18 mm Hg. Parameters for systolic blood pressure with this therapy are determined for each patient; they generally are higher than the patient's baseline and usually fall between 150 and 160 mm Hg. Because the hypervolemia also causes hemodilution, careful monitoring of HCT is essential. If the HCT level falls below 30%, packed RBCs often are given.

Nimodipine commonly is administered as an adjunct to hypertensive hypervolemic therapy for vasospasm. The mechanism of action of this calcium channel blocker is specific to the cerebral arteries and is believed to involve dilation of the cerebral microvasculature, promoting cerebral perfusion, and direct protection of the neurons by preventing massive influx of the calcium present in ischemic cell damage.

Administration of nimodipine should begin within 96 hours of the hemorrhage and should last for 21 days. The risk associated with nimodipine is the potential for a drop in blood pressure, which occurs in about 4% of patients treated with this agent. Other adverse reactions include headache, nausea, and bradycardia. To differentiate between the adverse reactions and complications of subarachnoid hemorrhage, the nurse must correlate these findings with any changes in the neurologic examination.

Appropriate nursing interventions include:
• Continually assess for signs of pulmonary congestion or heart failure.
• Titrate fluid therapy according to assessment findings within the ranges set by the physician. Clinical signs of vasospasm with a systolic pressure of 140 mm Hg and a CVP of 10 mm Hg may indicate the need to increase the fluid volume. It is essential to continually correlate the clinical assessment to the ordered parameters to ensure adequate therapy and prevent long-term neurologic complications.
• Monitor the patient's HCT level, and administer packed RBCs, if necessary.
• Administer nimodipine, as ordered; monitor for adverse reactions.

Surgical treatment

Surgical options include direct clipping of the aneurysm (the most desirable approach), wrapping (usually done for fusiform aneurysms with no neck), and endovascular obliteration with coils or balloons (a relatively new technique that is still being explored).

Currently, there are no absolute guidelines for the timing of aneurysm surgery. Proponents of early surgery assert that this approach eliminates the risk of rebleeding. Once the aneurysm has been eliminated from the cerebral circulation, vasospasm can be treated more aggressively. In patients who are considered poor surgical candidates, conservative medical treatment is continued in an attempt to optimize the neurologic grade. If the patient with a poorer grade improves with conservative treatment, surgery may be considered.

Postoperative nursing care includes routine postcraniotomy care and continued therapy for vasospasm (see *Postoperative care of patients undergoing aneurysm surgery,* page 199).

Monitoring for postoperative complications

Arrhythmias are seen in about 2% of the patients with subarachnoid hemorrhage. The most commonly identified rhythm disorders are supraventricular tachycardia, atrial flutter, and premature atrial and ventricular contractions. Unless the patient has underlying heart disease or is symptomatic as a result of the disturbance, antiarrhythmic agents are avoided.

Another complication that can occur after aneurysm surgery is the development of hydrocephalus, often caused by blood blocking the normal reabsorption process in the arachnoid villi. It may require the insertion of a ventriculoperitoneal shunt to facilitate drainage of the ventricular system and relieve the pressure caused by the dilated ventricles.

Because the large urine output is related to a lack of vasopressin, the patient is treated with DDAVP (desmopressin acetate), a synthetic vasopressin that promotes the reabsorption of water. The diabetes insipidus is generally self-limiting, so the patient may require vasopressin replacement only for a short period.

Another potential complication is pulmonary edema, which can occur as a result of the hypervolemic therapy.

Postoperative care of patients undergoing aneurysm surgery

Postoperative care following aneurysm surgery includes basic craniotomy care and measures to prevent vasospasm. Major nursing goals and interventions are listed below.

Goals	Nursing Interventions
Maintain airway patency	• Assess breath sounds. • Assess respiratory rate. • Position patient to maintain adequate airway. • Maintain airway adjuncts as necessary. • Suction patient as needed.
Control pain	• Assess for signs and symptoms of pain. • Administer analgesics, as ordered.
Reduce potential for permanent deficits from vasospasm	• Maintain hypertensive hypervolemia therapy. • Assess frequently for clinical signs of vasospasm. • Monitor fluid volume status carefully.
Maintain serum electrolyte levels within normal limits	• Monitor serum electrolyte levels. • Replace electrolytes as necessary. • Assess for symptoms of electrolyte imbalance.
Encourage improvement in level of consciousness; control increased intracranial pressure (ICP)	• Assess neurologic status frequently. • Report any signs of deterioration that may signify postoperative swelling, hemorrhage, increase in vasospasm, or hydrocephalus. • Prevent activities that are known to increase ICP.
Control hazards of immobility	• Assess for signs of deep vein thrombosis. • Apply elastic stockings, compression boots, or both. • Perform passive or active range of motion to extremities. • Change patient's position at least every 2 hours, maintaining good body alignment.

Careful monitoring of the response to the fluid load will prevent this syndrome. Treatment, if required, is the same as treatment for conventional acute pulmonary edema.

Important nursing interventions include the following:
• Monitor for ECG changes and arrhythmias.
• Assess for hydrocephalus.
• Monitor for signs of pulmonary edema.

• Continually monitor the patient's intake and output and serum and urine electrolyte levels; adjust fluid therapy to maintain desired goals.

Prognosis

Statistics for outcome after aneurysmal subarachnoid hemorrhage vary. The mortality rate from the initial hemorrhage ranges from 20% to 60%. For patients who survive the initial bleeding, the rebleeding rate is about 35% to 40% in the first 7 to 10 days. Mortality with rebleeding ranges from 40% to 60%.

For patients who are good surgical candidates, the outcome is better. Mortality and morbidity rates in some centers are as low as 10% for patients who are in good preoperative condition. This outcome worsens when the patient's presenting condition is graded at a 3 or higher on the Hunt and Hess Scale.

Discharge planning

As soon as the medical diagnosis and prognosis have been established, discharge plans can be modified and refined. A key component in aneurysmal subarachnoid hemorrhage is the continual assessment of patient needs. The goal is to return patients to the home environment at their previous level of function.

The need for rehabilitative services following hospitalization varies and often changes throughout the acute hospitalization. Inpatient rehabilitation should include physical therapy, occupational therapy, and cognitive retraining as necessary. Patients should be mobilized in the acute care setting as soon as their postoperative condition stabilizes, and their level of activity should be gradually increased as tolerance improves.

Cerebrovascular accident (CVA)

An infarction of brain tissue that ultimately leads to altered cognitive, sensory, motor, or emotional function, CVA is caused by partial or complete occlusion of a major cerebral vessel or a hemorrhage within the brain. This interruption of blood flow robs the vital brain tissue of needed oxygen and other nutrients, leading to long-term and often irreparable cerebral damage.

The causes of CVA can be divided into two broad categories: ischemic and hemorrhagic. Ischemic CVAs can be caused by either thrombosis or embolism, whereas hemorrhagic CVAs can be caused by bleeding anywhere within the cerebral circulation (see *Cerebral circulation,* page 202).

The third-leading cause of death in the United States, CVA continues to be a major ongoing health concern despite a decline in incidence over the past 20 years due to a reduction in smoking and better control of hypertension and diabetes in some populations. CVA afflicts both sexes equally but carries a higher mortality rate among African-Americans than Caucasians in the United States. Approximately 60% to 75% of all episodes occur in persons over age 65; the incidence increases dramatically in those over age 75. Two thirds of those who survive a CVA will be left with significant neurologic deficits.

Pathophysiology

Ischemic CVAs typically result from thromboses or embolisms (see *Predisposing factors for CVA,* page 203). With thrombosis, the most common cause of CVA, ischemia results when a blood vessel becomes occluded from atherosclerosis. Such a thrombosis may occur anywhere above the common carotid bifurcation or at the start of the branches from the aorta, innominate, and subclavian arteries.

With an embolism, the second-leading cause of CVA, ischemia results when atherosclerotic plaque, fat, bacteria, or other tissue breaks away from the heart's layer, enters the circulation, and lodges within a cerebral vessel, causing cellular necrosis and death of the tissue fed by the vessel. Most cerebral emboli originate from the endocardial layer of the heart. The embolism typically travels until it reaches a vessel too narrow to

Cerebral circulation

Cerebral circulation is maintained by a series of arteries that form the circle of Willis. From the aortic arch, two vertebral arteries meet to form the basilar artery, which feeds the posterior cerebral cortex. The common carotid arteries further subdivide into the internal carotid arteries to supply the anterior and middle brain with blood flow. This illustration provides a superior view of the major arteries involved.

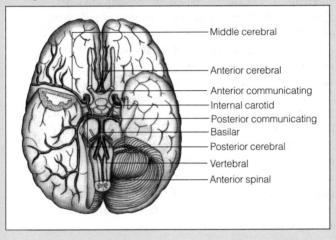

Middle cerebral

Anterior cerebral

Anterior communicating

Internal carotid

Posterior communicating

Basilar

Posterior cerebral

Vertebral

Anterior spinal

pass through. If the embolism is minute, the patient may experience a transient ischemic attack (TIA). Typically viewed as precursors to CVAs, TIAs are believed to be caused by microemboli that become lodged proximal to the ischemic site (see *Transient ischemic attacks,* page 204).

Underlying cardiac diseases contributing to the development of cerebral emboli include chronic atrial fibrillation, myocardial infarction, valvular disease, valve replacement, rheumatic heart disease, and infective bacterial endocarditis. Unlike thrombosis formation, which may take decades to form, cerebral embolism can affect any age group, with an increased incidence after age 40.

A hemorrhagic CVA occurs when a cerebral blood vessel ruptures, resulting in bleeding into the brain tis-

Predisposing factors for CVA

The following chart provides major predisposing factors for each of the different types of CVA.

Predisposing Factors	Thrombotic CVA	Embolic CVA	Hemorrhagic CVA
Age	Over 75	Over 40	Over 50
Sex	Male	Male	Female
Activity	May occur during or after sleep	Sudden onset; no relation to activity	Anytime during activity; one third occur during sleep
Major risk factors	• Diabetes mellitus • Atherosclerosis • Obesity	• Cardiac disease • Oral contraceptives • Smoking	• Hypertension • Emotional stress

sue. This type of CVA can occur spontaneously in those with hypertension or atherosclerosis of intracranial blood vessels because of the ensuing vessel changes. Blood leaking through a ruptured vessel forms a mass that displaces the surrounding brain tissue. If the lesion is extremely large, the brain may herniate, causing coma and eventual death. The mortality rate for this type of CVA is between 50% and 60%.

Clinical assessment

The presence and severity of symptoms in a patient with CVA depend on the location of brain involvement, typically the sensory-motor and speech centers in the brain, and on the amount of residual brain damage from tissue ischemia and edema. A timely, accurate assessment is necessary to establish a baseline of the patient's current status in the event of further deterioration of cerebral function.

Transient ischemic attacks

Often a precursor to CVAs, transient ischemic attacks pose additional challenges to the critical care nurse.

Causes	Signs and Symptoms	Treatment
• Atherosclerosis of extracerebral or cerebral arteries • Fibromuscular disease • Dissecting aneurysm of extracerebral vessels • Transient hypotension • Valvular stenosis or prosthetic vegetation • Atrial fibrillation • Right-left cardiac septal shunt • Intracardiac tumors • Abnormal coagulopathies: anemia, polycythemia, thrombocytosis	• Aphasia • Monocular blindness • Hemimotor deficit • Hemisensory deficit • Vertigo • Drop attacks • Bilateral visual loss or diplopia • Hemilateral or bilateral motor and sensory deficits	• Determine underlying cause and implement treatments to control cardiac arrhythmias and hypertension. • Administer anticoagulants with heparin until partial thromboplastin time is $1\frac{1}{2}$ to 2 times normal. • Maintain anticoagulation with aspirin or ticlopidine.

History
Because the patient with CVA may be unable to verbally communicate, the nurse should seek out and document the following information from the patient's family:
• time of occurrence
• precipitating factors, such as obesity, congenital anomalies, family history of CVA
• preexisting medical conditions
• smoking history
• use of medications and noncompliance with antihypertensive or anticoagulant regimens.

Physical findings
Because the associated signs and symptoms for thrombotic, embolic, and hemorrhagic CVAs are similar, it is important to differentiate the cause as quickly as possible. General signs and symptoms include:
• vomiting

• seizures
• fever (seen in hemorrhagic stroke as a signal of increasing intracranial pressure [ICP] and increasing pressure on the hypothalamus)
• ECG abnormalities (prolonged ST segment, indicating delayed ventricular recovery)
• cardiac arrhythmias (premature atrial contractions, atrial fibrillation, and atrial flutter seen as a cause of embolic CVA resulting in "showering" of emboli; ventricular arrhythmias seen with thrombotic or hemorrhagic CVA as a result of hypoxia)
• confusion and disorientation (see *Tracking level of consciousness using the Glasgow Coma Scale,* page 206)
• no loss of consciousness (with thrombotic or embolic CVA) to complete loss of consciousness (with hemorrhagic CVA)
• lethargy, apathy, or combativeness
• memory deficits
• loss of cough reflex, labored or irregular respirations, tachypnea, rhonchi, stertorous respirations or apneic periods
• hypertension (with thrombotic or hemorrhagic CVA)
• hemiplegia, spastic paralysis, and associated loss of protective reflex functioning of the affected side
• loss of gag reflex, bowel incontinence, decreased or absent bowel sounds
• urinary incontinence.
    Signs and symptoms commonly seen in CVAs caused by a thrombotic event usually follow the pattern of a "stroke in evolution" occurring over a period of several hours. Common findings include:
• progressive deterioration of motor and sensory functioning
• concurrent deterioration of speech functioning
• lethargy (not typically associated with a loss of consciousness).
    Patients with embolic CVAs may present with:
• sudden onset of motor and sensory deficits and speech pattern disturbance

Tracking level of consciousness using the Glasgow Coma Scale

Originally designed to help predict a patient's survival and recovery after a head injury, the Glasgow Coma Scale assesses level of consciousness (LOC). It minimizes the use of subjective impressions to evaluate LOC by testing and scoring three observations: eye response, motor response, and response to verbal stimuli.

Each response receives a point value. If the patient is alert, can follow simple commands, and is completely oriented to person, place, and time, the score will total 15 points. If the patient is comatose, the score will total 7 or less. A score of 3, the lowest possible score, indicates deep coma and a poor prognosis.

Many hospitals display the Glasgow Coma Scale on neurologic flowsheets to show changes in the patient's LOC over time.

Observation	Response Elicited	Score
Eye response	• Opens spontaneously	4
	• Opens to verbal commands	3
	• Opens to pain	2
	• No response	1
Motor response	• Reacts to verbal command	6
	• Reacts to painful stimuli:	5
	—Identifies localized pain	4
	—Flexes and withdraws	3
	• Assumes flexor posture	2
	• No response	1
Verbal response	• Is oriented and converses	5
	• Is disoriented but converses	4
	• Uses inappropriate words	3
	• Makes incomprehensible sounds	2
	• No response	1

• headache (may develop on the side in which the embolism is lodged)
• no associated loss of consciousness.

Patients with CVAs resulting from hemorrhage typically present with:
• severe headache at onset
• rapid onset of complete hemiplegia
• gradual loss of consciousness leading to coma
• nuchal rigidity.

The amount of brain damage from the CVA can be estimated by determining the side of the brain involved. Patients experiencing left-sided brain involvement typically exhibit:

• paralysis on right side
• speech and language deficits if left-brain dominant
• slow, cautious behavior
• language deficits
• astereognosis, autopagnosia, finger agnosia, and right-left disorientation
• distress and depression regarding disability.

Patients experiencing a right-sided CVA typically exhibit:

• paralysis on left side
• spatial-perceptual deficits leading to apraxia
• distractibility, impulsiveness
• performance deficits
• indifference or denial regarding disability.

Many of the neurologic deficits associated with CVA depend on the specific artery affected (see *Correlating neurologic deficits with location of CVA,* pages 208 and 209). A common residual effect is altered speech or language perception in the form of aphasia.

Diagnosis

The long-term prognosis for the patient with CVA depends on early identification of the cause and subsequent medical and nursing interventions. Because thrombotic, embolic, and hemorrhagic CVAs cannot be differentiated purely from the signs and symptoms, it is important to support the patient through the diagnostic tests as quickly and safely as possible (see *Confirming CVA,* page 210, for the most commonly ordered tests).

Additional diagnostic tests may include brain scan, electroencephalogram, skull X-rays, positron emission tomography scan, and digital subtraction angiography. Noninvasive studies used to evaluate blood flow include transcranial Doppler and oculopneumoplethysomography. A transesophageal echocardiogram may be used to define an embolic focus.

Correlating neurologic deficits with location of CVA

The neurologic deficits associated with CVA depend on the artery affected.

Type of Neurologic Deficit	Anterior Cerebral Artery	Middle Cerebral Artery
Sensory	Contralateral sensory alterations	Contralateral sensory alterations
Motor	Contralateral hemiparesis; more weakness in leg than arm; foot drop; gait disturbance; apraxia (unaffected side)	Hemiplegia
Visual and hearing	Eye deviation toward affected side	Homonymous hemianopia
Speech	Expressive aphasia	Dyslexia; aphasia
Cognitive	Confusion; flat affect; amnesia	None

Treatment and care

During the diagnostic testing phase, the patient's cardiovascular, respiratory, and neurologic status should be monitored continuously for developing or continuing cardiac arrhythmias, changes in respiratory pattern, and alterations in level of consciousness. Once the cardiac, respiratory, and neurologic systems have been stabilized, treatment goals are aimed at beginning the rehabilitative process.

Maximizing cerebral perfusion

Depending on the site of the lesion, the patient may be prepared for surgery and placement of an intracranial monitoring device. Antiembolitic therapy usually is not indicated; however, therapies aimed at reducing cerebral edema, stabilizing blood pressure, and controlling seizures usually are prescribed.

Posterior Cerebral Artery	Internal Carotid	Vertebral-Basilar Arterial System
Sporadic sensory loss	Contralateral sensory alterations; asymmetry	Tongue numbness
Contralateral hemiparesis; tremor	Contralateral hemiplegia; facial asymmetry	Ataxic gait; uncoordinated motor actions
Nystagmus; loss of depth perception; visual hallucinations	Hemianopia; Horner's syndrome	Double vision; nystagmus; tinnitus; hearing loss
Dyslexia	Dysphagia	Dysarthria
Memory loss	None	Memory loss; disorientation

Nursing interventions may include:
• Perform hourly neurologic checks; report evidence of deteriorating status.
• Administer corticosteroids, anticonvulsants, or both, as prescribed.
• Monitor vital signs, including blood pressure, every hour; administer antihypertensives as ordered.
• Administer anticoagulant therapy as prescribed; monitor partial thromboplastin time to achieve therapeutic level ($1\frac{1}{2}$ to 2 times normal).
• Maintain the head of the bed at the prescribed angle (typically 30 degrees).
• Following surgery, monitor for signs of intracranial bleeding.

Improving cardiopulmonary function
A patient who has experienced a CVA requires continuous monitoring of the cardiovascular and respiratory

DIAGNOSTIC TESTS

Confirming cerebrovascular accident (CVA)

This chart reviews select diagnostic tests useful in the diagnosis of CVA.

Test	Purpose	Findings for Thrombotic or Embolic CVA	Findings for Hemorrhagic CVA
Magnetic resonance imaging (MRI)	More sensitive than CT scan and viewed as the leading diagnostic tool for CVA. MRI visualizes location and extent of affected area and differentiates between a thrombosis, embolism, or hemorrhage.	• Accurately pinpoints site • Shows ventricular shift	• Affected site appears denser • Shows ventricular shift
Computed tomography (CT scan)	Used to rule out lesions during the admission of patient with a change in level of consciousness. CT scans can be normal up to 72 hours after infarction. Findings include increased density in areas of hemorrhage and decreased density in areas of infarction and ischemia.	• Accurately pinpoints site • Shows ventricular shift • Affected site appears less dense • May be normal up to 72 hours after infarction	• Determines exact location of bleeding • Affected site appears denser
Cerebrospinal fluid (CSF) analysis	Performed primarily to confirm subarachnoid hemorrhage. Fluid is evaluated for increased leukocytes or presence of blood, which may indicate a brain hemorrhage.	• Shows clear obstruction or narrowing	• Shows bloody vascular area surrounded by displaced veins and arteries
Cerebral angiography	Visualizes areas of cervical and cerebral vessel atherosclerosis, cerebrovascular malformation, and aneurysms. Accurately pinpoints location.	• Arterial obstruction or narrowing of circle of Willis	• Affected site appears as a vascular zone surrounded by stretched, displaced arteries and veins

systems. Medical therapies may include the use of anti-arrhythmics, diuretics, and tube feedings.

Key interventions include the following:
• Monitor intake and output; restrict fluids as ordered.
• Monitor heart and breath sounds every hour.
• Provide continuous cardiac monitoring; report changes in rhythm, rate, and ectopy; administer antiarrhythmics as ordered.
• Administer oxygen, as ordered.
• Provide nasotracheal suctioning as necessary.
• Administer osmotic diuretics (mannitol) as prescribed.
• Maintain head of the bed at a 30-degree angle.
• Aspirate gastric contents before the next scheduled tube feeding; withhold tube feeding for residual gastric contents as ordered.
• Monitor for signs of aspiration.

Rehabilitation therapies

Therapy is geared toward preventing further motor and sensory deterioration and restoring normal function. Besides the physician and nurse, the rehabilitative therapy team should include a physical therapist, speech therapist, occupational therapist, ophthalmologist, and social service worker.

Appropriate nursing interventions are listed below:
• Assess the patient's level of paresis.
• Consult a physical therapist for ways to progressively increase the patient's activity. Perform passive range-of-motion exercises every 2 hours, and apply a foot board to the foot of the bed to prevent foot drop. Support flaccid extremities by applying splints.
• Assess the patient's ability to speak and communicate.
• Consult a speech therapist to assist in determining the best method for communicating with the patient. Provide assistive devices, such as calendars and picture charts. A speech therapist also can evaluate the patient's ability to swallow via video fluoroscopy.
• Assess the patient's visual fields. Provide eye shields, if necessary.

• Assess for depression, which is common following a CVA and should be expected. Periods of euphoria followed by episodes of extreme depression do not have a purely psychological basis but rather correlate with the cerebral hemisphere injured by the CVA.

Prognosis

The long-term prognosis for CVA depends on the severity of cerebral damage and the speed with which medical treatment was implemented. For embolic CVA, the chance for recurrence decreases if the cause has been pinpointed and treatment started. In many cases, the patient must agree to lifestyle changes—involving diet, control of hypertension or diabetes, medication usage, exercise, and smoking—that can help reduce the chance for recurrence. For hemorrhagic CVA, the prognosis usually improves if the patient seeks medical attention while conscious. Unconscious or comatose patients have a smaller chance of survival and subsequent rehabilitation.

Discharge planning

Discharge planning should begin once the cause has been determined. Because the patient will have some residual effects from cerebral damage, a social service worker should help the family to determine the patient's likelihood of returning home after discharge. If the acute care therapy has not been sufficient for the patient to reach an optimal level of physical functioning, plans must be made for transfer to a rehabilitation facility. If the patient is returning home, the environment should be assessed for the number of stairs to climb and the location of bathroom and kitchen facilities; the patient's ability to provide self-care, including meal preparation, also should be evaluated.

Prior to discharge, the patient and family must comprehend and be willing to follow instructions regarding:
• diet and nutrition
• lifestyle changes
• medications (name, dosage, frequency, purpose)

• physical activity (limb exercises, limitations, use of assistive devices)
• home care visits (frequency, specific therapies).

Congestive heart failure (CHF)

The inability of the heart to pump an adequate amount of blood to meet the body's metabolic needs, heart failure can manifest as inadequate cardiac output to support vital organs or as pulmonary congestion (left-sided heart failure) or systemic venous congestion (right-sided heart failure). Because pump failure frequently results in vascular congestion, this condition is commonly called CHF.

CHF is the presenting symptom for most cardiac diseases, including myocardial infarction (MI), valvular heart disease, cardiomyopathy, congenital defects, hypertension, and inflammatory diseases of the heart. It also can be a symptom of myriad noncardiac diseases, including hypothyroidism, renal disease, and malnutrition.

CHF may be acute or chronic. Most patients experience a chronic form of the disorder associated with renal retention of sodium and water and cope through compensatory mechanisms; however, the acute form of CHF is more serious because pulmonary congestion may lead to pulmonary edema, a life-threatening emergency. Over 400,000 new cases of CHF are diagnosed in the United States each year, and the incidence is rising, partly due to the expanding elderly population and improved survival rate among those with underlying cardiac disease.

Pathophysiology

CHF denotes impaired ventricular function (systolic dysfunction, diastolic dysfunction, or both) and may be classified as isolated right ventricular failure, left ventricular failure, or biventricular failure.

Systolic dysfunction is an abnormality that results from impaired contractibility of the ventricular muscle or pressure overload to the muscle. Contractile impairment may be acute or insidious in nature, such as acute heart failure resulting from an MI or chronic heart failure secondary to cardiomyopathy. Regardless of the cause of the contractile dysfunction, decreased stroke volume and symptoms of impaired cardiac output result. Incomplete ventricular emptying ultimately follows, which impedes diastolic function.

Isolated diastolic dysfunction occurs in approximately one third of patients with heart failure and is demonstrated by impaired early diastolic relaxation, increased ventricular wall stiffness, or both. Diastolic relaxation is a dynamic, energy-requiring process that can be actively impaired (as in myocardial ischemia) or passively impaired (as in ventricular hypertrophy). The net effect of diastolic dysfunction is greater-than-normal ventricular diastolic pressure increases at any given volume of blood, ultimately producing signs of vascular congestion due to ventricular overdistention and backward congestion.

Left ventricular failure
In the early stages of heart failure, patients often present with isolated left ventricular failure. The right ventricle contracts vigorously, delivering normal amounts of blood to the pulmonary circulation; however, the left ventricle cannot deliver this volume to the systemic circulation due to systolic dysfunction. This results in:
• backup of blood into the pulmonary system with resultant pulmonary congestion (backward failure)
• decreased cardiac output to the systemic circulation with resultant hypoperfusion of the vital organs (forward failure).

Common causes of left ventricular failure include left ventricular infarction or ischemia, aortic stenosis or insufficiency, mitral stenosis or insufficiency, and cardiomyopathy. When diastolic dysfunction is present, the pulmonary congestive symptoms are intensified.

Right ventricular failure

Right ventricular failure is systolic or diastolic dysfunction of the right side of the heart resulting from either increased resistance to pulmonary forward blood flow or primary impairment of the ventricular muscle. The result of the higher pulmonary resistance to blood flow is amplified pulmonary vascular resistance, which increases the afterload that the right ventricle must pump against and increases the strain on the right side of the heart.

Common causes of right ventricular failure include:
• uncontrolled left ventricular failure, which causes the right ventricle to ultimately fail in response to the tremendous pulmonary pressure created by the backward failure of the impaired left ventricle
• right ventricular MI, which results in both systolic and diastolic dysfunction of the right side of the heart
• cor pulmonale, which is isolated right ventricular failure that occurs with severely increased pulmonary pressure in the absence of left-sided heart failure, commonly as a result of chronic obstructive pulmonary disease.

The physiologic consequences of right ventricular failure include decreased delivery of blood to the pulmonary bed and therefore the left ventricle (forward failure) and systemic venous congestion, especially into the portal system and lower extremities (backward failure).

Compensatory mechanisms

Several compensatory mechanisms, including the Frank-Starling mechanism, ventricular hypertrophy, and neurohormonal activation, are called into play to maintain systemic blood pressure in CHF. All of these mechanisms aim to maintain homeostasis; however, each has its limits and may ultimately fail and lead to worsening CHF.

The Frank-Starling mechanism involves cardiac output and diastolic stretching of ventricular muscle fibers (see *The Frank-Starling mechanism in heart failure,* page 216).

The Frank-Starling mechanism in heart failure

According to Frank-Starling's law, cardiac output increases with increased diastolic stretch on the ventricular muscle, within reasonable limits. When increased amounts of blood are delivered to the ventricle, the actin and myosin filaments achieve a greater degree of interdigitation (connection). This stretched muscle subsequently contracts with greater vigor, similar to how a rubber band contracts when stretched further and further. Because the stretched cardiac muscle is capable of contracting with greater force, the degree of arterial pressure (afterload) that the heart must pump against has minimal effect on the cardiac output, again within reasonable limits. Therefore, the most critical element in determining the cardiac output is the amount of blood delivered to the heart (preload), which creates the stretch of the muscle fibers.

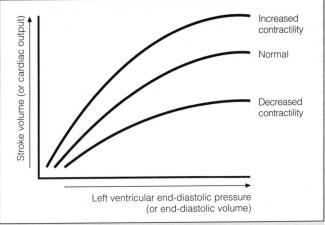

In CHF, blood flow to the myocardium is insufficient, contractility declines, and stroke volume and cardiac output fall, as illustrated.

Note that, on the normal curve, the stroke volume is increased with increasing amounts of preload. However, in states of increased contractility, the stroke volume is augmented above normal at any given measure of preload. Conversely, decreased contractility is characterized by a lower, flatter curve. This demonstrates that:
• stroke volume is reduced at the same preload in patients with heart failure as in normal individuals

• in early, compensated heart failure, the reduced stroke volume results in decreased systolic emptying of the ventricle, thus resulting in accumulation of more blood in the ventricle for diastole; the ultimate increase in end-diastolic volume is equated to an increase in preload, which induces a greater stroke volume on the subsequent contraction
• in late, uncompensated heart failure, excess amounts of preload serve only to increase the end-diastolic pressure without a concomitant increase in stroke volume (as noted on the flat portion of the curve).

Ventricular hypertrophy is caused by increased ventricular wall stress, a consequence of chronically elevated afterload or left ventricular dilatation, and results in increased muscle fiber mass, increased ventricular wall thickness, or both. The increased muscle fiber mass maintains ventricular contractility, and the increased wall thickness helps reduce stress on the ventricular wall. However, the end-diastolic pressure is subsequently elevated, which can worsen congestive symptoms. Additionally, the increased muscle fiber mass can cause compression of the coronary arteries and capillaries, resulting in angina.

Three neurohormonal systems—the sympathetic nervous system, the renin-angiotensin-aldosterone system, and antidiuretic hormone—are activated to ultimately increase cardiac output in the face of heart failure.

• The sympathetic nervous system directly increases cardiac output via the mechanisms of tachycardia, augmented contractility, and venous constriction (which generates greater preload). Systemic blood pressure is maintained by increased arterial constriction. Even though these mechanisms are compensatory early on, they may ultimately expend what little reserve a failing heart has and worsen the CHF.

• The renin-angiotensin-aldosterone system is activated when renin is released by the kidneys in response to reduced renal artery perfusion pressure caused by low cardiac output or to direct stimulation by the adrenergic nervous system. Renin stimulates the conversion of angiotensinogen into angiotensin I, which is converted into angiotensin II in the presence of angiotensin-converting enzyme (ACE). The end result is profound vasoconstriction and the release of aldosterone, both of which increase the blood pressure. Arterial baroreceptors and angiotensin II stimulate the posterior pituitary to secrete increased amounts of antidiuretic hormone. The water retention produced increases the circulating blood volume and provides more preload for the Frank-Starling mechanism.

• Unlike the case in the other mechanisms, atrial natriuretic peptide is secreted by the atria in response to increased intracardiac pressure. It causes sodium and water secretion, vasodilation, and inhibition of the renin-angiotensin-aldosterone system. However, its effects are often diminished by end-organ unresponsiveness and overpowering of the other mechanisms, and therefore it is not a primary compensatory mechanism in CHF.

Clinical assessment

CHF is a syndrome that produces signs and symptoms involving many organ systems and can occur secondary to numerous cardiac diseases.

History

A thorough patient history can help identify the etiology of heart failure. A history of chronic, progressive symptoms may indicate valvular heart disease, cardiomyopathy, or ischemic cardiac disease with dyspnea and fatigue as an anginal equivalent (a symptom that occurs with myocardial ischemia instead of typical anginal pain). The acute onset of severe dyspnea may indicate rupture of the chordae tendineae with mitral insufficiency or acute MI. Information should be elicited regarding:
• duration of symptoms
• presence of orthopnea, and how many pillows the patient sleeps on
• medications and regimen
• weight changes
• precipitating factors
• preexisting medical conditions
• recent change in diet or salt intake
• activity level and tolerance.

Knowing the patient's activity level and tolerance, as well as any accompanying symptoms, is necessary for categorizing the patient's symptoms according to the New York Heart Association classification of heart failure, a standard upon which many therapies are insti-

Heart failure classification system

Patients with heart failure often are categorized into functional classes based on activity level and presenting symptoms. The most commonly used system is the New York Heart Association classification, which is shown below. This classification system is used to identify the severity of the heart failure, evaluate the patient's response to treatment, compare patients in research studies, and provide a severity-of-illness scale for transplant lists.

Classification	Description
Class I	• No limitation of physical activity
Class II	• Slight limitation of activity • Dyspnea and fatigue with moderate physical activity (such as quickly walking up stairs)
Class III	• Marked limitation of activity • Dyspnea with minimal activity (such as slowly walking up stairs)
Class IV	• Severe limitation of activity • Symptoms present even at rest

tuted (see *Heart failure classification system,* page 219).

Physical findings

Physical findings of heart failure can be separated according to right ventricular failure and left ventricular failure (see *Clinical manifestations of CHF,* page 220).

Diagnosis

The diagnosis of right-sided versus left-sided heart failure is largely based on clinical findings. Determining the etiology of the failure, however, is imperative to provide appropriate treatment and usually requires more sophisticated tests. Likewise, differentiation of systolic versus diastolic dysfunction is difficult to make clinically and requires diagnostic procedures. (See *Diagnosing heart failure,* pages 221 and 222, for a description of the various tests used.)

Clinical manifestations of CHF

Signs and symptoms and physical findings often manifest according to the specific ventricle involved. Note that findings are more common with left ventricular failure.

Type of Failure	Signs and Symptoms	Physical Findings
Left ventricular failure	Dyspnea, paroxysmal nocturnal dyspnea, orthopnea, irritating cough, blood-tinged sputum, decreased daytime urine output (output may increase at night because peripheral tissue edema is reabsorbed into circulation with patient in supine position, thus increasing preload and ultimately renal blood flow)	Pulmonary edema, S_3 gallop, possibly loud P_2, possibly S_4, atrial fibrillation, tachycardia, pulmonary rales or wheezes, decreased cardiac output, hypotension
Right ventricular failure	Anorexia, weight gain from fluid retention, abdominal discomfort (especially right upper quadrant)	Jugular venous distention, hepatomegaly, peripheral edema

Treatment and care

Management of the patient with heart failure is directed toward optimizing cardiac output, managing fluid status, and preventing recurrence of acute episodes.

Pharmacologic therapy

Medications used to treat patients with systolic left ventricular failure include diuretics, inotropic agents, and vasodilators (see *Drugs used to manage CHF,* pages 223 and 224). Such patients generally require several medications to achieve the physiological goals of afterload reduction, preload reduction, and contractility enhancement.

Occasionally, patients with chronic CHF are electively admitted to the critical care unit for pulmonary artery catheter placement and trials of various medication regimens to individualize their therapy. Periodically these patients may be placed on intermittent, scheduled home intravenous dobutamine therapy based

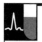

DIAGNOSTIC TESTS
Diagnosing heart failure

The diagnosis of congestive heart failure (CHF) is based on patient history and clinical findings combined with various diagnostic tests.

Chest X-ray
One of the most readily available and easily interpreted diagnostic tools for patients with CHF. X-ray findings of CHF result primarily from redistribution of pulmonary fluid. Resolution of acute CHF symptoms may precede chest X-ray resolution of abnormal findings. Typical findings in CHF include:
• Redistribution of pulmonary vasculature toward the upper lung zones from elevated hydrostatic forces
• Transudation of fluid out of the pulmonary vasculature and into the tissues
• Presence of Kerley B lines, which are short, thin transverse lines identified near the lung bases laterally at the costophrenic angle representing edematous interlobular septa
• Large cardiac silhouette secondary to left ventricular hypertrophy and left atrial distension
• Intra-alveolar pulmonary edema, identified as patchy, ill-defined, coalescent densities with air bronchograms
• Pleural effusion (may be a nonspecific finding associated with heart failure).

Pulmonary artery (PA) catheterization
The PA catheter is a useful guide for determining the severity of heart failure as well as the effectiveness of therapeutic measures. Patients with CHF generally present with the following hemodynamic alterations:
• Left ventricular failure and biventricular failure

—increased pulmonary artery systolic (PAS) pressure
—increased pulmonary artery diastolic (PAD) pressure
—increased pulmonary artery wedge (PAW) pressure
—decreased cardiac output (CO)
—increased systemic vascular resistance (SVR)
• Isolated right ventricular failure
—increased PAS
—increased PAD
—normal PAW
—decreased CO
—increased pulmonary vascular resistance (PVR)
—increased right atrial pressure (RAP)

Electrocardiography (ECG)
The ECG is useful in determining right-sided versus left-sided failure. Right or left axis deviation may be present, indicating right or left ventricular hypertrophy.

Echocardiography
A safe, noninvasive, readily available, and relatively inexpensive method of cardiac imaging that can yield sensitive information, echocardiography provides information on the cardiac chamber size, valvular structures and integrity, cardiac function (including ejection fraction, blood flow direction, turbulence, and velocity), and estimation of pressure gradients within the heart and great vessels. Chamber size is further delineated according to shape:
• Eccentric hypertrophy, an increase in the ventricular radius, results from a synthesis of new

(continued)

Diagnosing heart failure *(continued)*

sarcomeres in series with the old caused by chronic chamber dilatation from volume overload.
• Concentric hypertrophy, an increase in wall thickness without chamber dilatation, occurs from new sarcomere synthesis parallel to the old and is a consequence of chronic pressure overload.

Echocardiography also is useful in diagnosing pericardial effusion and the presence of thrombus in the atrium, often present in heart failure patients with atrial fibrillation.

on their individual response to therapy. More frequently, they are switched to oral medications. Patients who are controlled on oral medications most need diligent education because much of their home care is unsupervised by medical personnel.

Only the ACE inhibitors have been proven to improve survival in patients with mild, moderate, and severe CHF. Antiarrhythmic agents may be used if the patient has sustained or symptomatic arrhythmias. Anticoagulation, primarily warfarin, is used in patients with markedly reduced left ventricular function or chronic atrial fibrillation to prevent thrombus formation. Daily aspirin may also be used for patients who do not tolerate warfarin.

Specific nursing measures are listed below:
• Administer vasodilators, as ordered.
• Assist with insertion of an intra-aortic balloon pump.
• Monitor hemodynamic parameters (afterload reduction is evident in decreased systemic vascular resistance; preload reduction is evident in decreased pulmonary artery diastolic pressure and pulmonary capillary wedge pressure; improved contractility is evident with increased cardiac output and improved end-organ perfusion).
• Monitor blood pressure for excessive decreases and orthostatic hypotension in patients receiving afterload reduction agents.
• Administer diuretics, as ordered.
• Administer morphine, as ordered (causes transient arterial and venous dilatation).

MAJOR DRUGS

Drugs used to manage CHF

The following drugs commonly are used, often in combination, to manage CHF.

Drug	Action	Adverse Reactions
Vasodilators: angiotensin-converting enzyme inhibitors • captopril • enalapril • lisinopril • ramipril • benazepril • fosinopril • quinapril	• Provide arterial and venous dilatation • Prevent conversion of angiotensin I into angiotensin II, preventing hemodynamic sequelae of the renin-angiotensin-aldosterone system, such as the vasoconstrictive properties of angiotensin II • Prevent stimulation of aldosterone secretion from the adrenal cortex, decreasing renal sodium reabsorption • Provide potent afterload reduction • Decrease remodeling (dilatation, hypertrophy, and infarct expansion) after acute myocardial infarction • Increase cardiac output by afterload reduction • Improve left ventricular ejection fraction • May slow rate of intimal hyperplasia, reducing atherogenesis	• Elevated serum creatinine and blood urea nitrogen levels • Nephrotic syndrome with increased urinary protein • Hyperkalemia • Dry cough • Neutropenia
Vasodilators: venous vasodilators • nitrates • nitroprusside • morphine	• Increase venous capacitance, resulting in decreased preload • Decrease venous return to the heart (preload) • Decrease left ventricular end-diastolic pressure • Reduce pulmonary congestion	• May result in undesired drop in stroke volume, cardiac output, and blood pressure in severely compromised patients • Must be used with extreme caution in patients with severe aortic stenosis or hypertrophic cardiomyopathy
Vasodilators: arterial vasodilators • hydralazine	• Decrease systemic vascular resistance afterload • Increased ventricular muscle fiber shortening dur-	• Hypotension • Orthostatic hypotension *(continued)*

Drugs used to manage CHF *(continued)*

Drug	Action	Adverse Reactions
Vasodilators: arterial vasodilators *(continued)* • clonidine • minoxidil	ing systole • Augment stroke volume and cardiac output	• These drugs are dangerous in diastolic failure because they cause a drop in systemic vascular resistance
Diuretics • furosemide • bumetanide • ethacrynic acid	• Reduce intravascular volume and preload by promoting elimination of sodium and water • Decrease ventricular diastolic pressure • Treat and prevent pulmonary edema • Act on loop of Henle to produce potent diuresis	• Overdiuresis, producing decreased cardiac output • Hyponatremia • Hypokalemia • Hypomagnesemia
Inotropic agents • digitalis • dobutamine • dopamine • phosphodiesterase inhibitors (amrinone)	• Increase availability of intracellular calcium, increasing the force of ventricular contraction • Shift the Frank-Starling curve in an upward direction, increasing contractility • Increase stroke volume and cardiac output • Reduce cardiac enlargement (digitalis) • Reduce heart rate (digitalis)	• Tachycardia • Increased renal blood flow at low doses, increasing urine output • Decreased renal blood flow at high doses, decreasing urine output • Peripheral vasoconstriction • Hypertension

• Administer positive inotropic agents, as ordered.

Fluid management

Symptoms related to excess fluid volume cause the most discomfort for CHF patients. Typical symptoms include orthopnea, paroxysmal nocturnal dyspnea, hemoptysis, positional cough, and dependent edema. Management of fluid volume excess is primarily accomplished with diuretics. Vigilant follow-up of patients receiving diuretics is imperative to monitor the effectiveness of therapy, prevent excess diuresis with consequent dehydration, and prevent electrolyte disturbances, which may precipitate lethal arrhythmias.

Specific nursing measures include the following:
- Weigh the patient daily.
- Record intake and output.
- Assess pulmonary status.
- Administer oxygen as needed for dyspnea or hypoxemia.
- Monitor hemodynamic parameters for evidence of decreased preload.
- Assess skin turgor and mucous membranes.
- Assess blood urea nitrogen levels (elevation is an early sign of dehydration).
- Monitor for orthostatic blood pressure drops.
- Monitor serum electrolyte levels for signs and symptoms of hypokalemia, hypomagnesemia, or hyponatremia.

Prevention of recurrent acute episodes

After the patient is stabilized and at optimal functioning, the patient and health care team must take appropriate measures to prevent recurrences. This is best achieved through vigilant medical follow-up, meticulous education, and frequent communication between the patient and the health providers. Specific areas that should be reinforced include monitoring for adverse reactions to drug therapy, monitoring for fluctuations in fluid volume status, maintaining good nutrition, and participating in a cardiac rehabilitation program.

Specific nursing measures to accomplish these goals include the following:
- Monitor all laboratory levels, including electrolytes, carefully.
- Instruct the patient about the actions, doses, and adverse reactions to all medications.
- Instruct the patient to monitor daily weight at home and to report any increase over 2 pounds within 1 week to the physician.
- Provide a sodium-restricted diet, and instruct the patient about hidden sources of salt.

• Advise the patient to report any increase in peripheral edema or alteration in normal respiratory status.

• Instruct the patient to report excess thirst or postural light-headedness (signs of dehydration).

• If the patient is young and has coronary artery disease, restrict cholesterol intake.

• Encourage well-balanced, frequent, small feedings to combat anorexia and fatigue; consult a dietitian, if needed.

• Encourage participation in a cardiac rehabilitation program. Current research demonstrates that CHF patients who participate in cardiac rehabilitation programs experience significant improvement in their New York Heart Association functional class, increases in their peak exercise capacity, decreased resting heart rate, increased systemic arteriovenous oxygen (AVO_2) difference at rest and at peak exercise, increased skeletal muscle vascular conductance and oxygen extraction, decreased skeletal muscle lactate production, and decreased dyspnea and fatigue while performing activities of daily living.

Prognosis

The prognosis for patients with CHF has improved dramatically since the introduction of ACE inhibitors. However, the long-term survival for patients with no correctable underlying cause is still in the 50% range 5 years after diagnosis. Patients who are designated as Class III or IV have a 1-year survival rate of 40% when no correctable cause can be identified.

Discharge planning

Discharge planning should be initiated as soon as the cause is identified. Patients who undergo surgical correction have vastly different discharge planning needs than those patients who receive medical management. In addition to the instructions mentioned previously, factors to consider when planning discharge include determining the patient's social support and need for referrals and reviewing what the patient should do if severe symptoms recur.

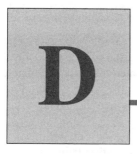

D

Diabetes insipidus

Diabetes insipidus (DI), a sometimes serious disease characterized by water imbalance, results from either a lack of antidiuretic hormone (ADH) or the kidneys' resistance to the effects of ADH, leading to water diuresis. DI may occur in one of two forms: central or nephrogenic. Central (neurogenic) DI is caused by a relative lack of ADH and responds favorably to vasopressin administration. Nephrogenic (vasopressin-resistant) DI results from failure of the kidney to respond to ADH, not to a deficit of the hormone.

DI may be partial or complete and permanent or temporary, depending on the severity of the disease and the patient's response to a dehydration test.

Pathophysiology

Urine concentration depends on the presence of ADH, which is produced in the hypothalamus and transported to the posterior pituitary gland for storage and release. The release of ADH is controlled by the osmolality of the extracellular fluid environment near the hypothalamus. As the plasma osmolality increases, the osmoreceptors are stimulated, resulting in release of ADH. ADH then is transported by the blood to the kidneys, where it binds to receptors on the surface of epithelial cells and reabsorbs water from the distal tubule and collecting ducts.

An absence of ADH or decreased responsiveness to ADH renders the cells of the distal tubule and collecting tubules impermeable to water and therefore unable to reabsorb water. Consequently, large volumes of dilute urine are excreted, even when the patient needs to conserve water.

As free water is lost from the body, the serum sodium level and osmolality rise, stimulating the osmoreceptors to release more ADH. As a result of a defect in either the production or activation of the renal tubules, this mechanism fails to correct the serum osmolality elevation. Osmoreceptor stimulation also increases the thirst sensation, causing the patient to ingest copious amounts of water, thereby diluting the serum and returning it to normal concentration. The inability to respond to these alterations in sodium levels, to the thirst sensation, or both results in DI.

In a few patients with DI, the thirst sensation also is abnormal. In the patient who has an impaired thirst sensation (common among the elderly) or who cannot respond to it because of decreased level of consciousness or immobility, severe hypernatremia and hyperosmolality can result in hypovolemic shock and death.

Neurogenic (central) DI

The most common cause of neurogenic DI is injury to the neurohypophysis from surgery or trauma. This occurs with basilar skull fractures or surgical procedures near the pituitary gland. Intracranial tumors are the second leading cause of decreased production of ADH. Most of the remaining causes are due to various granulomas (tuberculosis, sarcoidosis, eosinophilic granuloma) or local vascular problems (aneurysms, thrombosis, Sheehan's syndrome).

Local ischemia of the hypothalamus or pituitary also can cause neurogenic DI. This ischemia can result from decreased blood supply caused by ruptured aneurysm, hemorrhage, thrombus formation, or severe hypotension and can lead to impaired oxygen delivery to cells, with subsequent cellular dysfunction or cellular death. Certain medications, including ethanol, reserpine, morphine sulfate, chlorpromazine, and phenytoin, also may have a central effect, decreasing the amount of circulating ADH. Discontinuing the drug usually corrects the condition.

Traumatic DI often is transient and typically triphasic. Determining factors include the area of lesion and the amount of destruction produced. The condition usually begins with polyuria from insufficient ADH secretion by hypothalamic cells. A transient (1 to 7 days) second phase follows, with a relatively normal urine flow due to release of previously formed ADH from the posterior pituitary. In the third phase, central DI returns after the released hormone has been used, then gradually improves over a period of weeks or months as ADH-secreting cells gradually regenerate.

The ADH-secreting cells, located primarily in the hypothalamus, usually are not completely destroyed by trauma. ADH is transported to its storage chamber, the posterior pituitary, by the infundibular arteries. Their capillary tufts are contained in the infundibulum of the hypothalamus. Lesions of the hypothalamus and the axonal tract above the median eminence, the prominent lower segment of the infundibulum, produce permanent DI; lesions below this point, even involving total removal of the pituitary gland, result only in temporary cessation of circulating hormone.

Nephrogenic DI

Nephrogenic DI results when the kidneys, especially the collecting ducts, do not respond appropriately to ADH. The renal tubules are resistant to vasopressin and therefore do not reabsorb water. Nephrogenic DI may occur as a rare genetic disorder or may be acquired. Nephrogenic DI usually is less severe than central DI, with fluid loss averaging only 3 liters/day.

An intact thirst mechanism allows the patient to maintain an adequate fluid balance. Mild hypovolemia produces a negative salt balance that diminishes delivery of fluid to the distal tubules of the kidneys, minimizing free water loss. Nephrogenic and neurogenic DI usually present with identical urine and serum osmolality; however, nephrogenic DI does not respond to the administration of vasopressin.

The rare familial form, an X-linked recessive or autosomal dominant trait seen in male infants, presents as hypotonic urine, dehydration, and fever. This is a permanent form of nephrogenic DI and must be treated with dietary restrictions and drugs that reduce urine output. Females carrying the trait experience subclinical disease, which is evident only when challenged by fluid deprivation. In the dehydrated state, the urine osmolality decreases while the serum osmolality rises.

Acquired nephrogenic DI is more common than the primary form and may result from any renal disease in the advanced stages. Diseases affecting the papillary and medullary regions of the kidneys most severely limit the kidneys' concentrating ability. With damage to these regions, the kidneys are unable to control the amount of urine excreted. Common causes include polycystic kidney disease, medullary cystic disease, pyelonephritis, and renal transplantation.

Nephrogenic DI also may result from hypercalcemia or hypokalemia and can be reversed after correction of the imbalance. Severe hypercalcemia results in an increased urine output caused by blockage of ADH on the renal tubules, dehydration, and oliguria. Hypokalemia initially causes oliguria, then eventually dehydration because of the reduced ability to concentrate urine.

Many drugs, including lithium, demeclocycline, amphotericin, aminoglycosides, and vinblastine, can cause nephrogenic DI by interfering with the medullary concentrating mechanism. These drugs are believed to block the ADH receptor site in the distal tubule, resulting in increased excretion of dilute urine. The dose-related effect associated with these drugs usually is reversible, although not immediately. The effects on the kidney may last for several weeks after the drug is discontinued.

Malnutrition, especially caused by a severely restricted protein diet, can cause nephrogenic DI due to reduced availability of urea. Urea is responsible for a large portion of the medullary hypertonicity, which helps to pull water from the collecting duct and to concentrate urine. Sodium chloride levels also are important. If sodium intake is severely restricted, a larger amount of filtered sodium chloride is reabsorbed from the proximal tubule, leading to reduced delivery of sodium chloride to the loop of Henle. If less sodium chloride is available, the medulla is less hypertonic and smaller volumes of water are reabsorbed.

Clinical assessment

The priorities of assessment are to determine the cause of the DI and the severity of the fluid and electrolyte abnormalities. A thorough history and identification of signs and symptoms are required.

History

The patient usually has an abrupt onset of symptoms, the most prevalent being a large urine volume and intense thirst. During the health history, the nurse should question the patient regarding:
• neurologic surgery or trauma
• intracranial cancer
• neurologic ischemia (hemorrhage, thrombosis, or hypotension)
• advanced renal disease
• use of medications that can cause DI
• diet history, especially pertaining to protein and sodium chloride ingestion.

Physical findings

Common findings include:
• polyuria (neurogenic type produces from 3 to 24 liters/24 hours; nephrogenic, 3 to 4 liters/24 hours)
• intense thirst in the alert patient

- polydipsia
- inadequate I.V. fluid resuscitation resulting in signs of dehydration (dry skin and mucous membranes, constipation, confusion, sunken eyeballs) and hypernatremia (altered mental status, coma, symptoms specific to area of neuronal death); inadequate fluid resuscitation may arise secondary to impaired thirst mechanism
- fever
- dyspnea
- pale and voluminous urine
- poor skin turgor
- tachycardia
- muscle weakness, muscle pain
- hypotension
- weight loss
- lethargy.

Signs and symptoms of neurologic lesion are also possible.

Diagnosis

The patient history, physical findings, and laboratory tests help to identify DI and distinguish between central and nephrogenic types. However, the diagnosis is complicated by the degree of ADH insufficiency and resistance. A differential diagnosis involves the investigation of other possible causes of polyuria, such as hyperglycemia, diabetes mellitus, psychogenic polydipsia, chronic renal failure, excessive oral or parenteral fluid intake, and administration of corticosteroids or osmotic diuretics.

Laboratory tests aid in the diagnosis and treatment of DI. Common findings include urine specific gravity less than 1.005; urine osmolality less than 300 mOsm/liter; serum osmolality elevated (> 295 mOsm/liter) if water intake does not match output; and serum sodium greater than 145 mEq/liter. The serum osmolality and serum sodium may be much higher if the patient remains untreated.

The water deprivation test is the most commonly used test to help diagnose DI; other helpful tests include the vasopressin test, nicotine test, ADH immunoassay, and Hickey-Hare test.

Treatment and care

The primary goals for care of the patient with DI are to identify and correct the primary cause, maintain fluid and electrolyte balance, and prevent complications (see *Key nursing interventions for patients with DI,* page 234). The most common treatments and related nursing interventions are listed below.

Acute DI can be complicated by severe volume depletion, dehydration, hypovolemia, and hyperosmolality, possibly resulting in cerebral damage. These problems are more likely to occur if the thirst mechanism is absent or impaired. Patients with partial DI tolerate their disease well as long as they have an intact thirst mechanism and access to unrestricted fluid intake. Patients with permanent DI also fare well as long as exogenous vasopressin is administered.

Chronic complications result from prolonged high urine flow. The patient may develop enlarged calyceal, ureteral, and bladder capacities resulting in thin, weak bladder walls. Renal failure (postrenal origin) can occur in these situations. Renal insufficiency may result from chronic bladder reflux and hydronephrosis. Patients also can develop a resistance to vasopressin with prolonged use, producing nephrogenic DI.

Fluid resuscitation

Fluids, most commonly free water in the form of dextrose 5% in water (D5W), should be administered until the patient's polyuria is controlled by vasopressin therapy. Massive fluid losses must be replaced to prevent the patient from developing hypovolemic shock. In replacing fluid, careful attention must be paid to preventing overload and water intoxication (excessive retention of water with a low serum sodium level), a potential complication of vasopressin therapy that can be as serious as dehydration. Water intoxication can lead to symptomatic hyponatremia and pulmonary edema.

ESSENTIAL ELEMENTS
Key nursing interventions for patients with DI

The following flowchart highlights key interventions that typically are performed when a patient is diagnosed with DI.

Achieve optimal fluid and electrolyte balance

Identify and correct the primary cause.	Correct fluid and electrolyte imbalance.	Prevent complications.
• Monitor and report these signs and symptoms: —polyuria —polydipsia —intense thirst. • Identify the use of drugs that commonly cause DI: —neurogenic (ethanol, reserpine, morphine sulfate, chlorpromazine, phenytoin) —nephrogenic (lithium, demeclocycline, amphotericin, aminoglycosides, vinblastine). • Assist with diagnostic tests to differentiate types of polyuria. • Administer exogenous vasopressin to patients with neurogenic DI.	• Monitor ECG for signs of hypokalemia: —U waves, prolonged QT interval, depressed ST segment, and low amplitude T waves —arrhythmias, particularly bradycardia, first-degree and second-degree heart block, atrial arrhythmias, and premature ventricular contractions. • Administer fluids to replace loss: —Weigh patient daily. —Record intake and output. • Monitor for signs of hyperkalemia with dehydration. • Monitor for signs of hypokalemia with administration of vasopressin.	• Administer fluids to replace losses. • Monitor and report signs of hypovolemia. • Assess for signs of renal failure. • Monitor for signs of resistance to vasopressin.

The hypernatremia seen in DI responds to administration of water taken orally or D_5W given I.V.; however, correction of hypernatremia depends on giving enough water to overcome the water deficit and to compensate for continued urine water losses. Hypotonic dextrose and water solutions are preferred to normal saline unless the patient has severe circulatory failure or severe hypernatremia. In severe DI, urine volume can exceed 500 ml/hour, and with a severe water deficit, water may have to be given I.V. at rates exceeding 600 to 700 ml/hour.

The following nursing interventions should be incorporated into the plan of care:

• Monitor plasma and urine osmolalities, urine specific gravity, and serum sodium and electrolyte levels.

• Administer D_5W in amounts to replace urinary and insensible losses.

• Monitor for evidence of water intoxication (decreased urine output, increased weight, peripheral edema, shortness of breath, rales on auscultation, change in level of consciousness).

• Monitor hourly intake and output.

• Weigh the patient daily at the same time of day on the same scale.

Pharmacologic management

Central DI should respond to synthetic ADH compounds. Aqueous vasopressin (5 to 10 units, given 2 to 3 times daily) can be given subcutaneously. Alternatively, desmopressin acetate, which lacks vasopressor effects but retains ADH activity, can be given I.V. or subcutaneously (2 to 4 g/day) or by nasal spray. The dose should be adjusted on the basis of serum sodium levels, urine output, and urine osmolality. Ideally, urine output should be reduced to 2 to 4 liters/day, an amount that can be replaced readily by oral or I.V. administration of ADH.

Nephrogenic DI rarely is as severe as complete central DI and, during water deprivation, urine osmolality sometimes is as high as 300 to 400 mOsm/kg. Administration of enough water to maintain normal serum sodium levels usually can be achieved. If a reversible cause, such as lithium use, is found, the offending agent can be discontinued, though the effect on renal concentrating ability may persist for days.

Some patients have been given thiazide diuretics to induce a state of mild volume depletion. This leads to increased proximal tubular sodium reabsorption and decreased delivery of sodium and water to the distal diluting segment so that less water is lost. Thiazide diuretics may be used for all causes of nephrogenic DI. (See *Major drugs used to treat DI,* pages 237 and 238, for more information.)

The following nursing interventions should be incorporated into the plan of care:

• Monitor and report signs of inadequate treatment (polyuria, polydipsia, intense thirst).

• Administer vasopressin, desmopressin, or lysine to patients with neurogenic DI.

• Monitor for signs and symptoms of overtreatment (hyponatremia, weight gain, peripheral edema, headache, drowsiness, listlessness, seizures, cerebral edema, coma, and death).

• Assess for adverse effects to drugs.

Prognosis

Patients with partial or nephrogenic DI do well as long as their thirst mechanism is intact and they have unlimited access to fluid intake. Patients with complete DI require administration of exogenous ADH.

Discharge planning

Discharge planning should begin once the patient's life-threatening fluid and electrolyte imbalances have been corrected. All of the following should be considered to prepare the patient for discharge:

• emotional and physical support system

• medication regimen, including the purpose, name, dose, administration schedule, need for compliance, common adverse effects, and need for medical alert identification

MAJOR DRUGS

Major drugs used to treat DI

The following drugs may be used as part of the pharmacologic management to treat the neurogenic and nephrogenic forms of DI.

Drug	Dosage	Adverse Reactions and Precautions
NEUROGENIC DI		
1-deamino-8-D-arginine vasopressin Desmopressin acetate (DDAVP)	• 0.1 to 0.4 ml (single or divided into 2 to 3 doses) intranasally • Action begins within 1 hour • Controls polyuria for 8 to 24 hours	• Monitor for edema, hypertension, allergic reaction (hypotension and bronchoconstriction), drug resistance (polyuria and polydipsia), and vasoconstriction (angina, abdominal cramping, GI distress, headache). • Overdose can result in overhydration (pulmonary edema, drowsiness, hyponatremia, weight gain). • Nasal congestion can decrease effectiveness of drug, since it is given intranasally.
Pitressin tannate in oil	• 2.5 to 5 units (0.5 to 1 ml) I.M. every 48 hours • Onset is cumulative and cannot be determined for days • Average duration of action is 36 to 72 hours; therapeutic effects generally last 36 to 48 hours	• Monitor for same adverse reactions as with DDAVP (except, since drug is not given intranasally, nasal congestion has no impact on drug effectiveness).
Aqueous pitressin	• 2 to 4 units (0.1 to 0.3 ml) every 4 to 6 hours I.M., S.C., or intranasally • Controls polyuria for 1 to 8 hours	• Same adverse reactions as with DDAVP. • Monitor for signs of polyuria and polydipsia if I.V. discontinued (therapeutic effect decreases within minutes after infusion is discontinued).
Lysine vasopressin nasal spray (Diapid) Lypressin	• 5 to 20 units intranasally, 3 to 7 times/day • Action begins in 1 hour	• Same adverse reactions as with DDAVP. • Warn patient not to inhale spray. • If more than 2 sprays for each nostril are needed every 4 to 6

(continued)

Major drugs used to treat DI *(continued)*

Drug	Dosage	Adverse Reactions and Precautions
Lysine vaso-pressin na-sal spray *(continued)*	• Controls polyuria for 2 to 6 hours	hours to decrease urinary output, frequency of administration rather than number of sprays per dose should be increased.
Chlorprop-amide (Diabinese)	• 100 to 250 mg/day orally; dosage adjusted at 2-day or 3-day intervals if necessary, up to 500 mg daily • Action begins in 1 hour, peaks in 3 to 6 hours, and lasts 60 to 72 hours	• Monitor for signs of hypoglycemia (anorexia, nausea, vomiting, fatigue, drowsiness, muscle weakness). • Monitor for adverse reactions (headache, tinnitus, alcohol intolerance, GI disturbances). • Taking medication with meals minimizes GI effects.
Car-bamazepine (Tegretol)	• 400 to 600 mg/day orally • Peak serum levels in 2 to 8 hours • Serum half-life 14 to 16 hours	• Monitor for adverse reactions (bone marrow suppression, hepatotoxicity, headache, fatigue, mental depression).
NEPHROGENIC DI		
Hydrochloro-thiazide (Thiazide diuretic)	• 50 to 100 mg/day orally • Action begins in 2 hours, peaks in 4 hours, and lasts 6 to 12 hours	• Monitor for adverse reactions (hypokalemia, mild hypotension, nausea, fatigue). • Discourage liberal use of dietary salt, which decreases effectiveness of therapy.
Indometha-cin (Indocin)	• 100 mg/day orally • Action begins in 1 to 2 hours, peaks in 4 to 6 hours; half-life about 4½ hours	• Monitor for adverse reactions (decreased platelet aggregation, GI distress, headache, tachycardia, hematuria). • Contraindicated in patients allergic to aspirin. • Administer immediately after meals to minimize GI adverse reactions.

• the need to notify the physician of changes in fluid balance, including evidence of excessive water retention (weight gain, peripheral edema, right upper quadrant pain, shortness of breath) or evidence of inefficient water conservation (continued polyuria or polydipsia)
• the need to record daily weight on the same scale, at the same time of day, and in same state of dress
• the need to record intake and output (frequency of urination, amount of fluids ingested) and measurement of specific gravity.

Diabetic ketoacidosis

Diabetic ketoacidosis (DKA) is a disease characterized by profound hyperglycemia, severe metabolic acidosis, and fluid and electrolyte imbalance. It is the most serious metabolic complication of insulin-dependent diabetes mellitus (IDDM) and, to a lesser degree, non-insulin-dependent diabetes mellitus (NIDDM).

Possible causes of DKA include decreased exogenous insulin intake and increased endogenous glucose production. Decreased exogenous insulin intake can result from lack of knowledge, poor compliance, and use of phenytoin and thiazide and sulfonamide diuretics, which inhibit insulin secretion. Increased endogenous glucose production typically occurs with alterations in diet or exercise, with increased glucagon and growth hormone concentrations, and with the secretion of the catecholamines epinephrine and norepinephrine. This sympathetic stimulation generally occurs in stressful situations, such as injury, surgery, infections, and, on rare occasions, emotional trauma.

The most common etiologies of DKA are insulin withdrawal, infection, and undiagnosed diabetes during the initial presentation of the disease. Although DKA can occur in the absence of precipitating factors, a precipitating factor should be investigated.

Pathophysiology

The development of DKA depends on insulin deficiency combined with an excess of counterregulatory hormones (glucagon, cortisol, catecholamines, and growth hormone) that increase the blood glucose level—a condition very similar to the physiologic state of normal fasting. During the fed state, insulin is the predominant hormone, required for glucose delivery to the cells. During fasting, the body converts to endogenous sources of glucose for support of the brain and muscles, resulting in hormonal changes. Plasma insulin levels fall and glucagon levels rise, allowing the liver to become the major source of glucose during the fasting state.

Stored glycogen, protein, and fat are broken down as an alternative source of fuel. Concurrently, decreased insulin concentrations lead to lipolysis in fat deposits, providing a source of free fatty acids as a fuel for muscle and reserving glucose for use in the brain. Glucagon promotes the liver's conversion of free fatty acids to ketones, another alternative energy source for brain and muscle tissue.

In the search for energy from noncarbohydrate sources, the body begins breaking down large amounts of fat to obtain glucose in the form of glycerol and fatty acids. Glycerol is released and converted to glucose; fatty acids are converted to acetyl-coenzyme A (acetyl-CoA) by the liver. Accumulation of acetyl-CoA increases the number of ketone bodies, or keto acids. Acetone, which forms in urine and is detectable on the breath, is a spontaneous by-product of keto acids.

In DKA, the above process is greatly exaggerated as a result of severe insulin deficiency; however, insulin deficiency alone does not explain the elevated glucose seen in all cases of DKA. The effectiveness of circulating insulin also is reduced due to insulin resistance. Initially believed to result from massive doses of insulin used to treat DKA, insulin resistance is caused by elevated counterregulatory hormones, acidemia, hypertonicity of blood, phosphate depletion, elevated plasma free fatty acids, hyperaminoacidemia, and prolonged elevations of glucose.

DKA is characterized by large increases in the levels of stress hormones, including the glucose counterregulatory hormones cortisol, catecholamines, and growth hormone, which are responsible for hyperglycemia and ketonemia. Cortisol enhances gluconeogenesis by increasing delivery of fats and proteins to the liver to be converted into glucose. Prolonged hypersecretion of cortisol also decreases sensitivity to insulin. Catecholamines enhance lipolysis, providing substrate for ketogenesis. Growth hormone also contributes to increased lipolysis and insulin resistance.

Hyperglycemia

Hyperglycemia in the DKA patient is the result of excessive hepatic glucose production. Glucose clearance by insulin-sensitive tissues also is reduced. However, as long as the kidneys are well perfused, they allow glucose to leak from the extracellular space into the collecting duct to be excreted into the urine. This prevents severe hyperglycemia.

Ketosis and metabolic acidosis

Ketosis and metabolic acidosis are major manifestations of DKA. Ketosis is primarily due to increased synthesis of keto acids by the liver. An inability of the peripheral tissues to utilize excess ketones also contributes to the increased ketone levels. The ketone bodies dissociate to yield hydrogen ions that interfere with the normal serum hydrogen ion concentration (pH) and produce metabolic acidosis. The body attempts to buffer this acidosis with bicarbonate; however, body stores have already been depleted by osmotic diuresis.

If the acidosis in DKA is due only to ketosis and not to hypovolemia, the fall in serum bicarbonate is equal to the increase in anion gap. In many patients the reduction in serum bicarbonate concentration is greater than the increase in anion gap, indicating the presence of a non–anion gap hyperchloremic acidosis. Hyperchloremic acidosis appears to occur in patients who are less severely volume-depleted; correction is much more difficult, requiring increased regeneration of bicarbonate by the kidneys.

Hyperchloremia is related directly to the severity of azotemia. Patients with normal renal function and relatively little volume depletion have hyperchloremia and a low anion gap. Patients with significant azotemia have an elevated anion gap, and the increased serum ketones account for most or all of the decrease in bicarbonate levels. Patients with normal renal function have increased urinary losses of ketones with a compensatory chloride retention in excess of sodium retention. The loss of ketones in the urine without the accompanying loss of hydrogen ions has the same effect on acid-base balance as the loss of bicarbonate.

Another cause of acidosis in DKA is lactic acidosis, which results from decreased perfusion to the cells accompanying the hypovolemia produced by osmotic diuresis. Lactic acidosis contributes to a further increase in the anion gap, which decreases the serum bicarbonate level.

Fluid and electrolyte imbalances

Fluid and electrolyte imbalance is the third major feature of DKA. Fluid and electrolytes are lost in the osmotic diuresis caused by marked hyperglycemia and ketonemia seen in DKA. The large number of glucose molecules and increased ketone bodies result in hypertonicity of the intravascular space, pulling fluid from the interstitium and increasing the glomerular filtration rate. Fluid losses generally are 5 to 8 liters in a 70-kg patient. Depletion of sodium, potassium, and chloride may be 300 to 500 mmol or more at presentation. Magnesium and phosphate also are lost, but in smaller quantities.

Several electrolyte abnormalities are seen in the patient with DKA; however, serum electrolyte concentrations do not accurately reflect the large losses that occur in the DKA patient. This is especially true for potassium, which is at normal or even high serum levels on presentation. These levels result from a shift of potassium from the intracellular fluid to the extracellular fluid due to acidosis and the loss of water from the extracellular space. Hyperkalemia is quickly reduced as potassium is lost by vomiting, diarrhea, and osmotic diuresis. An initial low serum potassium concentration suggests severe total-body depletion, requiring aggressive management.

Hyponatremia occurs for two reasons: water shifting from the intracellular compartment to extracellular space due to hyperosmolality, and a total sodium deficit that results from osmotic diuresis and the fact that sodium accompanies ketone excretion in the urine. Serum chloride levels vary with volume status and fluid resuscitation. Hypochloremia due to sustained osmotic diuresis occurs most frequently. If the kidneys are working well, hypochloremia is less likely because chloride is not lost with urinary ketones and there is a high incidence of hyperchloremic acidosis.

The serum phosphorus level usually is normal on admission; however, total-body phosphate often is decreased in DKA from osmotic diuresis.

Clinical assessment

The priorities when assessing a patient with DKA are to determine the cause of DKA and the severity of the acidosis and fluid and electrolyte abnormalities. A thorough history and review of signs and symptoms are required. An individualized approach to patient management is determined according to laboratory findings and signs and symptoms.

History

The patient with DKA has a history of lethargy, polyuria, and polydipsia usually accompanied by weight loss. The symptoms may persist for as short as 24 hours before the patient seeks medical attention, but usually extend over several days; in newly diagnosed diabetes, symptoms often persist for weeks. During the health

history, the nurse should gather as much information as possible about the following:
• insulin intake (determine whether the patient is aware of or complies with the prescribed insulin regimen)
• use of phenytoin or thiazide and sulfonamide diuretics
• recent changes in diabetes management
• precipitating events (stressful events, infections, injury, surgery, emotional trauma)
• recent use of steroids, epinephrine, or norepinephrine.

Physical findings
Findings commonly associated with DKA include:
• polydipsia and polyuria (caused by osmotic diuresis induced by hyperglycemia)
• weakness, marked fatigue, anorexia, vomiting, and abdominal pain and tenderness (caused by extracellular volume depletion and ketoacidosis; more common in patients under age 40 with serum bicarbonate concentration 10 mEq/liter)
• altered mental status (stupor to coma related to hyperosmolality)
• tachycardia, orthostatic hypotension
• dry mucous membranes, flushed dry skin, poor skin turgor
• Kussmaul's respiration
• fruity, acetone breath
• urine ketones (signal insulin leakage or pump failure before it becomes serious and leads to DKA)
• normal or subnormal temperatures (if the patient has elevated temperature, suspect infection, the most common cause of DKA in the diagnosed diabetic).

Diagnosis
With a known diabetic patient, a diagnosis of DKA is determined by ketonuria and glycosuria in the presence of hyperglycemia and ketonemia. The diagnosis should be suspected even if serum glucose levels are not greatly elevated. This is important in patients who are fasting, patients who may have ingested alcohol, or pregnant women. For a nondiabetic patient, other caus-

es of metabolic acidosis must be differentiated before a course of therapy is begun. Starvation, alcoholism, lactic acidosis, and uremia can cause ketoacidosis, even in the absence of diabetes.

Laboratory findings can assist in identifying characteristic changes seen in DKA, such as ketoacidosis, dehydration, extreme catabolism (results from lack of glucose use by the cell, causing a breakdown of fats and proteins for a glucose source), and electrolyte abnormalities. (For a list of laboratory tests useful in diagnosing DKA, see *Confirming DKA,* page 246.)

Treatment and care

The goals of therapy for DKA include rapidly replacing life-threatening fluid and electrolyte deficits; restoring the insulin-glucagon ratio to promote cellular use of glucose, reduce the counterregulatory hormone glucagon, and stop the production of keto acids; identifying precipitating events; and preventing complications.

Fluid therapy

Volume replacement is a critical part of the initial management of DKA. The total water deficit in most patients is 6 liters but can approach 10 liters or more. Which type of replacement fluid to use—crystalloid or colloid, isotonic or hypotonic—remains controversial. Appropriate volume expansion will lower the glucose level even without the use of insulin by increasing glucose secretion by the kidneys. Reexpanding the intravascular volume also decreases the production of counterregulatory hormones and eliminates the tachycardia, peripheral constriction, and decreased organ perfusion seen in hypovolemic shock.

Most experts advocate the use of normal saline (isotonic) solution to be infused at the rate of 1 liter during the first hour, then at a rate adequate to maintain a stable blood pressure. An infusion rate of 300 to 500 ml/hour may be required to maintain hemodynamic stability. Normal saline solution also avoids a rapid fall in extra-

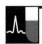

DIAGNOSTIC TESTS

Confirming DKA

Laboratory findings can assist in identifying metabolic changes seen in patients with DKA, who characteristically present with ketoacidosis, dehydration, extreme catabolism, and electrolyte imbalance. The laboratory findings often used to define these alterations are included below.

Ketoacidosis
• urine ketones positive
• elevated bedside fingerstick blood sugar level
• elevated serum glucose level (500 to 800 mg/dl)
• low arterial blood hydrogen ion concentration level (< 7.3)
• low plasma bicarbonate level (< 15 mEq/liter)

Dehydration
• increased serum osmolality level (usually < 333 mOsm/liter)
• elevated hematocrit level (depends on level of dehydration)
• marked leukocytosis (often > 25 mm^3 with a shift to the right)
• increased blood urea nitrogen level (depends on level of dehydration)
• high urine specific gravity (depends on level of dehydration)

Extreme catabolism
• hypertriglyceridemia (depends on level of dehydration)
• ketonemia
• ketonuria

Electrolyte abnormalities
• below-normal serum sodium level (< 135 mEq/liter)
• below-normal serum chloride level (< 99 mEq/liter)
• above-normal serum potassium level initially (> 5.5 mEq/liter)
• below-normal serum potassium level with administration of insulin and fluids, unless potassium supplement given (< 3.0 mEq/liter)
• below-normal serum phosphate level with administration of insulin and fluids, unless phosphate supplement given (< 1.5 mEq/liter)
• below-normal serum magnesium level (< 1.5 mEq/liter)
• below-normal serum calcium level (< 4.5 mEq/liter)

cellular osmolality, which can lead to cerebral edema. The goal is to replace one half of the calculated fluid deficit over the first 8 hours and the second half over the next 16 hours.

As the plasma glucose level approaches 250 mg/dl, 5% dextrose should be added to the replacement fluid to avoid hypoglycemia. Normal saline solution may be changed to 0.45% sodium chloride. The serum glucose level should be maintained between 200 and 300 mg/dl. During fluid replacement, assessments should include vital signs, level of consciousness, weight, input, and urine output.

The following nursing interventions should be incorporated into the plan of care:
• Monitor serum glucose levels hourly until level reaches 250 to 300 mg/dl.
• Monitor for signs and symptoms of dehydration and shock (tachycardia, hypotension, weak peripheral pulses, capillary refill time > 3 seconds, poor skin turgor, polyuria, and oliguria). Continuously monitor blood pressure and heart rate and rhythm.
• Monitor serum osmolality.
• Monitor intake and output hourly.
• Administer I.V. fluids, as prescribed.
• During the first 24 hours, monitor for signs and symptoms of pulmonary edema (crackles, dyspnea, cough, and frothy sputum).

Electrolyte replacement
Osmotic diuresis leads to total-body potassium depletion ranging from 5 to 10 mEq/kg of body weight. In the absence of anuria or life-threatening hyperkalemia, potassium replacement should begin at the onset of fluid therapy; however, potassium replacement should not be started when the patient's serum potassium level is above 5.8 mEq/liter. The average adult requires 80 to 160 mEq of potassium chloride over the first 12 hours to maintain an adequate serum potassium concentration.

Phosphorus replacement also is necessary in the patient with DKA and should be administered before levels become critical. Phosphate is important to tissue oxygenation, central nervous system (CNS) function, carbohydrate use, and leukocyte function. The total-body phosphorus is depleted as a result of osmotic diuresis; with fluid and insulin therapy, it is shifted intracellularly, resulting in a significant drop in phosphate levels. Severe hypophosphatemia (serum levels < 1 mg/dl) may result in serious organ dysfunction, including respiratory failure, rhabdomyolysis, and impaired cardiac function.

Potassium level is often critically low in the patient being treated for DKA. Some experts believe that one third of the potassium deficit should be replaced with potassium phosphate. Replacing phosphorus too rapidly can cause a significant decrease in calcium, resulting in tetany.

The following nursing interventions should be incorporated into the plan of care:
• Monitor serum electrolyte levels hourly.
• Monitor for signs and symptoms of electrolyte imbalances, including hyperkalemia in the first 1 to 4 hours of treatment, hypokalemia after the first 1 to 4 hours of treatment, hyponatremia early in treatment, and hypophosphatemia.
• Administer I.V. fluids and electrolyte replacements, as ordered.

Insulin therapy

Insulin is required to reverse the hyperglycemia and ketonemia of DKA. The goal is to provide an adequate amount to reverse these processes without causing hypoglycemia, hypophosphatemia, and hypokalemia. The route of choice is I.V., especially in volume-depleted patients with altered perfusion. Regular insulin should be used because of its rapid onset. Initially, a bolus of regular insulin (0.3 units/kg) is given as a loading dose to prime the tissue receptors. The current recommended infusion dose is 0.1 units regular insulin/kg/hour. This dose will result in a decrease in plasma glucose level by 80 to 100 mg/dl/hour in most patients.

Insulin also stops ketogenesis and reverses metabolic acidosis. The plasma glucose level will respond more quickly than the ketoacidosis. Often, insulin is stopped deliberately before ketogenesis has resolved, which can result in worsening DKA. The insulin infusion should be continued until the anion gap has normalized, the serum bicarbonate level is greater than 15 mEq/liter, the patient is able to eat, and the patient has been on a subcutaneous regimen for 1 to 2 hours.

The following nursing interventions should be incorporated into the plan of care:
• Administer a loading dose of regular insulin.

• Administer 0.1 units of regular insulin/kg/hour to decrease the blood glucose by 80 to 100 mg/dl/hour. Piggyback the insulin so that fluid replacement can be changed without interfering with the insulin delivery rate.

• Monitor blood glucose levels hourly; notify the physician when blood glucose levels are between 250 and 300 mg/dl.

• Monitor for signs and symptoms of medication-induced hypoglycemia (headache, confusion, irritability, restlessness, trembling, pallor, diaphoresis, and stupor). If these develop, notify the physician, obtain an immediate serum glucose level, and administer dextrose 50% in water, 1 amp I.V.

Bicarbonate therapy

Bicarbonate therapy in the treatment of DKA remains controversial. Its use is reserved for the patient whose pH is below 7.1 due to a primary bicarbonate deficit. Acidosis can result in cardiac arrhythmias and cardiac dysfunction, while bicarbonate therapy and the resultant alkalosis can lead to worsening pH in the CNS and decreased CNS function. Bicarbonate therapy may also shift the oxyhemoglobin dissociation curve to the left, resulting in decreased release of oxygen to the cells and cellular anoxia. Most authorities recommend the use of bicarbonate when arterial blood pH is 7.1 or less. Two ampules of sodium bicarbonate should be added to the initial liter of hypotonic saline solution and infused until the arterial blood pH is 7.2.

The following nursing interventions should be incorporated into the plan of care:

• Monitor respiratory status (respiratory rate and depth, breath odor, and breath sounds) hourly.

• Monitor arterial blood gas levels at least hourly.

• Administer I.V. sodium bicarbonate if pH is greater than 7.1 or bicarbonate is less than 10 mEq/liter.

• Monitor for hypokalemia, which occurs secondary to the rapid shift of potassium into the cells.

Prevention of complications

A number of metabolic complications can occur in the treatment of DKA, including hypoglycemia, hypokalemia, hypophosphatemia, and hypomagnesemia. DKA patients are also prone to thromboembolism as a result of increased platelet adhesiveness and hyperviscosity. Fluid replacement is sufficient therapy in the majority of patients to prevent thromboembolism.

A rare, often fatal complication of DKA is cerebral edema. It occurs most frequently in children; however, it also can occur in adults and usually presents within 12 hours after initiation of fluid therapy. There are no warning signs. The patient usually complains of headache, develops lethargy, and becomes unconscious. Physical examination reveals papilledema and fixed, dilated, or unequal pupils. A rapid fall in plasma glucose, as the result of overzealous administration of insulin, and aggressive replacement of fluids may cause intracellular movement of water, leading to brain swelling.

Crystalloid infusion, especially excess replacement, may also predispose the patient to adult respiratory distress syndrome. This is a rare complication of DKA, but carries a high mortality.

The following nursing interventions should be incorporated into the plan of care:
- Monitor serum electrolyte levels hourly.
- Monitor serum glucose levels hourly, and titrate insulin drip as ordered. Notify the physician of decreases in serum glucose greater than 50 to 100 mg/dl/hour, or as ordered.
- Cautiously administer fluid replacement.
- Evaluate pulmonary status (auscultation of breath sounds, widening alveolar-arterial gradient, dyspnea, and infiltrates on chest X-rays).
- Measure intake and output hourly.

Prognosis

Despite proper identification and treatment, the mortality of DKA remains at 10%. Most deaths result from

profound dehydration. Other factors that affect the patient's chances for recovery from DKA include:
• prompt treatment of electrolyte imbalances
• preexisting pathophysiology related to the diabetes
• correction of the acidosis.

Discharge planning

Discharge planning should begin as soon as the patient has been stabilized. All of the following factors should be considered:
• the patient's and family's understanding of diabetes, appropriate diabetic care and monitoring skills, signs and symptoms of hyperglycemia and hypoglycemia, and the importance of seeking early medical help when these signs and symptoms present
• the patient's and family's understanding of the importance of testing urine for sugar and acetone, as well as ketones in patients with signs of infection, or when finger capillary glucose level is unexpectedly high
• the patient's and family's ability to perform fingerstick measurement of serum glucose, administer insulin, and keep a record of weight, glucose levels, and insulin adjustments
• the patient's and family's understanding of when to notify the physician (if the patient is stressed, has an infection, or has any signs or symptoms of hypoglycemia or hyperglycemia)
• support systems and the need for referral to a diabetes education program.

Disseminated intravascular coagulation

Disseminated intravascular coagulation (DIC), a coagulation disorder that always occurs in conjunction with a defined disease process, is also referred to as hypofibrinogenemia, defibrination syndrome, and consumptive coagulopathy. Under normal conditions, the hematologic system is in a constant balance between two opposing forces: coagulation and fibrinolysis. However, in DIC, thrombosis occurs at a faster rate than clots can be lysed. Clotting factors are consumed, and bleeding, often in the form of massive hemorrhage, ensues.

A life-threatening acute condition, DIC can persist in a chronic, compensated state for years during which primarily thrombotic symptoms wax and wane. The mortality rate associated with DIC ranges from 50% to 80%, depending on the acuteness of onset and etiology.

Pathophysiology

DIC develops through a complicated series of events, beginning with an overwhelming trigger of the coagulation system (see *Events that can trigger DIC*, pages 253 and 254).

The initial events include the formation of excess soluble fibrin, which becomes trapped in the microvasculature along with platelets. Clotting results in decreased blood flow to the tissues, leading to acidemia, blood stasis, and tissue hypoxia. These three elements, plus excess fibrin and thrombin, trigger both the fibrinolytic and antithrombin systems, leading to anticoagulated blood. Additionally, platelets and coagulation factors are consumed, and massive hemorrhage can ensue (for an illustration of the pathologic process of DIC and a list of participating coagulation factors and fibrinolytic proteins, see *Pathogenesis of DIC,* pages 255 and 256).

Clinical assessment

DIC is a process of both thrombosis and hemorrhagic diathesis. Although the initial phase of DIC probably is thrombotic, often the focus of care and the first noticed event in acute fulminant DIC is bleeding. The cardinal signs of fulminant DIC include bleeding from three different sites, necrosis of fingertips or tips of the toes, thrombocytopenia, and hypofibrinogenemia. In evaluating the patient with DIC for response to interventions or disease progression, a comprehensive head-to-toe

Events that can trigger DIC

Below is a list of common events that can trigger DIC, along with their possible causes, mechanisms, and considerations.

Triggering Event	Possible Causes	Mechanisms and Considerations
Obstetrical emergencies	• Amniotic fluid embolism • Retained dead fetus • Placental abruption • Eclampsia • Abortion (saline-induced) • Retained placenta • Hydatidiform mole • Acute fatty liver of pregnancy	• Amniotic fluid embolism, the most common obstetric accident associated with DIC, carries an 80% mortality rate. • Retained dead fetus lasting > 5 weeks is associated with a 50% incidence. • DIC can be limited to the uterus and can lead to postpartum hemorrhage. • Placenta and amniotic fluid have high amounts of thromboplastin.
Neoplasms	• Adenocarcinoma • Acute leukemia • Giant cavernous hemangioma • Sarcoma • Polycythemia vera • Pheochromocytoma	• Incidence is 10% to 82%. • All chemotherapeutic agents may induce DIC by lysing a large number of cells. • Tissue factor is expressed on circulating tumor cells.
Hematologic problems or events	• Hemolytic transfusion reaction • Minor hemolysis • Massive transfusions • Sickle cell crisis • Thalassemia major	• Red cell lysis releases adenosine diphosphate or red cell membrane phospholipoprotein that may activate the coagulation cascade.
Trauma or surgery	• Burns • Head trauma • Surgery, especially if extracorporeal circulation is used • Multiple injuries • Transplant rejection • Fat emboli	• Large amount of tissue thromboplastin (factor VII) is released due to tissue injury. • Brain trauma carries the highest risk; thrombosis is more prevalent than hemorrhage. • The platelet count is the least abnormal value. • About 20% of those with DIC also have acute respiratory distress syndrome.

(continued)

Events that can trigger DIC (continued)

Triggering Event	Possible Causes	Mechanisms and Considerations
Infections	• Viremias • Gram-negative sepsis • Gram-positive sepsis	• Trigger by viruses is unknown; may be antibody-antigen activation of factor VII or endothelial damage. • Gram-negative sepsis and urosepsis are the most common causes. • Incidence in sepsis is 10% to 73%. • Endotoxins activate factor XII. • Shock leads to blood stagnatosis, acidosis.
Miscellaneous	• LeVeen shunt • Intra-aortic balloon device • Aspirin toxicity • Snake bite • Hypothermia • Liver disease	• May occur secondary to ascitic fluid with high concentrations of thrombin or secondary to platelet destruction that occurs with intra-aortic balloon devices. • Aspirin toxicity is associated with inhibition of platelet aggregation. • Snake poisoning, overdose, toxicity, and hypothermia are associated with hepatic necrosis.

assessment is necessary, and assessments should be conducted frequently.

History

The patient should be interviewed for information regarding one or more of the known etiologies for DIC, including neoplasm, recent surgery, trauma, infections, and pregnancy. Although the triggering event may not be obvious, a careful history can reveal health problems that should be addressed to enhance recovery from DIC. The nurse should ask about a history of:
• frequent nosebleeds
• bleeding gums
• vomiting blood or bloody diarrhea
• hematuria
• easy bruising
• cuts that fail to heal or stop bleeding

Pathogenesis of DIC

The pathologic processes involved in DIC are represented in this simplified illustration, which depicts the underlying mechanism as a vicious circle. Circulating thrombin activates both the coagulation cascade and fibrinolysis, leading to the paradoxical bleeding and clotting common in DIC. The coagulation factors and fibrinolytic proteins involved are included in the accompanying box.

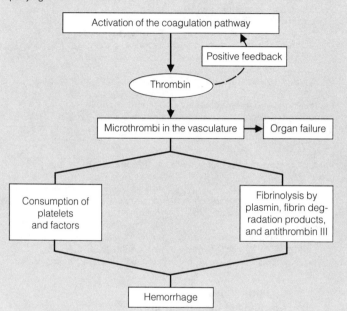

Coagulation factors

Factor I (fibrinogen) is a protein with six polypeptide chains (two alpha, two beta, and two gamma) that is produced in the liver. When acted upon by thrombin, this protein creates fibrin, which polymerizes with platelets and creates a fibrin clot.

Factor II (prothrombin), an inactive precursor to thrombin, is found in blood. An individual may lose 50% of blood volume and still clot normally. It is affected by Coumadin (warfarin sodium) and is vitamin K-dependent.

Factor III (tissue thromboplastin, tissue factor) initiates coagulation and is found on endothelium and in platelets. It is rich in lung, prostate, cerebral, and placental tissue.

Factor IV (calcium) normal values are 9 to 11 mg/ml. A person needs only a small amount for coagulation. Calcium-caused coagulopathies are rare, but can be seen in patients with massive hemorrhage or multiple myeloma.

Factor V (labile factor, accelerator globulin, proaccelerin) is found in plasma and manufactured by the

(continued)

Pathogenesis of DIC *(continued)*

liver. Consumed in coagulation, it forms prothrombin.

Factor VII (stable factor, pro-convertin) is vitamin K–dependent, manufactured by the liver, and active only with Factors III and IV.

Factor VIII (antihemophilic factor) maintains normal bleeding time. Its origin of production is unknown. About 30% to 50% of it is found in platelets. It is also activated by thrombin, creating a feedback mechanism in the coagulation system.

Factor IX (plasma thromboplastin component) is decreased by Coumadin; a lack of it causes hemophilia B. It is also vitamin K–dependent.

Factor X (Stuart-Prower factor, autoprothrombin) is a factor in the common pathway.

Factor XI (plasma thromboplastin antecedent, PTA) is a factor in the common pathway.

Factor XII (Hageman factor) is inactivated in blood by coagulation inhibitors; it has cytokine activity to maintain hemostasis.

Factor XIII (fibrin stabilizing factor) forms a covalent bond with fibrin polymers. About 50% of it is found in platelets. It stabilizes the clot.

Fibrinolytic proteins

Protein C circulates in plasma and is activated by thrombin in the presence of thrombomodulin and calcium. It degrades proteolytically Factors Va, VIII, and fibrin.

Thrombomodulin is a membrane protein, which is a cofactor in the activation of protein C. It inactivates thrombin by attracting it to antithrombin III.

Antithrombin III in combination with heparin inactivates thrombin. It also inactivates some coagulation factors.

Plasmin is an enzyme found in the plasma. When activated, it cleaves fibrin and inactivates fibrin and Factors V, VIII, and XIII.

- painful joints
- prolonged menstruation.

Physical findings

Bleeding symptomatology varies greatly but may include mucosal bleeding, spontaneous ecchymosis, petechiae, or massive GI, intracranial, or intrapulmonary bleeding (see *Manifestations of thrombosis and bleeding in DIC,* page 257).

Severe DIC can lead to hemorrhage, hypotension, shock, and death. The five systems most affected are the renal, pulmonary, cerebral, integumentary, and GI systems. Adrenal gland involvement in DIC causes adrenal hemorrhage (Waterhouse-Friderichsen syndrome), which is characterized by severe shock, cyanosis, and petechiae.

Manifestations of thrombosis and bleeding in DIC

The clinical manifestations of thrombosis and bleeding in DIC are broken down according to body system in the following chart.

Body System	Manifestations of Thrombosis	Manifestations of Bleeding
Cardiovascular	• Arrhythmias • Distal necrosis (acrocyanosis) • Absent or unequal pulses • Slow capillary refill	• Tachycardia • Hypotension • Shock • Low central venous pressure • Low pulmonary capillary wedge pressure
Pulmonary	• Hypoxia • Low lung compliance (acute respiratory distress syndrome) • Respiratory distress • Decreased breath sounds • Increased pulmonary artery (PA) pressures	• Decreased oxygenation • Decreased breath sounds or crackles • Bloody sputum • Increased airway and PA pressures
Neurologic	• Changes in strength • Aphasia • Unequal pupils	• Changes in level of consciousness • Convulsions • Coma • Increased intracranial pressure • Dilated pupils • Headache
Renal	• Increased creatinine and blood urea nitrogen levels • Decreased urine output, sometimes followed by high unconcentrated urine output (acute tubular necrosis)	• Hemorrhagic cystitis • Hematuria • Enlarged or tender kidney
Gastrointestinal	• Necrotic ulcers in mouth and around anus • Abdominal pain • Decreased bowel sounds	• Abdominal distention • Nausea • Guaiac-positive stool and emesis • Massive hemorrhage • Shock
Integumentary	• Necrosis of the extremities (acrocyanosis) • Possible odorous infection	• Oozing from 3 or more sites • Petechiae • Ecchymosis • Hemorrhagic bullae

Diagnosis

The diagnosis of DIC is primarily clinical: abrupt onset of bleeding, organ failure, and refractory shock are present with fulminant DIC. However, laboratory tests are necessary to confirm the diagnosis. Laboratory aberrations occur before clinical symptoms, and early diagnosis can prevent some of the damage.

DIC causes derangement in multiple hematologic tests, because its pathology affects all of the laboratory tests associated with the coagulation system. A typical DIC screen includes a complete blood count, partial thromboplastin time, prothrombin time, thrombin time, fibrinogen level, fibrin/fibrinogen degradation split products, and peripheral red blood smear; a newer test that assays D-dimer, a product specific to fibrinolysis, also may be used (see *Confirming DIC,* page 259).

Treatment and care

The primary treatment goal for DIC is to eliminate the triggering event or primary condition; therapy must be individualized, depending on the underlying disorder and on whether clinical manifestations are thrombotic or hemorrhagic. Other important goals include preventing and reducing hemorrhage, preventing complications, and promoting rest and comfort (see *Key nursing interventions for patients with DIC,* page 260).

Pain is present from the pressure of blood in the internal cavities, such as the abdomen, bleeding into the liver and spleen, joints, cerebral cortex, and lungs. Pain in extremities from necrosis and decreased blood flow also can be unbearable. Because heat relieves pain but also enhances bleeding, it should be used judiciously. Narcotics dull the pain, but care must be taken to prevent respiratory suppression. Morphine is the narcotic of choice because of its vasodilatory effect.

The unique combination of bleeding and random clot formation in DIC can lead to life-threatening complications, including shock, coma, acute renal failure, gangrene, and ARDS. The nurse should be vigilant of

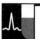

DIAGNOSTIC TESTS
Confirming DIC

The following tests may be used to help confirm DIC.

Platelet count
Platelets are consumed during thrombosis. Normal levels are 150 to 450 mm³; findings in DIC are < 150 mm³.

Activated partial thromboplastin time (APTT)
Measures intrinsic clotting; decreased when factors are consumed. Normal APTT is 25 to 35 seconds; abnormal is > 35 seconds.

Prothrombin time (PT)
PT is consumed with decreasing thrombin and fibrinogen levels; it measures extrinsic pathway. Abnormal in 90% of patient with DIC. Normal PT is 11 to 15 seconds; abnormal is > 15 seconds.

Thrombin time
Prolonged time can measure decreased fibrinogen. Normal time is 9 to 13 seconds ± 2 seconds; abnormal is > 15 seconds.

Fibrinogen
Consumed in clot formation; may be normal if underlying disease (hepatitis or pregnancy) elevates it. Normal level is 200 to 400 mg/dl; abnormal is < 200 mg/dl.

Fibrin degradation products (FDPs)
Excess fibrin clots are broken down by plasmin and produce increased FDPs. Normal level is < 10 g/ml; abnormal is > 10 g/ml.

D-dimer
A specific fibrin split product. Normal level is < 200 ng/ml; abnormal is > 200 ng/ml.

Antithrombin III
Tests functionality of the enzyme. Normal levels are 80% to 120%; abnormal are < 80%.

Peripheral blood smear
Red blood cells are sheared when passing multiple fibrin clots. Normal smear shows absence of schistocytes; abnormal smear shows schistocytes.

complications and knowledgeable about their causes and implications (see *Complications of DIC*, page 261).

Aggressive primary treatment
Primary treatment depends on the etiology. Sometimes surgery can remove the trigger (as in neoplasm or retained dead fetus), and antibiotics can destroy the insult of bacteria. Shock is treated to decrease activation of the coagulation system by the release of these procoagulants, acidosis hypotension, and hypoxia. Once the primary etiology is removed, a normal liver can

ESSENTIAL ELEMENTS

Key nursing interventions for patients with DIC

This flowchart highlights key interventions for a patient with DIC.

Maintain hemostasis

Prevent and reduce tissue ischemia

- Maintain vascular volume.
- —Monitor hemoglobin.
- —Monitor peripheral pulses.
- —Assess for changes in vital signs, including central venous and pulmonary artery pressures.
- —Document intake and output; notify physician if urine output is < 30 ml/hour.
- —Monitor weight and abdominal girth daily.
- —Assess distal pulses and perfusion, and document any acrocyanosis.
- Maintain oxygenation.
- —Promote rest and relaxation by administering anxiolytics as ordered.
- —Monitor level of consciousness, anxiety, and restlessness.
- —Assess breath sounds and respiratory distress every 4 hours; monitor oxygen saturation or ABG levels as needed.
- —Administer diuretics as ordered.
- —Administer oxygen as ordered; if necessary, assist during intubation
- —Monitor airway and cuff pressures.
- —Monitor continuous ECG for hypoxic arrhythmias.
- —Monitor daily blood urea nitrogen and creatinine levels.
- Counteract ischemic events due to immobility.

Minimize bleeding

- Avoid invasive procedures.
- —Use oxygen saturation monitor to assess oxygenation after baseline ABG levels.
- —Use a nasopharyngeal airway if NG suction is needed.
- —Organize blood sampling to prevent unnecessary sticks.
- —Do not administer enemas or suppositories; start bowel regimen.
- —Avoid I.M. and S.C. injections and rectal temperatures.
- Replenish lost blood products.
- —Monitor platelet counts and coagulation times; maintain a clot in the blood bank.
- —Administer packed RBCs, platelets, fresh frozen plasma, and cryoprecipitate as ordered.
- —Test all urine, stool, emesis, and secretions for heme.
- Prevent injuries likely to induce bleeding.
- —Use cuff pressures sparingly.
- —Monitor platelet counts and coagulation times before invasive procedures.
- —Lubricate skin, and help patient perform gentle mouth care every 1 to 2 hours.
- —Suction with care.
- Stop bleeding.
- —Apply pressure on I.V. sites, and administer topical hemostatics as ordered.
- —Administer drugs, such as heparin and Amicar (epsilon-aminocaproic acid), as ordered.

Complications of DIC

The causes and assessment findings for some of the most common life-threatening complications of DIC are listed below.

Complication	DIC-Related Causes	Assessment Findings
Hypovolemic shock	• Hemorrhage (GI, pulmonary, cerebral)	• Decreased hematocrit and hemoglobin • Tachycardia and decreased blood pressures • Frank blood in emesis and stool • Abdominal distention, decreased bowel signs • Change in level of consciousness and convulsions • Thready pulses, flat neck veins, dry mucosal membranes • Crackles and decreased lung compliance
Acute renal failure	• Microthrombi deposition in the renal capillaries • Hypoperfusion due to hemorrhage	• Urine output < 30 ml/hour • Increased blood urea nitrogen level > 21 and creatinine level < 1.3 • Acute tubular necrosis, large amounts of dilute urine after fluid resuscitation • Electrolyte disorders
Infection	• Tissue hypoxia from fibrin deposition especially in the extremities, leading to anaerobic bacteria growth	• Black extremities, especially tips of toes and fingers • Malodorous secretions from necrotic skin
Acute respiratory distress syndrome	• Microthrombi deposition in the lung leading to shunting • Pulmonary hemorrhage	• Shortness of breath • Ventilation-perfusion mismatches • Low lung compliance • Blood-tinged sputum • Crepitus • Tension pneumothorax

replenish clotting factors within 24 to 48 hours. The success of treatment strongly depends on elimination of the underlying cause.

Appropriate nursing interventions are listed below:

• Treat the underlying cause using aggressive nursing measures.
• Assist with surgical procedures, if necessary.
• Administer antibiotics, as ordered.
• Administer blood products and fluids, as ordered.
• Monitor the patient continuously.

Hemorrhage control and prevention

Coagulation components are replaced with platelets, packed RBCs, fresh frozen plasma (FFP), cryoprecipitate, antithrombin III, and volume expanders. The prothrombin time is followed to assess efficacy of clotting factor replenishment. Complete blood counts and coagulation times are monitored at least daily. A clot should be maintained in the blood bank at all times. Life-threatening hemorrhage must be prevented so the primary disease can be treated.

Transfusion reactions in these patients are dramatically problematic, since the lysis of RBCs is an etiology for DIC and increases risk of hemorrhage.

The following nursing interventions are necessary:
• Infuse platelets to plug bleeding sites and replace those consumed.
• Infuse packed RBCs to replace those lost in bleeding.
• Infuse FFP to replace lost clotting factors and antithrombin III.
• Administer cryoprecipitate to replace fibrinogen, antithrombin III, Factor VIII, Factor XIII, and protein C.
• Monitor for transfusion reactions.

Drug therapy

Drug therapy varies, depending on the primary cause of DIC. Commonly used drugs include heparin, low-molecular-weight heparin, epsilon-aminocaproic acid, antithrombin III, vitamin K, and gabexate mesilate.

Heparin therapy increases the inactivation of thrombin, which decreases thrombin's concentration in blood and decreases fibrinogen breakdown and fibrin deposition. Heparin also minimizes platelet aggregation, which decreases deposition of thrombi in the microvasculature. Heparin's efficacy in DIC is documented only anecdotally. It is contraindicated in patients with postoperative, GI, or central nervous system bleeding and is of no benefit in sepsis. It is used more often when thrombotic symptoms of DIC predominate.

Low-molecular-weight heparin inhibits Factor Xa and thrombin. This type of heparin has displayed some efficacy in DIC with less bleeding side effects, according to some studies. Epsilon-aminocaproic acid (Amicar) maintains thrombi in the vasculature and slows their breakdown. It is often given with concurrent heparin therapy to prevent hemorrhage.

Antithrombin III is used to prevent thrombotic complications. It does this by inhibiting the amount of thrombin. Vitamin K, which is consumed in DIC and not released in liver failure, is necessary for coagulation reactions. Antibiotics also affect vitamin K production. Gabexate mesilate inhibits thrombin and has been effective in clinical trials. Topical therapy also is commonly used to manage bleeding on the skin.

Prognosis

DIC is a life-threatening disease with a mortality rate between 50% and 90%, depending on the primary underlying disorder. For example, in sepsis the development of DIC indicates a mortality rate greater than 80%.

Discharge planning

Discharge planning is often not an option with these patients. If the patient recovers from the acute event, there are long-term implications associated with the hemorrhage, shock, and organ damage associated with clot formation. Some common deficits include:
• mental changes from neuronal damage due to a hypoxic event, cerebral bleeding, or cerebral clots
• blindness from retinal hemorrhage
• respiratory compromise due to pulmonary fibrosis from bleeding or ARDS

- chronic renal failure due to damage to the kidneys from microthrombi and hypoperfusion
- colostomy drainage from necrotic bowel resection
- loss of limb due to necrosis.

Helping the family and the patient cope with these deficits is quite a challenge. Discharge planning must be tailored to fit the patient's needs. Once the patient leaves the intensive care unit, rehabilitation may be long, and a full recovery may not be possible.

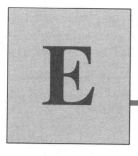

Electrolyte imbalances

Electrolytes play a vital role in maintaining electro-chemical and fluid balance within the body. Any alter-ation in the homeostasis of major electrolytes (sodium, potassium, calcium, magnesium, phosphorus, and phosphates) can disrupt normal bodily functions at the cellular, tissue, or organ level. Sodium and calcium are primarily extracellular electrolytes; potassium, magne-sium, and phosphates are primarily intracellular elec-trolytes (see *Plasma and intracellular levels of major electrolytes,* page 266).

The critical care nurse is constantly exposed to pa-tients with serious illnesses affecting more than one body system. Knowledge of which electrolytes can be affected by various disorders and an ability to quickly identify signs and symptoms of electrolyte imbalance can ensure prompt treatment, thereby circumventing more serious complications. (For a discussion of the effects of the major electrolytes, see *Major electrolytes: Normal function and pathophysiologic effects,* pages 268 to 273.)

Pathophysiology

Electrolytes are necessary to ensure the proper function of adenosine triphosphate (ATP), calcium-phosphorus bone matrix, cell wall sodium-potassium pumps, cardi-

Plasma and intracellular levels of major electrolytes

Electrolytes are measured by their combining power. In the United States, milliequivalents/liter (mEq/liter) traditionally have been the measurement of choice. The international unit (IU) of measure is provided in millimoles/liter (mmol/liter). Grams/liter is also stated as milligrams/liter (mg/liter) and milligrams/dilution (mg/dl or mg%). Dilution refers to 100 ml of solution. The following table compares the normal plasma and intracellular levels of the major electrolytes, in both traditional and IU measures. Note: Phosphoric compounds have different valences depending on their chemical composition. The phosphates measured in this table are primarily valence 2. Phospholipids are expressed in g% (g/dl) because of their ill-defined composition.

	Traditional		International	
Electrolyte	Plasma concentration	Intracellular concentration	Plasma concentration	Intracellular concentration
Potassium	4.2 mEq/liter	140 mEq/liter	4.2 mOsm/liter	140 mOsm/liter
Sodium	140 mEq/liter	10 mEq/liter	140 mOsm/liter	10 mOsm/liter
Calcium	5 mEq/liter	< 1 mEq/liter	2.5 mOsm/liter	< 1 mOsm/liter
Magnesium	3 mEq/liter	58 mEq/liter	1.5 mOsm/liter	30 mOsm/liter
Phosphates	4 mEq/liter	75 mEq/liter	2 mOsm/liter	37 mOsm/liter
Phospholipids	0.5 g%	2 to 95 g%	Not applicable	Not applicable

ac slow calcium channels, neuromuscular integration affecting the excitability of muscle cells, and acid-base balance. Alterations in sodium, potassium, calcium, and magnesium can affect muscle contraction and may result in cardiac arrhythmias, GI disturbances, central nervous system (CNS) changes, and altered muscle reflexes. Acid-base disturbances affect the flow of calcium, phosphorus, and potassium, which shift in response to hydrogen. Such disturbances may affect respiration, cardiac contraction, bone structure, reflexes, GI tract functioning, and the neurologic system.

One of the biochemical laws that affects electrolytes is the maintenance of electrical neutrality. Substances tend to combine in such a way that they cancel opposite charges. Thus, every cation (positively charged ion) has an anion (negatively charged ion) counterpart. Sodium, potassium, calcium, and magnesium are cations, whereas chloride, phosphate, and bicarbonate are anions. An action involving the active transport of one electrolyte may also take along its electrochemical counterpart. To maintain electrical neutrality, sodium is often coupled with chloride, phosphate, or bicarbonate.

Renal intrinsic mechanisms

Several mechanisms intrinsic to the kidney that are involved in the pathology of electrolyte balance and imbalance are discussed below.

Glomerular filtration rate (GFR), the volume of blood delivered to the glomerulus, is perhaps the chief electrolyte-altering mechanism intrinsic to the kidney. The amount of filtrate passed into the nephron's proximal tubular system depends on the ability of the glomerulus to maintain glomerular blood pressure close to 60 mm Hg. When cardiac output (CO) is low, constriction of the efferent arteriole is stimulated; conversely, a high CO stimulates constriction of the afferent arteriole. In each instance, the goal is to maintain the glomerular blood pressure at around 60 mm Hg. (Systemic systolic blood pressure may change 75 to 160 mm Hg with very little change in glomerular pressure and, subsequently, GFR.)

The tubuloglomerular feedback (TGF) mechanism involves autoregulation of GFR by rapid feedback between the distal tubules (upper end of the loop of Henle) and the afferent and efferent arterioles. The composition and volume of the tubular filtrate signal an increase in GFR by afferent arteriolar dilatation and

(Text continues on page 274.)

Major electrolytes: Normal function and pathophysiologic effects

The following chart highlights the normal function of the major electrolytes and identifies the underlying causes and assessment findings of electrolyte imbalances.

Electrolyte	Function	Imbalance
Sodium	Primary extracellular fluid cation that maintains fluid balance between intracellular and extracellular compartments and contributes to the contraction of soft tissue. Sodium is conserved in the kidney by reabsorption along all sections of the nephron. It is prominent in maintaining a negative electrical gradient across the cell wall.	Hypernatremia (Free loss of water in excess of sodium results in shrinkage of cells and excitation of sodium-potassium pump.)
		Hyponatremia (Retention of free water or excessive loss of sodium causes sodium to shift into cells, resulting in cellular swelling and a sluggish sodium-potassium pump.)
Potassium	Primary intracellular cation that has increased permeability across the cell wall. Potassium, which depends on sodium for extracellular fluid balance, facilitates contraction of skeletal and smooth muscles, including myocardial contraction. It figures prominently in nerve impulse conduction, acid-base balance, enzyme action, and cell membrane function. The kidney reabsorbs	Hyperkalemia (Results from reduced excretion of potassium by the kidneys or from failure to excrete excessive amounts of potassium infused I.V. or administered orally.)

Underlying Causes	Assessment Findings
• Watery diarrhea • High fever • Severe burns • Osmotic diuresis • Diabetes insipidus • Hypertonic parenteral intake • Hyperaldosteronism • Increased steroid administration • Cushing's syndrome	• Dehydration • Dry, sticky mucous membranes; dry, rough, red tongue • Thirst • Poor skin turgor • Weight loss • Low blood pressure • Tachycardia • Low-grade fever • Impaired cognition, disorientation, confusion • Hallucinations • Lethargy, coma, seizures • Hyperactive deep tendon reflexes • Oliguria
• Water intoxication • Burns • Diarrhea • Vomiting • Gastric suctioning or lavage • Hypothyroidism • Hypoaldosteronism • Cystic fibrosis • Oxytocin-induced labor • Therapy with nonsteroidal anti-inflammatory drugs • Alcoholism • Renal failure • Prolonged diuretic therapy	• Signs of congestive heart failure • Possible weight changes • Vomiting • Diarrhea • Headaches • Confusion, convulsions, coma • Muscle cramps, twitching • Possible high or low urine sodium and potassium levels • Hyperglycemia or hyperlipidemia (possible with pseudohyponatremia)
• Renal failure • Renal conservation of potassium • Acidosis • Cellular destruction • Hypoaldosteronism • Burns • Trauma • Catabolic states • Administration of old blood • Use of potassium-sparing diuretics	• Bradycardia • Low cardiac output • Weakness, lethargy • Confusion

(continued)

Major electrolytes: Normal function and pathophysiologic effects *(continued)*

Electrolyte	Function	Imbalance
Potassium *(continued)*	potassium in the proximal tubules and the descending loop of Henle, then secretes it in the distal tubules.	Hypokalemia (Results from excessive loss of potassium.)
Calcium	Plays an important role in cell permeability, tissue membrane firing, bone structure, blood coagulation and activation of complement, nerve impulse transmission, and normal muscle contraction. Primarily an extracellular ion, calcium is stored in great quantities in bone. It is integral to proper functioning of slow cardiac calcium channels.	Hypercalcemia (Results from increased bone reabsorption.)
		Hypocalcemia (Results from inadequate calcium intake or from impaired GI absorption or renal reabsorption of calcium.)
Magnesium	Essential for neuromuscular integration, enzyme systems, bone structure, and intracellular biochemical processes. Magnesium levels are regulated by renal reabsorption and GI absorption. Magnesium plasma levels, parathyroid hormone, vitamin D, thyrocalcitonin, lactose, sodium, and fluid	Hypermagnesemia (Results from renal failure and excessive magnesium intake.)

Underlying Causes	Assessment Findings
• Renal potassium wasting • Alkalosis • GI losses • Insufficient potassium intake • Parenteral support • Hyperinsulinemia • Hyperaldosteronism • Alcoholism • Prolonged diuretic therapy	• Tachycardia • Tremors, spasms • Cramping • Nausea and vomiting • Drowsiness
• Hypophosphatemia • Calcium-based phosphate binders • Hyperparathyroidism • Thyrotoxicosis • Prolonged inactivity • Metastatic carcinoma • Renal tubular acidosis • Use of thiazide diuretics	• Nervous system depression (lethargy, weakness) • Spastic, less effective heart contractions (tachycardia, decreased cardiac output) • Vasoconstriction of smooth muscle • Dehydration • Constipation • Nausea and vomiting • Polyuria • Personality changes
• Alkalosis • Hyperphosphatemia • Hypomagnesemia • Calcium and vitamin D deficiencies • Hypoparathyroidism • Parathyroidectomy • Acute pancreatitis • Autoimmune disorders • Hypoalbuminemia • Administration of large amounts of citrated blood • Renal failure	• Spasms, muscle cramps • Tetany • Bradycardia • Digital and perioral paresthesias • Seizures • Hyperactive reflexes • Positive Trousseau's and Chvostek's signs
• Prolonged parenteral and GI intake • Diabetic ketoacidosis • Hypoadrenalism • Hard water dialysis • Overuse of magnesium-containing antacids • Severe dehydration • Overdose of magnesium salts	• Hypotension • Bradycardia • Diffuse vasodilation • Heart block or cardiac arrest (with high magnesium levels) • Diminished deep tendon reflexes • Weakness, flaccid paralysis • Respiratory muscle paralysis (with *(continued)*

Major electrolytes: Normal function and pathophysiologic effect *(continued)*

Electrolyte	Function	Imbalance
Magnesium *(continued)*	balance affect magnesium absorption and reabsorption.	Hypermagnesemia *(continued)*
		Hypomagnesemia (Results from prolonged diuretic therapy, prolonged total parenteral nutrition without magnesium, low GI intake, and excessive calcium and vitamin D intake.)
Phosphorus	Primary intracellular anion and ATP building block that participates in renal acid-base buffering and is important in carbohydrate, protein, and lipid metabolism; it promotes oxygen release to the cells through 2,3-DPG. Phosphorus levels are maintained through diet, GI absorption, and renal regulation. Phosphorus has an inverse relationship with calcium but is similar to it in that both are stored in bone.	Hyperphosphatemia (Results from the kidneys' inability to excrete phosphorus. Contributing factors include all conditions that participate in phosphorus loading by intake, cellular release, or renal retention.)
		Hypophosphatemia (Results from malabsorption or renal wasting.)

Underlying Causes	Assessment Findings
	high magnesium levels) • Drowsiness, confusion • Possible coma
• Chronic alcoholism • Chronic diarrhea • Prolonged nasogastric suction • Malnutrition • Malabsorption • Ulcerative colitis • Hypoparathyroidism • Hypoaldosteronism • High steroid doses • Chemotherapy	• Tachycardia • Nausea • Anorexia • Leg and foot cramps • Chvostek's sign • Tremors • Tetany • Confusion, delusions • Seizures • Hypotension resulting from a sustained arrhythmia producing low cardiac output
• Rhabdomyolysis • Use of cytotoxic drugs • Hypoparathyroidism • Severe trauma • Acidosis	• Seizures • Muscle spasms or cramps • Tetany • Paresthesias • Soft tissue calcification • Oliguria • Conjunctivitis • Papular eruptions • Irregular heart rate
• Malabsorption syndromes • Prolonged parenteral nutrition without phosphorus • Prolonged use of thiazide diuretics • Prolonged diabetic ketoacidosis • Respiratory alkalosis • Glucose infusions • Hyperparathyroidism • Aldosteronism	• Anorexia • Memory loss • Muscle and bone pain, fractures • Chest pain • Apprehension • Paresthesias • Weakness or tremor in speaking voice and hand grasp • Confusion to coma • Seizures • Bruises and bleeding

efferent arteriolar constriction. Hyponatremia and hypernatremia often trigger this mechanism, causing appropriate and inappropriate regulation by the kidney.

The renin-angiotensin-aldosterone (RAA) mechanism, another mechanism affecting GFR, operates within the TGF mechanism that releases renin from the juxtaglomerular apparatus. The endproduct of this event is the conversion of angiotensin I to angiotensin II in the lungs and the release of aldosterone by the adrenal glands. Angiotensin II, one of the most powerful vasoconstrictors known, elevates both glomerular and systemic blood pressure. RAA hypertensive crisis may be triggered by hypovolemia, low CO, or renal artery stenosis. RAA causes the kidney to markedly reabsorb water, sodium, chloride, potassium, and other substances via efferent arteriolar resistance. Angiotensin also stimulates the secretion of aldosterone, which causes additional retention of sodium and chloride ions from the distal segments of the nephron.

Inflammation within the kidney, another intrinsic mechanism, affects the integrity of the cellular structure, the cell's ability to carry on normal transport, and intracellular metabolism. It may be triggered by antigens, autoimmune disorders, trauma, heat, or any phenomenon that injures the affected area. Dramatic secondary changes occur in the tissue and may include:
• vasodilation of the local vessels and increased permeability of local capillaries leaking large quantities of fluid into interstitial spaces
• clotting of interstitial fluid due to excessive amounts of fibrinogen and other proteins leaking from the capillaries
• swelling of the cells
• walling off of the affected area by the blood-clotting system.

The immune system is activated with macrophages, neutrophils, and monocytes that engage in the cleanup, devouring destroyed and living tissue. Pus eventually forms in the cavity created by the fluid and ingested tissue. If this process engulfs any part of the nephron, normal function ceases, and permanent damage (including necrosis and scar tissue formation) may ensue. If more than 90% of the nephrons are destroyed, electrolyte balance probably will be affected, as will other renal-dependent functions, such as acid-base balance, fluid balance, waste removal, blood pressure control, bone deposition, and red blood cell production.

Renal extrinsic mechanisms

Other electrolyte-altering mechanisms that are extrinsic to the kidney may target the kidney as their primary site of action or influence the way the kidney functions.

Two separate systems—the antidiuretic hormone (ADH)–thirst mechanism and the osmosodium-receptor-antidiuretic system—work together to regulate extracellular fluid volume, osmolarity, and thus sodium concentration. The ADH-thirst mechanism is the major feedback system for control of sodium concentration and adequate fluid balance. ADH (also called arginine vasopressin) causes the kidneys to retain water and is primarily stimulated by low blood pressure at the atrial stretch receptors. In high concentrations, it causes vasoconstriction and raises the blood pressure systemically. The thirst mechanism, although ill defined, is important for regulating body water and sodium, as are the osmoreceptors of the hypothalamus. A rise in the sodium level of 2 mEq/liter above baseline triggers thirst. When both thirst and the ADH system fail, the body becomes hypernatremic and dehydrated.

Aldosterone, the primary mineralocorticoid secreted by the adrenal cortex, affects sodium and water retention and potassium excretion in the distal tubules of the kidney. The primary function of aldosterone is to reabsorb sodium and excrete potassium. Potassium concentration depends on a direct aldosterone feedback mechanism that controls potassium levels within tenths of a point, even when intake varies as much as sevenfold. ADH and thirst can override aldosterone control of extracellular fluid sodium concentration during dehydration, salt loading, and aldosteronism.

Two pathological states that are responsible for inadequate potassium regulation are primary aldosteronism and Addison's disease. In primary aldosteronism, a tumor in the adrenal glands secretes large quantities of aldosterone. Potassium may become depleted to the point of impaired nerve conduction and subsequent paralysis, cardiac arrhythmias, and death. In Addison's disease, the adrenal glands have been destroyed by radiation, trauma, surgery, or a pathological process, and extracellular fluid potassium frequently rises to twice the normal level, leading to cardiac arrest in many patients.

Atrial natriuretic peptides (ANPs) are hormone-like substances found in the cell walls of the cardiac atria, especially the right atrium. When released into the circulation, they increase the renal excretion of sodium and water 3 to 10 times the normal levels. ANPs are part of a natriuretic (sodium uresis) vasodilatory system that opposes the vasoconstricting effects and subsequent water and electrolyte reabsorption of RAA and catecholamines. They are also short-acting (active from hours to days) and work to rid the body of extra fluid and salt and return the blood volume to normal.

The baroreceptor mechanism involves baroreceptors located in vessel walls (cardiac atria, pulmonary vasculature, aorta, carotid, and renal arteries), which are sensory nerve endings stimulated by changes in pressure. This feedback mechanism functions best between 60 and 200 mm Hg, where it is most needed. Rapid control of arterial blood pressure is mediated by baroreceptor-autonomic and CNS ischemic mechanisms that are activated within seconds and that lose their effectiveness within hours or days. Intermediate control is mediated by norepinephrine and epinephrine, vasopressin (ADH), renin and angiotensin, and capillary shifting of fluid in or out of tissue beds—a process that becomes fully active within 20 minutes. Long-term control is mediated by RAA, ADH, thirst, and TGF—a process that is activated within hours.

Another extrinsic renal mechanism involves diuretics, catecholamines, and osmolytes. Generally, the more blood the kidney receives, the greater the diuresis. Cardiac diuretics, hematopiesic (blood pressure–raising) diuretics, and catecholamines deliver greater blood pressure to the kidney by increasing CO or by raising systemic blood pressure. Loop diuretics, thiazide diuretics, potassium-sparing diuretics, osmotic diuretics, and osmolytes act by inhibiting or enhancing the absorption or secretion of potassium, sodium, magnesium, chloride, calcium, and phosphorus in the kidney. In a patient receiving maximum doses of vasoactive drugs, the kidney's blood supply may be compromised, resulting in lower urine output.

Clinical assessment

Assessment of a patient with suspected electrolyte imbalance requires a comprehensive review of the patient's overall condition. Typically, the patient has one or more of the following predisposing factors:
- age under 6 or over 60
- parenteral nutrition for more than 1 week
- gastric suction for several days
- multiple trauma and multiple blood transfusions
- prolonged nausea and vomiting, diarrhea, or dehydration
- adrenal disorder
- alcoholism
- autoimmune disorder
- cancer
- cystic fibrosis
- diabetes
- eating disorder
- parathyroid disorder
- prolonged diuretic therapy
- prolonged therapy with nonsteroidal anti-inflammatory drugs
- renal failure.

Assessment begins with addressing emergency conditions first, then proceeding to less acute but important factors that affect the patient's long-term quality of life. The nurse should evaluate the following conditions:

• Life-threatening conditions: Monitor heart rhythm; airway; breathing; lung sounds; presence of hemorrhage; presence of seizures; status of serum electrolyte levels, acid-base levels, and osmolality; and fluid status by checking central venous pressure, peripheral arterial pressure, CO, and peripheral perfusion.

• Acute conditions: Assess level of consciousness, cognition, muscular response and reflexes, urine output, fever, sensation, nausea and vomiting, and diarrhea.

• Chronic conditions: Assess for discomfort (headache), paresthesias, activity intolerance, cognitive impairment, eating disorders (anorexia), long-standing diarrhea, depression, poor adjustment to chronic disease, laxative abuse, diuretic abuse, enema abuse, alcohol abuse, and poor diabetic control.

(See *Major electrolytes: Normal function and pathophysiologic effects,* pages 268 to 273, for assessment findings associated with individual electrolyte imbalances.)

Diagnosis

Any patient in the critical care setting is at risk for electrolyte abnormalities. The diagnosis of electrolyte imbalances is straightforward in that there are specific laboratory ranges for normal values. The nurse's objective is to monitor signs and symptoms of electrolyte trends and patient response to treatment. Early diagnosis and prompt treatment are essential to prevent the more serious consequences of electrolyte disorders, which can include life-threatening arrhythmias (see *ECG changes related to electrolyte imbalances,* page 279).

Diagnostic levels for electrolyte imbalances are listed below:

• Hypernatremia: Indicated by a serum sodium level greater than 150 mEq/liter. Urine sodium may be greater than 20 mEq/liter or less than 10 mEq/liter, depending

ECG changes related to electrolyte imbalances

Electrolyte imbalances produce characteristic ECG changes that can aid in early identification and treatment. The ECG strips shown here indicate arrhythmias.

Potassium
Hyperkalemia
Produces tented T-waves, wide QRS complexes, long PR intervals, depressed ST segments, short QT intervals, and bradycardia.

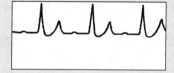

Hypokalemia
Produces flattened T-waves, prominent U-waves, and depressed ST segments on ECG. Premature atrial contractions and premature ventricular contractions are also possible.

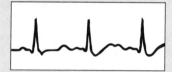

Calcium
Hypercalcemia
Produces short QT intervals and short ST segments. Supraventricular tachycardia, heart block, ventricular tachycardia, and fibrillation (excited muscle) are also possible.

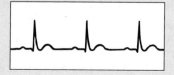

Hypocalcemia
Produces prolonged QT intervals and prolonged ST segments (flaccid muscle).

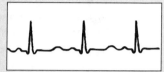

Magnesium
Hypermagnesemia
Produces prolonged PR intervals, wide QRS complexes, prolonged QT intervals, and elevated T-waves. Heart block and asystole are also possible.

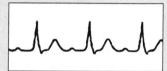

Hypomagnesemia
Produces prolonged PR intervals, prolonged QT intervals, wide QRS complexes, depressed ST segments, and inverted T-waves (often accompanies digitalis toxicity).

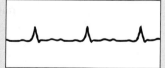

on the cause (salt loading, free-water diuresis, or sodium-wasting diuresis) of hypernatremia; serum osmolality may be greater than 295 mOsm/kg. ECG changes typically occur secondary to vascular collapse, usually when the serum sodium level exceeds 160 mEq/liter.

• Hyponatremia: Indicated by a serum sodium level less than 135 mEq/liter, although severe symptoms do not occur above 120 mEq/liter. Serum osmolality may be greater than 300 mOsm/kg with hyperglycemia and hyperlipidemia or normal (285 to 295 mOsm/kg). Serum osmolality is typically low (< 285 mOsm/kg) in true hyponatremia and usually is associated with hypovolemic states, congestive heart failure, autonomous ADH release, and salt depletion in the critical care setting (from loss of sodium with hypotonic replacement). Urine sodium levels may be high, low, or normal, depending on the cause of the condition. ECG changes typically occur secondary to total vascular collapse.

• Hyperkalemia: Indicated by a serum potassium level greater than 5.5 mEq/liter and an arterial hydrogen ion concentration (pH) less than 7.35.

• Hypokalemia: Manifested by a serum potassium level less than 3.5 mEq/liter, a serum pH greater than 7.4 (due to bicarbonate elevations), a urine specific gravity less than 1.010, and a slightly elevated serum glucose level.

• Hypercalcemia: Indicated by a serum calcium level greater than 10.5 mg/dl. Severe symptoms may occur with levels that exceed 15 mg/dl. May accompany pathologic bone fractures confirmed by X-ray, a positive Sulkowitch urine (heavy precipitation). Digitalis toxicity may also occur.

• Hypocalcemia: Indicated by a serum calcium level less than 8.5 mg/dl and an ionized calcium level less than 4 mg/dl. The patient may also have a positive Sulkowitch urine (light precipitation) and prolonged prothrombin time and partial thromboplastin time.

• Hypermagnesemia: Indicated by a serum magnesium level greater than 3 mEq/liter.

• Hypomagnesemia: Indicated by a serum magnesium level less than 1.5 mEq/liter. Clinical symptoms occur

with levels less than 1 mEq/liter. May accompany hypercalcemia, hypokalemia, or hypophosphatemia. Hypomagnesemia may be related to digitalis toxicity.
• Hyperphosphatemia: Indicated by a serum phosphorus level greater than 4.5 mg/dl and a serum calcium level less than 8.5 mg/dl. Chronic elevated phosphorus levels will lead to elevated parathyroid hormone levels. Usually associated with hypocalcemia. ECG changes typically occur secondary to low calcium levels.
• Hypophosphatemia: Indicated by a serum phosphorus level less than 2.5 mg/dl, hypercalciuria, and elevated creatine phosphokinase (when phosphorus is 1 mg/dl for a day or longer). Severe hypophosphatemia may cause heart failure. It often is associated with hypokalemia, hypomagnesemia, and hypercalcemia.

Treatment and care
A sudden, significant change in electrolyte values or a slow, continuous, significant change requires prompt diagnosis and treatment. A significant change is one in which the patient ceases to compensate for electrolyte shifts and begins to demonstrate physical responses.

Treatment and care of the patient with an electrolyte imbalance generally focuses on:
• stabilizing the patient's life-threatening conditions
• assessing laboratory values and signs and symptoms
• administering or restricting fluids, electrolytes, diuretics, insulin, exchange resins, laxatives, and steroids
• instituting dietary adjustments
• treating the underlying cause
• monitoring the patient's response to treatment.

For treatments and nursing interventions specific to each electrolyte imbalance, see *Treating electrolyte imbalances,* pages 283 to 287.

Prognosis
The prognosis for patients with electrolyte imbalances depends on successful management of the underlying
(Text continues on page 286.)

Treating electrolyte imbalances

The following treatments and nursing considerations are crucial to successful management of electrolyte imbalances. Note that treatment of the underlying cause is often the most beneficial action and that slow correction is generally the rule.

Disorder	Treatment
Hypernatremia	• For acute development, lower plasma level to no faster than 2 mEq/liter/hour (prevents cerebral edema). Rule of thumb is slow correction; however, may correct faster for first half of treatment. • Administer hypotonic and isotonic saline treatment of choice. Dextrose 5% in water (D5W) may be used cautiously only with free-water loss and true sodium overload (dehydration). • May use loop diuretics to eliminate sodium.
Hyponatremia	• Treat underlying cause. • For sodium levels < 120 mEq/liter, correct with 3% or 5% saline solution at the rate of 2 mEq/liter/hour. Correction is slowed when plasma levels reach 125 mEq/liter. • Diuretics may be added or discontinued depending on the need for sodium conservation or free-water loss. • Restrict fluid intake.
Hyperkalemia	• Treat underlying cause. • Administer the following treatments: dextrose 10% with insulin, Kayexalate (sodium polystyrene sulfonate) (orally or enema), dialysis, hemofiltration (continuous venovenous hemodiafiltration, continuous arteriovenous hemodiafiltration), I.V. calcium (if myocardium is depressed), and sodium bicarbonate (if acidotic).
Hypokalemia	• Treat underlying cause. • Administer oral, parenteral, or dialysis supplementation of potassium. • Provide conservative insulin therapy until potassium level is normal (slows cellular uptake of potassium). • Reduce or stop potassium-wasting diuretics. • Correct alkalosis.

Nursing Intervention

- Monitor intake and output, urine sodium levels, and daily weights.
- Monitor for signs and symptoms of hypotension.
- Monitor level of consciousness, central nervous system irritability, and skin integrity.
- Evaluate response to I.V. fluids and regulate as necessary.
- Provide a quiet environment.
- Institute necessary accident and seizure precautions.
- Provide frequent oral care.

- Restrict fluids.
- Institute necessary accident and seizure precautions.
- Administer I.V. fluids cautiously.
- Monitor intake and output, and daily weights.
- Monitor vital signs for signs of fluid overload or aspiration.
- Maintain skin integrity; assess edema and pressure points.
- Monitor plasma sodium level and assess for hypokalemia (develops with loop diuretics).

- Avoid rapid infusion of I.V. solutions containing potassium; use a volumetric infusion pump whenever possible.
- Monitor ECG for hyperkalemia.
- Monitor vital signs and blood sugar levels.
- Assess for weakness, drowsiness, and confusion.
- Ensure that urine output is > 30 ml/hour before giving I.V. potassium in normokalemic patients.
- Be prepared to give calcium I.V. (watch for digitalis toxicity), dextrose 10% with insulin I.V., $NaHCO_3^-$ I.V., Kayexalate P.O., or enema (if not excreted in 24 hours, give soapsuds enema). Patient may need emergency dialysis.
- Repeat sample hyperkalemic blood obtained with tight tourniquet, rapid aspiration, or delayed (> 30 minute) testing. All of these cause hemolysis.

- Monitor ECG for hypokalemic changes; consult physician about reducing digitalis.
- Caution patient about taking potassium-wasting diuretics.
- Monitor intake and output and vital signs; ensure that urine potassium loss does not exceed 10 mEq/liter.
- Assess for alkalosis, decreased cardiac output, congestive heart failure (CHF), and postural hypotension.
- Administer I.V. potassium cautiously; assess site for pain and inflammation; dilute, never give bolus; give through two sites if necessary.
- Assess for muscle weakness frequently.
- Have emergency equipment ready if potassium level is < 3 mEq/liter.

(continued)

Treating electrolyte imbalances *(continued)*

Disorder	Treatment
Hypercalce-mia	• Treat underlying cause. • The following treatments may be ordered: —I.V. 0.9% or 0.45% normal saline solution, 200 to 500 ml/hour (6 to 12 liters in 24 hours if renal function is good) —D_5W if patient has CHF or hypernatremia —loop diuretics every 4 to 6 hours to prevent fluid overload to excrete calcium —calcitonin 4 IU/kg S.C. or I.M. every 6 hours to lower plasma calcium levels —phosphate salts if phosphate level is low —glucocorticoids to reduce GI uptake and bone resorption —low calcium hemodialysis —parathyroidectomy.
Hypocalce-mia	• Treat underlying cause. • Give P.O. or I.V. calcium and vitamin D (I.V. calcium not to exceed 50 mg/minute. A total dose of 2 g not to be exceeded without repeating calcium level.)
Hypermagne-semia	• Treat underlying cause. • Treatments may include: —volume expansion if dehydrated —lowering magnesium intake (diet, medications) —calcium administration in emergency (magnesium antagonist).
Hypomagne-semia	• Treat underlying cause. • Magnesium salts may be given P.O., I.V., or I.M. —for seizures, may give magnesium 500 mg I.V. bolus, then 10% magnesium I.V. at rate of 1.5 ml/minute —decrease magnesium dosage with renal insufficiency.

Nursing Intervention

• Watch for signs and symptoms of dehydration, CHF, renal failure, renal calculi, and digitalis toxicity.
• Monitor urine output, ECG changes, and plasma calcium, phosphate, and sodium levels.
• May give phosphorus P.O., rectally, or I.V. Note that I.V. administration may precipitate and cause extravascular deposition, renal failure, or death.
• Monitor for increased neuromuscular excitability.
• Institute safety precautions for confused patients.
• Provide family support during patient personality changes.
• Provide skin care; sedate for severe itching.
• Assess home medication use of vitamin D, calcium supplements, thiazides, or digitalis.
• Use at least two large-bore I.V. lines.

• Monitor ECG; stop or slow infusion if ventricular irritability or heart block develops.
• Administer calcium at the bedside after thyroidectomy or parathyroidectomy, massive transfusions, or immediately after plasmapheresis.
• Monitor I.V. sites for necrosis, especially with calcium chloride administration.
• Use I.V. calcium cautiously with digitalis.
• Institute seizure precautions.
• Monitor for airway spasm, obstruction, stridor, or respiratory arrest.
• Monitor for numbness, tingling, cramps, spasms, and changes in mentation, mood, and memory.

• Administer I.V. calcium (not to exceed 50 mg/minute, even in emergencies).
• Question use of magnesium-containing medications, antacids, enemas, and test preparations.
• Monitor ECG (some sources say that ECG changes do not occur until magnesium level is 15 mEq/liter).
• Assess for dehydration; position patient and increase fluids as needed.
• Monitor for respiratory distress (magnesium level > 7 mEq/liter places patient at risk for respiratory arrest).
• Have calcium and resuscitation equipment ready.
• Assess frequently for muscle weakness, absence of deep tendon reflexes, and impaired breathing.
• Monitor for magnesium imbalances associated with hypocalcemia.

• Monitor for changes in ECG, urine output, blood pressure, and level of consciousness.
• Assess for dysphagia, laryngeal stridor, and airway obstruction.
• Monitor plasma potassium, calcium, and magnesium levels (hourly during acute magnesium replacement).
• Institute seizure precautions.
• Note that rapid magnesium administration may cause respiratory or cardiac arrest.
• Assess for sudden loss of deep tendon reflexes in patient on long-term magnesium replacement.   *(continued)*

Treating electrolyte imbalances *(continued)*

Disorder	Treatment
Hyperphos-phatemia	• Treat underlying cause. • Give phosphate-binding antacids. • May give calcium (withhold if plasma calcium × phosphorus levels > 72). • Give phosphorus-wasting diuretics (acetazolamide). • Use dialysis.
Hypophos-phatemia	• Treat underlying cause. • Administer phosphorus replacement therapy.

condition. Electrolyte abnormalities are symptoms of major body system failures and the lack of successful treatment and response. An electrolyte imbalance can easily cause death, although it may not be the underlying cause. All of the electrolyte imbalances previously discussed can be associated with fatal cardiac arrhythmias. A poor prognosis is associated with the following values:
• plasma sodium less than 105 mEq/liter
• plasma sodium greater than 160 mEq/liter
• plasma potassium less than half the individual norm
• plasma potassium greater than 2 to 3 times the individual norm
• plasma calcium (ionized) less than 2 mg/dl
• plasma calcium (ionized) greater than 16 mg/dl
• plasma magnesium less than 1 mg/dl
• plasma magnesium greater than 8 mg/dl
• plasma phosphorus less than 1 to 1.5 mg/dl
• plasma phosphorus greater than 5 mg/dl uncorrected (may not cause immediate problems but may contribute to bone reabsorption and spontaneous fractures beginning in about 10 years).

Nursing Intervention
• Monitor for neuromuscular irritability and ECG changes associated with hypocalcemia. • Institute seizure precautions. • Avoid phosphorus-based enemas, laxatives, and preparations. • Administer calcium supplements cautiously. • Severe itching is common. Lightly rub area and avoid scratching (clip patient's fingernails). Use topical anesthetics and oil-based soaps. Sedate if necessary.
• Monitor for tingling and numbness around mouth, rising $PaCO_2$, infection, muscle weakness, and poor tissue oxygenation. • If patient is confused, institute safety precautions. • Give parenteral phosphorus slowly to prevent hypocalcemic reaction. • Administer phosphorus during extubation and ventilation weaning. • Administer analgesics after parathyroidectomy for 2 to 3 days. • Limit activity to conserve strength.

Discharge planning

Discharge planning should begin when the patient is admitted. Often, precipitating factors for electrolyte imbalances include behaviors related to lack of social support, lack of knowledge, noncompliance, poor social adjustment, poor adjustment to chronic disease, or spiritual and psychiatric disorders.

The patient's final discharge plan should cover the following areas:
• home management (home health care, nursing home, family support, and need for assistive devices)
• instructions for managing personality changes, muscle weakness, constipation, and anorexia
• outpatient services, such as diabetic, dialysis, psychiatric, medical clinics, and physical therapy
• need for follow-up blood work if diuretics or steroids are prescribed
• assistance with decisions, family support, lifestyle changes, financial support, dialysis access care, treatment options (if patient has renal failure)
• social services and support groups
• rehabilitation

- dietary and fluid intake instructions
- medication instructions
- skin and wound care instruction
- activity instructions
- patient and family education related to terminal conditions.

Encephalopathy

The nonspecific term encephalopathy describes any abnormality in the structure or function of the brain. The hallmark of all encephalopathies is diffuse cerebral dysfunction manifesting as alterations in mentation and level of consciousness (LOC). Although similar in clinical manifestations, encephalopathies are quite varied etiologies. Encephalopathies most often encountered by critical care nurses fall into three broad categories: metabolic, hypoxic-ischemic, and infectious.

Pathophysiology

The pathophysiologic processes underlying metabolic, hypoxic-ischemic, and infectious encephalopathies vary greatly, as described below.

Metabolic encephalopathy

The most common type of encephalopathy, metabolic encephalopathy arises when an organ other than the brain fails. For example, when the kidneys or liver fail, the brain is affected adversely by the accumulation of toxins normally controlled by those organs. The most common metabolic encephalopathies are hepatic, Wernicke's, uremic, hypoglycemic or hyperglycemic, and hyposmolar or hyperosmolar.

Hepatic encephalopathy commonly develops over a period of days or weeks as a complication of portal-systemic shunting or liver failure, probably as a result of increased blood ammonia levels. However, recent investigations have also raised the possibility that excessive gamma-aminobutyric acid (GABA) causes hepatic encephalopathy. Found in high concentrations throughout the brain, GABA is a major inhibitory neurotransmitter. Patients with hepatic encephalopathy have increased plasma GABA levels, a factor that could cause neural inhibition and cerebral dysfunction.

Wernicke's encephalopathy, most commonly associated with chronic alcoholism, is caused by a vitamin B_1 (thiamine) deficiency. Thiamine is required for the metabolism of carbohydrates by all cells. Because the brain depends almost entirely on glucose metabolism to meet cellular energy requirements, a deficiency of thiamine severely reduces the brain's ability to utilize glucose. The cause of thiamine deficiency in alcoholics is a diminished intake of thiamine combined with impaired absorption and utilization by the liver.

Thiamine-deficit encephalopathy also may occur in patients receiving total parenteral nutrition (TPN) without thiamine, or as a result of malnutrition or malabsorption. Additionally, the administration of dextrose solutions to patients with thiamine deficiency can precipitate Wernicke's encephalopathy.

Uremic encephalopathy is associated with either the consequences or treatment of renal failure. Little is known about its pathogenesis except that it is linked to a reduction in cerebral blood flow and metabolism. The most consistent abnormality is an increased concentration of intracerebral calcium, which may result in altered neurotransmission.

Two other encephalopathies, dialysis disequilibrium and dialysis dementia, also occur in uremic patients. Dialysis disequilibrium, an acute syndrome that occurs during or immediately after dialysis, appears to be related to the development of cerebral edema. Dialysis dementia, a progressive, often fatal disorder associated with chronic hemodialysis, occurs sporadically in patients who have been dialyzed for at least 2 years, or as an epidemic affecting many patients receiving treatment at a particular dialysis unit. The dementia results from an accumulation of trace elements, especially aluminum, within the gray matter of the brain.

Hypoglycemic and hyperglycemic encephalopathies result from insufficient or excessive glucose levels. Hypoglycemic encephalopathy, caused by severe glucose deprivation, can result from overdosage of hypoglycemic agents, insulin-secreting tumors, end-stage hepatic disease, severe malnutrition, or fasting. Although the brain can tolerate an excess of glucose better than a deficit, hyperglycemic encephalopathy can result in hyperosmolality and cellular dehydration.

Hyperosmolar and hyposmolar encephalopathies result from fluid imbalances. The most common causes of hyperosmolality are hyperglycemia, dehydration, and hypernatremia. The most common cause of hyposmolality is hyponatremia. Acute hyponatremia is often an iatrogenic event, precipitated by parenteral overhydration, diuresis, or a GI loss of electrolytes. Another common cause is syndrome of inappropriate antidiuretic hormone secretion. The encephalopathy of hyposmolality is related to the development of cerebral edema and marked shifts in intracellular electrolytes, especially sodium and potassium.

Hypoxic-ischemic encephalopathy

Hypoxic-ischemic encephalopathy is caused by decreased cerebral perfusion and diminished oxygen delivery, which occurs with catastrophic cardiopulmonary events (cardiac arrest and respiratory failure). Other causes include carbon monoxide poisoning, suffocation, prolonged and profound hypotension, and septic shock.

Hypoxia alone is tolerated surprisingly well, because a low PaO_2 produces cerebral vasodilation, which increases blood flow and provides some compensation for the oxygen deficit. However, in acute ischemia, adequate circulation is not maintained. Total ischemia persisting beyond 6 to 8 minutes leads to irreversible neurologic damage.

Infectious encephalopathy

Infectious encephalopathies are caused by viruses or viral particles known as prions. Three infectious processes producing encephalopathy are acquired immune deficiency syndrome (AIDS), subacute spongiform encephalopathy, and progressive multifocal leukoencephalopathy.

At least half of all patients with AIDS develop an encephalopathy known as AIDS dementia complex (ADC). The pathophysiology of ADC is directly related to infection of the brain by human immunodeficiency virus. Brain cells most adversely affected are the macrophages and microglial cells. Following infection, these cells release cytokines and other toxic substances that destroy brain tissue and microvasculature. Significant loss of neurons and diffuse demyelination result, producing the characteristic clinical manifestations of ADC.

The spongiform encephalopathies are a group of neurodegenerative diseases caused by prions. The name "spongiform" is derived from the widespread neuronal loss and spongy state of the cerebral and cerebellar cortices of these patients. The most common of these rare infections, Creutzfeldt-Jakob disease (CJD), is transmissible. Inadvertent transmission of CJD has occurred following administration of contaminated human pituitary growth hormone, by transplantation of corneas from infected individuals, and from the use of improperly sterilized neurosurgical instruments.

Progressive multifocal leukoencephalopathy (PML) most commonly affects immunosuppressed persons, including transplant recipients, those treated for lupus and chronic neoplastic diseases, and those with AIDS. PML is caused by a papovavirus, which targets oligodendrocytes, cells whose primary function is the production of myelin. Accordingly, PML is characterized by diffuse demyelinative (white matter) lesions of the cerebrum, brain stem, and cerebellum.

Clinical assessment

Although various laboratory and radiologic studies are useful for confirming the diagnosis of encephalopathy, the most important clues are obtained from a thorough history and physical examination.

History

Even though an encephalopathy reflects diffuse cerebral dysfunction, the culprit is usually not the brain. Almost invariably, some other organ is involved. Therefore, obtaining a thorough history from the patient or family members is essential.

The critical care nurse should ask about:

• presence of hepatic disease, such as cirrhosis or hepatitis

• history of surgical portal-systemic shunting, Reye's syndrome, alcohol abuse, GI bleeding, and recent benzodiazepine use

• history of renal disease and uremia, including any relationship between the development of symptoms and dialysis or use of aluminum-containing phosphate binders in the treatment of renal failure

• endocrinopathy, such as Type I or II diabetes mellitus or pancreatic cancer

• use of drugs that can cause hypoglycemia (insulin, sulfonylureas, alcohol, salicylates, beta blockers, pentamidine) or hyperglycemia (diuretics, chlorpromazine, glucocorticoids, phenytoin)

• recent central nervous system events (head trauma, subarachnoid hemorrhage, intracranial neoplasms)

• severe cardiac or pulmonary disease

• recent carbon monoxide exposure

• history of AIDS

• corneal, renal, cardiac, or other organ transplantation

• use of immunosuppressive agents or human growth hormone

• diet, use of vitamins, and amount of carbohydrates and protein consumed.

The nurse also should be aware that patients may develop encephalopathy while in the intensive care unit. Especially vulnerable are those admitted for hepatic or renal failure, head injury, subarachnoid hemor-

rhage, cardiac or respiratory arrest, or severe fluid, glucose, or electrolyte disorders.

Physical findings

Despite their myriad etiologies, most encephalopathies
have remarkably uniform major clinical manifestations. The distinguishing feature of encephalopathy is a
generalized depression of the cerebral hemispheres.
The onset of symptoms may be slow and subtle, or
dramatic and rapidly progressive (see *Manifestations of
encephalopathy,* pages 294 and 295).

The hallmark of any encephalopathy is abnormal
mental status, which manifests as mental slowing and
impaired information processing; deficits in concentration, memory, attention, and judgment; disorders of
perception, including hallucinations; changes in personality and affect, including irritability and emotional
lability; and lethargy. Other signs and symptoms include headache, malaise, nausea, vomiting, muscle
weakness, and cramps.

Common physical findings include:
- decreased LOC, ranging from confusion to coma
- agitation, dementia, or delirium
- normal or diminished respirations
- small, equal, and reactive pupils (preservation of pupillary responses occurs even with deep coma, except
with severe hypoxic encephalopathy)
- conjugate or slightly disconjugate ocular movements
- normal oculocephalic and oculovestibular responses
(except with severe anoxic encephalopathy)
- increased muscle tone
- brisk, deep tendon reflexes
- movement abnormalities, including myoclonic jerks,
asterixis, and seizures
- hypothermia.

Diagnosis

The diagnosis of encephalopathy depends chiefly on
the patient's history, clinical manifestations, and physi-
(Text continues on page 296.)

Manifestations of encephalopathy

The following chart details the signs and symptoms and physical assessment findings for each of the major types of encephalopathy.

Encephalopathy	Signs and Symptoms	Physical Findings
Hepatic	Attention deficits, mental dullness, sleep disturbances (early signs); delusions, hallucinations (late signs)	Delirium progressing to decreased level of consciousness (LOC) and coma, hyperventilation and metabolic alkalosis, abnormal eye movements, asterixis, hyperreflexia, myoclonic jerks, extension posturing, generalized seizures (rare)
Wernicke's	Rapid onset of symptoms, including inattention, apathy, memory loss, drowsiness, polyneuropathy	Confusion, dementia, ataxia, hypothermia, tongue redness, postural hypotension, nystagmus, ophthalmoplegia
Uremic	Muscle cramps, headache, nausea, vomiting, lethargy, impaired memory and concentration, hallucinations	Obtundation, tremor, twitching, asterixis, myoclonus, focal or generalized seizures
Dialysis disequilibrium	Headache, acute fatigue, nausea, muscle cramps, restlessness, tremulousness	Confusion progressing to obtundation and coma, muscle twitching, seizures
Dialysis dementia	Personality changes, memory impairment, stuttering	Dysarthria, dysphasia, facial grimacing, asterixis, myoclonus, generalized tremors, seizures, progressive dementia
Hypoglycemic	Malaise, hunger, pallor, nervousness, tremor, restlessness, sweating, mental slowing (early manifestations often blunted in diabetics)	Tachycardia, ataxia, decreased LOC, hypothermia, coma, seizures
Hyperglycemic	Nausea; polydipsia, polyuria, and polyphagia (early signs); anorexia (late sign)	Hyperventilation and acetone breath with diabetic ketoacidosis (DKA) dehy-

Manifestations of encephalopathy *(continued)*

Encephalopathy	Signs and Symptoms	Physical Findings
Hyperglycemic *(continued)*		dration, dry mucous membranes, poor skin turgor, hypotension, sunken eyes, low urine output, disorientation, obtundation, coma, focal and generalized seizures
Hyperosmolar	Same as with hyperglycemia from DKA or hyperglycemic hyperosmolar nonketosis	Same as for hyperglycemic (see above)
Hyposmolar	Impaired cognition, headache	Confusion, delirium, psychosis, asterixis, ataxia, seizures
Hypoxic-ischemic	Headache, lethargy, impaired cognition, brief loss of consciousness (mild form); anterograde amnesia, hallucinations (moderate form)	Decreased LOC (confusion to coma), seizures, posturing, absent brain stem reflexes, myoclonus, asterixis (severe form)
AIDS dementia complex	Headache, incoordination, apathy, withdrawal, irritability, depression (early symptoms); loss of concentration, short-term memory deficits, intellectual slowing, emotional lability (later symptoms)	Slowly or rapidly progressive dementia, presenting as impaired cognitive and behavioral function and confusion; motor symptoms (ataxia, weakness, incontinence, myoclonus, seizures, paralysis)
Spongiform	Fatigue, depression, weight loss, sleep and appetite disorders, visual disturbances, hallucinations	Exaggerated startle response, slowly progressive ataxia and dementia, confusion, agitation, diffuse myoclonus, twitching, dysarthria, stupor, coma
Progressive multifocal leukoencephalopathy	Weakness and visual loss	Dementia, ataxia, blindness, hemiparesis progressing to quadriplegia, aphasia, coma

cal examination. Neuroimaging and laboratory data are useful for confirming the diagnosis and serve as a guide for treatment. (For a listing of diagnostic tests specific to each type of encephalopathy, see *Diagnostic tests for encephalopathy,* pages 297 and 298.)

Treatment and care
Although the specific treatment and care of patients with encephalopathy depend on the etiology, some general principles apply to all cases, including preventive measures, monitoring for and treating laboratory abnormalities, ensuring optimal nutrition, and dialysis therapy, as discussed below. More specific treatments are included in *Treating encephalopathy,* pages 299 to 301.

Preventive measures
The best treatment of encephalopathy is to prevent it from developing. Early recognition of precipitating factors is of utmost importance, especially because half of all encephalopathies are iatrogenic. Related nursing interventions are included below:
• Monitor neurologic function, especially mentation and LOC, and report changes immediately. Changes in LOC may be subtle at first and may progress to confusion, delirium, and obtundation. Observe for difficulty concentrating and problem solving, short attention span, and memory deficits.
• Observe for behavioral and psychological changes, such as irritability, emotional lability, delusions, and hallucinations.
• Promptly report any motor abnormalities, such as asterixis, tremors, myoclonus, or seizures. Also report any signs of lethargy, weakness, or hypothermia.
• Monitor for and report signs of GI bleeding, especially in patients with liver disease.
• Avoid administering benzodiazepines to patients with hepatic dysfunction.
• Avoid the use of drugs that induce hypoglycemia or hyperglycemia in susceptible patients.

DIAGNOSTIC TESTS

Diagnostic tests for encephalopathy

The following are common tests used in the diagnosis of encephalopathy.

Type of Encephalopathy	Diagnostic Tests and Findings
Hepatic	• Elevated arterial ammonia level, serum bilirubin, and hepatic enzyme levels • Low serum albumin and clotting factor levels • Abnormal EEG
Wernicke's	• Immediate, dramatic improvement following parenteral administration of thiamine (thiamine test) • Decreased serum thiamine level • Computed tomography (CT) and magnetic resonance imaging (MRI) showing atrophy of mammillary bodies
Uremic	• Creatinine clearance < 10% of normal • Elevated blood urea nitrogen and creatinine levels • Diffuse EEG slowing
Dialysis disequilibrium	• Increased serum osmolality and CSF pressure • EEG slowing and disorganization
Dialysis dementia	• Increased levels of serum aluminum and other trace minerals • Distinctive EEG changes
Hypoglycemia	• Low serum glucose and insulin levels • Unchanged CT (early); CT changes including diffuse areas of decreased density and ventricular dilation (late)
Hyperglycemia	• Elevated serum glucose level (may be as high as 2,000 mg/dl in hyperosmolar nonketotic coma) • Elevated serum osmolality • Electrolyte abnormalities • With diabetic ketoacidosis, low hydrogen ion concentration, $PaCO_2$, and bicarbonate levels
Hyperosmolality	• Elevated serum osmolality and, depending on cause, elevated glucose level, sodium level, or both
Hyposmolality	• Low serum osmolality and low sodium level
Hypoxic-ischemic	• Hypoxemia • Abnormal or isoelectric EEG

(continued)

Diagnostic tests for encephalopathy *(continued)*

Type of Encephalopathy	Diagnostic Tests and Findings
AIDS dementia complex	• CT showing widened sulci and enlarged ventricles • MRI showing diffuse white matter changes • CSF positive for human immunodeficiency virus
Subacute spongiform	• Distinctive EEG changes in most patients • Normal blood and CSF findings
Progressive multifocal leukoencephalopathy	• CT and MRI showing extensive multifocal lesions in white matter

• Ensure that patients at risk for thiamine deficiency receive thiamine supplements.

• Carefully monitor serum electrolyte and glucose levels, osmolality, and urine output of patients with renal or liver insufficiency or acute intracranial disease.

• Assess for and promptly treat hypotension or hypoxemia.

• Encourage pulmonary hygiene, and instruct the patient to use an incentive spirometer.

• Maintain patient safety by preventing falls and accidental tube dislodgment. Use the least restrictive restraints when such devices are necessary.

Correction of abnormal laboratory values

The correction of abnormal laboratory values should be carried out judiciously. Because the brain has adapted to the abnormal state, rapid correction of abnormalities can have negative consequences. As long as the patient is stable and not experiencing seizures, remediation of abnormalities should be aimed at achieving a 50% correction over a period of 24 to 48 hours. Appropriate nursing interventions include the following:

• Monitor laboratory values carefully, and report abnormalities promptly.

• Evaluate the patient's response.

Treating encephalopathy

Specific treatments and prognoses for the various types of encephalopathy are presented in the chart below.

Type of Encephalopathy	Treatment	Prognosis
Hepatic	• Treat precipitating factors (GI hemorrhage, infection, excessive dietary protein, use of benzodiazepines). • Reduce ammonia absorption with oral lactulose 20 to 30 g 3 to 4 times daily to induce diarrhea. • Decrease ammonia production with neomycin 1 g every 6 hours. • Maintain a low-protein (40 to 80 g) diet.	The condition is potentially completely reversible, but prolonged and repeated episodes are associated with increased mortality. Mortality is 80% to 85% in patients with severe hepatic coma.
Wernicke's	• Administer thiamine promptly to prevent progression. • Initially give 50 mg I.V. and 50 mg I.M., then 50 mg daily until good nutrition is resumed.	Mortality rate is 20%. Complete recovery occurs in 20% of surviving patients; partial recovery in 60%.
Uremic	• Administer dialysis and proceed with transplantation, if possible. • Administer anticonvulsants, such as phenytoin or phenobarbital, for seizures.	Condition is potentially reversible; symptoms usually dissipate with dialysis.
Dialysis disequilibrium	• Administer mannitol, albumin, or glycerol. • Slow the rate of dialysis.	Condition is potentially fatal, but outcome is usually good when the rate of dialysis is slowed or dialysis is instituted before uremia becomes severe.
Dialysis dementia	• Avoid aluminum-containing oral phosphate binders, and eliminate aluminum from dialysate. • Administer I.V. deferoxamine, an aluminum chelator, for symptoms.	Treatment is associated with limited success; the condition is often fatal.

(continued)

Treating encephalopathy *(continued)*

Type of Encephalopathy	Treatment	Prognosis
Hypoglycemia	• Treat signs and symptoms promptly. • Initiate treatment with oral glucose, parenteral glucose, or both. • Discontinue drugs that induce hypoglycemia.	Permanent brain damage and death occur without prompt treatment. Chronic and repeated episodes are associated with neurologic deficits, especially of intellectual functions.
Hyperglyce-mia	• Prevent diabetic ketoacidosis (DKA) and hyperosmolar hyoperglycemic nonketotic syndrome (HHNS). • Avoid use of phenytoin and glucocorticosteroids in susceptible patients.	A 50% mortality occurs with HNK; 5% to 10% mortality with DKA. In other patients, good outcomes are associated with prompt recognition and treatment.
Hyperosmolal-ity	• Replace fluids, orally if possible, parenterally if necessary.	Hyperosmolality is responsible for the 50% mortality associated with HNK. Outcome is better with early recognition and treatment.
Hyposmolality	• Administer hypertonic saline judiciously. • Limit free water and diuretics. • Replace urine output with normal saline solution.	The condition readily responds to treatment, and the mortality rate increases as serum sodium level declines. Serum sodium 112 mEq/liter is associated with a 50% mortality rate.
Hypoxic-isch-emic	• Treat promptly to restore cerebral blood flow and oxygenation. • Maintain blood pressure at normal or slightly higher levels. • Control hyperthermia and seizure activity. • Avoid steroids (they have no value in treating this condition).	Condition frequently produces permanent brain damage, persistent vegetative state, or death. Survival is inversely related to duration of coma. Better outcomes occur in patients who are arousable within 72 hours.
AIDS dementia complex	• Administer azidothymidine (AZT, zidovudine), which may temporarily improve cognition.	Severe dementia develops within 2 to 7 months after diagnosis. Survival

Treating encephalopathy *(continued)*

Type of Encephalopathy	Treatment	Prognosis
AIDS dementia complex *(continued)*	• Dideoxyinosine (ddI) may also be effective in improving cognitive deficits.	following onset of severe dementia ranges from 1 to 6 months.
Subacute spongiform	• No treatment is available. • Avoid transmission by autoclaving surgical instruments and washing thoroughly with soap.	The vast majority of patients die within 1 year.
Progressive multifocal leukoencephalopathy	• No treatment is available.	Most patients die within 6 months of symptom onset.

Nutritional measures

Like all other critically ill patients, those with encephalopathy require optimal nutrition. However, to decrease ammonia and urea loads, patients with hepatic or uremic encephalopathy may require protein-restricted diets. Nursing responsibilities related to maintaining dietary restrictions are listed below:
• Explain the purpose of the dietary restrictions to the patient and family.
• Monitor the patient's dietary intake carefully.
• Administer vitamin supplements, including thiamine, especially if the patient is on TPN, is an alcoholic, or has liver dysfunction.
• Assess the patient's compliance with protein-restricted or carbohydrate-restricted diets.
• Prevent aspiration by elevating the head of the bed 45 degrees and positioning the patient on the side.
• Check tube feeding residuals; withhold feedings if the residuals are greater than 50% of the previous hour's feeding (if continuous) or the last feeding volume (if bolus).
• Obtain a nutritional consultation.

Fluid therapy or restrictions

Because most patients with metabolic encephalopathy are prone to circulatory collapse, optimal hydration is a priority. Among these patients, the I.V. fluid of choice is normal saline solution. Conversely, patients with uremic or hyposmolar encephalopathy require fluid restriction (both parenteral and oral). The I.V. fluid of choice for hypernatremic patients is dextrose 5% in water. For those with severe hyponatremia, hypertonic saline solution is administered. Appropriate nursing interventions include:

• Ensure that the correct I.V. fluid is infusing at the proper rate.

• Provide meticulous assessment and documentation of intake and output, including daily weight.

• Monitor laboratory values carefully, especially the serum electrolyte levels and osmolality.

Dialysis

The definitive treatment of uremic encephalopathy is dialysis (usually hemodialysis). Although nurses usually are not responsible for dialyzing the patient with uremic encephalopathy, the patient must be monitored before and after treatments. Related nursing interventions include:

• Monitor laboratory values, especially serum electrolyte, blood urea nitrogen, creatinine, and glucose levels and osmolality, and report critical values.

• Assist the dialysis nurse in monitoring the patient during the procedure, especially if pulmonary artery values are being evaluated.

• During dialysis, monitor the patient for signs of dialysis disequilibrium. Keep in mind that this syndrome is more common in young patients who have very high serum urea levels.

• During or after dialysis, evaluate the patient for dialysis dementia. Keep in mind that this condition occurs most commonly in patients who have been receiving dialysis for more than 2 years.

Prognosis

The prognosis of any encephalopathy depends upon the patient's underlying condition. For example, end-stage liver or renal disease is associated with a poor prognosis independent of the actual encephalopathy. Also, the development of encephalopathy often serves as a measure of the severity of the underlying disorder.

Discharge planning

Because many of the encephalopathies are at least potentially preventable, patient and family education is essential to prevent recurrences. Specific areas to cover in the discharge planning include:

• dietary and nutritional education, which may include glucose and protein restriction and use of vitamins
• avoidance of specific medications and drugs that may precipitate encephalopathy, especially alcohol
• the importance of keeping follow-up appointments
• the need to seek prompt treatment for precipitating factors, such as GI bleeding, infection, respiratory distress, chest pain, and other physiologic stressors
• the importance of seeking prompt treatment for early manifestations of encephalopathy, especially changes in mental functioning or LOC.

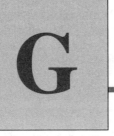

Gastrointestinal hemorrhage

Acute gastrointestinal (GI) hemorrhage occurs when large or small amounts of new or old blood are lost from the GI tract. The bleeding can range from minor and temporary to severe and constant; loss may be via emesis (hematemesis), stool (hematochezia), or both. About 85% of all GI hemorrhages involve the upper GI system; upper GI hemorrhage is responsible for more than 300,000 hospital admissions every year. If blood loss is sudden and severe enough, death may occur from circulatory failure and shock.

Pathophysiology

The GI tract is a highly vascular area, with arterial and venous blood supplies located very close to the mucosal surface. When the integrity of the mucosal surface is breached, gastric juices, such as hydrochloric acid and pepsin, can cause erosion through and into the vascular system. Whether the bleeding is caused by a breached mucosal-epithelial barrier or by an exposed artery or ruptured vein, the result is hemorrhage, accumulation of blood within the GI tract, and potential for cardiovascular compromise and collapse.

The most common cause of upper GI hemorrhages is peptic ulcers, although the percentage of patients who present with GI hemorrhage from ruptured esophageal varices is increasing. Lower GI hemorrhage can result from multiple disorders, including diverticular disease, angiodysplasia, tumors, acute mucosal tears, and ulcerative colitis. Patients who have experienced significant trauma, burns, renal failure, increased intracranial pressure, or other physically demanding situations are at increased risk for GI hemorrhage secondary to the increased catecholamine and acid production associated with the systemic response to stress. The continued systemic response leads to tissue ischemia, thought to be one of the principal causes of GI hemorrhage. Patients with bleeding abnormalities, such as disseminated intravascular coagulation or leukemia, also present with complications of acute GI bleeding.

For some patients, the GI bleed that brings them in for medical attention may be the first hint of an underlying process. Prescribed drug therapies (such as heparin or Coumadin [warfarin sodium]), as well as accidental or intentional ingestion of rat poison, alter the coagulation profile and leave the patient at risk for bleeding. Similarly, patients with severe liver disease and vitamin K deficiencies that affect clotting factor production and platelet performance are more prone to upper or lower GI bleeds, especially if comorbid chronic inflammatory bowel disease, ischemic colitis, or infectious colitis exists. (For an overview of common causes, see *Common causes of upper and lower GI hemorrhages,* pages 306 to 308.)

Small GI hemorrhages (characterized by a 15% blood loss or less) typically result in outward signs secondary to vasoconstriction and fluid retention. These reflect the activation of the sympathetic nervous system (SNS) to compensate for the volume loss. Unless the patient is elderly or anemic, or the loss is very rapid, a blood loss of less than 500 ml usually does not result in significant symptomatology.

A larger hemorrhage (up to 40% blood loss) typically overwhelms the SNS response and results in
(Text continues on page 309.)

Common causes of upper and lower GI hemorrhages

Ulcers are areas of breakdown in the GI tract that have significant depth, usually extending through the muscularis mucosa, while erosions, such as gastritis and esophagitis, are more superficial. Acid-peptic disease is usually confined to the distal esophagus, stomach, and proximal duodenum, unless the patient has a rare condition such as Zollinger-Ellison syndrome that could affect the small bowel. The following chart describes the most common causes of upper and lower GI hemorrhage, along with the major pathophysiologic changes that occur.

Cause of Hemorrhage	Description	Pathophysiologic Changes
Upper GI hemorrhages		
Peptic ulcer	• A deep erosion that occurs in the GI tract where pepsin collects or is secreted • Accounts for 80% of all upper GI hemorrhages • Most common type is duodenal ulcer • Patients at risk include those taking corticosteroids and those with significant trauma (such as sepsis, shock, or physical trauma), who may develop ulcerations of the stomach, esophagus, or duodenum • Stress ulcers occur in 40% of patients at risk, including long-term intensive care unit or trauma patients	• An inflammatory response involving histamine release is initiated, which causes more pepsin and hydrochloric acid to be released, resulting in increased capillary permeability and leakage of fluid and proteins. Mucosal edema, breakdown, and capillary bleeding result. • Rebleeding in patients with peptic ulcers has been associated with *Helicobacter pylori* infections, regardless of where the ulceration is found.
Gastritis	• Diffuse superficial erosion of the gastric mucosal layers • Associated with chronic alcohol use, anti-inflammatory drug use, major physical or mental stress, and recent surgery • The most common type of gastric erosion in critically ill patients without a history of GI illness; constitutes 15% of all upper GI hemorrhages	• Massive bleeding in a patient with confirmed gastritis may be an indication that the erosion has deepened and that ulcerations are causing the bleeding. • Diffuse gastritis may result in bleeding when large areas of the gastric mucosa "leak" blood.

Common causes of upper and lower GI hemorrhages *(continued)*

Cause of Hemorrhage	Description	Pathophysiologic Changes
Esophageal or gastric varices	• Constitute 5% of all upper GI hemorrhages • May be found in the esophagus, duodenum, or rectum • Commonly associated with alcohol abuse, liver disease (infectious or mechanical disruption), hepatitis B and C, and cirrhosis	• Portal hypertension compromises the integrity of the low-pressure venous system, which supplies the intestine; increased portal pressure causes the development of collateral channels (varicosities), which are more fragile than the systemic veins. • Within the esophagus, varicosities are especially sensitive to vomiting, retching, and enzymatic irritation; with sufficient pressure or erosion, they will burst and cause sudden, profuse bleeding. This appears to be related more to pressure within the vessel than to irritation of the mucosal layer.
Mallory-Weiss tear	• A mucosal tear occurring at the gastroesophageal junction, usually following constant or severe retching or emesis, which causes the tissue disruption • Most tears will stop bleeding spontaneously, and seldom recur	• The esophageal and gastric tissues separate, exposing vessels.
Esophagitis, esophageal carcinoma, hiatal hernia	• Relatively uncommon causes of upper GI bleeding • May also occur in patients with infections that have invaded the esophageal wall (cytomegalovirus, herpes simplex, *Candida albicans,* histoplasmosis, tuberculosis); presentation is usually more chronic than acute	• Esophagitis is caused by reflux of hydrochloric acid from the stomach that results in diffuse or localized erosion of the protective mucosa, usually in the presence of a hiatal hernia, incompetent lower esophageal sphincter, or increased abdominal pressure. • Continued reflux may lead to esophageal stricture, Barrett's esophagus, bleeding, and aspiration of acidic juices into the pulmonary tree. *(continued)*

Common causes of upper and lower GI hemorrhages *(continued)*

Cause of Hemorrhage	Description	Pathophysiologic Changes
Lower GI hemorrhages		
Diverticular hemorrhage	• Diverticula are usually located in the colonic wall where the wall is penetrated by nutrient vessels • One of the most common causes of lower GI hemorrhage • Less than 5% of patients with diverticulosis will have bleeding, but it will persist in 20% of those affected • Meckel's diverticulum, a congenital defect, is found in 2% of children and young adults, and is a significant cause of acute hemorrhage	• The etiology of diverticular bleeding is uncertain. The bleeding is from an arterial source (vasa recta) and most cases of diverticular bleeding show no association with inflammation. • When diverticula perforate, sudden and massive GI bleeding may ensue; the sigmoid colon is the most common source of this complication. • Meckel's diverticulum results in the development of a diverticulum on the ileum close to the ileocecal valve.
Arteriovenous malformations	• Very small mucosal lesions, most commonly diagnosed by endoscopy; also called angiodysplasia • Usually found within the ascending colon • Can be a source of acute and chronic bleeding in elderly patients and patients with chronic renal failure • Carcinomatous lesions within the colon may also precipitate lower GI bleeds	• These lesions are commonly seen in the stomach, small bowel, and colon. • They are mucosal vascular lesions consisting of a group of small arteries and veins that have become dilated and fragile and that tend to bleed.
Anal and rectal lesions	• Includes hemorrhoids (dilated and tortuous veins found in the anorectum), anal fissures, and fistulas • Can be either internal or external, and often have small amounts of bleeding after the passage of a hard stool	• Trauma to the rectum, found when foreign objects are inserted into the rectal vault, may result in perforation and acute rectal hemorrhage, which requires immediate attention.

hypovolemic shock (a smaller hemorrhage in a patient already compromised by an underlying disease will also cause this effect). Hemodynamic parameters fall (decreased diastolic blood pressure and cardiac output, pulmonary capillary wedge pressure and central venous pressure); tachycardia, hypotension, tachypnea, and cool, clammy extremities are typical signs of a 40% blood loss. Confusion, restlessness, and anxiety, as well as decreased urine output, show the effects of decreased tissue perfusion. In some cases, increases in peripheral vasoconstriction, heart rate, myocardial oxygen demand, and force of contraction are great enough to result in ischemia and further cardiac compromise. If the cycle is not broken, decreased blood flow and oxygen delivery will cause widespread ischemia, anaerobic activity, systemic failure (such as acute myocardial infarction or renal failure), and complete collapse.

Clinical assessment

Detailed and thorough clinical assessment and patient history are the mainstays of caring for the patient with an acute GI hemorrhage.

History

Although stabilizing the acutely ill patient may take priority over the acquisition of a detailed history, it should be obtained as soon as possible. Many of the causes of GI bleeding can be determined by the occurrence and timing of symptoms. The following points are important to cover when obtaining the history:
• frank, bloody stools without change in vital signs or hematocrit (HCT) (anorectal or left colonic source); melena (black, tarry stools usually indicate bleeding proximal to the cecum); maroon stools (usually found with bleeding from the distal small bowel or right colon)
• vomiting or retching of blood or coffee-ground material (may indicate Mallory-Weiss tear)
• trauma to the torso

• abdominal cramping (may indicate lower GI bleeding or blood accumulation)
• medication use: over-the-counter anti-inflammatory agents, prescription drugs (including anticoagulants), illicit drugs (especially steroids)
• recent illnesses or stressors
• alcohol use (may indicate gastritis or varices)
• prior history of GI bleeding
• history of liver disease and vitamin K deficiency (may indicate varices or coagulation disorders as source of the bleeding); active hepatitis infections, obstructive liver disease, chronic active hepatitis B and C, and so on (may be the source of the liver compromise)
• history of bruising (may indicate liver disease or coagulation disorders)
• history of GI lymphoma or other carcinomatous disease
• anorexia or weight loss
• allergy to medications, especially radiologic contrast
• previous blood transfusions or reactions
• religious preferences, especially as they relate to blood transfusions.

Physical findings

Common manifestations of a significant GI hemorrhage correspond with volume loss, inadequate perfusion, and pain related to the bleeding:
• orthostatic hypotension (diastolic drop of > 10 points, pulse rise of > 15 beats/minute), hypotension, tachycardia (> 110 beats/minute), vasoconstriction
• low HCT, hemoglobin (Hb), and red blood cell (RBC) count; elevated reticulocyte count
• thirst, sweating, decreased urine output, oliguria
• hypernatremia, hyperosmolality, hypocalcemia, hyperkalemia, metabolic acidosis
• increased bleeding or bruising, abnormal coagulation profile
• dyspnea, cyanosis, temperature fluctuation
• substernal burning, seen with bleeding esophagitis
• abdominal, stomach, or esophageal pain

• bloody emesis (hematemesis): usually indicates bleeding above the duodenum

• coffee-ground emesis: indicates bleeding above the duodenum, where blood that has been held in the stomach has iron dissociated from Hb

• melena: from breakdown of blood as it passes through the GI tract

• bright red, bloody stools (hematochezia): indicates lower GI hemorrhage, or rapid, large upper GI hemorrhage

• frequent stools; blood or bloody stool with digital examination of rectum

• stigmata of liver disease (spider angiomas, distended abdominal veins, jaundice, ascites)

• pallor, poor skin turgor, decreased capillary refill

• pain of the stomach or esophagus, or upon palpation of the abdomen; hyperactive bowel sounds

• decreased level of consciousness, confusion, disorientation related to decreased cerebral perfusion and decreased oxygen carrying capacity with volume loss; may also reflect hypoglycemia, increased blood urea nitrogen (BUN) and ammonia production from prolonged hemorrhages and liver compromise.

Diagnosis

The patient with severe GI bleeding typically presents with signs and symptoms of general shock. Cardiogenic failure, sepsis, hypovolemia from dehydration, and hemorrhage from another source must be ruled out. The patient presenting with visible bleeding from the GI tract should be evaluated for secondary or contributing factors; comorbid disease requires a tailored approach to diagnosis and treatment. Focusing on diagnostic procedures after the patient's circulatory function and oxygenation have been stabilized will assist in determining appropriate treatment regimens.

Confirming GI hemorrhage, pages 312 and 313, highlights diagnostic tests used to identify and evaluate potential sources of GI bleeding and laboratory studies

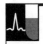

DIAGNOSTIC TESTS
Confirming GI hemorrhage

The following procedures and studies may be performed to establish the exact site and the impact of the GI hemorrhage. Additionally, X-rays are utilized in the diagnosis of GI bleeding if suspicion of cause is secondary to perforation, obstruction, or trauma. Surgery may be used in patients with life-threatening hemorrhage who do not have access to angiographic or endoscopic temporizing measures.

Nasogastric (NG) tube placement
Hematemesis or bloody gastric aspirate via NG tube indicates bleeding above the jejunum and is considered positive if gastric contents contain a significant amount of blood (bright red, dark coffee-ground material, or strongly positive on the testing strip). If bleeding is intermittent or within the pylorus without regurgitation to the body of the stomach, a false-negative aspirate may result.

Laboratory values
Hemoglobin (men: 14 to 18 g/dl, women: 12 to 16 g/dl) and hematocrit (men: 37-47%, women: 42-52%)
Hematocrit and hemoglobin will fall as the blood is lost from the circulation. However, the fall will be delayed approximately 6 hours or more from the time of the bleeding, because dilution occurs as extracellular fluid is pulled back into the circulation and as volume resuscitation is initiated.

Platelet count (130,000 to 370,000 mm³)
Decreased platelet count may indicate an underlying disease process, such as leukemia or marrow suppression, as well as an indication of the utilization of the platelets to stop the bleeding.

Prothrombin time (PT) (men: 9.6 to 11.8 seconds, women: 9.5 to 11.3 seconds) and partial thromboplastin time (PTT) (30 to 45 seconds)
These tests are designed to evaluate coagulation abnormalities. PT is prolonged in patients with vitamin K deficiency and alcoholic cirrhosis. PTT is prolonged in patients with hemophilia A or B, vitamin K deficiency, or alcoholic cirrhosis.

Serum electrolyte (Na⁺ = 135 to 145 mEq/L, K⁺ = 3.5 to 5 mEq/L, Ca⁺ = 8.8 to 10.0 mg/dl, Mg = 1.3 to 2.1 mEq/L), blood urea nitrogen (BUN) = 7 to 18 mg/dl
Baseline serum electrolyte values to determine how well the kidneys are working and any other abnormalities that may affect the patient's presentation are essential. An increased BUN level may reflect absorption and breakdown of blood proteins within the GI tract; it is usually higher in upper GI bleeding than lower, as protein breakdown occurs in the upper GI tract.

Liver function tests (amylase: 50 to 150 U/L, aspartate aminotransferase: 8 to 20 U/L, alkaline phosphatase: 20 to 70 U/L, alanine aminotransferase: 7 to 24 U/L, total bilirubin: 0.2 to 1.0 mg/dl)
Elevated liver enzymes reflect a disturbance in liver function, as seen with alcohol abuse and cirrhosis, hepatitis, and liver failure. Bilirubin levels can be followed to evaluate the ability of the liver to handle the

Confirming GI hemorrhage *(continued)*

blood proteins and factors presented for processing.

Esophagogastroduodenoscopy (endoscopy)

Endoscopy is the first choice in the diagnostic evaluation of upper GI hemorrhages, as it allows the examiner to have direct visualization of the esophagus, stomach, and duodenum. It is best performed within the first 12 to 24 hours of the bleeding, but may well be performed in the midst of the early resuscitative efforts because it can be not only diagnostic but therapeutic (cautery, sclerotherapy).

Arteriography

When bleeding is so brisk or diffuse that it is not possible to clear the GI tract sufficiently for endoscopic evaluation, selective angiography may pinpoint the bleeding site. It can be the best initial test for the patient with massive bleeding.

Barium studies

Barium studies may help in the recognition of mucosal lesions, but are not able to confirm active bleeding from a specific site. These studies offer little to the practitioner and can interfere with future studies (endoscopic or colonoscopic, arterio-

graphic), which require direct visualization of the GI tract. Retained barium also makes arteriographic investigation of the roentgenographic view difficult.

Bleeding scans

Technetium-99^m labeled red blood cell scanning (^{99m}TcRBC) is useful in the examination of patients who have active but slower bleeding rates, as found in lower GI hemorrhages. Sites that are bleeding as little as 0.1 ml/minute can be identified by this study, and it can be repeated over a prolonged period to look for collections of extravasated fluids. If no site is seen, but clinical signs still confirm the potential of a lower GI hemorrhage, this should be followed by colonoscopy for direct visualization of the GI tract.

Sigmoidoscopy, colonoscopy

This test is reserved for those with suspected lower GI bleeding but negative bleeding scans. Optimal examinations follow good oral lavage to clear the GI tract. Colonoscopy facilitates identification of lesions that are no longer actively bleeding. Tissue can be biopsied via the scope for diagnosis of mass lesions.

that are used to evaluate the patient's response to and tolerance of bleeding.

Treatment and care

The primary goals in the patient with a GI hemorrhage are to achieve an adequate blood pressure and to maintain tissue perfusion and oxygenation. Prolonged hypotension or hypoperfusion results in ischemia and infarction, causing what may be irreparable damage.

Treatment will focus on replacing lost fluids, finding the hemorrhagic source, and preventing complications or further deterioration.

Maintaining hemodynamic stability

For a patient who is hemodynamically compromised by GI bleeding, the most important action is constant monitoring of vital signs and restoration of blood volume. GI bleeding and utilization of fluid replacement can compromise a patient's oxygenation and must be continually assessed. Fluid volume replacement utilizing normal saline, lactated Ringer's solution, or hetastarch may be ordered. Blood transfusions may also be ordered to maintaining an HCT greater than 25%. RBCs, fresh frozen plasma (FFP), platelets, and cryoprecipitate may be utilized to correct coagulopathies and support blood pressure.

The following nursing interventions should be incorporated into the plan of care:

• Establish I.V. access. Active bleeding requires two 16G to 18G lines, which may be placed peripherally; central access is recommended but not required.

• Collect samples for blood typing and crossmatching, complete blood count, and prothrombin and partial thromboplastin times.

• Administer oxygen therapy as indicated by mentation, respiratory evaluation, arterial blood gas analysis, and oxygen saturation readings.

• Insert a urinary catheter; monitor intake and output.

• Initiate fluid volume replacement. Titrate replacement to vital signs and hemodynamic status.

• Assess vital signs every 5 to 15 minutes during the acute stage; institution protocol should be followed if the patient is receiving vasoactive drugs.

• Initiate vasoactive drugs to support blood pressure (ensuring that volume IV fluid has been administered, because it is ineffective to constrict empty capillary beds); phenylephrine to vasoconstrict (pure alpha adrenergic agent), dopamine or Levophed (norepinephrine) for beta and alpha effects.

• Administer blood transfusions, as ordered. Monitor for transfusion reactions.
• Monitor Hb, HCT, and arterial oxygen pressures.
• Monitor clotting factors, which may decrease with the transfusion of large amounts of blood products: administer FFP as needed.

Identification of active bleeding

Attempts to identify the source of bleeding may be initiated during fluid resuscitation; they must not prohibit appropriate resuscitation efforts. The source must be identified as soon as possible to determine the most effective treatment and curative regimen. Invasive procedures may be performed to locate and treat the source of the GI bleeding. (For a description of these procedures, see *Invasive treatment regimens for GI hemorrhage,* pages 316 to 318.)

The following nursing interventions should be incorporated into the plan of care:
• Ensure immediate placement of nasogastric (NG) tube.
• Lavage the stomach with room-temperature fluid to clear the clots from the stomach, as well as to assess the rate of bleeding.
• Put NG tube to intermittent suction or straight drainage for continued assessment.
• Check stool and emesis for blood quality and quantity.
• Prepare the patient, as needed, for diagnostic testing and invasive procedures.

Prevention of complications

Prolonged hypovolemia and hypotension may precipitate multiple organ dysfunction and compromise. Careful monitoring of the patient may prevent further insults to the system, as well as limiting the sequelae of the initial injury.

The following nursing interventions should be incorporated into the plan of care:
• Maintain airway support; monitor and prevent aspiration secondary to bypassing of the gastroesophageal sphincter.

(Text continues on page 318.)

Invasive treatment regimens for GI hemorrhage

The patient with a GI hemorrhage will often require concomitant resuscitation, stabilization, and treatment activities. The patient must be prepared for multiple invasive activities occurring simultaneously. Frequent and detailed patient assessment should continue throughout the treatment period, with special attention given to the evaluation for rebleeding, whether from the original site or a fresh site.

Treatment	Description	Nursing Actions
Therapeutic endoscopy	Bleeding is controlled by electrocoagulation and laser therapy directed at the bleeding site; recommended for patients with clinical evidence of major bleeding, endoscopic evidence of an ulcer with major bleeding, or a nonbleeding visible vessel	• Inform the patient that analgesia, sedation, and lubrication will be used. Explain that the patient will be positioned on the left side during the procedure and that oral intake is prohibited before and after (until the gag reflex returns). • Apply a pulse oximeter, cardiac monitor, and blood pressure measurement equipment during the procedure. • Inform the patient that cauterization may require placement of a sticky grounding pad on the patient's thigh and that insufflation of air to facilitate visualization may result in a full and "gassy" feeling.
Endoscopic sclerotherapy	Direct injection of caustic agents into the base of an ulcer or other bleeding lesion via a retractable sclerotherapy needle through the biopsy channel of an endoscope; commonly used to treat esophageal varices	• Inform the patient that analgesia, sedation, and lubrication will be used. Explain that the patient will be positioned on the left side during the procedure and that oral intake is prohibited before and after (until the gag reflex returns). • Apply a pulse oximeter, cardiac monitor, and blood pressure measurement equipment during the procedure. • Explain that repeated endoscopies and therapies probably will be required over a prolonged period to prevent rebleeding. • Monitor temperature following sclerotherapy. Fevers are common in 40% of patients in the first 48 hours.

Invasive treatment regimens for GI hemorrhage *(continued)*

Treatment	Description	Nursing Actions
Endoscopic sclerotherapy *(continued)*		• Monitor for complications following the procedure, including ulcerations, stricture formation, perforation, sepsis, pleural effusions, and acute respiratory distress syndrome. • Inform the patient of the potential for transient chest pain related to the sclerotherapy; it is not indicative of cardiac problems.
Arterial angiography	Allows the angiographer to instill medication (vasopressin) or to embolize the bleeding artery with absorbable gelatin sponge, metal coil springs, or other agents	• Monitor for adverse reactions, including bradycardia, vasoconstriction, myocardial ischemia, and abdominal pain or cramping. • Monitor for adverse reactions related to the cannulizing of an arterial vessel. • Monitor for distant vessel or organ embolization.
Balloon tamponade	Tamponade of bleeding vessels above the gastroesophageal junction; associated with moderate, temporary success	• Prepare the patient for placement of a large 3-port to 4-port tube through one of the nares. • Advance the tube until gastric placement is confirmed; the gastric balloon of the tube is then inflated and pulled back against the gastroesophageal junction. If bleeding is above this junction, the second balloon is inflated in the esophagus to compress bleeders in this area. The tube is then anchored in place by an external fixator, such as a football helmet–type device to which the tube is secured. • Provide careful maintenance of the traction so the balloons and tube do not advance. Nares may become ischemic or necrotic. • Some balloon catheters have ports for aspiration of stomach contents; regardless, aspiration precautions must be instituted. • Periodically deflate the balloons according to medical and manufacturers recommendations. *(continued)*

Invasive treatment regimens for GI hemorrhage *(continued)*

Treatment	Description	Nursing Actions
Surgery	Removal of bleeding or intractable peptic ulcer; may involve shunt surgery (to decrease variceal bleeding by bypassing portions of portal circulation and releasing portal pressures), severing of portions of the vagus nerve (to decrease acid production), or ligation of esophageal varices	• If emergency surgery is required, perform a rapid assessment and provide any instruction required. • If no emergency exists, perform a standard preoperative workup. • Prepare the patient for the possibility of "dumping syndrome" (rapid transit through the gut following meals, sometimes accompanied by vasomotor symptomatology), which can be controlled by dietary measures. Some patients will experience postvagotomy diarrhea, which can be partially controlled by diet. • When ligation of the esophageal varix has been performed monitor the patient closely for signs and symptoms related to portal hypertension, including bleeding at a new site. This procedure will relieve the acute bleeding episode but will not relieve the portal hypertension that caused the varices.
Transjugular intrahepatic portosystemic shunt (TIPS)	Nonsurgical procedure that results in stent placement between the systemic and portal venous systems; results in decreased portal venous pressures, decreased variceal pressures, and control of bleeding	• Monitor the patient for the development of or an increase in hepatic encephalopathy, because the blood flow shunted past the liver is not cleansed appropriately. • Monitor for bleeding and infection following the procedure. • Administer lactulose therapy, as ordered, to decrease ammonia production and treat increased encephalopathy.

• Evaluate for pulmonary edema and congestive heart failure with volume resuscitation; notify the physician of rales, dyspnea, shortness of breath, peripheral edema, or distended neck veins.

• Evaluate for complications resulting from massive transfusions (transfusion reactions, calcium binding with citrate in banked blood, potassium increasing with hemolysis and degradation of blood).

• Monitor the patient's safety:

—If a Sengstaken-Blakemore tube is used to compress esophageal varices, ensure that the tube is correctly secured and balloons are intact;

—Evaluate NG tube placement every shift and before administration of drugs or feedings; evaluate mucous membranes for erosion of nares with long-term use of an NG tube;

—Restrain limbs to protect the patient and lines according to need and institutional protocols.

• If vasopressin is administered, monitor the ECG for signs and symptoms of cardiac ischemia (elevation of the ST segment) and hemodynamic compromise (decreased cardiac output, bradyarrhythmias); also monitor for abdominal cramping (mesenteric ischemia, with potential for infarction). Consider administration of nitroglycerin (continuous infusion or paste patch) to vasodilate the coronary arteries.

• Monitor BUN (increased with protein breakdown in the gut, dehydration) and ammonia level (increased with protein breakdown in the gut and in patients with hepatic disorders).

• Provide constant assessment for evidence of rebleeding; check NG tube aspirate, stools, emesis.

• Provide consistent oral care to control breakdown and risk of infection.

• Provide rectal skin care (blood within the GI tract acts as a cathartic agent and will lead to significant diarrhea and increase the risk of infection from skin breakdown).

• Administer medication, as needed, to alcoholic patients to tolerate symptoms of withdrawal.

Pharmacologic treatment

Most patients can expect to be on long-term pharmaceutical therapies that require vigilant self-medication (see *Major drugs for GI hemorrhage,* pages 320 and 321). Meeting nutritional requirements (decreasing

MAJOR DRUGS

Major drugs for GI hemorrhage

Therapy for GI hemorrhage is less definitive than for other diseases. Below is a sampling of medications that may be used when caring for the patient with a GI hemorrhage.

Medication	Effect	Nursing Considerations
Antacids (Maalox, Mylanta)	Used to neutralize gastric acidity and decreased the rate of gastric emptying; to decrease the erosive effect of hydrochloric acid	• Monitor for constipation (with Amphojel [aluminum hydroxide]) or diarrhea (with Maalox and Mylanta). • Monitor for elevated magnesium in patients with renal failure (from GI absorption of magnesium found in magnesium hydroxide formulations) or for hypophosphatemia (phosphate is bound to and excreted with aluminum hydroxide agents).
Histamine blockers (famotidine, ranitidine, cimetidine)	Block gastric secretion of hydrochloric acid; will not stop an active GI hemorrhage, but may help prevent rebleeding from ulcerations	• Monitor for adverse reactions including dizziness, headache, constipation, neutropenia, thrombocytopenia, and GI distress. • Monitor dosing of cimetidine in patients who are elderly or with a compromised hepatic system; it may cause mental status changes. • Cimetidine also impairs metabolism of warfarin anticoagulants, theophylline, and phenytoin.
Vasopressin	Constricts mesenteric and coronary vessels; decreases blood flow to the mesentery	• Monitor for cramping, nausea, pain, and increased GI inflammation caused by mesenteric constriction. • Monitor for signs of cardiac compromise, including angina, ischemia, bradyarrhythmias, or myocardial infarction. Maintain continuous ECG monitoring and monitor vital signs frequently. • Frequently assess the infusion site for extravasation. • Monitor for adverse reactions, including bowel infarction, syndrome of inappropriate secretion of antidiuretic hormone and related electrolyte/fluid balance disturbances, diarrhea, and tremors.

Major drugs for GI hemorrhage *(continued)*

Medication	Effect	Nursing Considerations
Sucralfate	Coats stomach lining	• Do not administer immediately before or after histamine blockers, because it alters their efficacy.
Antibiotics (metronidazole, bismuth, erythromycin, amoxicillin, fluoroquinolones, omeprazole, nystatin, acyclovir, ganciclovir [DHPG])	Combination therapy is used to eradicate *Helicobacter pylori* from peptic ulcers (monotherapy probably not effective); antibiotics are also used to fight infectious sources of esophagitis and gastritis	• Monitor antibiotic levels in patients with hepatic or renal compromise; their ability to clear the drugs may be diminished. • Monitor albumin levels in the patient with hepatic disease, because the drug is usually bound to or carried by albumin. • Evaluate the patient for secondary or opportunistic infections.

protein intake for patients with compromised liver function, bland foods for patients who are hyperacidic, and so on) or limitations often are difficult.

Prognosis

About 80% of all episodes of GI bleeding stop spontaneously. Mortality is approximately 10% and has not changed in the last 30 years, despite medical and surgical advances. The prognosis is grimmer (23% to 30% mortality), however, if the patient is already in the hospital with a preexisting condition. Variceal bleeding alone is associated with a 41% mortality, with up to one third dying during the initial hospitalization; duodenal ulcers carry a 5.5% mortality rate. Mallory-Weiss tears have a very low mortality rate, with most stopping spontaneously and seldom recurring.

Overall prognostic factors include age, liver disease, organ failure, bleeding site, degree of bleeding, extent of resuscitation required, concomitant disease process, and vital signs at the initiation of bleeding.

Discharge planning

The patient who has survived an episode of either upper or lower GI bleeding will require careful follow-up. All of the following factors should be considered to prepare the patient for discharge:

• Reinforce lifestyle changes (stress reduction, alcohol counseling, nutritional support) necessary to prevent recurrence.

• Consult with psychiatric, nutritional, and substance abuse counselors.

• Encourage smoking cessation, as smoking is associated with an increased rate or recurrence of peptic ulcer disease.

• Teach the patient the signs and symptoms of recurrent bleeding (occult blood, light-headedness, syncope, abdominal pain, bloating).

• Teach which drugs to avoid or to take consistently in keeping with the therapeutic regimen.

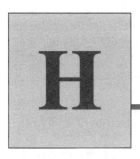

Head trauma

Head injury will affect over 10 million people this year. Trauma is a major cause of death and disability in the under-45 age group, and many of these deaths are associated with head injury. Most head injuries result from motor vehicle accidents; other causes are falls, sports injuries, and violent crime. Not only does head injury carry with it a high mortality rate (20% to 50%) (Ross 1992), but the morbidity associated with survival also is a long-term problem. Of the 75,000 people who will suffer head injury this year, 2,000 will be left in a persistently vegetative state, and another 6,000 will have hemiplegia, paraplegia, or quadriplegia (Testani-Dufor 1992). Deficits such as memory difficulty, decreased attention span, and inability to concentrate, along with personality changes that affect most victims of head injury, add to the high morbidity rate.

Pathophysiology

Head injuries occur as a result of dynamic forces within the intracranial cavity. The brain is semi-solid and easily torn and bruised as it moves inside the very rigid and irregular skull. Primary injury to the brain occurs at the time of impact, results in tissue or vascular disruption, and generally is irreversible. Most primary head injuries are a result of an acceleration-deceleration impact. In this type of injury the head hits a rigid structure and the brain rotates and moves laterally inside the skull, producing internal stress on the tissue. The result of this is compression of tissue, tension or stretching of the fibers, and shearing of the neurons.

The velocity of the impact plays a major role in the severity of the injury. This mechanism of injury often produces a primary lesion (coup) and a contrecoup lesion, one opposite the area of impact, as a result of the brain's rapid movement inside the skull.

Recognized for years in head injury but only recently being understood is the secondary injury that occurs hours or days after injury to the brain. Secondary injury often is the result of hypoxia, hypotension, hypercarbia, edema, ischemia, and increased intracranial pressure (ICP). These conditions cause inadequate oxygenation of tissue, which contributes to ischemia. Patients who suffer mild head injury are at great risk for poorer outcome as a result of secondary injury.

Cellular derangements also are being further explored to explain this phase of head injury. When cerebral perfusion falls, impulse transmission is lost. Because membrane potential cannot be maintained, energy-dependent transport mechanisms fail. As a result, "toxic" levels of neurotransmitters such as glutamate and aspartate circulate in the extracellular fluid, increasing tissue ischemia.

Head injuries usually are classified as focal injuries, diffuse injuries, or fractures. Focal injuries occur at a specific site in the cranial vault and account for more than half of all brain injuries seen, most often as a result of acceleration-deceleration injuries. Lesions that fall into the category of focal injuries include cerebral contusion and epidural, subdural, and intracerebral hematomas (for further information, see *Focal head injuries,* page 325). A focal lesion can become an expanding-mass lesion and can cause symptoms of increased ICP. Neurologic dysfunction can progress rapidly, leading to herniation of the brain.

Focal head injuries

Focal injuries, a common finding in head injury, present a neurologic picture of injury to a specific area of the brain. The common classifications, management, and outcomes for focal injuries are listed below. For specific information on the Glasgow Coma Scale (GCS), refer to the entry on Cerebrovascular Accident.

Type and Mechanism of Injury	Management	Outcome
Contusion Acceleration or deceleration injury creating tissue necrosis, pulping, and infarct. Most common in the frontal and temporal lobes.	Monitor for signs of increased intracranial pressure (ICP). Extensive contusions require surgical evacuation.	Mortality 25 to 60%. Good outcome is associated with no coma under age 50.
Epidural hematoma Usually results from falls, motor vehicle accidents, or assaults. Usually associated with temporal bone fracture.	Surgical evacuation of hematoma.	Depends on severity. GCS 3 to 5 = 40%, GCS 6 to 8 = 90% mortality.
Subdural hematoma Results from falls, motor vehicle accidents, or assaults. May be acute, chronic, or subacute, depending on timing of symptom presentation.	Surgical evacuation of hematoma.	Acute = 90% mortality.
Intracerebral hematoma Acceleration or deceleration injury. Also can result from penetrating injury.	Monitor for signs of ICP. Surgical removal sometimes indicated if in a location that will not lead to increased deficits.	High morbidity.

Diffuse brain injuries involve multiple areas of the brain, resulting in more widespread neuronal injury. The damage occurs in the white matter of the brain and is microscopic in nature. It results from shearing forces as the brain moves within the skull, stretching nerve fibers. Diffuse injuries range from mild to severe and are classified on the basis of the neurologic dysfunction exhibited by the patient. (For a discussion of the various types, see *Diffuse brain injuries,* page 326.)

Diffuse brain injuries

Diffuse brain injuries are a result of a more global injury without lateralizing signs. Patients with a diffuse injury often have no specific findings on diagnostic studies yet present with a picture of severe neurologic damage. The degrees of diffuse injuries are listed.

Type	Presentation	Outcome
Concussion	Clinical diagnosis based on degree of symptoms. Transient loss of consciousness followed by varying degrees of memory disturbances	• There generally are no deficits. • Postconcussion syndrome, characterized by headache and memory difficulty, can last up to 1 year after the injury; treatment is symptomatic.
Mild diffuse axonal injury	Deep coma without focal lesion on computed tomography (CT), lasting 6 to 24 hours; involves both hemispheres, reticular activating system, and brain stem	• As level of consciousness (LOC) improves, can leave damage commonly cognitive or memory deficits.
Moderate diffuse axonal injury	Deep coma lasting more than 24 hours; no mass lesion on CT, but often diffuse white-matter swelling is seen	• Mortality is 20%. • Significant morbidity with wide variation in LOC and ability to perform activities of daily living. Most patients require lengthy rehabilitation and some assistance with daily routine.
Severe diffuse axonal injury	Deep, prolonged coma, often accompanied by spontaneous posturing; signs of significantly increased intracranial pressure	• Mortality is 57%. • Significant morbidity; many patients remain in the persistent vegetative state and require long-term nursing home care.

Skull fractures are a very common type of head injury. Statistics on skull fractures vary because many fractures occur at the base of the skull and are undetected by X-ray. In addition, many fractures that occur with other types of head injury remain unclassified. Fractures are divided into several categories, including linear, compound or depressed, comminuted, and basilar. The type of fracture depends on the velocity, direction, and momentum of the object on impact. (For a description of the most common fractures and treatment, see *Defining skull fractures,* page 328).

Clinical assessment

Assessment of the patient with a head injury should include as much history information as possible along with a physical examination that substantiates the neurologic injury. Diagnostic studies help to confirm the injury.

History

Routine history information (past medical history, family history, social history, and current medication) should be obtained from a reliable source as soon as possible. Other historical information that will help to evaluate the kind of injury sustained includes:
* mechanism of injury
* whether the patient was restrained if involved in a motor vehicle accident
* whether the air bag was deployed in a motor vehicle accident
* if applicable, whether the patient was wearing a helmet
* estimated speed at impact
* whether the object hit was stationary or moving
* recent alcohol or recreational drug use
* whether the patient lost consciousness
* the position in which the patient was found.

Physical findings

Signs and symptoms of head injury are related to the area of the brain involved and the magnitude of the injury. The most sensitive indicators of increased ICP are changes in level of consciousness (LOC) and pupil size, shape, and response to light. It is important to obtain good baseline values on these indicators early so that any deterioration in neurologic status can be measured. Assessment for focal signs can help localize the lesion. General findings include:
* depressed LOC ranging from lethargy to unarousable

Defining skull fractures

Skull fractures are a common head injury. The amount of neurologic dysfunction associated with a fracture depends on the damage to the underlying brain. Many fractures do not require any specific intervention. Types of fractures and treatment concerns are listed below.

Type	Defining Characteristics	Treatment
Linear	• Account for 70% of skull fractures • Characterized by a single clean break and no displacement of bony fragments • If along the temporal bone, associated with a laceration of the middle meningeal artery, which can contribute to the development of an epidural hematoma	• No medical intervention generally is needed. • Patient may be observed for 24 hours to assess for underlying brain injury. • Mild analgesic may be needed for headaches.
De-pressed	• Can cause an inward depression of the bony fragments that can tear the dura, resulting in neurological sequelae • Seriousness of the fracture determined by the damage to underlying brain structures	• Often requires surgical elevation of the depression and repair of dural tear. • Postoperatively, monitor for signs of increased intracranial pressure from the development of cerebral edema.
Comminuted	• Open fracture in which the bone splinters or crushes as it is displaced inward	• Repaired surgically with debridement of the underlying brain tissue. • Major risk is infection; monitor closely for signs of meningitis. • Often requires cranioplasty to repair the defect after risk of infection has passed.
Basilar	• Can arise as the extension of a linear fracture into the base of the skull in the anterior or middle fossa • 75% involve the petrous process of the temporal bone • Because of fragility of the bones in this area and how the dura adheres to it, cerebrospinal fluid (CSF) leak either from the nose or the ear is common	• Medical management varies, but patient may be on bed rest with head of the bed elevated. • Antibiotics may be administered for the risk of meningitis caused by a dural tear. • CSF leaks usually resolve without surgical intervention in about 7 to 10 days.

- nausea or vomiting
- headache
- motor dysfunction (observe for lateralization—dysfunction limited to one side), flaccid extremities
- abnormal or absent brain stem reflexes (cough, gag, corneal)
- abnormal respiratory pattern
- pupils sluggish or unreactive to light (unilateral or bilateral)
- large oval pupil (unilateral or bilateral)
- hemiplegia (usually associated with a focal lesion)
- deviation of one or both eyes
- abnormal posturing (decorticate, decerebrate)
- seizure activity
- absence of cough, gag, and oculocephalic reflexes
- abnormal respiratory patterns: Cheyne-Stokes, central neurogenic hyperventilation, apneustic, cluster, ataxic
- Battle's sign
- raccoon's eyes
- cerebrospinal fluid (CSF) rhinorrhea or otorrhea (CSF leaking from the nose or ear).

Diagnosis

Presumptive diagnosis of head injury is based on the clinical presentation of the patient and the circumstances of the traumatic event. Definitive diagnosis often is made by radiologic examination.

The type of procedure used depends upon the type of injury suspected. If a focal injury is suspected, a computed tomography (CT) scan or an arteriogram is performed. For suspected fractures, skull films, CT bone windows, and physical findings (most common with basal fractures) are evaluated. History, physical examination, and the absence of a treatable lesion on CT provide evidence in a diffuse injury.

CT remains the imaging of choice in the acute phase of head injury because the scan time is shorter and the patient can be more easily monitored throughout the test. Magnetic resonance imaging often is used to confirm the diagnosis of diffuse axonal injury once

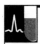

Confirming head injury

The following diagnostic studies are performed to confirm a diagnosis of head injury. Once the patient's condition has been stabilized and the presence of an injury is verified, studies such as positron emission tomography or evoked potential studies may be performed to provide further information that can be utilized as a prognostic indicator.

Skull X-rays
Determines the presence of fractures.

Computed tomography (CT)
Determines the presence of a hematoma or contusion of the brain. Also can identify cerebral edema and hydrocephalus.

Arteriogram
Identifies the cerebral blood vessels and any malformation or aneurysms.

Magnetic resonance imaging
Identifies structural lesions, presence of infarct, or shearing injuries not visible on CT.

the patient has stabilized. (For additional information, see *Confirming head injury,* page 330).

Treatment and care
Following a head injury, the immediate treatment goals are to promote hemodynamic stability and to quickly identify the type of injury so that a treatment plan can be developed. Initial treatment may require surgical intervention as well as continued assessment of neurological status to promote and improve neurologic function. Other goals include preventing further deterioration of status and secondary brain injury, such as increased ICP, and preventing complications that result from immobility.

Neurologic function regulation
Initial medical management is focused on treating the injury, promoting improvement in neurologic function, and preventing further deterioration in neurologic status. If diagnostic procedures identify a space-occupying lesion, surgical removal of the lesion may be required. The prompt evacuation of a hematoma increases the likelihood of survival from head injury. In

addition to routine postoperative care, the patient also requires the same monitoring as a patient whose closed head injury does not require surgical intervention.

Monitoring neurologic status is essential to optimizing the patient's outcome. The key to the assessment is to establish a firm baseline and note any deviations that may indicate a worsening status. Frequent assessments often identify subtle changes that may indicate increased ICP, which must be treated promptly. The follow nursing interventions should be incorporated into the plan of care:

• Perform frequent neurologic assessments, including the evaluation of the following: LOC; pupil size, shape, and reaction to light; extraocular movements and deviations of gaze; presence or absence of brain stem reflexes; motor response, including normal, random, purposeful, non-purposeful, decorticate or decerebrate posturing; and symmetry of motor response or presence of weakness.

• Monitor ICP and its correlation with the clinical assessment whenever possible.

• Maintain normovolemic to slightly hypovolemic fluid status.

• Maintain mean arterial pressure (MAP) to promote a cerebral perfusion pressure (CPP) of 60 to 70 mm Hg.

• Monitor serum electrolyte levels, especially sodium and potassium.

• Maintain pulmonary function and adequate oxygenation.

Management of ICP

All head trauma victims require care focused on prevention of secondary brain injury and increased ICP. Increased ICP associated with head injury is usually caused by cerebral edema. Brain edema occurs rapidly after head injury and usually peaks within 72 hours. Pharmacologic management may be initiated based on the ICP findings. (See the section entitled Pharmacologic Management, page 333, for further information.)

Treatment aimed at reducing CO_2 may be utilized to decrease venous engorgement. Reduction of partial pressure of carbon dioxide by hyperventilation promotes cerebral vasoconstriction but usually is effective only during the first 2 days after injury. This treatment must be instituted with care because vasoconstriction decreases cerebral blood flow, which could contribute to secondary brain injury through infarction of cerebral tissue. The degree of hyperventilation is based on individual patient response, but the general range is between 25 and 30 mm Hg.

If an ICP monitor is not in place, treatment will be initiated based on changes in the neurologic examination. ICP monitoring is used to provide a continuous trend of the pressure in the cranial cavity throughout this critical period. The intraventricular catheter is one of the most commonly used ICP monitors because it does not require a special monitor. (For further discussion, see *Types of intracranial pressure (ICP) monitors,* page 333). Drainage of CSF effectively reduces ICP and with the ventricular catheter in place can be accomplished repeatedly. The physician will order the height of the drainage collection chamber and parameters for drainage. A new monitoring technique, jugular bulb oxygen saturation (SjO_2) monitoring, also is being used to provide information about the metabolic state of the brain. (For additional information, see *Jugular bulb oxygen saturation (SjO_2) monitoring,* page 334.)

The following nursing interventions should be incorporated into the plan of care:
• Perform frequent neurologic assessments.
• Maintain ICP monitoring device.
• Drain ventriculostomy as necessary.
• Administer medications, as ordered. (See the section entitled Pharmacologic Management, page 333, for further information.)
• Incorporate strategies to minimize the effects of routine care on the patient's ICP, such as keeping environmental stimuli to a minimum, promoting rest periods between interventions, performing routine pulmonary care including suctioning, maintaining the neck in a neutral position, and avoiding extreme hip flexion. To

Types of intracranial pressure (ICP) monitors

ICP monitoring has become standard to the critical care phase of management of head injury. Several types of monitors are available, each with specific advantages and disadvantages.

Type	Advantages	Disadvantages
Intraventricular catheter	• Rapid access to the ventricles for cerebrospinal fluid (CSF) drainage and sampling • Allows for assessment compliance • Considered most accurate	• High risk of infection, hemorrhage, or CSF leak • Requires frequent zero balancing • Inadvertent loss of CSF • Can cause subdural empyema
Subarachnoid bolt or screw	• No penetration of brain • Lower risk of infection	• At high pressure can be inaccurate • Brain may herniate through the bolt • Requires frequent zero balancing
Epidural sensor	• Easy to insert • No fluid system • No zero balancing after insertion	• No access to CSF • Measurement is less reliable
Intraparenchymal sensor	• Easy to insert • No fluid system • Good waveform even with significant cerebral edema • No zero balancing after insertion	• No access to CSF • Relationship between volume and pressure cannot be measured • Higher infection risk because system is placed directly into brain tissue

promote good venous drainage, keep the head of the bed elevated between 30 and 45 degrees as long as MAP is not compromised.

Pharmacologic management

Cerebral edema in traumatic brain injury most often is the vasogenic type, in which fluid from the intravascular space leaks into the brain tissue because of a breakdown of the blood-brain barrier. As cerebral edema

Jugular bulb oxygen saturation (SjO_2) monitoring

SjO_2 monitoring provides information about the metabolic state of the brain, which is especially helpful in head-injured patients. Monitoring requires the placement of a fiberoptic catheter. The SjO_2 monitor is placed in the jugular bulb where the venous outflow of the brain drains. Measuring O_2 content at this point allows a determination of how much O_2 is being utilized by the brain and therefore of cerebral metabolism and blood flow. Normal SjO_2 is thought to be in a range of 60% to 80% when the partial pressure of carbon dioxide is normal. Oligemic cerebral hypoxia is present when the SjO_2 falls below 50%. It is important for the nurse to rule out systemic factors such as anemia or hypotension as a cause when the SjO_2 falls. Monitoring of SjO_2 gives additional information about the effects of increased intracranial pressure and allows for rapid changes in treatment plan in response to the changes in this dynamic parameter.

builds, diuretic therapy is used to reduce cerebral water, which can help to reduce ICP.

The treatment regimen also may include muscle relaxants, sedatives, or paralytic agents to control increased ICP. This will decrease the response to noxious stimuli known to increase thoracic and venous pressures, and also decrease cellular muscle activity, which in turn will promote a decrease in ICP and a decrease in O_2 consumption. The most commonly used drugs, vecuronium and morphine sulfate, can be given as hourly boluses or as continuous infusions. In the early phases of treatment, continuous infusion often provides better control. Prior to any procedure, the patient not receiving continuous sedation should receive a sedative and analgesic medication, if necessary. ICP that does not respond to conventional therapy may be managed by utilizing barbiturate coma therapy. Therapy usually consists of initiating a loading dose of pentobarbital, followed by a continuous infusion.

The following nursing interventions should be incorporated into the plan of care:

• Administer mannitol, 0.5 to 1.5 g/kg, which is given by I.V. bolus for an acute rise in ICP or given as a continuous infusion.

• Obtain baseline and serial urine and serum osmolarities prior to administering Mannitol and during the duration of mannitol therapy.

• Notify the physician if the serum osmolarity rises above 315 mOsm/liter. Therapy generally is discontinued.

• Monitor serum sodium level, as hypernatremia often is a concurrent result of this osmotic diuretic therapy.

• Titrate muscle-blocking agents, such as vecuronium, to the lowest dose possible by using a train-of-four response, which involves using a peripheral nerve stimulator to stimulate the ulnar nerve by giving four successive stimuli. The ideal response, single thumb adduction, represents 92% blockade of neuromuscular function and correlates clinically with absence of movement. This is interpreted as a 1:4 train-of-four thumb adduction.

• Maintain a consistent therapeutic barbiturate level by continuous infusion, as ordered. The dosage usually is a 3 to 10 mg/kg loading dose, followed by an infusion at about 2 to 3 mg/kg/hour.

• Monitor electroencephalogram (EEG) to be sure the patient is at the desired level. If a burst suppression is noted on the EEG, the barbiturate dose is deemed therapeutic.

• Monitor for side effects of barbiturate therapy such as cardiovascular failure by evaluating pulmonary artery catheter pressures during therapy.

Prevention of complications

Other care administered to the patient with a head trauma is directed at preventing secondary injury and involves support of other body systems. Measures may be instituted to prevent alterations in temperature or blood pressure and seizures. The patient also is monitored for any adverse effects from prolonged immobility. Both hyperthermia and seizures will increase cerebral metabolic demand and subsequently increase ICP. Research in head injury is challenging the traditional management of the patient with increased ICP. Because early

Cerebral perfusion pressure (CPP) management

Investigational research done by Dr. Michael Rosner of the Division of Neurosurgery, University of Alabama, suggests that CPP can be managed by augmenting the systemic arterial pressure in patients with increased intracranial pressure (ICP). The goal is to maintain the CPP (mean arterial blood pressure [MABP] – ICP) above 70; in some patients the desired CPP may be higher.

Achieving the desired CPP is accomplished by the use of pressors to raise the systemic blood pressure to a level that will achieve the desired CPP in the face of an elevated ICP. Thus, if the desired CPP is

90 and the ICP is 20, the MABP should be 110. The most commonly used pressor is phenylephrine, which often is used with low-dose dopamine to protect renal function.

Other differences in this method of management include:
• Normovolemia is maintained.
• Mannitol is used for its positive hemodynamic effects on hemodilution, decreasing blood viscosity and improving oxygen delivery.
• The patient is maintained in a flat position.

The results of his studies have shown a decrease in mortality by 50%, with a corresponding increase in quality-of-life measures.

reports suggest a better outcome, critical care nurses may see the management of these patients change (see *Cerebral perfusion pressure (CPP) management,* page 336).

The following nursing interventions should be incorporated into the plan of care to prevent complications:

• Observe for signs of infection or elevated temperature.

• Treat hyperthermia promptly with acetaminophen and cooling blankets.

• Avoid rapid changes in temperature, because hypothermia can cause shivering, which will increase cerebral metabolic demand as well.

• Administer anticonvulsant medications such as phenytoin prophylactically, as prescribed.

• Maintain skin clean and dry.

• Turn, reposition, and provide range of motion for the patient every 2 hours.

• Use functional splints as needed.

• Initiate rehabilitation care or consultation as soon as possible.

Prognosis

Most studies that have evaluated recovery from severe head injury agree that the greatest degree of recovery is achieved in the 6 months after the injury and that any subsequent recovery generally is not significant. Most patients with severe head injury have a poor outcome, with persistent motor, sensory, and cognitive disabilities. Patients who have experienced moderate head injury most often report difficulty with persistent headache, memory difficulty, and problems with activities of daily living. In the category of minor head injury, 80% complain of headache and slightly more than half complain of memory difficulty. On cognitive evaluation, mild head injury patients are found to have significant problems with attention, memory, concentration, and judgment.

Discharge planning

A multidisciplinary team approach is required to continually assess the patient's changing needs and make the appropriate referrals. The nurse's role is to assess both patient and family needs and to coordinate the efforts of all the disciplines. Discharge needs to be addressed include:
• identification of inpatient rehabilitation services for the severely head-injured patient
• availability of support services, including occupational, speech, cognitive, and physical therapy
• possible placement to a skilled nursing facility
• outpatient rehabilitation services for the moderate to mild head-injured patient
• referrals to home and community service agencies.

Hepatic failure

Hepatic failure is characterized by the loss or disruption of one or more of the liver's four major functions: glucose and lipid metabolism, drug and toxin metabolism, protein synthesis, and phagocytic clearance of organisms and cellular debris. As a result of these disruptions, the body is unable to meet metabolic demands, remove cellular or metabolic by-products, produce the building blocks of the clotting cascade and transport proteins, and protect the body from various organisms. The hepatocellular disruption and functional loss may be the result of a sudden and acute insult (infection, inflammation, direct injury), a chronic condition that slowly compromises hepatocellular organization, or complete destruction such as seen with cirrhosis.

Pathophysiology

In hepatic failure, the liver functions are compromised and energy regulation is significantly altered. The result can be overwhelming hyperglycemia when the glycogen stores are released indiscriminately, followed by hypoglycemia from exhaustion of energy stores and subsequent inability to replenish them. Acetyl coenzyme A, produced during fat metabolism and transported as ketones for energy supply at distant sites, is not produced when liver function is disrupted. Therefore, energy stores are compromised in areas outside the liver itself.

With hepatocellular destruction and flow abnormalities, the phagocytic Kupffer cells cannot function appropriately. As a result of hepatic compromise, bacterial phagocytosis is impaired secondary to the decreased synthesis of complement, neutrophil adherence is diminished, and polymorphonuclear leukocyte function is compromised. Without the ability to degrade toxins and convert substances into less toxic forms, cellular by-products and ingested toxins are left to collect and circulate throughout the body. Inability to process the ammonia that is created during the deamination of proteins and fats for energy is just one of the side effects of diminished clearance of endogenous toxins. Consequently, these toxins are responsible for changes in mental status and alteration in cognitive function of the hepatic patient. (For additional discussion, see *Grades of hepatic coma,* page 340.)

Plasma proteins, such as albumin and gamma globulins, are not produced in adequate quantities in the patient with liver disease. As a result, the plasma oncotic pressure is altered and fluid tends to be pulled out of the vessels instead of remaining in the circulation. The displaced volume results in edema and ascites, as evidenced by weight gain in the presence of intravascular volume depletion. Substances that rely on the proteins and albumin for transport are severely affected in hepatic compromise.

The liver is responsible for creation of all clotting factors except factor VIII (von Willebrand's factor). Without these factors, normal hemostatic mechanisms no longer are functional. Thrombocytopenia is common. Platelet disruption can occur because of functional problems (alteration in platelet adhesion and adherence properties) or because the count and morphology have been altered. Fibrin levels increase, as do the levels of fibrin split products. These products, normally degraded by the liver, accumulate in liver failure.

Inappropriate clotting may result from diminished production of endogenous heparin and antithrombin III, a coagulation inhibitor. At the same time, because the patient cannot absorb and store vitamin K from the GI tract, coagulation factors and pathways that depend on the use of vitamin K do not function appropriately, and the patient is at increased risk for initiation and continuation of bleeding.

Bile production is markedly decreased in the patient with hepatocellular disease, and prolonged dysfunction can lead to vitamin deficiencies and excess bile salts that normally are used to form bile. It is the inability of the liver to combine glucuronic acid and

ASSESSMENT TIP
Grades of hepatic coma

Clinical signs and symptoms of hepatic failure often are measured along a continuum. The patient with severe hepatic disease may progress into hepatic coma. The following descriptions of clinical findings can be used to assess the patient's condition.

Grade	Patient Characteristics
I	Restless, euphoric, confused (mild), depressed; asterixis, reversal of sleep cycle
II	Drowsy, using inappropriate behavior or speech, having difficulty with fine motor movement, confused; asterixis
III	Stuporous but arousable, without fine motor coordination, very confused, incoherent speech; asterixis
IV	Comatose, responsive to noxious stimuli but will become unresponsive; no asterixis

bilirubin that is equated with increased bilirubin counts and clinical jaundice.

Acute hepatic injury

Acute infectious and inflammatory disorders, trauma, and toxic and drug-induced hepatic injury may antedate severe functional disruption of hepatic function. Exposure to an injurious agent causes inflammation, cellular damage, necrosis, or hyperplasia with phagocytic infiltration into the hepatic tissue. Edema, lobular disorganization, and functional compromise result in the clinical symptomatology. The extent of injury can be as mild as infiltration and inflammation or as severe as necrosis and lobular collapse.

Infectious hepatitis

Infectious sources of hepatitis include protozoa, bacteria, and viruses. Most cases of infectious hepatic disease result from a viral infection; the most common are listed in *Summary of viral hepatitis A–E,* pages 342 and 343. Other viruses include coxsackievirus, cytomegalovirus, adenovirus, Epstein-Barr, herpes simplex, infectious mononucleosis, rubella, and yellow fever.

Drugs and toxins

Drugs that are known to precipitate liver disease include acetaminophen, halothane, isoniazid, methyldopa, monamine oxidase inhibitors, rifampin, tetracycline, valproic acid, and nonsteroidal anti-inflammatory agents. Some patients develop idiosyncratic hepatic failure after exposure to a drug not commonly associated with hepatotoxic drug reactions; these patients have "hypersensitivity" reactions, postulated to be the result of an immune-mediated reaction to the drug or its metabolites. Each toxin produces its own form of hepatocellular and lobular damage that often can be identified on direct cellular examination.

The most common ingested toxin is alcohol. The liver will preferentially degrade alcohol before carbohydrates and glucose. In the process, fats that would have otherwise been used as nutrient energy are deposited in the liver cells and cause hepatocellular destruction. Cells begin to balloon, degenerate, and necrose. Oxygen demand is increased because of the use of alternate metabolic pathways, leaving the liver more susceptible to ischemia. Production of triglycerides increases, the process of gluconeogenesis is impaired, and glucose supplies within the liver are reduced.

Certain plants (for example, *Amanita phalloides* mushrooms) cause hepatic damage, as do many industrial toxins. Other injurious agents include paint, paint-removal products, and chemicals used for developing photographs, especially when used in enclosed or poorly ventilated areas.

Hypoperfusion of liver

Obstruction of flow through and out of the liver increases hepatocellular swelling and venous congestion. Budd-Chiari syndrome is defined as interruption of normal blood flow out of the liver, usually by obstruction of one or more of the hepatic veins or the inferior

Summary of viral hepatitis A–E

The following chart compares and contrasts the possible causes of viral hepatic disease.

Feature	Hepatitis A	Hepatitis B
Incubation	15 to 45 days (mean 30)	30 to 180 days (mean 60 to 90)
Onset	Acute	Insidious
Age preference	Children, young adults	Any age
Transmission	Fecal-oral, sexual (especially oral-anal contact), nonpercutaneous (sexual, maternal-neonatal), unusual percutaneous	Nonpercutaneous, percutaneous
Severity	Mild	Often severe
Prognosis	Generally good	Worse with age, premorbid debility
Progression to chronicity	None	Occasional

vena cava. It can be caused by thrombosis, tumors, venal caval web, or right-sided heart failure serious enough to produce congestion. Whatever the cause, the result is sinusoidal dilatation, decreased perfusion, cellular ischemia, cellular necrosis, and hepatic failure. Similar effects are found in patients with veno-occlusive disease, in which obstruction occurs at the hepatic venule level. Initiating factors for veno-occlusive disease are some chemotherapy regimens, irradiation, and some pyrrolizidine alkaloids, which are contained in bush teas.

Hepatitis C	Hepatitis D	Hepatitis E
15 to 160 days (mean 50)	14 to 64 days	14 to 60 days (mean 40)
Insidious	Acute and chronic	Acute
More common in adults	Any age	Young adults (20 to 40)
Blood-borne, unknown fecal-oral transmission ability	Parenteral route; must be infected with hepatitis B also, as it lives in the hepatitis B viral shell	Primarily fecal-oral
Moderate	Can be severe; may lead to fulminant hepatitis	Very virulent with frequent progression to fulminant hepatitis failure, especially if pregnant
Moderate	Fair; worse in chronic cases; can lead to chronic hepatitis D virus and chronic liver disease	Good, unless pregnant
10% to 50% of cases	Occasional	None

Regardless of the perfusion it receives, the liver has a constant oxygen requirement. When flow diminishes to the extent that oxygen supply is reduced while demand remains constant, hepatocellular ischemia and injury result. This occurs when patients present with volume deficits caused by hypovolemia or third-space fluid shifts, or in cases of cardiogenic shock. In early shock, the liver can compensate slightly by mobilizing volume reserves and directing flow. After the initial shock period (usually less than 24 hours), the liver is unable to maintain its compensatory response, and perfusion becomes consistently less than required. The results are ischemia and central liver necrosis.

Chronic hepatic injury

Chronic hepatic disease is characterized by long-term, progressive disease processes. Complications such as portal hypertension, ascites, bleeding, and varices plague the patient and may result in cirrhosis and death.

Chronic hepatitis

Hepatic inflammation, necrosis, or dysfunction that continues for more than 6 months is considered chronic hepatitis. Chronic hepatitis has the same causes as acute hepatitis, excluding hepatitis A, which does not progress to chronic disease. While medications, metabolic disorders, and autoimmune diseases often can be identified as the precipitator of chronic hepatitis, in some patients its cause may never be identified.

Cirrhosis

Cirrhosis results from massive, irreversible liver injury. The most common cause is alcohol abuse, although it may result from a variety of infections, medications, and metabolic and hereditary factors. The injury leads to destruction of the support structures for the healthy cells and lobes. The liver tries to regenerate the tissue by depositing collagen in the injured area. In the cirrhotic liver, these collagen deposits are organized into bands of fibrotic tissue, which, when connected, cause reorganization of the liver's basic structure. The vascular structures upon which the liver depends now are compressed and twisted by the collagen bands, increasing the pressure within the liver itself. If blood flow is not maintained or regained, ischemia and necrosis will result.

Clinical assessment

Assessment of the patient with hepatic disease should focus on identifying the possible cause of hepatic injury, as well as the extent of systemic effects.

History

In taking the history of a patient with probable liver disease, the nurse should elicit the following information:
- recent travel
- amount and frequency of alcohol consumption
- history of liver disease
- duration of current problems
- sexual behavior and patterns
- recent use of prescription and nonprescription drugs
- exposure to chemicals or toxic substances
- previous medical history.

Physical findings

The health care team caring for a patient with hepatic failure will assess for symptoms associated with the actual disease process. Specific symptoms of fulminant hepatic failure can be found in *Fulminant hepatic failure*, page 346. The patient may present with mental status changes associated with the liver's inability to convert ammonia and its diminished capacity to clear endogenous toxins from the body. The patient may present with GI bleeding related to a loss of normally functional hemostatic properties of the liver. The physical findings associated with acute hepatitis include:
- asterixis
- jaundice
- pruritus (itching, irritated skin)
- clay-colored stool
- elevated temperature
- fatigue.

Vague, flu-like symptoms that have a relatively insidious onset, including the following:
- anorexia, nausea, weight loss
- headache
- cough, low-grade fever
- right upper quadrant pain.

Patients with chronic hepatitis may be asymptomatic, but with exacerbation can exhibit signs of acute hepatitis, including anorexia, fatigue, and occasional nausea and vomiting.

Fulminant hepatic failure

Fulminant hepatic failure is defined as the acute onset of hepatic failure with the development of encephalopathy in the absence of chronic liver failure. It can follow any process that initiates hepatocellular destruction. Most commonly caused by viral hepatitis, especially in patients who are coinfected with hepatitis D, it also is seen with increasing frequency as a result of acetaminophen overdose. It is least prevalent with hepatitis A infections.

The signs and symptoms of fulminant liver failure are similar to those of any other form of liver compromise, except that they exacerbate rapidly and will lead to death if not promptly controlled. Full-blown fulminant hepatic failure is characterized by:

• jaundice, tachycardia, vasodilation, hypotension
• fluid retention, mild to extreme ascites, decreased urine output
• spider nevi, palmar erythema (from excess circulating hormones)
• bleeding (as a result of increased prothrombin time and fibrin degradation products)
• electrolyte and glucose abnormalities (decreased sodium, potassium, calcium, magnesium, and glucose levels), intolerance of protein intake
• arrhythmias, secondary to electrolyte imbalances
• fetor hepaticus (sweet, musty odor on the breath)
• asterixis
• hyperventilation (neurologic) and respiratory distress (from ascites and swollen liver)
• renal failure (prerenal azotemia, hypotension, or functional renal failure)
• alterations in level of consciousness, ranging from mild confusion to nonresponsive coma
• cerebral edema and increased intracranial pressure, unequal pupils (anisocoria), decerebrate posturing, myoclonus, abnormal oculocephalic and oculovestibular reflexes
• acid-base imbalance, secondary to inability to clear organic anions (lactic acid, pyruvate, acetoacetate, free fatty acids) and electrolyte imbalances
• sepsis (peritoneal, pancreatitis)
• portal hypertension.

The hallmarks of cirrhosis are coagulation deficits, metabolic and nutritional compromise, ascites, peripheral venocongestion, portal hypertension, hepatic encephalopathy, electrolyte imbalances, and alterations of glucose metabolism. (For further information, see *Signs and symptoms of cirrhosis,* page 347.)

Details of differences between the presentations of acute, alcoholic, and toxic or drug-induced hepatic disease are discussed in *Presentations of hepatic disease,* page 348.

Signs and symptoms of cirrhosis

The following table correlates the patient's signs and symptoms with the form of deterioration or injury caused by cirrhosis.

Cause	Signs and Symptoms
Prerenal kidney failure	• Azotemia
Loss of coagulation factors	• Bruising (impaired vitamin K uptake) • Bleeding
Circulatory compromise	• Clubbing of fingers
Disturbance of hormone metabolism	• Decreased body hair (men) • Gynecomastia (men) • Menstrual irregularities • Palmar erythema • Spider angiomas • Testicular atrophy • Virilization (women)
Nutritional abnormalities	• Hemolytic anemia (hypercholesterolemia) • Weakness, fatigue • Weight loss, loss of muscle • Hypokalemia • Bone pain, osteomalacia (impaired vitamin D uptake) • Dermatitis (impaired vitamin E uptake) • Xanthelasmas, xanthomas (elevation of serum lipids) • Glucose intolerance
Electrolyte imbalances	• Hypokalemia (hyperaldosteronism) • Hypomagnesemia (urinary losses, dietary deficiency)
Impaired bilirubin metabolism	• Jaundice, dark skin • Pruritus • Steatorrhea
Pulsatile liver	• Tricuspid regurgitation
Severe right upper quadrant pain	• Stretching of Glisson's capsule • Cholangitis, biliary colic
Respiratory alkalosis	• Central hyperventilation

Presentations of hepatic disease

The following table provides a comparison of acute, alcoholic, and toxic or drug-induced presentations.

Acute (viral)	Alcoholic	Toxic or Drug-induced
Presenting symptom		
• Flu-like symptoms, fatigue, anorexia, nausea, and tiredness; abdominal pain and vomiting	• Pain, fevers, anorexia, vomiting; fever < 39.4° C	• Depends upon source and patient hypersensitivity: fever, rash, eosinophilia, 2 weeks to 2 months after exposure to agent
Laboratory tests		
• Transaminase: 10 times greater than normal (peak 400 to 4,000) • Bilirubin: 5 to 20 mg/dl • Albumin: Normal to low early • Prothrombin time: Normal to 1 to 2 times normal	• Transaminase: Mild increase, aspartate aminotransferase (AST) > alanine aminotransferase (ALT) • Bilirubin: 2 to 10 mg/dl • Albumin: Normal to low early, low if late in the process • Prothrombin time: Prolonged (3 to 4.0 times normal)	• Transaminase: Slightly elevated to 5,000 IU/liter; > 5,000 IU/liter, suspect drug injury • Albumin: Normal to low early • Prothrombin time: Varies depending on source and extent of injury
Other		
• Splenomegaly in 20%; leukopenia, lymphopenia, and neutropenia • Hepatitis A: low-grade fever (38° to 39° C) • Hepatitis B: arthralgia, high fever, urticarial rash; stable hepatitis B with sudden onset of worsening symptoms: suspect hepatitis D superinfection	• Splenomegaly in some patients; anemia and leukocytosis, glucose abnormalities • If bilirubin and alkaline phosphatase are both elevated, consider cholestatic complications in patients with a history of alcohol abuse • May be unresponsive to vitamin K therapy	• Blood levels of acetaminophen will correlate with level of injury • Extent of injury from isoniazid probably related to increasing age

Diagnosis

Aside from clinical signs and symptoms, the best method of diagnosing hepatic dysfunction is by laboratory testing and radiologic examination. The patient's reports of alterations in elimination, nutritional intake or tolerance, exposure to injurious agents, pain, bleeding, and decreased physical abilities, combined with laboratory test results, will help to determine the source and scope of the hepatic disease. (For a detailed discussion, see *Confirming hepatic disease,* page 350.)

Treatment and care

Hepatic failure impacts upon all organ systems and requires that the nurse recognize, integrate, and respond quickly to multiple subtle signals. For those caring for critically ill patients with hepatic compromise, the treatment goal is to manage and minimize the disease's clinical side effects and to continually evaluate the patient's progress toward healing.

Removal of stressors and agents of injury

If the cause of the hepatic injury can be identified, a specific antidote may be administered, if appropriate. For example, N-acetyl cysteine may be administered for acetaminophen overdose. Efforts also are made to prevent further exposure to injury-causing agents, including administering medications, such as morphine, which are cleared by the liver. Nursing interventions to aid in removing stressors or agents of injury that should be incorporated into the plan of care include:

• Administer lactulose and neomycin, as prescribed, to remove or decrease ammonia production.
• Minimize medications to decrease the liver workload.
• Limit intake of protein, amino acids, and fat.
• Prevent exposure to further physiologic stressors (alcohol cessation).
• Encourage rest and carefully space stressing activities.

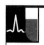

DIAGNOSTIC TEST

Confirming hepatic disease

Diagnostic testing can aid in the diagnosis of hepatic dysfunction as well as pinpointing the cause. Radiological studies such as abdominal X-rays, computed tomography scan, and magnetic resonance imaging, liver-spleen scan, ultrasonography, and arteriography can be used to evaluate organ placement, size, and filling processes, as well as to evaluate for extrahepatic or intrahepatic obstruction. A liver biopsy may be performed to evaluate for histologic changes caused by hepatic disease. An electroencephalogram (EEG) may indicate diffuse slowing or alpha wave changes associated with hepatic encephalopathy. Laboratory studies also will provide vital information to aid in the assessment of the extent of liver disease. Some of the typical tests are identified below. Normal values are found within parentheses.

Test	Serum Measurements
Liver function	Increased alanine aminotransferase (ALT) (7 to 53 IU/liter) and aspartate aminotransferase (AST) (11 to 47 IU/liter) measure the amount of hepatocellular destruction. Gamma-glutamyltransferase and alkaline phosphatase (38 to 126 IU/liter) increases are correlated with cholestatic processes.
Coagulation panel	Prothrombin time (11.4 to 14.0 seconds), activated prothrombin times (25 to 36 seconds), fibrinogen (150 to 360 mg/dl), fibrin split products (< 8 mg/dl), d-dimer levels, and clotting factors reflect synthesis and functional ability of the liver.
Miscellaneous	Decreased glucose levels (65 to 110 mg/dl) reflect depleted glycogen stores. Cholesterol, bilirubin (total: .2 to 1.3 mg/dl; direct: 0 to 0.2 mg/dl), albumin (3.6 to 5.0 g/dl), and ammonia (19 to 43 μmole/liter) levels provide information related to the functional ability of the liver.

Hepatic workload reduction

Several aspects of care are geared toward decreasing the hepatic workload caused by the disease process or injury. Efforts are made to decrease external factors that may increase the workload. In addition, careful monitoring is required to detect any evidence of disease progression that could result in an increased workload with increased clinical side effects. The following nursing

interventions to promote a reduction in the hepatic workload should be incorporated into the plan of care:
• Limit nutritional intake of protein, fat, and amino acids in patients with oral intake.
• Administer osmotic cathartics via nasogastric or rectal tube to clear blood from the GI tract; administer cathartic agents to clear urea and ammonia from the GI tract.
• Administer antibiotics to decrease breakdown of protein in the GI tract.
• Titrate nutritional supplementation to liver status, especially if the patient has a history of prolonged liver disease; avoid the use of amino acids, which are converted to ammonia.

Managing symptoms

Hepatic failure impacts all organ systems. Managing the subsequent symptoms associated with the disease process may entail addressing and treating acid-base and fluid imbalances, such as reversing alkalosis to promote conversion of ammonia to ammonium, which cannot cross the blood-brain barrier. The patient's hemodynamic instability, encephalopathy, and coagulopathies will need to be confronted and appropriately treated. Ascites can contribute to respiratory compromise and may need to be tapped. Infection, pain, and neurological sequelae will all need to be managed.

The following nursing interventions should be incorporated into the plan of care:
• Monitor hemodynamic stability, including evaluation of central venous pressure (CVP), pulmonary capillary wedge pressure (PCWP), and urine output.
• Monitor serum drug levels, especially those that are bound to albumin or cleared by the liver; alter dosage as required.
• Monitor laboratory tests, including coagulation panel and chemistry levels, for evidence of disease progression and functional changes.
• Initiate fluid and electrolyte support, replacing volume lost through bleeding or overzealous fluid removal as required, usually with normal saline.

• Hemodialysis or continuous renal replacement therapy may be necessary to maintain a fluid balance and treat hyperkalemia associated with advanced failure.
• Monitor ECG; evaluate for ECG changes related to electrolyte disturbances and accumulation of ammonia and by-products.
• Maintain glucose levels; supplement with glucose infusions if low, or control with insulin bolus or infusions, if high, as ordered.
• Administer thiamine to alcoholics to prevent Wernicke's encephalopathy.
• Minimize needle sticks and invasive procedures to decrease bleeding risks; administer vitamin K and clotting factors for prolonged prothrombin times.
• During a peritoneal tap, limit removal to 1 liter at a time and allow an adequate period to assess physiologic changes (potential for hypovolemia and hypotension) that may occur with fluid shifts.
• Administer pain medications to patients with severe pain, tailoring the dose to renal and hepatic status.
• Monitor for increased intracranial pressure and cerebral edema and evaluate for intubation and hyperventilation to establish a PCO_2 of 28 to 32 mm Hg to promote cerebral vasoconstriction.
• Administer an osmotic diuretic (such as mannitol) to decrease cerebral edema.
• Monitor level of consciousness (LOC); reorient the patient to person, time, and place, as necessary.
• Apply restraints to patients with alterations in LOC, if ordered.

Preventing further injury

Preventing any further injury to the liver is important so as to prevent further functional cell loss. Treatment is aimed at prolonging the function of the compromised liver. Immune-mediated chronic active hepatitis may be treated with glucocorticoids to prolong survival. Immune globulin–containing hepatitis A antibodies may be given early in the incubation to decrease the damage associated with hepatitis A.

Prophylaxis for hepatitis B with a vaccine to confer surface antibody immunity is appropriate when the individual is at risk for development of hepatitis B. If exposure has already occurred, treatment with immune globulin is used to limit the extent of the disease process. Patients with severe hepatic disease may undergo shunt bypass placement to alleviate pressure within the portal system.

The following nursing interventions to prevent further injury should be incorporated into the plan of care:
• Administer glucocorticoids as ordered for immune-mediated chronic active hepatitis.
• Administer immune globulin–containing hepatitis A antibodies, as ordered.
• Encourage prophylaxis with hepatitis B vaccine.
• Prepare the patient and family for bypass shunt placement, if indicated.

Prognosis
Death from chronic active hepatitis within the first 2 years usually results from liver failure and coma; 80% will survive 5 years. Fulminant hepatic failure carries a 60% to 90% mortality rate, usually from the irreversible complications that accompany liver failure.

Discharge planning
Discharge planning for the patient with hepatic failure should include the following components:
• evaluation of the physical, psychological, and social support systems that are available to the patient
• nutritional counseling, including monitoring of daily fat and protein intake
• alcohol counseling, regardless of the source of the hepatic compromise
• education of the signs and symptoms of infection or bypass shunt failure, both of which require immediate intervention
• education regarding medication use, and expected outcomes of the current disease process

• education of the patient and family about the use of universal precautions, and preventing retransmission of the disease.

Hyperosmolar hyperglycemic nonketotic syndrome (HHNS)

HHNS, which results from an insulin deficiency, is a condition characterized by hyperglycemia with a blood sugar level greater than 800 mg/dl, serum osmolality level greater than 330 mOsm/kg, absent or minimal serum ketones, an arterial hydrogen ion concentration (pH) higher than 7.30, serum bicarbonate level greater than 20 mEq/liter, and moderate to severe mental obtundation. The most common etiology is undiagnosed type II diabetes accompanied by a delay in seeking medical treatment after an associated illness. Common coexistent illnesses and other factors that may predispose a patient to HHNS are listed in *Etiologies of HHNS,* page 355.

Metabolic acidosis in HHNS usually is mild and is attributed to poor tissue perfusion and lactic acidosis. It has been suggested that in diabetic ketoacidosis (DKA), acidosis makes the patient feel more ill and thus prevents the syndrome from going undiagnosed for prolonged periods. Because of the absence of severe metabolic acidosis in HHNS, the prodrome of this syndrome is prolonged and greater deficits of body water develop, leading to more severe hyperglycemia. The older age of these patients also may predispose them to greater water deficits than in DKA, because of altered thirst sensation, impaired renal conservation of water, and limited access to water as a result of limited mobility. The severity of symptoms, plus the minimal or absent ketosis, distinguishes HHNS from DKA.

Etiologies of HHNS

HHNS has three major types of causes: insufficient circulating insulin, increased endogenous glucose, and increased exogenous glucose.

Insufficient circulating insulin
- Diabetes mellitus
- Pancreatic disease
- Pancreatectomy
- Pharmacological
—phenytoin
—thiazide or sulfonamide diuretics

—infection
- High-calorie enteral feedings
- Pharmacological
—glucocorticoids
—steroids
—sympathomimetics
—thyroid preparations

Increased endogenous glucose
- Acute stress
—extensive burns
—myocardial infarction

Increased exogenous glucose
- Hyperalimentation
- Hemodialysis
- Peritoneal dialysis

Pathophysiology

Insulin is released from the pancreas in the postprandial state (within the first 2 hours after a meal) and facilitates the uptake of glucose by hepatic, muscle, and adipose tissue. Within the liver, insulin promotes the formation of glycogen, the storage form of glucose, which can be readily mobilized in the fasting state. In addition, insulin inhibits gluconeogenesis, which is not required in the fed state, thus sparing amino acids and glycerol for protein and fatty acid synthesis.

Insulin promotes glycogen synthesis in muscle and stimulates amino acid uptake in muscle and liver, augmenting protein synthesis and inhibiting proteolysis. Fat metabolism is affected by insulin in several ways. Insulin stimulates the synthesis and secretion of lipoprotein lipase by fat and muscle cells. This enzyme is responsible for hydrolyzing fatty acids from chylomicron (lipid droplet) and very-low-density lipoproteins, which are then taken up by adipose tissue and converted into triglycerides. Insulin inhibits lipolysis of triglycerides stored in adipose tissue while it increases the supply of glycerol for esterification (removal of a water molecule when an acid and alcohol are combined) of fatty acids and stimulates synthesis of fatty acids from glucose and other substrates.

In the fasting state the body must maintain the plasma glucose concentration, because glucose is the primary source of energy for the central nervous system (CNS). During fasting, there is a decrease in insulin and an increase in the glucose counterregulatory hormones (glucagon, catecholamines, cortisol, and growth hormone). The alteration in the ratio between glucose and glucagon during fasting inhibits the peripheral uptake of glucose as well as protein synthesis and lipogenesis. Glycogenesis is inhibited in favor of glycogen breakdown as an immediate source of glucose.

The type II diabetic has a "relative" deficiency in insulin production. Reduced insulin levels prevent the movement of glucose into the cells. Glucagon release is triggered by the decreased insulin, and hepatic glucose from glycogenolysis accumulates in the systemic circulation. Glucagon also stimulates the metabolism of fat and protein through gluconeogenesis in an attempt to provide cells with an energy source. The end products of fat and protein metabolism also accumulate in the bloodstream with the excess glucose, leading to hyperosmolality. In an effort to decrease the serum osmolality, fluid is drawn from the intracellular compartment into the vascular bed. Profound intracellular volume depletion occurs if the patient's thirst sensation is absent or decreased, if the patient is unable to respond to thirst, or if fluids are inaccessible.

Hemoconcentration, the result of increased renal excretion secondary to hyperglycemia, is evidenced by extremely elevated hematocrit. Hemoconcentration persists despite removal by the kidney of large amounts of glucose through glycosuria. The hyperosmolality and reduced blood volume stimulate the release of antidiuretic hormone (ADH) to increase tubular reabsorption of water. ADH, however, is powerless in overcoming the osmotic pull exerted by the glucose load. Excessive fluid volume is lost at the kidney tubule, with simultaneous loss of potassium, sodium, and phosphate in the urine. Hypovolemia reduces renal circulation, and oliguria develops. Although this conserves water and preserves the blood volume, it prevents further glucose loss, and hyperosmolality increases.

Ketoacidosis is absent or very mild in HHNS, despite the level of free fatty acids resulting from gluconeogenesis. The lack of ketosis has been explained by several possible mechanisms:

• Beta cell function is adequate to produce sufficient insulin levels to prevent lipolysis but not hyperglycemia. This is supported by the fact that less circulating insulin is required to inhibit lipolysis than to promote glucose uptake or inhibit gluconeogenesis. However, no significant differences have been found between circulating insulin levels in DKA and HHNS.

• There is some evidence that portal vein insulin levels are higher in HHNS than in DKA, thus inhibiting lipolysis in the liver in the former condition.

• Hyperosmolality itself may inhibit lipolysis and ketone formation. Hyperosmolality depresses pancreatic insulin secretion, inhibits adipose tissue lipolysis, and impairs CNS control of growth hormone and cortisol response.

• Glucose counterregulatory hormones that promote lipolysis are lower in HHNS than in DKA.

Failure of the body to regain homeostatic balance further accelerates the life-threatening cycle brought about by hyperglycemia, hyperosmolality, osmotic diuresis, and profound dehydration. In an effort to restore homeostasis, the sympathetic nervous system reacts to the body's stress response. Epinephrine, a potent stimulus for gluconeogenesis, is released and additional glucose is added to the bloodstream. The intracellular dehydration affects fluid and oxygen transport to the brain cells. CNS dysfunction may result and lead to coma. Hemoconcentration increases the blood viscosity, which may result in clot formation, thromboemboli, and cerebral, cardiac, and pleural infarcts.

Clinical assessment

The priorities in assessment of the patient with HHNS are to determine the probable etiology of the disease and the severity of the fluid and electrolyte imbalance. A thorough history and careful analysis of laboratory findings are essential.

History

Although HHNS can occur in any diabetic patient, it usually occurs in type II patients and rarely occurs in children. The patient with nonketotic coma typically is an elderly person (the average age of patients with HHNS is 60 years) with a prior history of non-insulin-dependent diabetes mellitus, which may not have been previously diagnosed. The patient is severely dehydrated, is often in a coma, and has severe associated diseases and a poor outcome. HHNS has a slow, subtle onset. Initially, the symptoms may be nonspecific and may be ignored or attributed to concurrent disease processes.

While taking the health history, the nurse should question the patient or family members regarding the following:
• medication knowledge and compliance
• medication use, with special attention to cimetidine, phenytoin, thiazide or sulfonamide diuretics, thyroid preparations, glucocorticoids, steroids, and sympathomimetics
• increased exogenous glucose resulting from hyperalimentation, hemodialysis, or peritoneal dialysis
• increased endogenous glucose caused by stress
• concurrent illness, including renal disease, such as chronic renal insufficiency, gram-negative pneumonia or sepsis, and cardiovascular disease, such as myocardial infarction.

Physical findings

Because of the lack of ketosis, symptoms such as Kussmaul's respiration, abdominal discomfort, nausea, and vomiting are absent. This often delays seeking medical attention. Findings commonly associated with HHNS include:

- evidence of osmotic diuresis induced by hyperglycemia
    —polydipsia, polyuria (present over a longer period than with DKA)
    —weight loss and extracellular volume depletion
    —weakness and anorexia, vomiting
    —altered mental status
- hyponatremia
    —confusion, lethargy, or seizures
    —weakness, paralysis
- tachycardia, hypotension or orthostatic hypotension
- tachypnea (not Kussmaul's respiration)
- dehydration exhibited by dry skin and mucosa with leathery tongue, eyeballs sunken and soft under finger pressure
- positive Babinski reflex
- nystagmus
- seizures and neurologic deficits, including decreased level of consciousness, focal deficits, hemiparesis or hemisensory loss.

Diagnosis

Laboratory results in HHNS differ from those in DKA in several respects. Hyperglycemia is more profound, while plasma osmolality is higher. Ketosis generally is absent or mild, and serum electrolyte concentrations may be low, normal, or elevated and do not reflect the profound total-body electrolyte losses. A list of laboratory findings in the patient with HHNS is found in *Laboratory findings in HHNS,* page 360.

Treatment and care

Immediate goals of therapy for the HHNS patient include rapid replacement of life-threatening fluid and electrolyte deficits, correction of intermediary metabolism, recognition of precipitating events, and avoidance of complications of therapy. (For more information, see

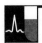

DIAGNOSTIC TESTS
Laboratory findings in HHNS

The diagnosis of HHNS is made by identification of clinical symptoms consistent with the disease and laboratory findings. The laboratory findings are used to confirm the diagnosis of HHNS.

Increased serum glucose level often > 1,000 mg/dl; maximum 2,000 mg/dl **(70 to 110 mg/dl)**
Increased serum osmolality > 330 mOsm/kg **(280 to 300 mOsm/kg)**
Serum sodium level < 145 mEq/liter **(135 to 145 mEq/liter)**
Absent or minimal ketones, serum and urine **(absent)**
Increased blood urea nitrogen (BUN) level, mean of 65 mg/dl **(8 to 25 mg/dl)**
Increased creatinine level **(0.6 to 1.2 mg/dl)**
Increased BUN/creatinine ratio > 20:1 **(10 to 15:1)**
Increased hemoglobin level **(12 to 18 g/dl)**
Increased hematocrit level **(36% to 54%)**
Decreased serum potassium level **(3.5 to 5.5 mEq/liter)**
Hydrogen ion concentration > 7.3 **(7.35 to 7.45)**

Key nursing interventions for patients with HHNS, page 361.)

Fluid therapy

Intravascular volume expansion is the treatment of choice for HHNS. As in DKA, electrolytes must be replaced, but smaller insulin doses are needed.

The fluid volume deficit may be as much as 25% of the patient's total body water. Administration of isotonic solutions would expand the extracellular fluid and treat hypotension, but it could compound the serum osmolality and exceed the body's requirement for sodium. Administration of hypotonic solutions would reduce the serum osmolality and provide free water for excretion, but this could result in hypotonic expansion of the cells.

A common consequence of administration of hypotonic normal saline in these patients is the development of cerebral edema and worsening neurologic function. Cerebral edema can occur from 4 to 16 hours after initial therapy and frequently may occur following biochemical improvement. The patient will complain of

ESSENTIAL ELEMENTS

Key nursing interventions for patients with HHNS

The following flowchart highlights key interventions that typically are performed when a patient is diagnosed with HHNS.

ACHIEVE OPTIMAL METABOLIC FUNCTION

Identify fluid volume deficit

- Assess vital signs hourly.
- Maintain hourly intake and output.
- Assess and document hydration status.
- Monitor central venous pressure (CVP) hourly.
- Administer I.V. fluid replacement.
- Observe for central venous overload and pulmonary edema:
—jugular venous distention
—auscultated S_3 heart sound
—increasing pulse rate, CVP, or pulmonary artery wedge pressure (PAWP)
—dyspnea
—breath sounds for crackles.
- Monitor for inadequate central perfusion:
—decreased CVP. PAWP, and urine output
—lowered blood pressure, elevated heart rate

Correct alteration in nutrition

- Monitor insulin infusion.
- Monitor serum glucose hourly.
- Assess and document for signs and symptoms of hyperglycemia:
—polydipsia or polyuria
—drowsiness
—flushed dry skin.
- Assess and document for signs and symptoms of hypoglycemia:
—weakness
—hunger
—slurred speech.

Correct electrolyte abnormalities

- Assess and document neurologic status:
—level of consciousness
—pupil size, equality, and reaction to light
—response to verbal and tactile stimuli.
- Monitor electrolyte values as ordered
- Assess for symptoms of K^+ imbalance.
- Assess for symptoms of sodium imbalance.
- Administer electrolytes as ordered.

headache, develop lethargy, and become unconscious. Physical examination reveals papilledema and fixed dilated or unequal pupils. The rapid fall in plasma glucose causes water to move intracellularly, resulting in brain swelling. CNS hypoxia and altered cerebral pH with paradoxic cerebrospinal fluid acidosis occur. Avoiding rapid falls in the serum osmolality by maintaining plasma glucose levels above 250 mg/dl during the first few hours of therapy may help avoid osmotic gradients contributing to cerebral edema.

Appropriate initial volume expansion will result in lowering the plasma glucose concentration independent of insulin. This occurs as adequate urine flow is reestablished, promoting glycosuria. Reexpanding the intravascular volume also will decrease the counterregulatory hormone production.

In the patient with profound shock, rapid expansion of the intravascular space is needed and isotonic saline, or in some cases colloid, is required. Isotonic saline usually is administered at a rate of 1 liter/hour until the blood pressure is stable and urine output of 60 ml/hour has been established. Use of normal saline solution as the initial replacement fluid may prevent a rapid fall in the extracellular osmolality, which may contribute to the complication of cerebral edema.

After initial intravascular repletion, hydration should continue with either isotonic saline or hypotonic saline (0.45% normal saline solution) with the goal of replacing one half of the calculated fluid deficit over the first 8 hours and the second half over the subsequent 16 hours. Since the overall loss of water is relatively greater than that of salt, the use of 0.45% normal saline solution will help prevent the development of hyperchloremic metabolic acidosis. The use of half-normal saline may be most appropriate when the serum osmolality is elevated. As the plasma glucose level approaches 250 to 300 mg/dl, 5% dextrose should be added to the replacement fluid to avoid hypoglycemia.

If hypotension occurs during therapy, 0.9% saline should be substituted for 0.45% saline. Isotonic saline should be used in patients with normal or reduced serum sodium concentrations, and 0.45% saline should be used in hypernatremic patients unless they are hypotensive.

When the initial plasma sodium value is normal or elevated, correction of the hyperglycemia and simultaneous infusion of 0.9% saline may be associated with the development of significant hypernatremia (plasma sodium of 160 to 170 mEq/liter). This may be beneficial, since it buffers rapid changes in extracellular osmolality. Frequent measurements of the sodium concentration and hemodynamic evaluation should allow the proper use of 0.9% and 0.45% saline.

The nurse is responsible for the administration of the fluid and evaluation of the patient's response to the therapy. The following interventions should be incorporated into the plan of care:
• Monitor hourly intake and output and daily weight.
• Monitor for blood pressure changes (orthostatic hypotension and pulse pressure).
• Assess pulse rate (character and rhythm).
• Assess neck vein filling.
• Assess skin turgor and moisture.
• Monitor central venous pressure and pulmonary artery wedge pressure.

Electrolyte replacement

Osmotic diuresis in HHNS results in total-body potassium depletion ranging from 400 to 600 mEq (5 to 10 mEq/liter/kg of body weight). In the absence of anuria or life-threatening hyperkalemia, potassium replacement should begin at the onset of fluid therapy. Between 20 and 40 mEq of potassium chloride may be added to each liter of fluid. The average adult will require 80 to 160 mEq potassium chloride over the first 12 hours to maintain a normal serum potassium concentration.

Total-body phosphorus is depleted as a result of osmotic diuresis, and with fluid and insulin therapy phosphorus is shifted intracellularly, resulting in a fall in the serum phosphorus concentration that requires replacement. Phosphate replacement should not be used in patients with renal failure, as hyperphosphatemia may develop.

HHNS also is associated with significant urinary losses of magnesium. Initial magnesium levels may be normal or elevated and subsequently fall with fluid and insulin therapy. Magnesium replacement may be required.

The following nursing interventions should be incorporated into the plan of care when providing electrolyte replacement:

• Monitor laboratory tests for hypokalemia, hypophosphatemia, hypernatremia, and hypomagnesemia.

• Monitor ECG continuously.

• Administer potassium chloride and potassium phosphate to correct hypokalemia and hypophosphatemia.

• Monitor for signs and symptoms of hypokalemia, such as diminished reflexes, irregular pulse, thirst, hypotension, ECG changes (U wave, premature ventricular contractions), muscular weakness, or irritability.

• Monitor for signs of hypophosphatemia, such as deep-bone or flank pain, lethargy, nausea, and vomiting; severe hypophosphatemia may be identified by signs of organ dysfunction, including respiratory failure, rhabdomyolysis, and impaired cardiac function.

• Monitor for complications of phosphate replacement, including hypocalcemia, hyperphosphatemia, and metastatic calcifications.

• Administer 0.45% saline to correct hypernatremia.

• Monitor for signs of hypernatremia, such as thirst, dry mucous membranes, weakness, fever, warm, flushed skin, and muscle pain.

• Monitor for signs of hypomagnesemia, such as tetany, lethargy, nausea, vomiting, tachyarrhythmias, hypotension, confusion, seizures, CNS depression, and hyperactive reflexes; administer 1 to 2 g magnesium sulfate 10% solution I.V. over 15 to 30 minutes for the patient with tetany or seizures. If less emergent, administer 2.5 to 5 ml of a 50% solution intramuscularly.

Insulin therapy

The goal of insulin therapy is to provide enough insulin to reverse the hyperglycemia while avoiding the complications of excessive insulin: hypoglycemia, hypokalemia, and hypophosphatemia. The recommended initial dose of regular insulin is 0.1 units/kg/hour. This dose will result in a decrease in plasma glucose level by 80 to 100 mg/dl/hour in most patients.

When plasma glucose levels fall to 300 mg/dl, it is advisable to change the I.V. fluid to a solution containing 5% dextrose, which will allow for continuing the insulin infusion. It is recommended that plasma glucose levels be maintained at 300 mg/dl for the first 24 hours. Insulin infusion should be continued until the anion gap has normalized, the serum bicarbonate level has normalized, and the patient is able to eat. The insulin infusion should not be stopped until 1 to 2 hours after the patient has been given a subcutaneous insulin regimen. Since most patients with HHNS have some endogenous insulin available, the insulin requirements needed to correct hyperglycemia usually are less than those in DKA.

The following nursing interventions should be incorporated into the plan of care:
• Administer regular insulin as described above.
• Monitor blood glucose levels hourly.
• Notify the physician when blood glucose levels are between 250 and 300 mg/dl.
• Monitor for signs and symptoms of medication-induced hypoglycemia, such as headache, confusion, irritability, restlessness, trembling, pallor, diaphoresis, and stupor.

Prognosis

Mortality associated with HHNS can be as high as 60% to 70%. Mortality often is caused by coexistent serious medical problems and complications (for more information, see *Complications of HHNS,* page 366).

Complications of HHNS

Serious and sometimes fatal complications can follow HHNS. Prevention of complications and early intervention are essential to provide the best possible outcome. Some common complications are listed here.

- Cerebral ischemia
- Cerebral bleeding
- Thromboembolism
- Acute tubular necrosis
- Myocardial infarction
- Metabolic disorders (for example, hypoglycemia, hypokalemia)

- Noncardiogenic pulmonary edema
- Disseminated intravascular coagulation
- Rhabdomyolysis

Discharge planning

Discharge planning should begin as soon as the patient has stabilized. All of the following guidelines should be considered to prepare the patient for discharge:

• Ensure that the patient and family demonstrate an understanding of diabetes, signs and symptoms of hyperglycemia and hypoglycemia, when to notify the physician, and precipitating events (for example, infection, stress, signs and symptoms of hypoglycemia and hyperglycemia).

• Confirm that the patient and family can assess serum glucose levels, administer oral hypoglycemic agents or insulin, and keep a record of appropriate information, including weight and glucose levels.

Hypertensive crisis

Hypertensive crisis, a sudden and sustained increase in the diastolic blood pressure (BP) above 140 mm Hg, is seen in approximately 1% of the population with hypertension. Of the 60 million Americans diagnosed with hypertension, 600,000 will experience a crisis annually. If left untreated, the increase in pressure and corresponding stress to the vessels leads to vascular necrosis and subsequent damage to the kidneys, eyes, heart, and brain.

Primary or essential hypertension accounts for 90% of those diagnosed with hypertension and has no known cause. Patients with this hypertension, which often is termed idiopathic, do not have any specific organ defect that causes the pressure elevation. The increased pressure is caused by a combination of increased vascular resistance, elevated cardiac output, and increased extracellular fluid volume. Secondary hypertension, which is seen in the other 10% of the population, is caused by a specific metabolic or organ deficit that leads to hypertension. In these cases, treatment of the hypertension depends upon the timely diagnosis of the underlying medical condition and subsequent medical or surgical intervention (see *Secondary causes of hypertensive crisis,* page 368).

Hypertensive crisis is seen in patients with chronic primary hypertension with a peak occurrence at 40 to 50 years. Men have a higher incidence than women, and blacks have a higher incidence than whites. If a hypertensive crisis occurs in a person less than 30 years old or more than 60 years old with no previous history of hypertension, a secondary cause of the hypertensive crisis must be ruled out.

Pathophysiology

Hypertensive crisis is believed to be caused by chronic uncontrolled hypertension. Because of the unrelenting pressure on the vasculature, the vessels undergo structural and reactivity changes. Vessels that once responded to the vasoactive mechanisms of renin-angiotensin, catecholamines, and vasopressin no longer sufficiently respond, and the hypertensive crisis cycle is set in motion.

Systemic vascular resistance of the renal efferent arterioles increases, thought to be caused by an abrupt elevation of circulating vasoconstricting substances (angiotensin II, antidiuretic hormone, or norepinephrine). With the rise in glomerular capillary pressure, there is diuresis and corresponding volume depletion. Because hypovolemia causes a further release of vasoconstricting substances, there is further narrowing and

Secondary causes of hypertensive crisis

Although not seen as a common cause of hypertensive crisis, secondary causes may precipitate an acute rise in diastolic blood pressure. When a secondary cause is suspected, specific testing performed to confirm it may include renal ultrasound and renal arteriography to rule out renal disease; blood glucose levels to rule out diabetes mellitus or other endocrine causes; urine catecholamine levels to evaluate for pheochromocytoma; and serum cholesterol and triglyceride levels to evaluate the possibility of atherosclerosis.

System or Area	Causative Condition
Cardiovascular	• Acute left ventricular failure • Acute myocardial infarction • Dissecting aortic aneurysm • Unstable angina pectoris
Catecholamine-associated	• Antihypertensive therapy • Withdrawal syndrome • Monoamine oxidase inhibitors and tyramine interaction • Pheochromocytoma • Spinal cord disease (Guillain-Barré syndrome) • Spinal cord injury • Sympathomimetic agents
Miscellaneous neurologic	• Scleroderma crisis • Cerebrovascular accident • Eclampsia • Head injury • Hypertensive encephalopathy • Intracranial or subarachnoid hemorrhage
Renal	• Acute glomerulonephritis • Renal parenchymal disease • Renovascular hypertension • Vasculitis

endothelial damage to the renal arteries. Vascular lesions, believed to be the result of fibrin leaking into the arteriolar wall, create an obstruction that reduces the blood flow into the organ involved. As this vicious cycle continues, systemic vascular resistance and arterial BP increase, leading to organ damage. The organs most susceptible to damage, often termed end organs, include the kidneys, brain, heart, and eyes.

Hypertensive crisis can be of three types. In the case of simple hypertensive crisis, the episode occurs without any signs or symptoms of end-organ damage. Complicated hypertensive crisis is evidenced by altered cardiac or central nervous system (CNS) functioning. In the case of decompensated hypertensive crisis, life-sustaining interventions are indicated to reverse the BP and preserve end-organ functioning.

Untreated hypertensive crisis can lead to hypertensive encephalopathy. As cerebral vessels dilate, blood flow increases, forcing fluid into the cerebral tissue and causing cerebral edema. Cardiac vessel damage can lead to acute left ventricular failure or acute myocardial infarction (MI). As a result of the increase in cardiac afterload, there is an increase in myocardial oxygen demand, leading to ischemia and infarction.

Even though all organs are at risk of damage with hypertensive crisis, the kidneys and eyes are particularly susceptible. With the obstruction of renal vessels by fibrin lesions, renal blood flow is impeded, leading to renal parenchymal damage. Retinal vessels respond to increases in intracranial pressure caused by spasm or hemorrhage. Grade IV retinal changes, or papilledema, are indicative of a hypertensive crisis.

Clinical assessment

The successful treatment of hypertensive crisis depends upon the speed of diagnosis and subsequent interventions aimed to decrease BP, replace lost fluid, and reduce the release of vasoconstricting substances.

History

Because hypertensive crisis often is seen in patients with a history of chronic primary hypertension, information on the duration, severity, and level of control of the disorder should be obtained. In addition, the following must be documented:

• family history of hypertension, cardiovascular disease, or diabetes mellitus

• history of underlying diagnosed diseases such as angina, dyspnea, claudication, kidney failure, MI, or congestive heart failure that indicate a weakened systemic vasculature that may be magnified during the current hypertensive crisis episode
• recent changes in weight, sodium intake, exercise level, or alcohol use
• smoking history
• use of prescribed medications to control hypertension and time and date of last dose
• use of other prescribed medications that may interfere with the effectiveness of prescribed antihypertensives or cause an increase in BP, such as oral contraceptives, steroids, cyclosporine, tricyclic antidepressants, or monoamine oxidase inhibitors
• use of over-the-counter medications, such as nonsteroidal anti-inflammatory agents, weight control agents, or cold remedies, and time and date of last dose (these medications are known to interfere with the mechanisms of action of antihypertensives and may exacerbate the crisis or magnify complications)
• any use of nonprescription drugs such as amphetamines, cocaine, or cocaine derivatives (cocaine potentiates the effects of norepinephrine, leading to the cardiovascular effects of increased BP, tachycardia, and possibly ventricular fibrillation)
• any recent emotional stress.

Physical findings
Hypertensive crisis often begins insidiously, with the patient experiencing only vague discomfort, fatigue, dizziness, and a mild headache. Over time, the symptoms worsen, causing the patient to seek medical treatment. The patient should be evaluated for evidence of the following:
• a persistent severe headache that is more intense in the morning, focused on the occipital region, and often accompanied by nausea, vomiting, and restlessness; possibly leading to confusion and coma

• markedly elevated diastolic BP, over 120 mm Hg, accompanied by elevated systolic BP, orthostatic dizziness
• increased heart rate of over 120 beats/minute (apical heart rate auscultated at the left anterior axillary line instead of the midclavicular line)
• presence of S_3 and S_4 heart sounds
• presence of crackles (rales), shortness of breath at rest, dyspnea on exertion
• distended neck veins
• neurologic changes such as hemiparesis, hemiplegia, ataxia, confusion, or alterations in cognitive status
• alteration in vision affecting ability to read and view objects and people
• diaphoresis and palpitations
• nausea and vomiting
• sudden onset of pedal edema with unequal or absent pulses
• complaints of chest pain or exacerbation of angina
• onset of hematuria, complaints of increasing nocturia
• increasing irritability, bouts of confusion, drowsiness, or increasing fatigue
• transient blurred vision or temporary blindness, funduscopic examination findings of hemorrhagic sites, fluffy cotton exudates, or arterial-venous nicking of the vessels.

Diagnosis

Definitively diagnosing hypertensive crisis is contingent upon the diastolic BP. For a listing of tests performed for primary hypertension see *Confirming hypertensive crisis,* page 372. Once hypertensive crisis has been established, further diagnostic testing is focused on the presence and extent of organs damaged and on ruling out any secondary causes of the disorder to begin treatment. This testing may include the following:
• renal ultrasound and renal arteriography—performed to rule out renal disease and renal artery stenosis as secondary causes

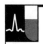

Confirming hypertensive crisis

The following tests may be performed to definitively diagnose hypertensive crisis. The findings commonly seen in hypertensive crisis are listed.

Test	Findings
Blood pressure measurement	• Mild with diastolic pressures between 90 and 114 mm Hg • Moderate with diastolic pressures between 115 and 130 mm Hg • Severe with diastolic pressures > 130 mm Hg
ECG	• Increased voltage in leads V_5 and V_6 indicates left ventricular hypertrophy • A strain pattern of ST-segment depression and T-wave inversion suggests repolarization abnormalities due to endocardial fibrosis accompanying hypertrophy
Echocardiogram	• Increased left ventricle thickness with or without dilatation or increase in left chamber size
Chest X-ray	• Enlarged heart if left ventricular hypertrophy is present • Widened silhouette of thoracic aorta or widened mediastinum suggests aortic dissection, which may be associated with hypertension
Urinalysis	• A low specific gravity (< 1.010) with proteinuria suggests renal impairment • Granular or red cell casts or hematuria, which suggests acute glomerulonephritis and renal-induced hypertension
Blood urea nitrogen	• > 20 mg/dl
Serum creatinine level	• > 1.2 mg/dl for men and > 1.1 mg/dl for women is a cardinal sign of acute hypertensive nephropathy
Serum potassium level	• < 3.5 mEq is secondary to high renin levels
Serum sodium level	• < 135 mEq due to the loss of water and salt through the urine

• blood glucose level—fasting blood glucose levels greater than 120 mg may indicate diabetes mellitus or a less common endocrine cause such as Cushing's syndrome

• urine catecholamine levels—epinephrine levels greater than 20 g/day or norepinephrine levels greater than 100 g/day in a 24-hour collected urine sample indicate pheochromocytoma

• serum cholesterol and triglycerides levels—cholesterol level greater than 220 mg and triglycerides level greater than 150 mg indicate atherosclerosis, a contributing factor in the development of hypertension.

Treatment and care

The overall treatment goal for hypertensive crisis is to reduce the diastolic BP while maintaining cardiac, respiratory, cerebral, and renal functioning.

Blood pressure management

Pharmacologic therapy is the main focus of initial medical treatment for the patient in hypertensive crisis. Through various pharmacologic agents, attempts are made to decrease the diastolic BP to 100 to 110 mm Hg over several hours. If the BP drops too low or too fast, the CNS's autoregulation mechanism may not be able to respond quickly, leading to inadequate cerebral perfusion. The hypertensive crisis may, at this time, be compounded by cerebral ischemia or stroke.

Any efforts to reduce the pressure to normotensive levels should be undertaken slowly, over several days to weeks, unless a secondary cause for the crisis has been determined. Should the patient have a dissecting aortic aneurysm, the pressure should be lowered as quickly as possible to stop the progressive dissection. For patients with cerebral infarctions or intracerebral or subarachnoid hemorrhages, aggressive antihypertensive therapy usually is contraindicated because of the potential for cerebral hypoperfusion. However, a reduction in BP for these patients may prevent further bleeding and ischemia and usually is instituted with frequent neurological evaluations as the guide for pressure reduction.

The vasodilator of choice for hypertensive crisis is sodium nitroprusside (Nipride, Nitropress) delivered at the rate of 0.25 to 10 g/kg/minute intravenously. By working directly on the vessels, this medication has instantaneous effects.

Additional vasodilators commonly used in the treatment of hypertensive crisis include (in order of rapidity of action) nitroglycerin, diazoxide (Hyperstat), hydralazine (Apresoline), enalaprilat (Vasotec IV), and nicardipine (Cardene). The usual dosage, onset of action, and any adverse effects can be found in the table *Hypertensive crisis medication management,* pages 375 and 376.

Adrenergic inhibitors also aid in the safe treatment of this disorder. These medications block beta receptors in the heart and peripheral vessels to reduce peripheral vascular resistance. Those commonly used include phentolamine (Regitine), trimethaphan (Arfonad), esmolol (Brevibloc), propranolol (Inderal), and labetalol (Normodyne).

The eventual medication regimen used to treat hypertensive crisis will depend upon the presence or absence of secondary causes. Should the patient also have an MI or unstable angina, nitrates will be given in addition to calcium channel blockers. In this case, hydralazine and diazoxide would be avoided because both increase the heart rate and subsequent myocardial oxygen demand.

If the patient has left ventricular failure, sodium nitroprusside is indicated in addition to diuretics to treat pulmonary edema. Again, hydralazine, diazoxide, and other beta blockers are contraindicated because of reflex tachycardia.

With aortic dissection, sodium nitroprusside usually is given in addition to a beta blocker. Both hydralazine and diazoxide may worsen the dissection and are not traditionally given.

MAJOR DRUGS
Hypertensive crisis medication management

Hypertensive crisis is a medical emergency, and any delay in initiating medication therapy can be detrimental to the patient's outcome. The following parenteral and oral medications most commonly are used to treat hypertensive crisis; they are listed in order of rapidity of action.

Drug	Dosage/Response Time	Adverse Effects
Sodium nitroprusside Provides immediate reduction in blood pressure	0.25 to 10 g/kg/minute Response time: immediate	• Hypotension • Diaphoresis • Nausea and vomiting • Thiocyanate toxicity
Nitroglycerin Dilates coronary vessels; decreases cardiac workload	5 to 10 g/minute Response time: 2 to 5 minutes	• Tachycardia • Headache • Flushing
Enalaprilat (angiotensin converting enzyme inhibitor) Limits the production of angiotensin II and aldosterone production	1.25 to 5 mg every 6 hours Response time: 15 minutes	• Hypotension • Fever • Rash • Stomatitis
Nicardipine (calcium channel blocker) Causes arteriolar vasodilation and decreases peripheral vascular resistance	5 to 10 mg/hour I.V. Response time: 10 minutes	• Tachycardia • Headache • Flushing • Local phlebitis
Trimethaphan (ganglionic blocker) Blocks transmission in autonomic ganglia; exerts a direct peripheral vasodilator effect Note: Contraindicated in eclampsia	0.5 to 5 mg/minute I.V. Response time: 1 to 5 minutes	• Bowel and bladder paresis • Blurred vision • Respiratory paralysis
Esmolol (beta and alpha blocker) Antiarrhythmic with antihypertensive qualities, primarily used for intraoperative and postoperative hypertension	500 g/kg/minute for 1 minute, then 50 to 300 g/kg/minute I.V. for 4 minutes; repeat Response time: 1 to 2 minutes	• Hypotension

(continued)

Hypertensive crisis medication management *(continued)*

Drug	Dosage/Response Time	Adverse Effects
Propranolol (beta blocker) Reduces peripheral vascular resistance	1 to 10 mg load; 3 mg/hour Response time: 1 to 2 minutes	• Bronchospasm • Decreased cardiac output • Congestive heart failure • Hypoglycemia
Labetalol (beta and alpha blocker) Reduces peripheral vascular resistance; useful for chronic care	2 mg/minute I.V. Response time: 5 to 10 minutes	• Vomiting and nausea • Postural hypotension • Bradycardia • Bronchospasm

In those patients with imminent renal failure, sodium nitroprusside should be used cautiously because of the risk of thiocyanate toxicity. Once the BP has been lowered to a level that can be managed by other medications, such as labetalol or a calcium channel blocker, sodium nitroprusside should be discontinued to decrease the risk of compromising renal blood flow or glomerular filtration.

The following nursing interventions should be incorporated into the plan of care when caring for a patient receiving pharmacologic therapy for BP reduction:

• Administer antihypertensive agents, titrating according to the target pressure, as ordered.

• Monitor BP and mean arterial pressure (MAP) every 1 to 5 minutes while titrating the prescribed antihypertensive medication. (See *Calculating mean arterial pressure (MAP),* page 377.)

• Continue to monitor BP and MAP every 15 to 30 minutes as pressure begins to stabilize.

• Cover prepared sodium nitroprusside with a light resistive covering (it is light-sensitive and stable in solution for 24 hours).

• Monitor the patient receiving sodium nitroprusside for adverse effects, including hypotension, nausea, dia-

ASSESSMENT TIP
Calculating mean arterial pressure (MAP)

MAP can be calculated from indirect systolic and diastolic blood pressure measurements by using the following formula:

$$\text{MAP} = \frac{\text{Systolic pressure} + 2\,(\text{diastolic pressure})}{3}$$

phoresis, headache, restlessness, confusion, and muscle twitching.
• Perform blood cyanide levels on the patient receiving sodium nitroprusside therapy. A metabolite of sodium nitroprusside is thiocyanate. High-dose sodium nitroprusside therapy can lead to elevated blood cyanide levels. A safe thiocyanate blood level for this patient would be less than 10 mg/dl.
• Monitor the patient for signs and symptoms of early thiocyanate toxicity, including giddiness, headache, anxiety, tachycardia, hyperpnea, mild hypertension, and palpitations. Late signs of thiocyanate toxicity are nausea, vomiting, tachycardia or bradycardia, hypotension, generalized seizures, coma, apnea, dilated pupils, ischemic ECG changes, supraventricular or ventricular tachyarrhythmias, atrioventricular blocks, and asystole.
• Decrease or discontinue (as per physician's guidelines) medication if BP drops below target level.
• Begin administering oral medication regimen as ordered with BP monitoring every 1 to 4 hours.

Preservation of end-organ function
In addition to pharmacologic therapy, the treatment regimen is focused on preserving end organs. Ongoing evaluation of the patient's end-organ function and recognition of pending end-organ damage are essential. Nursing interventions to incorporate into the plan of care to identify signs of impending end-organ damage include:
• Assess the eyes for retinal arteriolar narrowing, hemorrhages, exudates, and papilledema.

• Assess the neck for vein distention, carotid bruits, and enlarged thyroid.

• Assess the heart for increased heart rate, arrhythmias, enlarged heart, precordial impulses, murmurs, and S_3 and S_4 heart sounds.

• Assess the abdomen for bruits, aortic dilation, and enlarged kidneys.

• Assess the extremities for diminished or absent peripheral pulses, edema, and bilateral inequality of pulses.

• Assess the neurologic status for signs of cerebral thrombosis or hemorrhage.

• Monitor intake and output every hour and report urinary output of less than 30 ml/hour for 2 consecutive hours.

• Monitor serum laboratory values and report increases in blood urea nitrogen level (> 20 mg/dl) and creatinine level (> 1.2 mg/dl for men and > 1.1 mg/dl for women).

Pain control and anxiety reduction

The patient in hypertensive crisis may have pain from the increase in pressure. Any anxiety preexisting or secondary to the treatment for the hypertensive crisis can actually worsen the patient's condition. The following nursing interventions should be incorporated into the plan of care to control pain and reduce anxiety:

• Monitor severity of pain (pain scale of 1 to 10).

• Provide analgesics as prescribed and monitor their effectiveness.

• Explain all procedures and reasons for implementing them.

• Monitor the patient's ability to comprehend his or her environment and explain the need for being in the intensive care unit.

• Maintain a quiet environment and place the patient in a private room if possible.

• Administer anxiolytics as prescribed and appropriate.

• Reassure the patient that efforts are being taken to safely reduce BP.

• Reassure the patient of a timely transfer to a non–critical care area as soon as his or her physical condition warrants.

Prognosis

The prognosis of a patient with acute hypertensive crisis is good if appropriate diagnosis and medical intervention are instituted in a timely manner. If efforts to safely reduce the pressure while preserving end-organ functioning are effective, and secondary causes have been appropriately treated, organ damage will be minimal. Once the crisis has passed, attention to the long-term control of the hypertension will reduce the likelihood of future episodes. Without treatment, hypertensive crisis results in a 90% mortality rate within 1 year secondary to renal or congestive heart failure, cerebrovascular accident, MI, or aortic dissection.

Discharge planning

Prevention of future episodes of hypertensive crisis depends upon successful patient compliance with the prescribed medication regime and lifestyle changes. The following should be included in discharge planning:

• Review all prescribed medications. Remind the patient to take the prescribed medication even if he or she is asymptomatic.

• Explain why the patient should notify the physician if symptoms recur and before stopping any prescribed medication. Stress the importance of follow-up visits.

• Initiate a social services consultation to evaluate the patient's financial resources for the purchase and use of medications, if needed.

• Provide information on smoking cessation and stress reduction.

• Initiate a dietary consultation for a sodium-restricted diet.

• Review how the patient can keep a record of BP and medication regime for monitoring at home.

Hypoglycemia

Although hypoglycemia usually is defined as a drop in blood glucose levels below 50 mg/dl, it may occur at higher glucose levels with symptoms often dependent on how quickly the patient's glucose levels drop. Hypoglycemia is most prevalent in patients with insulin-dependent diabetes mellitus and is much more common than ketoacidosis; it has a more rapid onset and variable manifestations. If the low glucose level is not treated, severe hypoglycemia may result in coma, irreversible brain damage, and even death.

Because hypoglycemia can result from too much insulin, too little food, or excessive physical activity, its onset varies with the type of insulin administered, injection site, and time of last meal. Hypoglycemia may occur 1 to 3 hours after a dose of regular insulin, 4 to 18 hours after NPH or Lente insulin, or 18 to 30 hours or more after Protamine Zinc or Ultralente insulin.

Hypoglycemia may occur at any time, but usually takes place before meals. In addition to causing permanent neurologic damage, it also may impair diabetic control, because release of counterregulatory hormones results in rebound hyperglycemia, occasionally accompanied by mild ketosis. Recurrent hypoglycemia can be caused by:
- onset of pregnancy
- renal failure
- exercise
- failure to adjust an insulin dose after recovery from an illness.

There are two forms of spontaneous hypoglycemia: fasting and postprandial. Fasting hypoglycemia can be subacute or chronic and usually manifests principally with neurologic symptoms. Postprandial hypoglycemia is a hypoglycemic reaction occurring within 2 hours after a meal. It is relatively acute and often is heralded by symptoms of adrenergic discharge, including sweating, palpitations, anxiety, and tremulousness.

Hypoglycemia has many potential causes and contributing factors. The episode may be related to excessive insulin therapy or to a change in insulin absorption. It may be the result of insufficient nutritional intake or of decreased need for exogenous insulin (for example, removal of a stressor, such as infection). Medications and drugs that can precipitate this episode include excessive oral hypoglycemic agents and alcohol, which inhibit gluconeogenesis by the liver. Finally, other health problems, such as liver disease (depleted glycogen stores) and adrenal insufficiency (insufficient glucocorticoids), may be contributing factors (see *Common causes of hypoglycemia,* page 382).

Pathophysiology

During oral nutritional intake, insulin is the predominant hormone required for the uptake of glucose, the body's chief energy source. During fasting, the body uses endogenous sources of fuels to support the brain and muscles; this results in hormonal changes. There is a decrease in insulin and an increase in the glucose counterregulatory hormones glucagon, catecholamines, cortisol, and growth hormone. The alteration in the ratio of glucose to glucagon inhibits the peripheral uptake of glucose as well as protein synthesis and lipogenesis. Glycogenesis is inhibited in favor of glycogen breakdown as an immediate source of glucose.

As the plasma insulin levels fall and glucagon levels rise, the liver becomes the major source of glucose during the fasting state. Concurrently, decreased insulin concentrations lead to lipolysis in fat deposits, providing a source of free fatty acids as fuel for muscle and reserving glucose for use in the brain. Under the influence of glucagon, the free fatty acids are converted by the liver to ketones, which are an alternative energy source for brain and muscle tissue.

Glucagon, epinephrine, growth hormone, and cortisol assist in glycogenolysis and gluconeogenesis and encourage utilization of fatty acids instead of glucose as fuel by most body tissues. However, because the brain

Common causes of hypoglycemia

Hypoglycemia is a disease process characterized by the presence of low blood glucose. Some of the most common causes are outlined below.

Fasting hypoglycemia
• Hyperinsulinism
—pancreatic beta-cell tumor
—surreptitious administration of insulin or oral hypoglycemic agents
• Extrapancreatic tumors
• Stress

Postprandial (reactive) hypoglycemia
• Early hypoglycemia (alimentary)
—postgastrectomy
—functional (increased vagal tone)
• Late hypoglycemia (occult diabetes)

—delayed insulin release caused by beta-cell dysfunction
• Counterregulatory deficiency
• Idiopathic

Alcohol hypoglycemia

Immunopathologic hypoglycemia
• Idiopathic anti-insulin antibodies (which release their bound insulin)
• Antibodies to insulin receptors (which act as agonists)

Pentamidine-induced hypoglycemia

cannot utilize long-chain free fatty acids and lacks glucose stored as glycogen, a certain level of circulating glucose must be delivered to the brain.

In hypoglycemia, there is either too much insulin or too little glucagon. An insulinoma of the pancreas leads to increased production of insulin, which allows rapid transport of glucose from the blood into the cell. This transport increases protein synthesis, glucose conversion to glycogen in the liver, and fat storage, resulting in hypoglycemia.

With alpha-cell destruction in the pancreas, production of glucagon is decreased. This results in decreased gluconeogenesis in the liver and decreased glycolysis, also leading to hypoglycemia. If glucose levels continue to drop, starvation ketosis can occur, resulting in cerebral hypoxia and cerebral edema.

Other signs seen in hypoglycemia involve the autonomic nervous system. Hypoglycemia stimulates release of the catecholamines epinephrine and norepinephrine. These hormones cause tachycardia, pallor, diaphoresis, cool skin, and tremors, with potential seizure activity. A larger stress response that includes release of large quantities of the counterregulatory hormones (such as glucocorticoids, growth hormone, and glucagon) attempts to drive the blood sugar back up, primarily by stimulating hepatic glycogen breakdown.

Some diabetic patients appear to have decreased insulin requirements or a decreasing need for oral hypoglycemic agents. If adjustments in the dose of the oral hypoglycemic agent are not made, hypoglycemia can result.

Decreased insulin resistance
Weight loss, which may occur before or during an acute illness, is known to reduce insulin resistance in diabetes mellitus. Small decreases in weight often are sufficient to substantially decrease the requirement of insulin or other hypoglycemic agents. Another cause of decreased insulin resistance is a deficiency of one of the glucose counterregulatory hormones. Adrenal or pituitary insufficiency may be part of an preexisting disease process. Decreased growth hormone or cortisol can diminish the need for hypoglycemic agents by enhancing peripheral insulin sensitivity and decreasing gluconeogenesis.

Decreased clearance of insulin or oral hypoglycemic agents
The liver and kidneys are the primary organs involved in the metabolism of insulin and oral hypoglycemic agents. Development of renal or hepatic failure is associated with a delay in drug clearance, which may result in hypoglycemia. In patients who take oral hypoglycemic agents, this may be associated with the onset of severe, prolonged hypoglycemia and coma.

Concomitant use of other drugs may also influence the metabolism of oral hypoglycemic agents (see *Drugs that influence the metabolism of oral hypoglycemic agents,* page 384).

A relatively common cause of unexpected hypoglycemia occurs during acute episodes of congestive heart failure (CHF) in insulin-dependent patients. Liver con-

Drugs that influence the metabolism of oral hypoglycemic agents

The following table outlines the commonly prescribed drugs that can affect the metabolism of an oral hypoglycemic agent.

Drug(s)	Mechanism of Action
Clofibrate Salicylates Sulfonamides	Displace the sulfonylurea from plasma proteins
Chloramphenicol	Reduces hepatic sulfonylurea metabolism
Allopurinol Phenylbutazone Salicylates Sulfonamides	Decrease urinary excretion of oral hypoglycemic agents or their metabolites
Insulin Beta-adrenergic agonists Salicylates	Cause intrinsic hypoglycemic activity

gestion and possibly impaired hepatic blood flow cause a transient decrease in insulin requirements. Hypoglycemia in hospitalized patients occurs most commonly in those with diabetes and usually is the result of a decrease in caloric intake related to illness or hospital routine and maintenance of hypoglycemic drugs.

Concomitant diseases play an important role in increasing the risk of hypoglycemia in patients with diabetes. Renal insufficiency, malnutrition, and sepsis are associated with hypoglycemia even in nondiabetic hospitalized patients. Alcohol ingestion, liver disease, shock, pregnancy, and malignancy also can lead to hypoglycemia. A high mortality rate has been reported in nondiabetic critically ill patients who develop hypoglycemia, and in some this may represent a terminal phenomenon associated with malnutrition or kidney and liver disease. During end-stage disease the patient's release and function of counterregulatory hormones are altered, putting the patient at risk for developing hypoglycemia.

Pentamidine, used for the treatment of *Pneumocystis carinii* infection, is associated with hypoglycemia, probably as a result of the acute increase in insulin release that accompanies drug-related destruction of pancreatic islet cells.

Clinical assessment

The signs and symptoms of hypoglycemia are nonspecific and very often confused with several other conditions seen in the critical care setting. A detailed patient history and physical examination assist in accurate diagnosis and treatment.

History

The patient with hypoglycemia usually has an abrupt onset of symptoms. During the health history, the nurse should question the patient about the following:
• history of alcohol intake (amount and frequency)
• presence of preexisting illness
  —diabetes
  —CHF
  —hepatic failure
  —renal insufficiency
  —malnutrition
  —sepsis
• use of medications
  —oral hypoglycemic agents
  —clofibrate
  —salicylates
  —sulfonamides
  —chloramphenicol
  —allopurinol
  —insulin
  —beta agonists.

Physical findings

Insufficient supply of glucose to the brain cells results in cerebral changes, because the brain does not utilize alternative energy sources as well as do other tissues. Patients usually will first experience an inability to concentrate, apprehension, or light-headedness. Often they are aware of these symptoms, yet unable to verbalize their need for help. They often present with slurred speech, trembling, or staggering gait, which may be mistaken for alcohol-induced signs. Unless treatment is initiated, the central nervous system (CNS) signs will progress to coma within minutes to an hour.

Any patient taking insulin whose behavior becomes inappropriate or uncharacteristic should be suspected of having an insulin reaction and treated accordingly. The index of suspicion should be particularly high if the changes are episodic or occur when the particular form of insulin used is expected to have its maximum activity.

As the hypoglycemia persists and worsens, consciousness is progressively impaired, leading first to stupor, then coma (see *Serum glucose levels and associated signs,* page 387). Severe hypoglycemia that lasts more than 15 to 30 minutes often results in at least some symptoms that persist after glucose is given.

Any one or a combination of the following findings may be observed:
- anxiety, tremors
- diaphoresis, pallor
- dilated pupils
- increase in systolic pressure
- seizures
- tachycardia.

Diagnosis
The diagnosis of hypoglycemia should be relatively simple and clear-cut; however, because of extreme nonspecificity of its manifestations and the great variation in response to low blood sugar levels, the diagnosis is often subtle and complex (see *Confirming hypoglycemia,* pages 388 and 389).

A serum sugar level below 25 mg/dl always is responsible for accompanying symptoms. In the range

Serum glucose levels and associated signs

The chart below outlines the signs typically found in patients with low serum glucose levels.

Glucose Levels	Signs
50 to 70 mg/dl	• Central nervous system excitability and hallucinations • Extreme nervousness • Tremors and slurred speech
20 to 50 mg/dl	• Clonic convulsions • Loss of consciousness • Pupil dilation
< 20 mg/dl	• Coma

from 25 to 45 mg/dl, the symptoms may not always be attributable to the hypoglycemia, especially in spontaneous or reactive hypoglycemia. When the serum glucose level is between 45 and 65 mg/dl, the cause of symptoms is even more difficult to distinguish.

Diagnosis of hypoglycemia is based on correlation of signs and symptoms with a low plasma glucose level and on prompt reversal of symptoms upon administration of glucose. Patients generally respond rapidly and dramatically to glucose administration.

Treatment and care

Treatment of hypoglycemia focuses on prompt identification of the condition (see Clinical Assessment, page 385), improvement of cellular function by correcting metabolic defects, and avoiding complications of hypoglycemia.

Restoration of normal cellular function

If the patient is alert enough to swallow, 5 to 10 g of a rapidly absorbable carbohydrate, such as fruit juice, candy, or a carbonated beverage containing sugar, may be ordered. This allows the glucose to move quickly through the stomach and into the intestine, where it is

Confirming hypoglycemia

The following laboratory studies typically are performed to help confirm a diagnosis of hypoglycemia.

Serum glucose

Glucose is formed from dietary carbohydrates and is stored as glycogen in the liver and skeletal muscles. Insulin and glucagon, two hormones from the pancreas, affect the blood glucose level. **A normal blood glucose level is 70 to 110 mg/dl.** Hypoglycemia, low blood sugar, is a blood sugar level < 70 mg/dl.

Glucose tolerance test (GTT)

An oral GTT can be done to detect hyperinsulinism. Starting 3 days before the test, the patient should consume 200 to 300 g of carbohydrate daily and should take nothing by mouth (except for water) for 12 hours before the test. Blood and urine samples are collected in the fasting state. If the fasting blood sugar is more than 200 mg/dl, the test is not performed. A glucose load of 1.75 g/kg is given orally. Blood and urine specimens are collected at 0.5, 1, 2, and 3 hours after glucose intake. **A normal response is a blood glucose level of 70 to 110 mg/dl fasting; < 160 mg/dl at 0.5 hour; < 170 mg/dl at 1 hour; < 125 mg/dl at 2 hours; and fasting level at 3 hours.** In a patient with hyperinsulinism, the blood glucose level is usually lower than in the fasting blood sugar test.

C-peptide level

Proinsulin is cleaved into insulin and a biologically inactive protein, C-peptide. The principal use of C-peptide is in the evaluation of hypoglycemia. Patients with insulin-secreting neoplasms have high levels of both C-peptide and endogenous insulin. Patients with factitious hypoglycemia will have low C-peptide levels in the presence of elevated exogenous serum insulin. C-peptide also is useful in evaluating residual beta-cell function in insulin-dependent diabetics. Glucagon-stimulated C-peptide concentration has been shown to be a good discriminator between insulin-requiring and non-insulin-requiring diabetic patients. **Normal values for fasting C-peptide levels are 0.5 to 2.5 ng/ml.** The diagnosis of islet cell tumor is supported by elevation of C-peptide above 2.5 ng/ml when serum glucose is 40 mg/dl or less.

Plasma glucagon

Glucagon is a hormone secreted by the alpha 2 cells of the pancreatic islets. It exerts a counterbalancing effect to insulin in regulation of glucose metabolism. It is secreted in response to hypoglycemia. **Normal values for glucagon levels are 30 to 210 pg/ml.** Patients with hypoglycemia due to decreased levels of glucagon will have values < 30 pg/ml.

Plasma insulin

Insulin is a hormone secreted by the beta cells of the pancreatic islets in response to elevated glucose levels. Insulin levels can be drawn to diagnose the different forms of hypoglycemia. **The normal range for serum insulin is 20 to 30 µU/ml.** Suspect islet cell tu-

> ### Confirming hypoglycemia *(continued)*
>
> mor when a fasting serum insulin is > 30 µU/ml with glucose level < 50 mg/dl. The diagnosis of insulinoma is established when the serum insulin and C-peptide levels are significantly increased and the symptoms of hypoglycemia are present and plasma glucose is low.

absorbed. Supplemental slowly metabolized carbohydrates should be given as the patient improves, to restore glycogen and prevent recurring hypoglycemia. If the patient is unresponsive, 50 ml of 50% dextrose, I.V., may be administered. A patient with hypoglycemia will respond within a few minutes to the administration of I.V. glucose.

Some experts suggest that glucagon be administered instead. Glucagon mobilizes liver glycogen stores and can arouse a comatose patient to the point where he or she can accept food. Glucagon is given as 0.5 to 1 mg I.V. The half-life of glucagon is 3 to 6 minutes; therefore, if the patient fails to respond to treatment after 20 minutes, another dose of I.V. glucose or glucagon can be given. Patients with low glycogen stores will not respond within 20 minutes, so the only effective treatment is glucose. When the patient regains consciousness, complex carbohydrates may be administered to replenish glycogen stores and ward off further hypoglycemia.

The following nursing interventions should be incorporated into the plan of care:
• Assess the patient frequently for signs and symptoms of hypoglycemia. Be aware that tachycardia, diaphoresis, anxiety, and trembling are masked in the patient on beta blockers.
• Monitor serum glucose levels hourly.
• Administer 50 ml of 50% dextrose to the patient who is unresponsive and unable to take fluids by mouth.
• Administer 5 to 10 g of fruit juice, candy, or carbonated drinks sweete· ˙d with sugar to a conscious patient.

Prevention of hypoglycemic complications

Insulin administration may be adjusted during hospitalization to avoid hypoglycemic episodes in the patient with diabetes. Patients with insulin-controlled diabetes who are not being fed do not need to receive the bolus injections of regular insulin that are required to maintain glucose homeostasis postprandially. Instead, they should receive insulin in a continuous I.V. infusion. This is especially necessary in the patient receiving total parenteral nutrition (TPN), because of the large load of calories associated with TPN formulations.

Insulin-dependent patients who are acutely ill and experiencing some vomiting or those with decreased food intake should be managed differently. Longer-acting insulins are inappropriate because of the difficulty in predicting insulin needs for more than a few hours in advance. Regular insulin should be given before each meal and at midnight.

If a patient is receiving pentamidine, a life-threatening hypoglycemic reaction may occur. Therefore, close glucose monitoring is required.

The following nursing interventions should be incorporated into the plan of care:

• Monitor and report signs of hypoglycemia.
• Identify peak insulin levels and document the time at which the patient should be observed closely.
• If the patient is receiving TPN, monitor blood glucose levels at 2- to 3-hour intervals.
• If the patient is receiving pentamidine, monitor glucose hourly for the first 6 hours after the initial dose, and at least every 6 hours even after the drug is discontinued.
• Perform routine glucose monitoring, as ordered, for all hospitalized patients with diabetes.
• Provide extensive teaching to the patient and family on signs and symptoms of hypoglycemia, diet restriction, medications, and contributing factors in the development of hypoglycemia.

Prognosis

Prognosis in hypoglycemia is good if therapy is prompt. In patients with delayed treatment, irreversible CNS sequelae such as lethargy, stupor, and coma may occur.

Discharge planning

Discharge planning must begin as soon as the patient has stabilized. All of the following guidelines should be considered to prepare the patient for discharge.

• Teach the patient and family to recognize signs and symptoms of impending hypoglycemia.

• Provide information on diet modifications and education, including restriction of simple sugars, small frequent meals (for alimentary hypoglycemia), restrictions of caffeine-containing beverages and cigarettes in emotionally labile patients, and the restriction of candy to use in an emergency for severe hypoglycemic reaction.

• Teach the patient and family about glucose monitoring techniques.

• Instruct the patient and family to report the following to the physician: hemiplegia, blurred vision, persistent dizziness, slurring of speech, hypoglycemia or hyperglycemia not controlled by diet.

• Advise the patient and family to reduce the risk that hypoglycemia will recur by avoiding excessive use of alcohol or the administration of drugs such as aspirin, propranolol, and sulfonamides.

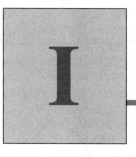

Immunosuppression

Abnormal immune system function can be classified as either hyperreactive or suppressed. Suppressed immunity is further subdivided into conditions that represent unintentional suppression (such as congenital immunodeficiency disorders or acquired immune deficiency syndrome [AIDS]) or suppression as a planned adverse effect of a therapeutic regimen (such as with treatment of autoimmune disease or an antirejection plan following a transplant).

Immunosuppression, defined as a deterioration in the function of the nonspecific or specific immune activities of the body, can encompass a wide variety of clinical syndromes. In its most abstract form, immunosuppression may represent an abnormality in the anatomy or physiology of the immune system, which implies only an increased risk for clinical diseases such as infection or cancer. For consistency, this text will use the term immunosuppression to encompass both temporary and permanent incompetence of the immune system.

Primary (genetic) immunosuppression disorders are hereditary or congenital defects of the immune system and represent the rarest disorders of immune function. Secondary immunosuppression, which is acquired after birth, is a more common presentation in the critically ill. This type of immunosuppression will be the focus of the treatment and care section within this text.

It is estimated that virtually all critically ill patients develop some degree of secondary immunosuppression due to altered defensive barriers or cellular responses. In the critical care area numerous examples of invasive procedures result in a route of entry for microbes. Nutritional deficit is another common cause of acquired immunosuppression among the critically ill. Many medications and diseases also alter quantity or function of white blood cells (WBCs) or immune organs, resulting in immunosuppression. The populations most likely to develop complications of immunosuppression include patients with cancer, bone marrow disease, organ transplant, AIDS, diabetes mellitus, hepatic failure, or splenectomy, or those receiving steroids. A summary of immune structure and function abnormalities, disease states, and pharmacologic agents that cause immunosuppression are outlined in *Physical consequences of abnormal immune functions,* pages 394 and 395.

Pathophysiology

The body's two immune systems (nonspecific and specific) aid in recognition and destruction of pathogens, malignant cells, and foreign tissue and in responding to tissue injury. The three levels of immune defense include: (1) barrier defense, (2) nonspecific cellular activity, and (3) specific immune reactions. Disruptions of the barrier defenses or granulocytes often lead to bacterial infection or an exaggerated inflammatory response. In immunosuppression of the specific immune system, inadequate B and T lymphocyte activity results in viral or opportunistic infections, cancer growth, and nonrecognition of foreign tissue (for example, a transplanted organ).

Primary (genetic) immunodeficiencies represent the rarest disorders of immune function. The most common syndromes of immune suppression in the critically ill are secondary immunosuppressive disorders such as AIDS, neutropenia, and medication- or disease-in-

Physical consequences of abnormal immune functions

The normal integrated immune response involves a variety of mechanisms and body organs. This chart provides an overview of the physiological consequences when immune activities are not normal.

Barrier	Dysfunction
Skin	• Break in the barrier or lack of the normal flora changes the hydrogen ion concentration (pH) and alters ability to resist pathogens. • Extended use of broad-spectrum antibiotics kills normal flora. • Destruction of normal flora allows colonization of pathogenic organisms on skin and orifices, which may provide an entry to the bloodstream.
Eye	• Absence of eyelashes increases risk of ocular infection. • Dry eyes decrease ability to protect against eye infections.
Respiratory tract	• Smoking can damage the cilia on the epithelial cells. • Cancer and other degenerative diseases interfere with coughing and sneezing. • Bone marrow or immune suppression decreases neutrophil and macrophage phagocytic activity. • Pulmonary disease reduce quantity and effectiveness of lysozyme. • IgA deficiency places patient at risk for pulmonary infections.
GI tract	• Antacids or histamine$_2$ blocker agents change stomach pH and alter resistance to pathogens; GI suction removes protective acids. • Anticholinergics and opiates slow bowel motility and increase risk of bacterial translocation into the bloodstream. • Nasogastric tube causes direct damage to the stomach's mucosal surface and increases risk of infection. • Immunosuppression decreases phagocytic activity. • IgA deficiency causes increased risk of GI infections.
Genitourinary (GU) tract	• Antimicrobial therapy, administration of bicarbonate, and hyperglycemia increase the urine pH and place patients at risk for GU infections. • Renal failure reduces urine flow and decreases flushing activity. • Immunosuppression decreases phagocytosis by neutrophils and macrophages. • Prostate removal decreases available immunoglobulins (Workman, 1993) • IgA deficiency causes increased risk of GU infections.

Physical consequences of abnormal immune functions *(continued)*

Barrier	Dysfunction
Inflammatory response	• Neutropenia impairs the inflammatory response. • Chronic infections affect the bone marrow's capacity to synthesize and release mature neutrophils. Immature neutrophils cannot function well in phagocytosis and inflammation, and cannot complete their maturation outside the bone marrow. This leads to increased risk for new and recurrent bacterial and fungal infection.
Phagocytosis	• Neutropenia impairs phagocytosis. • Impaired neutrophil activity predisposes patients to bacterial infections. • Solid tumors impair quantity and function of neutrophils.
Complement immunity	• Secondary complement deficiency can occur with immune complex diseases (for example, glomerulonephritis). • Angioedema is an example of a complement deficiency syndrome.
Immunoglobulins created by B lymphocytes	• Deficiencies cause bacterial and viral infection. • Multiple myeloma is a cancer involving an abnormal immunoglobulin, M protein. Other immunoglobulins function abnormally. • Non-Hodgkin's lymphoma can impair humoral immunity when it involves B cells.
Cytokines created by T-lymphs	• Tumors such as Hodgkin's lymphoma, non-Hodgkin's lymphoma, and hairy cell leukemia can suppress T cells. • Acquired immune deficiency syndrome causes the reduction of CD4 (helper lymphocytes). • Antineoplastic agents and corticosteroids are among the most prominent pharmacological agents to suppress T cells. • Impaired cell-mediated immunity occurs with some solid tumors.

duced immunosuppression (Allen, 1993). Other variables known to influence an individual's immune competence include the degree of physiologic or emotional stress, age (very young or very old), nutritional status, and amount of sleep and rest. An overview of specific immunosuppressant medications used to prevent organ-graft rejection during transplantation can be found in the entry "Organ Transplantation" (page 457), and

AIDS-related immunosuppression is addressed in the entry "Acquired Immunodeficiency Syndrome" (page 25). Other common disorders of immunosuppression are described on the following pages.

Neutropenia

Neutropenia refers to a decrease in the absolute neutrophil count (ANC) to less than $1,000/mm^3$. A decreased number of circulating neutrophils leads to diminished recognition and ability to destroy bacteria and fungi. The consequence is an increased risk of infection with these organisms. Causes of neutropenia include bone marrow suppressants such as cancer, antineoplastic drugs, certain antimicrobials (such as ganciclovir), immunosuppressive agents (such as azathioprine or methotrexate), antiretroviral agents (for example, zidovudine), radiotherapy or radiation exposure, chronic infection, nutritional disorders, and older age. Infections become more frequent and serious when the ANC falls below $100/mm^3$. The majority of patients who are neutropenic for more than 21 days develop infection.

Acute phases of neutropenia lead to an increase in the bacterial infection rate; however, prolonged neutropenia is associated with an increased incidence of fungal infections. Most infection-causing organisms in the neutropenic host are part of the patient's normal flora. In prolonged neutropenia, systemic fungal infections are common problems and often require critical care intervention.

Because neutrophils are the primary cell responsible for the inflammatory reaction, when they are decreased in quantity, there is less inflammatory reaction at the site of infection. Erythema, edema, and exudate formation (for example, pus or sputum) are diminished in this patient population. A fever may be the single symptom of life-threatening infection. With temporary neutropenia, as in the case of cancer chemotherapy–related neutropenia, a return of the WBCs (particularly as the ANC increases) will produce a dramatic increase in symptoms near the location of infection. This should subside as the neutrophils effectively destroy the pathogens, but may produce a short-lived critical illness such as severe and rapid-onset pneumonia requiring mechanical ventilation.

Medication- or disease-induced immunosuppression

Acquired immune compromise has been reported in patients with a variety of other diseases or therapies used in the intensive care setting. In some, the pathophysiologic mechanism alters phagocytic function; others have altered antibody production; and other clinical situations alter T-cell recognition of non-self and viri. The pathophysiology involved will predict infectious complications. Many patients have one of the following risk factors for immune compromise:

• protein-calorie malnutrition—can lead to protein deficiency, resulting in a reduction of the number and quality of T cells. The critically ill patient has impaired nutritional status caused by impaired use of the GI system, the presence of catabolic disorders, and limited I.V. fluids due to cardiovascular or renal system deterioration.

• diabetes mellitus—impairs neutrophil function.

• hepatic disease—damage to hepatocytes alters immunoglobulin storage and decreases fibrinogen production needed to localize the inflammatory process.

• dysfunctional spleen (repeated sickle cell crises)—injury to the spleen alters ability to filter encapsulated organisms (for example, streptococcus, mycobacteria).

• renal disease—breaks the acid barrier of urine because the amount of urine passing through the bladder and urethra is reduced.

• burns—disrupt the skin barrier and depress phagocytic activity.

• autoimmune disease (for example, glomerulonephritis or systemic lupus erythematosus)—antibodies are produced against body tissues. Autoimmune disease is associated with hypersensitivity type II and often is treated with immunosuppressive agents.

• disruption of the blood-brain barrier (for example, head trauma)—increases the risk of deep-seated neurologic infection.

• exposure to illicit I.V. drug use—needles break the skin barrier and reach the bloodstream.

• post-transplant immune suppression medications.

• high-dose corticosteroid therapy—affects skin turgor; inhibits activity of complement system and of neutrophils, eosinophils, monocytes, and B cells; reduces serum immunoglobulin level; and inhibits or depresses the activity of T cells.

• receiving antimicrobial therapy that suppresses normal flora and enhances overgrowth of opportunistic infections can cause leukopenia and suppress immune function.

• recent anesthesia, especially accompanying major surgery—anesthetic agents suppress T-lymphocyte function and depress phagocytosis; endotracheal intubation disrupts the natural barrier and may cause respiratory infection.

• cancer treatment—antineoplastic agents suppress bone marrow function, leading to immunosuppression; radiation contributes to B- and T-cell destruction.

• age—infants have immature immune systems. Deterioration of cell-mediated immunity occurs in elderly persons.

Clinical assessment
A thorough health and social history that is reviewed in conjunction with signs, symptoms, and laboratory tests serves to guide patient management.

History
The patient's health history is important in identifying potential risk factors for the development of immunosuppression. Investigation into the following information will offer some clues for recognizing immune dysfunction:

• age

• current diet, evidence of weight loss, or malnutrition

• medications taken currently or within the past 2 months (glucocorticoids, antibiotics, immunosuppressants: suppress T-lymphocyte immune function, which can lead to various infections)
• recent surgeries
• history of cancer or treatment with cancer therapy
• alcohol use—alcohol destroys stomach mucosa and changes stomach hydrogen ion concentration, leading to infection via GI route; alcohol consumption usually leads to malnutrition, compromises the immune function, damages the hepatocytes, and alters immunoglobulin storage
• drug use—narcotics suppress the immune system
• sexual history—sexual intercourse with others who have multiple partners increases the risk of contracting immune-suppressing viral infections and human immunodeficiency virus
• recent travel outside the United States
• recent physical and emotional stressors—serum levels of endogenous steroids have been noted to increase in patients responding to stress; steroids can interfere with normal function of the immune system by reducing the inflammatory response, thus increasing the development of infection
• living conditions—poor sanitation or crowded conditions may predispose the patient to more unusual communicable diseases such as salmonella and tuberculosis.

Physical findings

Although the signs and symptoms of immunosuppression may not be overtly visible, immunosuppressed patients usually present suddenly with frequent and severe infections. Because neutropenic patients have a reduced inflammatory response, the classic inflammatory signs may be absent. Assessment findings in the immunosuppressed patient that indicate infection or sepsis include:
• altered mental status
• crackles, sputum production, diminished breath sounds, egophony, tachypnea, labored breathing

• full bounding pulses, systolic ejection murmur, low diastolic blood pressure, low central venous pressure, low pulmonary capillary wedge pressure
• concentrated or cloudy urine, decreased urine output, back pain, dysuria
• hypoactive bowel sounds, abdominal distention, abdominal tenderness, anorexia, nausea or vomiting, diarrhea
• unhealed wounds, abnormal wound drainage
• temperature 38° C or 36° C for more than 12 hours
• severe fatigue, arthralgias, myalgias, headache, or other flu-like symptoms
• altered mucous membranes (oral ulcerations, shiny tongue, reddened gums, bleeding gums, rashes, skin lesions, abnormal vaginal or penile drainage)
• lymph node enlargement, hepatomegaly, and splenomegaly.

Diagnosis

The most important and frequently used test to detect immune suppression is the total WBC count and differential. Obtaining the total amount of WBCs is essential to identify any leukocytosis or leukopenia. The diagnosis and management of immunosuppressive states is given in *Evaluating immune function,* pages 401 and 402.

Treatment and care

The prioritization of treatment goals in the immunosuppressed patient will depend in part upon the etiology of immunosuppression. In patients who are unintentionally suppressed, the goal is to enhance immune function. Conversely, in those patients who are immunocompromised for therapeutic intent, the primary goal is to prevent serious infections. These two goals give rise to the key elements or desired outcomes of nursing and medical care of the immune-compromised patient—preventing infections, minimizing infections that do occur, and enhancing immune system functioning.

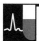

DIAGNOSTIC TESTS

Evaluating immune function

The diagnosis of immunosuppression involves evaluation of white blood cell (WBC) development and activity, as well as function of various protein components of the immune response. This chart identifies the diagnostic tests that may be performed when initially evaluating the immune response. Depending on the results, further testing for specific disorders may be performed, including the measurement of immunoglobulin levels and electrophoresis, and complement proteins; tissue anergy panels; bone marrow aspiration; or bone marrow or lymph node biopsy.

Diagnostic Test and Normal Values	Implications of Abnormal Findings
Total WBCs 5,000 to 10,000/mm^3	• Elevated WBC count can indicate infection, inflammation, or tissue necrosis. The total WBC count also is used to monitor response to therapy in these conditions. • A reduced WBC count indicates a lack of production or depletion outside the bone marrow. Decreased WBCs are expected with older age, infancy, chronic illness, long-term infections, and malnutrition. Certain medications (for example, antiretroviral agents or antineoplastic drugs) also are associated with leukopenia and may require dose modification. Reduced total WBC counts predispose the patient to infection.
WBC differential —Neutrophils 35% to 75% —Eosinophils 1% to 4% —Basophils 2% to 5% —Lymphocytes 15% to 45% —Monocytes 1% to 9%	• Leukocytosis with neutrophilia is called a left shift and is considered a normal response to infection. Elevations of other specific cells may indicate particular infections or allergic reactions. For example, eosinophilia often indicates a pulmonary inflammation (viral, bacterial, or allergic) or dermatologic conditions. Elevations of lymphocytes and monocytes often indicate a viral or opportunistic infection. • Decreases in any of these specific WBC subtypes are indicative of specific disorders. For example, decreased lymphocyte counts occur in the patient with acquired immune deficiency syndrome (AIDS). • An absolute neutrophil count (ANC) less than 1,000 is considered critical and needs further investigation and intervention unless it has been anticipated in a particular antineoplastic regimen and has been predetermined to last only 2 to 3 days.
Albumin levels 3.0 to 5.0 mg/dl	• Decreased plasma proteins (particularly albumin) occur with malnutrition, liver diseases, and capillary permeability problems. Albumin loss affects the body's ability to recognize pathogens and produce antibodies. *(continued)*

Evaluating immune function (continued)

Diagnostic Test and Normal Values	Implications of Abnormal Findings
Lymphocyte helper/ suppressor ratio T4:T8/2:1	• Increased T8 level indicates suppressed immune function. Human immunodeficiency virus (HIV) is associated with low T4 levels, but no actual increase in T8 levels. • The T-cell subpopulation ratio (T4:T8) is used as an indicator of immune status, particularly in AIDS patients.
CD4 count (approximately correlates to number of T-helper cells) > 500 cells/mm^3	• Decreased CD4 count is used in conjunction with T-cell count as an indicator of immune status for HIV infection.

Prevent infections

A major goal in the treatment of immunosuppressed patients is to control environmental and iatrogenic risks for infection. This begins with enforcement of general infection control guidelines such as frequent hand-washing between contacts with patients or between clean and dirty procedures. It also includes screening visitors for communicable diseases. Health care team members should be carefully assigned and additional shielding precautions (for example, use of gowns) undertaken to prevent the risk of cross infection among patients, particularly if resistant organisms are problematic. The following nursing interventions to prevent infection in the immunosuppressed patient should be incorporated into the plan of care:
• Use sterile technique for invasive procedures and dressing changes.
• Meticulously access injection ports and cover stopcocks with sterile dead-end caps.
• Apply skin protectant to prevent skin breakdown.
• Encourage frequent incentive spirometry or coughing and deep breathing to prevent pulmonary infection.

• Treat open skin areas with topical antimicrobials and cover with a dressing.
• Assess for early detection of infection, including monitoring temperatures at least every 4 hours and inspecting body orifices and wounds every shift for localized tenderness, abnormal exudate, or lesions, which can signal infection.
• Inspect all excretions (urine, stool, emesis) for evidence of infection or WBCs.
• Perform frequent evaluation of mental status and auscultation of breath sounds and report abnormal findings.

Minimize infection dissemination and severity

Hyperglycemia is common during critical illness but should be aggressively controlled, since high blood glucose levels reduce the phagocytic activity of neutrophils. Other physiologic problems that increase the risk of infection dissemination in the immunosuppressed patient include renal and hepatic compromise, reduced cardiac output, nutritional deficits, and sleep deprivation. Early detection and appropriate intervention for infectious complications will reduce the risk of life-threatening crises such as septic shock. The following nursing interventions should be incorporated into the plan of care:
• Perform urine, sputum, and blood cultures when appropriate. Blood cultures should be from two different sites and should be from existing venous or arterial access devices, if possible. If diarrhea is present, perform stool cultures daily for 3 days.
• Ensure that additional diagnostic testing is performed, when ordered, including chest X-ray and cultures of the nose, mouth, and rectum.
• Assess breath sounds.
• Administer antimicrobial therapy within 30 minutes of fever, after cultures are taken to reduce the risk of septic shock. The most important antimicrobial medi-

(Text continues on page 406.)

MAJOR DRUGS

Therapeutic agents to enhance immune function

In the treatment of immunosuppressed patients, enhancement of existing immune function occasionally is desirable and possible. In these circumstances, the following agents may be employed.

Medication	Administration Guidelines
Granulocyte colony-stimulating factor (G-CSF, Filgrastim, Neupogen)	• Single I.V. dose of 5 g/kg every day for up to 2 weeks based on post-therapy nadir absolute neutrophil count (ANC). • Should not be used 24 hours before to 24 hours after the administration of cytotoxic chemotherapy. • Therapy must be continued until the postnadir ANC is greater than 10,000/mm^3 after the expected chemotherapy nadir has passed.
Granulocyte- macrophage colony-stimulating factor (GM-CSF, Leukine, Prokine)	• Daily infusion of 250 μg/m^2 • Initiate 2 to 4 hours after autologous bone marrow infusion and not less than 24 hours after the last dose of chemotherapy or 12 hours after the last dose of radiation. • Reduce dose in impaired renal or hepatic function. • Each 250 or 500 μg vial must be diluted with 1 ml preservative-free sterile water for injection. • If the final concentration will be below 10 μg/ml, add albumin to normal saline (1 ml of 5% albumin to each 50 ml normal saline) before addition of medication.
Interleukin-2, Aldesleukin (IL-2, Proleukin)	• Used experimentally with immune-deficient states, but not licensed for use. • Dosage is 1 million IU S.C. 3 times/week.
Alpha-interferon (Roferon-A)	• Dose of Roferon-A is 36 million IU daily for 10 to 12 weeks.
Immune globulin intravenous (IGIV, Gammagard, Gammar-I.V., Iveegam, Sandoglobulin, Venoglobulin-1, Venoglobulin-S)	• I.V. administration of a single dose of 100 to 200 mg/kg (2 to 4 ml/kg). • Dose may be repeated monthly if adequate IgG levels in serum or clinical response is not achieved.

Nursing Implications

- Complete I.V. administration of the single dose in 1 minute or less.
- Use extreme caution in myeloid malignancy; can act as tumor growth factor.
- Use caution in patients with preexisting cardiac disease.
- Discontinue therapy and notify physician immediately if allergic reactions (itching, redness, swelling at injection site) occur.
- Discontinue therapy after ANC surpasses 10,000/mm^3 and chemotherapy nadir has occurred.

- Administer each single dose over 2 hours.
- Reduce rate or discontinue therapy if allergic reactions occur.
- Should be clear and colorless.
- Use caution when administering for any malignancy with myeloid characteristics.
- Monitor complete blood count (CBC) and differential before and twice weekly thereafter to detect any leukocytosis (white blood cell [WBC] count > 50,000 cells/mm^3 or ANC > 20,000 cells/mm^3).
- Reduce dose or discontinue therapy if leukocytosis is detected.
- Observe for fluid retention (peripheral edema, pleural or pericardial effusion).
- Use caution in individuals with a history of renal or hepatic dysfunction.

- Injection site induration and redness may be relieved with hot or cold compresses.
- Fever 4 to 8 hours after injection is common. Advise patients to take acetaminophen at the time of injection, 4 hours later, and 8 hours later.
- Other fevers should be reported to the physician.
- Monitor CBC with CD4 count weekly during therapy.

- Contraindicated in patients with hypersensitivity to alpha interferon, mouse immunoglobulin, or any component of the product.
- Use with caution in patients with severe preexisting cardiac disease, severe renal or hepatic disease, seizure disorders, or compromised central nervous system function.
- Use with caution in individuals with myelosuppression or when administering in combination with other agents that suppress immunity.

- Administer I.V. only, through a central venous access.
- Do not skin test; can cause a localized chemical skin reaction.
- Use caution in patients with isolated IgA deficiency.
- Observe vital signs frequently during infusion; hypotension or anaphylaxis may occur.
- Emergency equipment should be available at bedside.
- IgG level should exceed 300 mg/dl after infusion.

(continued)

Therapeutic agents to enhance immune function *(continued)*

Medication	Administration Guidelines
Cytomegalovirus (CMV)-IgG (CMV-IGIV)	• 150 mg/kg I.V. as a single dose given every 2 weeks after transplant (until week 8), then monthly for 2 additional doses. • For treatment of probable CMV infection, administer 150 mg/kg every week until conclusion of ganciclovir therapy. • Begin infusion at 15 mg/kg/hour, increase to 15 mg/kg/hour every 30 minutes until maximum infusion rate of 60 mg/kg or 75 ml/hour. • Dilute with 50 ml sterile water before transfer.
Granulocyte transfusions	• Premedicate with acetaminophen 625 mg and Benadryl (diphenhydramine hydrochloride) 25 to 50 mg. • Hang on blood infusion set, but without microaggregate filter. Have normal saline available for flushing. • Administer slowly, approximately 5 ml/minute for first 5 minutes. Increase rate as ordered by blood bank, because WBCs should be transfused as a certain number of cells/minute and the blood bank has determined how much diluent is in cells.

cations used in the treatment of immunosuppressed patients are listed in *Antimicrobial therapy for opportunistic infections* (found in the entry on "Acquired Immunodeficiency Syndrome," page 25).

• Obtain antimicrobial peak and trough blood levels to optimize the drug dose for effective organism destruction and to determine if doses are excessive and toxic. Toxicity monitoring most commonly is used for aminoglycoside levels.

• Initiate prophylactic antifungal therapy (such as oral nystatin) to treat potential for fungal superinfection after broad-spectrum antibiotics.

Enhance immune system functioning

While preventing infection is the optimal goal, and minimizing infection is the reality, enhancing immune functioning throughout critical illness supports both

Nursing Implications

- Administer only clear and colorless, without foam.
- Do not use I.V. filter.
- Use caution in patients with isolated IgA deficiency.
- Observe vital signs frequently during observation; hypotension or anaphylaxis may occur.
- Emergency equipment should be available at bedside.

- Reserved for individuals with overwhelming sepsis and little hope of return of their WBC function during the crisis.
- Take baseline vital signs.
- Be certain that patient has an additional patent intravenous access for possible emergency medication administration.
- Monitor for anaphylaxis or severe allergic reactions, including respiratory distress, wheezing, hypotension, pain at I.V. site, and chest pain.
- Agitate bottom of bag every 15 minutes to ensure mixing of cells in solution. (Cells will settle to bottom of bag and infuse rapidly if not agitated.)
- Draw postinfusion WBC count 2 to 4 hours after infusion.
- Observe for inflammatory symptoms at site of suspected infection.

goals. The following nursing interventions should be incorporated into the plan of care:

- Ensure that nutritional and sleep needs are being met to enhance healing and resistance to infection.
- Assess liver and kidney function and report any abnormal findings. Intact function can preserve immunoglobulin function that the patient needs for recovery.
- With specific immune deficits such as neutropenia or immunoglobulin deficiency, administer agents used for replacement or immune stimulant activity to enhance the patient's existing immune system function. Agents used for this purpose are summarized in *Therapeutic agents to enhance immune function,* pages 404 to 407.

Prognosis

The prognosis of a patient with immunosuppression is directly related to the length of time the patient must remain in this compromised state and the extent of exposure to potential pathogens. The past two decades have demonstrated almost continuous technologic advancements in pharmacologic management and noninvasive monitoring techniques. As recently as 1993, new broader-spectrum antimicrobial agents, bone marrow growth factors, immunosuppressive agents for the post-transplantation patient, and immunoglobulin replacement therapy have been licensed for use in managing immunosuppressed patients. Patients with prolonged suppression of the immune system are more likely to develop infections with resistant microorganisms. They also are reported to have a higher incidence of cancer, probably secondary to a decreased ability to provide immune surveillance protection against malignant cells (Barrett, 1993).

Discharge planning

In planning for the discharge of an immunocompromised patient, the nurse should:
• Evaluate the home environment for cleanliness and infection risks.
• Assess financial resources available for obtaining clean and sterile supplies, equipment, and medications.
• Teach the patient and family infection precautions.
• Describe symptoms that should be reported, including a temperature greater than 38.4° C or less than 36° C, chills, dizziness when standing, and abnormal body drainages.
• Encourage general health maintenance to enhance immune function, including adequate rest and sleep, balanced nutrition, and stress reduction.
• Advise patients undergoing periodic bone marrow aspirations not to drive on days when this test is planned, because of the effects of sedation.

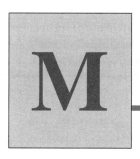

Myocardial conduction defects

Myocardial conduction defects represent abnormalities in conduction of the electrical impulse from the atria to the ventricles or in conduction through the ventricles. These defects include heart blocks, bundle branch blocks (BBBs), hemiblocks, and pre-excitation syndromes. The clinical effects of myocardial conduction defects depend on the resulting heart rate and the ability of the patient's cardiovascular system to compensate for any loss in cardiac output.

Heart blocks involve an abnormality in conduction of the electrical impulse from the atria to the ventricles, consisting of delay or complete absence of conduction in the atrioventricular (AV) node or the bundle of His. As a result, impulse conduction to the ventricles is delayed, occurs inconsistently, or does not occur at all. Failure of some impulses to reach the ventricle causes the heart rate to drop, which may result in significant decrease in cardiac output.

BBB results from failure of either the right or left bundle branch to conduct the impulse to the respective ventricle. Conduction proceeds normally to the unaffected ventricle, but then the impulse is conducted from one myocardial cell to the next until the entire affected ventricle is depolarized. Because this cell-to-cell conduction is 10 times slower than the conduction along the bundle branches and Purkinje fibers, depolarization and subsequent contraction of the affected ventricle are delayed. The presence of BBB indicates an area of the conduction system that is not functioning normally, leaving the patient at higher risk for advanced heart blocks.

Hemiblocks (also called fascicular blocks) occur when either the left anterior fascicle or left posterior fascicle (the two main branches of the left bundle branch) fails to conduct the electrical impulse. Conduction will proceed normally across the nonaffected fascicle and from one myocardial cell to the next to complete depolarization of the myocardium normally depolarized across the blocked fascicle. Hemiblocks represent damage to an area of the conduction system and a risk for the patient to progress to more significant conduction defects. The presence of a left posterior hemiblock indicates a particular risk for progression to complete heart block, and the incidence of such progression is even greater if the patient also has a right BBB.

Pre-excitation syndromes are abnormalities in myocardial conduction caused by the presence of accessory pathways between the atria and ventricles. These accessory pathways allow rapid conduction of atrial impulses to the ventricles and can participate in tachycardias as part of a macro-reentry circuit (see *Reentry mechanisms,* page 90, in the "Arrhythmias" entry). The most common type of pre-excitation syndrome is Wolff-Parkinson-White (WPW), occurring in 57% of patients with symptomatic supraventricular tachycardia (SVT) (Marriott & Conover, 1989). Criteria for differentiating among different types of heart blocks, BBBs, and pre-excitation syndromes are presented in *Identifying myocardial conduction disorders,* pages 411 and 412.

Pathophysiology

Myocardial conduction defects can result from ischemia or infarction of portions of the conduction system,

Identifying myocardial conduction disorders

The following criteria are used to diagnose heart blocks and bundle branch blocks (BBBs) on the ECG.

Heart Block	ECG Criteria
First-degree 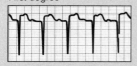	• Regular • One P per every QRS • PR > 0.20 second; constant for each beat • Atrial and ventricular rates equal • QRS usually normal (0.04 to 0.10 second)
Second-degree Type I (Wenckebach) 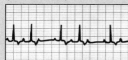	• Irregular QRSs • PR gradually gets longer with consecutive QRSs until finally drops a QRS • Regular P waves • Atrial rate > ventricular rate • QRS usually normal
Second-degree Type II 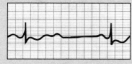	• Irregular QRSs • PR may be normal or long, but is constant for all conducted beats • Regular P waves • Atrial rate > ventricular rate • QRS usually wide (> 0.10 second) *Note:* Regular P-P differentiates this from non-conducted premature atrial complex (PAC)
2:1 second-degree 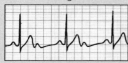	• Regular (P waves and QRSs) • 2 Ps per every QRS • PR constant for all conducted beats; may be normal or long • Atrial rate twice ventricular rate • QRS normal or wide • If QRS narrow, probably second-degree Type I; if QRS wide, probably second-degree Type II
Third-degree (complete heart block) 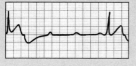	• Regular (P waves and QRSs) • PR varies, with no pattern, indicating total lack of communication between chambers • Atrial rate > ventricular rate • QRS normal or wide depending on subsidiary ventricular pacemaker *Note:* Some P waves may be hidden in QRSs and T waves

(continued)

Identifying myocardial conduction disorders *(continued)*

Heart Block	ECG Criteria
Right BBB 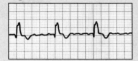	• QRS wide • In V₁ the last deflection of the QRS complex is positive
Left BBB 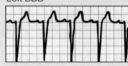	• QRS wide • In V₁ the last deflection of the QRS complex is negative

Hemiblock *(Note: A 12-lead ECG would be required to evaluate for hemiblocks)*

Left anterior hemiblock	• Small Q wave in lead I with large R wave • Small R wave in lead III with large S wave • Left axis deviation (axis ≥ 40°) • Bifascicular block present when ECG shows left anterior hemiblock + right BBB
Left posterior hemiblock	• Small R wave in lead I with large S wave • Small Q wave in lead III with large R wave • Right axis deviation (axis ≥ +120°) • Bifascicular block present when ECG shows left posterior hemiblock + right BBB

Pre-excitation

Wolff-Parkinson-White (WPW) in sinus rhythm (SR) 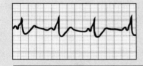	• Short PR interval (< 0.12 second) • Delta wave (widening and slurring of initial portion of QRS) *Note:* In nonevident WPW, criteria may be seen only with a PAC. Do not confuse a delta wave (first part of QRS wide) with an aberrantly conducted PAC (last part of QRS wide)
WPW and supraventricular tachycardia (SVT) 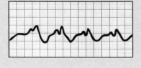	• Narrow or wide complex tachycardia; often precipitated by PAC; may be precipitated by premature ventricular complex • Cannot be differentiated from other kinds of SVT during the tachycardia; diagnosis of evident WPW can be made in SR; of nonevident WPW in SR with PACs; of concealed WPW only with electrophysiologic study

degenerative changes in the conduction system, congenital anomalies, or surgical or procedural injury. Heart blocks also can be seen as the result of adverse effects of some medications. Pre-excitation syndromes occur in individuals who have accessory pathways between the atria and ventricles.

Ischemia and infarction

The anaerobic process of ischemia results in a buildup of waste products and toxins within the cell. As a result, the adenosine triphosphate (ATP) pump required to repolarize cells is impaired; affected cells repolarize more slowly and may not return to a normal resting membrane potential. Consequently, affected cells may be incapable of responding to the next cardiac stimulus or may have a weaker response, resulting in decreased speed of impulse conduction. Clinically, this can cause temporary or transient BBB and heart blocks.

With infarction, cell necrosis has occurred. Myocardial cells no longer are capable of participating in electrical activity; the clinical result is permanent hemiblock, BBB, or heart block. First-degree and second-degree Type I AV blocks can result from ischemia or infarction at the AV node or AV junction. This also may result in third-degree AV block with the AV junction serving as the subsidiary pacemaker. Ischemia or infarction at the level of the bundle of His and bundle branches may produce second-degree Type II AV block or third-degree AV block in which the subsidiary pacemaker is the Purkinje fibers.

Degenerative changes

The normal aging process appears to be associated with a decrease in the number of conducting cells in the AV node, bundle of His, and bundle branches; changes in some tissues begin as early as age 40. Fibrous scarring may permanently block the bundle of His or bundle branches. Clinical findings related to aging include increased AV nodal refractory times, which can contribute to slower or impaired conduction.

Congenital anomalies

Besides structural congenital anomalies, anomalies of the conduction system may occur. Congenital complete heart block may be due to an AV node that does not conduct. In such cases, the patient may have a reasonable heart rate and adequate cardiac output if the ventricular escape rhythm originates in the AV junction. However, if the ventricular escape rhythm originates in the Purkinje system, the rate is significantly slow and a permanent pacemaker is needed.

Surgical or procedural injury

Occasionally during cardiac surgery, particularly involving replacement of valves or closure of a ventricular septal defect, the conduction system is inadvertently damaged, resulting in BBB or heart block. If the injury involves tissues adjacent to the surgical site and the conduction system is not physically disrupted, the block may be temporary. In cases in which a portion of the conduction system is severed, permanent block occurs. Similar disruption of the conduction system can occur from radiofrequency ablation if ablation energy is delivered close to the AV node, bundle of His, or bundle branches. (For a more detailed discussion, see *Radiofrequency ablation,* page 415.)

Drugs

Antiarrhythmic drugs affect repolarization and depolarization in specific tissues. Excessive drug dosage or an exaggerated response to a drug can cause or compound a tendency to heart block. The more common drugs known to cause or exacerbate heart blocks include digoxin, beta blockers, and calcium channel blockers.

Accessory pathways

In some individuals, an extra or accessory pathway exists between the atria and ventricles, consisting of tissue that can conduct impulses rapidly. In such an individu-

Radiofrequency ablation

Radiofrequency ablation is a fairly new nonsurgical treatment to permanently disrupt reentry pathways. During the prolonged procedure (which can last up to 12 hours), the patient is sedated and electrode catheters are introduced utilizing a vascular access. An ablation catheter, which can be flexed in small increments in any direction, also is introduced. Pacing stimuli are delivered to induce the reentry tachycardia, and the ablation catheter is manipulated until ECG recordings from its tip indicate that the catheter is located at one of the tissues participating in the reentry circuit. Radiofrequency energy (similar to electrocautery) is delivered through the ablation catheter for several seconds. A small area of tissue is damaged, and if the catheter has been correctly placed, this damage will permanently disrupt the reentry circuit. Disruption of the reentry circuit will permanently prevent recurrence of the tachycardia and is the goal of this treatment.

al, an electrical stimulus from the atria has another route to reach the ventricles.

Depending on the location and size of the bypass tract, the impulse can reach and depolarize part of the ventricular myocardium before the ventricle is fully depolarized through the normal conduction system. The most common accessory pathway is called a bundle of Kent; patients with this pathway have WPW pre-excitation syndrome. Reentry tachycardias often are precipitated by an early ectopic atrial impulse, which finds the AV node not repolarized. Although in a normal heart this would result in a nonconducted premature atrial contraction, in the WPW patient this impulse can conduct across the accessory pathway (which repolarizes rapidly), depolarize the ventricle, and, after reaching the AV node, find it capable of conducting retrograde to the atria. On reaching the atria, the impulse can be conducted again to the accessory tract and thereby establish a reentry tachycardia. Alternatively, an ectopic atrial impulse originating near the AV node may depolarize the entire ventricular myocardium across the normal conduction pathways and, on reaching the accessory pathway, conduct retrograde to the atria, back down the AV node, and so cause a reentry tachycardia. (For more information see *Reentry mechanisms,* page 90, in the "Arrhythmias" entry.)

Clinical assessment

As with all cardiac rhythm disorders, it is important to treat the patient, not the arrhythmia. Assessment of the individual patient precedes and guides treatment.

History

The patient with a suspected myocardial conduction defect should be asked about:
• current medications
• history of myocardial infarction (MI), cardiac surgery, or ablation
• history of symptoms, including alleviating factors.

The signs and symptoms experienced by the patient and the physical assessment findings associated with various myocardial conduction defects are identified on page 417 in *Clinical assessment findings with myocardial conduction defects.*

Diagnosis

To identify heart blocks and BBB, the nurse should analyze the ECG tracing. Evaluation of the PR interval and the relationship of the P wave to the QRS complex is the most critical step in diagnosing heart blocks. Note that in BBB, the terminal portion of the QRS complex is wide, while the initial portion is narrow. This differs from the delta wave in WPW, where the initial portion of the QRS is wide and the terminal portion is narrow.

If the heart block is intermittent, 24-hour Holter monitoring or event monitoring may be needed to "catch" the disturbance. Some patients develop BBB (most commonly right BBB) with an increase in heart rate. This represents an inability of that bundle branch to repolarize rapidly enough to participate in conduction at the higher rate. The BBB will resolve as the heart rate decreases.

Hemiblocks are diagnosed using the 12-lead ECG and require calculation of the electrical axis for the frontal plane (limb leads). Right BBB may occur with

Clinical assessment findings with myocardial conduction defects

The following findings *may* be seen with the various myocardial conduction defects.

Conduction Defect	Signs and Symptoms	Assessment Findings
Heart block	• Irregular beating or skipped beats • Slow rate • Dizziness, lightheadedness, syncope • Dyspnea • Chest discomfort	• Hypotension • Irregular or slow pulse • Irregularity in auscultated heart rhythm (pattern of S_1 and S_2 varies) • Dyspnea • Diaphoresis • Change in level of consciousness (LOC) • Pallor
Bundle branch block	• None	• Fixed split S_2 heart sound
Hemiblock	• None	• None
Pre-excitation syndrome	During tachycardia: • Palpitations • Fast rate • Dizziness, lightheadedness, syncope • Dyspnea • Chest discomfort	During tachycardia: • Hypotension • Rapid pulse • Dyspnea • Diaphoresis • Change in LOC • Pallor

either hemiblock, in which case the conduction disturbance is called bifascicular block. Left anterior hemiblock and right BBB is not unusual following MI, as these tissues share common circulation from the left anterior descending (LAD) coronary artery. Occurrence of left posterior hemiblock with right BBB following MI is a serious indication of the extent of infarction, as the distribution of both the LAD and of the posterior descending artery are involved and the infarction therefore involves a significant amount of myocardium.

In pre-excitation the early depolarization spreads cell to cell through the ventricular myocardium (slow conduction). The terminal portion of the QRS complex represents the remainder of the ventricle, depolarizing across the normal conduction system. The short PR interval is due to this early start of ventricular depolarization.

If a delta wave with a short PR interval is observed on the ECG, the diagnosis of WPW can be made. In some patients (nonevident WPW), the delta wave is seen only with premature atrial complexes. In other cases, the accessory tract may not participate in pre-excitation of the ventricle, but may conduct retrograde to participate in reentry tachycardia (concealed WPW). For these patients, electrophysiologic (EP) testing is needed for diagnosis. EP testing also is required to direct treatment if other than drug therapy is planned. Although the location of the pathway and degree of ventricular pre-excitation will determine the clinical effects, the patient typically is subject to episodes of SVT.

Treatment and care

BBBs and hemiblocks are not treated; the patient is observed for development of heart blocks. For the other myocardial conduction defects it is essential to assess the patient's current response to the rhythm, which will be based on the degree of compromise of cardiac output. Interventions are focused on restoring and maintaining adequate cardiac output, permanently restoring an adequate heart rate, and treating accessory pathways.

Cardiac output maintenance

Immediate restoration of adequate cardiac output in the compromised patient with a myocardial conduction defect is a priority. Treatment may include the administration of medication, such as atropine or Isuprel (isoproterenol hydrochloride), or the use of a pacemaker, depending on the patient's rhythm, in an effort to improve hemodynamic status. Nursing interventions that should be incorporated into the plan of care for the patient with a heart block include:

• Maintain continuous ECG monitoring; assess vital signs frequently and perform ECG analysis.

• Assess the patient for signs of decreased cardiac output, including decreased level of consciousness (LOC), decreased pulses, and decreased renal perfusion.

• Administer atropine, as ordered, to improve AV conduction and to increase sinus rate.

• Assist the patient in preparing for temporary pacemaker placement. (See "Restoration of adequate heart rate and rhythm," below, for additional interventions.)

• Administer Isuprel, as ordered. Use with caution, as it will increase myocardial oxygen demand and ischemia, and may expand the area of an acute infarction.

Restoration of adequate heart rate and rhythm

As noted, a temporary pacemaker may be placed to aid in improving cardiac output. Temporary pacemakers use either epicardial or transvenous wires or transcutaneous patches. Some patients may require the placement of permanent pacemakers. Today, various pacemakers and pacing modalities are seen in the critical care setting. To identify capabilities for pacemakers and pacing modes regardless of manufacturer, a generic code is used (see *Generic code for pacemakers,* page 420).

A limited number of problems can occur with paced rhythms. The challenge in identifying them is in knowing what is normal or expected function for the particular pacemaker in question. See *Problems associated with pacemakers,* page 421.

The following nursing interventions should be incorporated into the plan of care for the patient with a pacemaker:

• Examine the temporary pacing system for exposed wires or damaged cable insulation.

• Touch a metal object to ground any static electricity on your skin before touching any exposed wires, and wear gloves to protect the patient from conducted electricity.

• In the patient with temporary epicardial wires, cover the exposed wires with a nonconductive material (such as a needle cover) before dressing the site if the wires are not currently connected to the pacemaker cable.

Generic code for pacemakers

A generic code is used to identify the function of a pacemaker, no matter what manufacturer produced the device.

The following three-letter code is most widely used:
• Chamber-paced (where the pacemaker delivers pacing stimuli)
—V = Ventricle
—A = Atrium
—D = Dual (both atrium and ventricle)
• Chamber-sensed (where the pacemaker looks for intrinsic beats)
—V = Ventricle
—A = Atrium
—D = Dual (both atrium and ventricle)
—O = None (pacing mode with no sensing of intrinsic cardiac events)
• Mode of response (how pacemaker reacts to a sensed intrinsic event)
—I = Inhibited (pacemaker does not deliver stimulus)
—T = Triggered (pacemaker triggered to deliver a stimulus)
—D = Dual (inhibited in one chamber, triggered in the other)

—O = None (no response in pacing modes where there is no sensing).
   Using this code, a VVI pacemaker is one that paces in the ventricle, senses in the ventricle for QRSs, and is inhibited from pacing by a sensed QRS. Two other pacing modes are commonly seen in critical care: DVI (paces both chambers but senses only in the ventricle) and DDD (sensing and pacing in both chambers).
   A fourth symbol (R = rate) is added in the code when describing a rate-responsive pacemaker, one that can sense activity and increase the pacing rate accordingly. A pacemaker capable of sensing physical activity and increasing the ventricular pacing rate to correspond is labeled VVIR. A DDDR pacemaker has all the functions of a DDD pacemaker with the added ability to sense physical activity and increase the rate accordingly.

• If temporary wires are not attached to a pacemaker, label atrial and ventricular wires to avoid confusion when they are needed.
• When applying transcutaneous pacing pads, make sure there are no air bubbles under the pads, as this can cause arcing of electrical energy and burns to the patient.
• If applicable, discuss signs and symptoms that might indicate the need for reprogramming, such as lightheadedness, dizziness, increased swelling of the feet, or palpitations. If the problem is the result of a defect in the lead wire or pulse generator, surgery will be needed to replace the defective item.

Problems associated with pacemakers

The following problems may occur with either temporary or permanent pacemakers. The chart names and describes the problem, defines the ECG criteria for identifying the problem, and identifies possible causes and the steps taken to address the problem.

Pacemaker Problem	Possible Causes	Interventions
Failure to capture—a pacemaker stimulus falls at a place where it should result in a beat, and no paced beat occurs ECG criteria: Some or all pacemaker spikes do not result in P waves	• Output (measured in milliamperes, mA) too low to adequately stimulate myocardium • Lead wire in poor contact with myocardium or malfunctioning • Low battery energy	• Increase the output. • Turn the temporary transvenous pacemaker patient on the right side to facilitate lead wire contact with the myocardium. • Check transcutaneous pacemaker patches and replace if necessary.
Undersensing—the pacemaker fails to sense a cardiac event that it was programmed to sense ECG criteria: Some or all pacemaker spikes occur too soon after cardiac events	• Sensitivity set too high (measured in millivolts, mV) • Lead wire in poor contact with myocardium or malfunctioning	• Adjust the sensitivity to a smaller number, thus causing the pacemaker to "see" a smaller waveform. • Reposition the temporary transvenous pacemaker patient to the right side.
Oversensing—the pacemaker senses and responds to electrical activity other than the event it was intended to sense (often the T wave) ECG criteria: Pacing slower than programmed rate	• Sensitivity set too low	• Adjust the sensitivity to a larger number to eliminate sensing of events other than the QRS.
Lack of pacemaker output—the pacemaker does not produce a stimulus at the proper time, allowing a longer interval after the last cardiac event than programmed ECG criteria: Heart rate drops below the programmed pacing rate	• Loose connections of pacemaker lead wires to the cable • Loose cable connections at the pacemaker • Low battery energy	• Check connections. • Replace cables if insulation is damaged. • Check or replace the battery.

Treatment of accessory pathways

Verapamil, diltiazem, or adenosine can be given I.V. to terminate this tachyarrhythmia. If the patient with accessory pathways is in atrial fibrillation, verapamil and diltiazem are contraindicated because potential blocking of the AV node could allow all atrial impulses to conduct over the accessory pathway. The resulting rapid ventricular rate can deteriorate to ventricular fibrillation.

The physician may perform carotid sinus massage in an effort to stop the reentry tachycardia. It does, however, carry a risk of causing emboli if atherosclerotic plaque is present in the carotid arteries.

Long-term medical management with quinidine or Pronestyl (procainamide hydrochloride) is successful in suppressing the accessory pathway and avoiding reentry tachycardia in some patients. Digoxin has been used in some patients, but studies differ regarding the effects of digoxin on the accessory pathway, with some indicating a slowing and others a quickening of repolarization.

Surgical intervention has been found to be effective in interrupting the accessory pathway, either by cutting these tissues or freezing them with a cryoprobe (cryoablation). Radiofrequency ablation provides a permanent, nonsurgical treatment for these patients.

In some patients, more than one accessory pathway exists. While the secondary pathway may not be evident before treatment, such patients may continue to exhibit tachycardia after surgical or ablation treatment, requiring detection and treatment of this additional pathway.

The following nursing interventions for the patient with an accessory pathway should be incorporated into the plan of care:
• Maintain continuous ECG monitoring.
• If appropriate, instruct the patient to perform vagal maneuvers (cough or bear down).
• Administer medications, as prescribed, to terminate the reentry pathway.

• Prepare the patient for procedures, such as electrical cardioversion, radiofrequency ablation of pathway, or surgical clipping or cryoablation of pathway.
• Administer quinidine and Pronestyl (procainamide hydrochloride) as ordered, monitoring for signs or symptoms of increased blood levels. Monitor laboratory results for blood levels above the therapeutic range.

Prognosis

Third-degree heart block and 2:1 second-degree heart block may result in significant reduction in cardiac output and so constitute life-threatening rhythms in some patients. Permanent pacemakers restore life expectancy in these patients. The combination of left posterior hemiblock and right BBB carries a mortality of 71% in hospital, due to the significant area of myocardial damage needed to produce this bifascicular block. The other heart blocks and BBB do not affect mortality of themselves; rather, their prognosis is related to the underlying process that caused the conduction defect. Patients with pre-excitation syndromes and accessory pathways are at risk for reentry tachycardias or atrial fibrillation that can result in sudden cardiac death. If the condition is untreated, risks depend on the rate of the arrhythmia and degree of cardiac decompensation. If the condition is successfully treated, the patient's life expectancy returns to normal.

Discharge planning

The following discharge instructions should be given to a patient with BBB or heart block:
• Report the following symptoms to the physician: sensations of slow or irregular heart rhythm, light-headedness, near-syncope or syncope, changes in LOC.

For the patient with a permanent pacemaker, provide instructions regarding the schedule and procedures for telephone-tracing follow-up of pacemaker function. Other discharge instructions that should be given include:
• Inspect the skin at the pacemaker site weekly, reporting redness, irritation, and skin breakdown.

• Avoid contact sports or other activities that may cause an impact over the pacemaker.
• Avoid objects and activities that can interfere with the pacemaker's function, including microwave ovens with faulty shielding, and power transmitters such as at radio or television stations and power plants; if light-headedness, dyspnea, or chest discomfort are experienced near electrical equipment, move away and rest until symptoms subside. Contact the physician if symptoms persist.

The following discharge instructions should be given to the patient with an accessory pathway:
• If symptoms experienced in the past with tachycardia occur, attempt to terminate the rhythm by bearing down or coughing forcefully.
• Call 911 when the symptoms begin (for the patient with a history of loss of consciousness with tachycardia).

Myocardial infarction

Myocardial infarction (MI), a state of irreversible tissue necrosis, is caused by prolonged inadequate oxygenated blood flow through the coronary arteries. Such a disruption in the amount of oxygen available to the myocardial cells ultimately leads to permanent tissue injury and cellular death.

A leading cause of death in North America and western Europe, MI carries a mortality rate of about 25%. Over half of all sudden deaths attributed to MI occur within 1 hour after onset of signs and symptoms. The American Heart Association estimates that about 300,000 people in the United States die each year from MI prior to reaching the hospital. Consequently, early detection and treatment are the cornerstones of successful health care.

Pathophysiology

MI typically is caused by prolonged blockage or constriction of a coronary artery that leads to a decreased supply of oxygen to the myocardium. Such obstructions typically result from coronary artery disease (also known as atherosclerotic heart disease), coronary artery thrombus or embolism, or arterial spasm.

Coronary artery disease can result from a diffuse buildup of fatty plaque in the intimal layer of the coronary artery, with subsequent narrowing of the arterial lumen. According to one theory, injury to the endothelial lining of the coronary arteries causes platelets, white blood cells, fibrin, and lipids to converge at the injured site. Foam cells, or resident macrophages, congregate under the damaged lining and absorb oxidized cholesterol, gradually thickening the intimal layer and narrowing the arterial lumen. To compensate for the decreased blood flow, collateral circulation may develop. At the lesion site (where the coronary artery lumen narrows), further obstruction may result from continued atherosclerotic buildup, hemorrhage into the intimal wall, thrombus formation (as a result of the narrowed lumen), or embolism (from rupture of the lesion itself).

The exact cause of coronary arterial spasm is unknown, although some precipitating factors have been suggested. One factor involves the release of a potent vasoconstrictor, thromboxane A2, following stimulation of the sympathetic nervous system, such as occurs when a person experiences physical or emotional stress. Other possible factors include cigarette smoking, alcohol ingestion, and cocaine use.

Other conditions and events that can alter the blood volume supply or limit myocardial perfusion, thereby decreasing the oxygen supply, include shock, hemorrhage, hypotension, myocardial hypertrophy, severe dehydration, and intense physical activity.

When myocardial demand for oxygen is more than collateral circulation can supply, myocardial metabolism shifts from aerobic to anaerobic. This leads to the production of lactic acid, which stimulates pain nerve endings. Myocardial cells die from lack of oxygen, resulting in decreased myocardial contractility, stroke volume, and blood pressure. Hypoperfusion stimulates baroreceptors, which in turn stimulate the adrenal glands to release epinephrine and norepinephrine. These catecholamines increase the heart rate and cause peripheral vasoconstriction, further increasing myocardial oxygen demand.

Damaged cell membranes in the infarcted area allow intracellular contents into the vascular circulation. Elevated serum levels of potassium, creatine phosphokinase (CPK), CPK-MB (cardiac isoenzyme), aspartate aminotransferase (formerly serum glutamic oxaloacetic transaminase), and lactate dehydrogenase result, and ventricular arrhythmias may develop.

Infarction sites

Although MIs can occur in any area of the heart, most occur in the left ventricle. Only about 10% of MIs occur in the right ventricle, usually in conjunction with a left ventricular infarction; an isolated right ventricular infarction is rare. The actual site of an MI depends on the coronary artery affected and on how well the area is perfused by collateral circulation (for a detailed illustration of coronary artery blood flow and typical MI sites, see *Coronary arteries and myocardial infarction sites,* pages 427 and 428.)

A higher morbidity is associated with infarctions of the anterior or lateral portion of the heart because of the increased incidence of conduction defects and congestive heart failure that typically follow an infarction in these areas.

During an MI, three pathologic changes occur: an area of necrotic tissue (zone of infarction) develops, a zone of injury envelops the necrotic area, and an outer zone of ischemia forms. Characteristic ECG changes are directly related to each area and can pinpoint the extent of an MI.

The zone of ischemia produces characteristic T-wave inversions caused by altered repolarization. The zone of injury results in characteristic ST-segment elevations caused by severe ischemia. The zone of infarction pro-

Coronary arteries and myocardial infarction sites

The primary area of myocardial infarction (MI) and its ensuing structural damage depend on which major coronary artery is occluded and on how well the affected area is perfused by collateral circulation.

Coronary artery disease stimulates the development of collateral circulation, possibly through the release of vasodilators. Collateral circulation is especially well developed in patients with a 75% or greater reduction in the lumen of the coronary artery. During recovery from acute MI, nearly 40% of patients develop collateral circulation.

Collateral circulation seems to reduce myocardial necrosis in patients with coronary artery occlusion. In those with extensive collateral vessel development, collateral vessels can perfuse the area even if the artery is totally occluded as long as no stress is placed on the heart.

The chart below correlates the major regions and structures supplied by coronary arteries with the areas of infarction associated with obstruction.

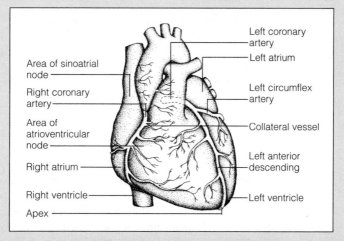

Coronary Artery	Major Areas and Structures Supplied	Primary Infarction Area
Right	• Sinoatrial (SA) node • Atrioventricular (AV) node • Bundle of His • Right atrium and right ventricle • Inferior and diaphragmatic surface of left ventricle • Posterior third of septum • Posteroinferior division of left bundle branch	• Inferior wall • Inferoposterior wall • Right ventricle

(continued)

Coronary arteries and myocardial infarction sites *(continued)*

Coronary Artery	Major Areas and Structures Supplied	Primary Infarction Area
Left	• Massive left ventricular area	• Left ventricle
Left anterior descending	• Anterior wall of left ventricle • Anterior two-thirds of septum • Bundle of His • Right bundle branch • Anterosuperior division of left bundle branch • Posteroinferior division of left bundle branch	• Anterior wall • Septum • Anterolateral wall • Inferoapical wall • Apex A_6
Left circum-flex	• SA node • AV node • Inferior and diaphragmatic surface of left ventricle • Lateral wall of left ventricle • Left atrium • Posteroinferior division of left bundle branch	• Lateral wall • Inferolateral wall • Posterior wall • Inferoposterior wall

Source: *Responding to Patients in Crisis.* Advanced Skills Series. Springhouse Corporation, 1993.

duces pathologic Q waves, indicating developing myocardial necrosis and true infarction. (A pathologic Q wave has a duration of 0.04 second or an amplitude measuring at least one-fourth to one-third the height of the entire QRS complex.) If treatment is begun immediately, necrosis can be minimized and the ischemic zone can recover. If not, this zone also may become necrotic, thereby extending the infarction site and further depressing myocardial function. (For examples of ECG changes, see *Pinpointing the zone of injury,* page 429.)

Traditionally, MIs have been classified as either transmural or nontransmural, depending on the extent of necrosis to the myocardial muscle layers. In a transmural MI, the area of necrosis extends through all of the myocardial layers; in a nontransmural MI, one or more (but not all) of the layers are damaged. Complications

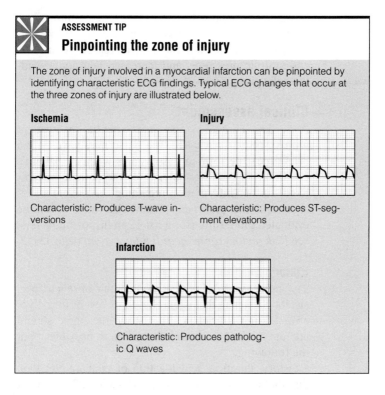

ASSESSMENT TIP
Pinpointing the zone of injury

The zone of injury involved in a myocardial infarction can be pinpointed by identifying characteristic ECG findings. Typical ECG changes that occur at the three zones of injury are illustrated below.

Ischemia

Characteristic: Produces T-wave inversions

Injury

Characteristic: Produces ST-segment elevations

Infarction

Characteristic: Produces pathologic Q waves

are more likely to observed with a transmural MI because of the multilayer involvement. Some settings use an alternative classification system, referring to MIs as Q-wave and non–Q-wave MIs based on the appearance or absence of these waves on ECGs.

The myocardium begins to heal itself if the infarction is not fatal. Within 24 hours, leukocytes infiltrate the infarcted area, beginning at its periphery. The injured myocardial cells release characteristic enzymes that can be measured in serum to help gauge the extent of tissue damage. Also, within 24 hours, degradation and removal of necrotic tissue begins. Within 3 weeks, scar tissue begins to form; tissue removal causes thinning of the heart wall, which may rupture if the removal occurs too rapidly. After 4 to 6 weeks, scar tissue is completely formed. This nonelastic tissue can affect the heart's performance by causing reduced contractility, altered ventricular wall movement, reduced stroke volume, reduced ejection fraction, increased ventricular end-systolic pressures, and increased ventricular end-diastolic pressures.

Clinical assessment

A thorough clinical assessment is essential for a patient with suspected acute MI. The nurse may have only a brief time to perform this assessment when the patient's condition appears unstable. Once the patient is stabilized, further information regarding the patient's lifestyle and the presence of any risk factors can be evaluated more fully (for a list of predisposing factors, see *Risk factors for myocardial infarction,* page 431).

History

The patient with MI typically complains of severe, persistent chest pain that is unrelieved by rest or nitroglycerin. During a brief health history, the nurse should attempt to elicit as much information as possible about the following:
• history, duration, and location of pain. (Note: Pain distribution varies from patient to patient. The patient may have no pain, pain in one area, or pain in multiple areas, such as the jaw, left arm, or back.)
• precipitating factors
• medication use
• preexisting medical conditions
• palpitations.

Physical findings

Besides those noted during the health history, other findings commonly associated with MI include:
• nausea or vomiting
• fatigue
• diaphoresis, cool extremities
• dyspnea, new onset or worsening of crackles
• jugular vein distention (when right ventricular failure is present)

Risk factors for myocardial infarction

- Family history of coronary artery disease
- Hypertension
- Smoking
- Elevated serum triglyceride, low-density lipoprotein, or cholesterol levels
- Decreased serum high-density lipoprotein level
- Diabetes mellitus
- Obesity
- Excessive intake of saturated fats, carbohyarates, or salt
- Lack of exercise (sedentary lifestyle)
- Aging
- Stress
- Aggressive or suppressed anger
- Drug use, especially cocaine or amphetamines
- Oral contraceptive use

- bradycardia or tachycardia; palpitations
- hypotension or hypertension; dizziness
- S_4, S_3, paradoxical splitting of S_2, or decreased heart sounds (when ventricular dysfunction is present)
- systolic murmur indicating mitral insufficiency (when papillary muscle dysfunction is present)
- low-grade fever (typically occurs a few days after onset of MI)
- restlessness, anxiety, or a feeling of impending doom.

Diagnosis

Although other conditions, such as anxiety, hiatal hernia, or pulmonary embolism, may mimic some signs and symptoms of MI, diagnostic test results can confirm the occurrence of an MI. Because some physical conditions may alter the results of these tests, a review of all the clinical information in conjunction with the test results is required.

Electrocardiogram

A serial 12-lead ECG is performed whenever an MI is suspected. An ECG may show no abnormalities or may prove inconclusive within the first few hours after an MI occurs. By observing changes in the ECG tracings during the patient's hospital stay, the health care team can track the progression of the MI.

Characteristic ECG abnormalities include ST-segment elevations, T-wave inversions, and the presence of pathological Q waves. Additionally, reciprocal (mirror image) changes may be present. Reciprocal changes (most commonly, ST-segment depression or tall R waves) occur in the leads opposite those reflecting the area of ischemia, injury, or infarction. Other ECG changes may occur in specific leads and may pinpoint the location of the MI (for a listing of ECG changes in specific leads, see *Infarction sites and ECG characteristics,* pages 433 and 434).

Diagnostic tests

An increase in serum laboratory enzyme and isoenzyme levels reflects the release of enzymes from inside the myocardial cell when the cellular membrane is destroyed by tissue necrosis. Imaging studies may evaluate further the extent of tissue necrosis and its effect on myocardial functioning. (For a complete listing of common diagnostic tests, see *Confirming a myocardial infarction,* pages 435 and 436.)

Treatment and care

The primary goals of treatment for the patient with an MI are to relieve chest pain, stabilize cardiac rhythm, and reduce the cardiac workload (see *Key nursing interventions for patients with myocardial infarction (MI),* page 437). The most common treatments and related nursing interventions are listed below.

During the initial stages of recovery, the patient should be monitored continuously for cardiovascular and respiratory complications (for a discussion of common complications, see *Identifying serious complications,* pages 438 and 439). The nurse should provide emotional support and instructions to the patient and family about the disorder and its prevention and treatment. A dietary consultation also should be initiated. The patient experiencing nausea should receive a clear liquid diet. Once the nausea has subsided and the patient is stable, the diet can advance to a low-cholesterol,

Infarction sites and ECG characteristics

Site	Characteristic Changes
Anterior	• Pathologic Q waves in leads V_1, V_2, V_3, V_4, I, and V_L • Loss of R-wave progression in the precordial leads • T-wave changes that may occur hours or weeks after the infarction • Initially, upright and peaked T waves • Subsequently, T waves inverted in leads V_2, V_3, V_4, I, and aV_L • Reciprocal changes (tall and symmetrical T waves) in leads II, III, and aV_F • ST-segment elevation a few hours after onset of myocardial infarction (MI) in leads V_1, V_2, V_3, V_4, and V_L • ST-segment depression in leads II, III, and V_F
Anterolateral	• Pathologic Q waves in leads I, aV_L, V_4, V_5, and V_6 • T-wave changes that may occur hours or weeks after the infarction • Initially, upright and peaked T waves • Subsequently, T waves inverted in leads I, aV_L, V_4, V_5, and V_6 • Reciprocal changes (tall and symmetrical T waves) in leads II, III, and aV_F • ST-segment elevation a few hours after onset of MI in leads I, aV_L, V_1, V_2, V_3, V_4, V_5, and V_6 • ST-segment depression in leads II, III, and aV_F
Anteroseptal	• Pathologic Q waves in leads V_1, V_2, and V_3 • Loss of R waves in lead V_1 • T-wave changes that may occur hours to weeks after the infarction • Initially, upright and peaked T waves • Subsequently, inverted T waves in leads V_1, V_2, and V_3 • ST-segment elevation that occurs a few hours after onset of MI in leads V_1, V_2, and V_3
Apical wall	• Pathologic Q waves in leads V_2, V_3, V_4, V_5, and V_6 • Loss of R-wave progression in leads V_3, V_4, V_5, and V_6 • T-wave changes that may occur hours to weeks after the infarction • Initially, upright and peaked T waves • Subsequently, inverted T waves in leads V_3, V_4, V_5, and V_6 • ST-segment elevation that occurs a few hours after onset of MI in leads V_3, V_4, V_5, and V_6

(continued)

Infarction sites and ECG characteristics *(continued)*

Site	Characteristic Changes
Inferior wall	• Pathologic Q waves in leads II, III, and aV$_F$ • T-wave changes that may occur hours to weeks after infarction • Initially, upright and peaked T waves • Subsequently, inverted T waves in leads II, III, and aV$_F$ • Reciprocal changes (tall and symmetrical T waves) in leads I and aV$_L$ • ST-segment elevation that occurs a few hours after onset of MI in leads II, III, and aV$_F$ • ST-segment depression in leads I and aV$_L$
Lateral wall	• Pathologic Q waves in leads I and aV$_L$ • T-wave changes that may occur hours to weeks after the infarction • Initially, upright and peaked T waves • Subsequently, inverted T waves in leads I and aV$_L$ • Reciprocal changes (tall and symmetrical T waves) in leads V$_{i1}$ and V$_{i2}$
Posterior wall	• Reciprocal changes (tall, broad R waves) in leads V$_1$ and V$_2$ • Reciprocal changes (ST-segment depression) in leads V$_1$ and V$_2$ • Possibly elevated T waves in leads V$_1$ and V$_2$

low-sodium one without caffeine-containing beverages.

Thrombolytic therapy

The first 6 hours after onset of signs and symptoms are crucial because, during this time, prompt intervention may result in reperfusion of the myocardium and a decrease in the size of the actual infarction. Revascularization therapy may involve the administration of thrombolytic agents. The earlier the patient receives thrombolytic therapy, the greater the chances for survival. Thrombolytic therapy may be used except when the patient has a history of a cerebrovascular accident, GI ulcers, marked hypertension, recent surgery, or chest pain persisting over 6 hours, or is over 70 years of age.

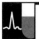

DIAGNOSTIC TESTS
Confirming a myocardial infarction

Besides serial ECGs, several diagnostic laboratory and imaging studies typically are performed to help confirm a diagnosis of MI.

Creatine phosphokinase (CPK)

An enzyme located in muscle cells and brain tissue, CPK reflects tissue catabolism. Total serum CPK previously was widely used to detect MI; however, an elevated serum CPK level caused by skeletal muscle damage reduces the test's specificity for MI. **The normal serum CPK level determined by the most commonly performed assay in North America ranges from 60 to 175 U/liter for men and 40 to 150 U/liter for women.** These levels may be higher in muscular individuals and may vary depending on the institution's measurement method.

Isoenzyme levels

CPK-MB, cardiac isoenzyme, can be isolated from CPK and is found primarily in cardiac muscle. (A small amount also resides in skeletal muscles.) The measurement of this isoenzyme is specific for MI as it typically will increase with an MI. **The normal value of CPK-MB ranges from 0 to 7 IU/liter.** The CPK-MB level rises within 2 to 4 hours, peaks within 12 to 24 hours, and typically returns to normal 24 to 48 hours after an MI.

Lactate dehydrogenase (LDH)

LDH is used to aid in the differential diagnosis of MI, pulmonary infarction, anemia, and hepatic disease. It can support CPK-MB results or confirm diagnosis when CPK-MB samples are obtained too late to display elevation. LDH is present in almost all body tissues; however, five tissue-specific isoenzymes can be identified and measured. Two of these isoenzymes, LDH_1 and LDH_2, appear primarily in the heart.

The myocardial LDH level rises after the CPK level rises, peaks in 2 to 5 days, and returns to normal in 7 to 10 days if tissue necrosis does not persist. The concentration of LDH_1 is greater than LDH_2 within 12 to 48 hours after onset of symptoms. This is a reversal of the normal LDH isoenzyme pattern and is typical of myocardial damage. **Normal LDH_1 levels are 18.1% to 29% of total LDH; normal LDH_2 levels are 29.4% to 37.5% of total LDH. The normal value for LDH ranges from 48 to 115 IU/liter.**

Aspartate aminotransferase (AST)

AST (formerly serum glutamic oxaloacetic transaminase), an enzyme found primarily in the liver, heart, skeletal muscles, kidneys, pancreas, and, to a lesser extent, red blood cells, is released into serum in proportion to the cellular damage. The levels may be transient and slightly elevated early in the disease and extremely elevated during the most acute phase. Because of its relatively low organ specificity, AST is not used routinely as the sole identifying test result for diagnosing a MI. **Normal levels are 10 to 30 U/liter.**

Complete blood count (CBC)

Patients with MI typically have an increased leukocyte count and erythrocyte sedimentation rate. Polycythemia, which increases blood viscosity and the heart's workload, also may be identified in a CBC.

(continued)

Confirming a myocardial infarction *(continued)*

Multiple-gated acquisition scanning (MUGA)

Also called radionuclide ventriculography, blood pool imaging, gated heart study, or wall motion study, MUGA is used to help:
• assess left ventricular function
• determine the extent of muscle impairment after MI
• evaluate the general level of cardiac function
• assess the extent of cardiac muscle damage
• diagnose congestive heart failure
• evaluate the patient's response to therapy.

Coronary angiography

This procedure may be performed early in the treatment of MI to determine the status of coronary artery occlusion, to evaluate left ventricular

function, and to measure cardiac heart pressures and oxygen saturation. It also is used during administration of intracoronary streptokinase, if required.

Echocardiography

The ultrahigh-frequency sound waves used in this test help evaluate heart chamber size, wall thickness, and valvular motion and structures. It also evaluates overall left ventricular function.

Chest X-ray

This test may reveal abnormalities resulting from atherosclerosis or its complications (such as cardiac enlargement, congestive heart failure, ventricular aneurysm, and pulmonary congestion).

Various thrombolytic agents are used in revascularization therapy; for a listing of the most commonly used drugs, see *Thrombolytics used in myocardial infarction,* pages 440 and 441.

The following nursing interventions should be incorporated into the plan of care:
• Perform continuous cardiac monitoring to assess for any arrhythmia that may develop as coronary artery blood flow is reestablished.
• Monitor frequently for hypotension.
• Assess the patient frequently for signs of ecchymosis or bleeding, including observing for signs of bleeding at I.V. or arterial catheter insertion sites, at the gums, in the retroperitoneal cavity, and in the GI tract.
• Monitor for signs of hypersensitivity, including urticaria, fever, flushing, and arrhythmias.
• Assess for changes in the patient's neurologic status that suggest evidence of intracranial hemorrhage, in-

ESSENTIAL ELEMENTS

Key nursing interventions for patients with myocardial infarction (MI)

The following flowchart highlights key interventions that typically are performed when a patient is diagnosed with MI.

ACHIEVE OPTIMAL CARDIOVASCULAR STATUS

Identify myocardial dysfunction	Decrease myocardial oxygen consumption	Increase myocardial oxygen supply
Monitor and report these signs and symptoms: • chest pain • crackles upon auscultation • abnormal heart sounds (S_3, S_4, or murmurs) • restlessness. Monitor ECG continuously for arrhythmias or electrical conduction defects. Assess and report unstable vital signs or hemodynamic variables. Monitor serum potassium and cardiac enzyme levels.	As prescribed, administer these drugs: • anxiolytics • beta blockers • vasodilating agents • calcium channel blockers • antiarrhythmics. Maintain intra-aortic balloon pump (IABP) or left ventricular assist device (LVAD) if in place. Maintain bed rest and enforce activity restrictions. Discourage use of Valsalva's maneuver.	As prescribed, administer these drugs: • dobutamine • thrombolytic agents. Administer oxygen, as prescribed. Monitor and report signs of hypoxemia. Maintain IABP or LVAD if in place. Prepare patient for coronary reperfusion procedures.

cluding headache, altered level of consciousness, nausea, vomiting, and paralysis.

• Avoid giving I.M. injections and obtaining a blood sample for arterial blood gas (ABG) analysis for 24 hours after thrombolytic therapy is discontinued.

• Administer anticoagulant therapy, as prescribed.

Identifying serious complications

Serious, sometimes fatal complications can follow a myocardial infarction (MI). Prevention of complications and early detection of signs and symptoms of complications are essential to afford the MI patient an optimal chance for recovery. Some common complications are discussed in the chart below.

Complication	MI-Related Causes	Assessment Findings
Arrhythmias	• Ischemia • Metabolic imbalances • Hypoxemia • Autonomic nervous system influences (such as bradycardia-induced vagal reflex) • Electrolyte imbalances (including hypokalemia and hypomagnesemia) • Hemodynamic abnormalities • Cardiac glycoside therapy • Ventricular rupture	• Abnormal ECG rhythm • Decreased or elevated electrolyte and metabolic levels • Abnormal cardiac index or pulmonary artery wedge pressure (PAWP) • Hypotension
Cardiogenic shock	• Loss of at least 40% of left ventricular function • Progressive hemodynamic deterioration (falling cardiac output causes hypotension, which triggers compensatory mechanisms; if compensatory mechanisms fail to maintain arterial blood pressure or perfusion of vital organs, blood pressure falls below a critical level, resulting in ischemia of all organs)	• Decreased cardiac output, increased pulmonary artery systolic and diastolic pressures, decreased cardiac index, increased systemic vascular resistance (SVR), and increased PAWP • Decreased level of consciousness • Decreased urine output • Neck vein distention
Congestive heart failure and pulmonary edema	• Left ventricular failure • Inability to expel blood adequately at the end of systole, resulting in increased ventricular volume and pressure • Escape of fluid into the interstitial spaces and alveoli, resulting in impaired gas exchange	• Venous congestion and cardiomegaly on chest X-ray • Increased pulmonary artery systolic and diastolic pressures, PAWP, central venous pressure, and SVR

Identifying serious complications *(continued)*

Complication	MI-Related Causes	Assessment Findings
Ventricular septal defect or rupture	• Necrosis of the interventricular septum from extensive coronary artery disease, which may lead to a rupture of the septal wall and shunting of blood from the left ventricle to the right ventricle, resulting in reduced ventricular output and increased pulmonary congestion	• Harsh, holosystolic (heard throughout systole) murmur and thrill on auscultation • Increased pulmonary artery pressure (PAP) and PAWP, as well as increased oxygen saturation of the right ventricle and pulmonary artery
Ventricular aneurysm and rupture	• Commonly associated with transmural infarction (involves the anterior or apical wall in 80% of cases)	• Increased PAP and PAWP • Increased oxygen saturation of right ventricle and pulmonary artery • With ventricular aneurysm: possible ventricular arrhythmias, chronic congestive heart failure, and release of mural thrombi into the systemic circulation • With ventricular rupture: cardiac tamponade and electromechanical dissociation and a sudden decrease in cardiac output following the rupture
Pericarditis and Dressler's syndrome	• Autoimmune reaction resulting in inflammation of the pericardium precipitated by the occurrence of an MI (typically within 1 week after an MI)	• Chest pain that commonly radiates to the left shoulder and becomes aggravated with deep inspiration (pain may subside when the patient sits and leans forward) • Possible pericardial friction rub upon auscultation

Arrhythmia control

Arrhythmias typically occur during an MI as a result of altered electrical conduction of the myocardium secondary to injury and necrosis of the myocardial tissue. Lidocaine commonly is prescribed for ventricular ar-

MAJOR DRUGS

Thrombolytics used in myocardial infarction

Different thrombolytics are used with varying degrees of success in the treatment of MI. The following table provides the usual adult dosages for these agents when used for lysis of thrombi, as well as the adverse drug reactions that may occur. This table can be used to individualize patient care when administering thrombolytic therapy.

Thrombolytic Agent	Dosage	Adverse Drug Reactions
Streptokinase (Kabikinase, Streptase)	• Loading dose of 20,000 IU via coronary catheter infusion followed by a maintenance dosage of 2,000 IU/minute for 60 minutes for a total infusion of 140,000 units. • Alternatively, 1.5 million IU I.V. infused over 60 minutes.	• *Blood*—bleeding, low hematocrit • *Cardiovascular (CV)*—transient increase or decrease in blood pressure • *EENT*—periorbital edema • *Local*—phlebitis at injection site • *Other*—hypersensitivity, fever, anaphylaxis, musculoskeletal pain, minor breathing difficulty, bronchospasms, angioneurotic edema
Alteplase [tissue plasminogen activator, recombinant; t-PA] (Activase)	• 100 mg I.V. infused over 3 hours as follows: 60 mg in the first hour, of which 6 to 10 mg is given as a bolus over the first 1 to 2 minutes; then 20 mg/hour for 2 hours. • For adults (who weigh less than 143 lb [65 kg]), 1.25 mg/kg in a similar fashion (60% in the first hour, with 10% as a bolus; then 20% of the total dose per hour for 2 hours).	• *Blood*—severe, spontaneous bleeding (cerebral, retroperitoneal, genitourinary, or GI) • *Central nervous system (CNS)*—cerebral hemorrhage, fever • *CV*—hypotension, arrhythmias • *GI*—nausea, vomiting • *Local*—bleeding at injection site • *Other*—hypersensitivity, urticaria
Urokinase (Abbokinase, Win-Kinase)	• A bolus dose of heparin ranging from 2,500 to 10,000 IU, then infuse 6,000 IU/minute into the occluded artery for up to 2 hours.	• *Blood*—bleeding, low hematocrit • *Local*—phlebitis at injection site • *Other*—hypersensitivity (not as common as in strep- *(continued)*

Thrombolytics used in myocardial infarction *(continued)*

Thrombolytic Agent	Dosage	Adverse Drug reactions
Urokinase *(continued)*	• Average total dose is 500,000 IU.	tokinase use), musculoskeletal pain bronchospasm, anaphylaxis
Anistreplase [anisoylated plasminogen-streptokinase activator complex; APSAC] (Eminase)	• 30 units I.V. over 2 to 5 minutes by direct injection.	• *Blood*—bleeding, eosinophilia • *CNS*—intracranial hemorrhage • *CV*—arrhythmias, electrical conduction disorders, hypotension • *EENT*—hemoptysis, gum or mouth hemorrhage • *GI*—bleeding • *GU*—hematuria • *Skin*—hematomas, urticaria, itching, flushing, purpuric rash (after 2 weeks of therapy) • *Local*—bleeding at injection site • *Other*—anaphylaxis (rare)

rhythmias. Other agents that may be given include procainamide, quinidine, bretylium, and disopyramide. If bradycardia or heart block develops, I.V. atropine may be administered or a temporary pacemaker may be inserted. (For details on arrhythmias and current treatment methods, see the entry on "Arrhythmias.")

Research indicates that magnesium sulfate may be beneficial for MI patients during the early treatment stages, when serum levels have been demonstrated to be low. Traditionally, magnesium sulfate has proved to be an effective agent in arrhythmia control, coronary artery vasodilation, and platelet inhibition. More and more hospitals are including magnesium sulfate in their protocols, while researchers continue to investigate the clinical effectiveness and appropriate dosage in treating MI.

The following nursing interventions for arrhythmia control should be incorporated into the plan of care:
• Administer antiarrhythmic therapy, as prescribed.
• Perform continuous ECG monitoring; frequently assess cardiac rhythm strips for changes.
• Assess vital signs frequently, reporting any abnormal findings.
• Monitor serum electrolyte levels, because arrhythmias can result from potassium or magnesium imbalances.

Cardiac function regulation

Because myocardial tissue necrosis may decrease actual cardiac function, interventions are geared toward decreasing the cardiac workload and improving cardiac function.

Typically, morphine is prescribed to alleviate or reduce pain and to decrease preload and myocardial oxygen consumption. Nitroglycerin, calcium channel blockers, or isosorbide dinitrate may be administered to relieve pain (by redistributing blood to the ischemic area of the myocardium), to increase the cardiac output, and to reduce cardiac workload. A positive inotropic agent may be administered to increase contractility or blood pressure. Also, oxygen typically is administered.

Pulmonary artery catheterization may be performed to detect left or right ventricular failure and to monitor the patient's response to treatment. An intra-aortic balloon pump or a left ventricular assist device may be used to decrease the cardiac workload or to prevent cardiogenic shock.

The following nursing interventions should be incorporated into the plan of care to help improve cardiac function:
• Frequently monitor and record ECG readings, blood pressure, temperature, and heart and breath sounds; notify the physician if abnormalities occur.
• Obtain baseline ABG and mixed venous oxygenation values, as prescribed.
• Assess for pain, and administer analgesics as prescribed. Record the severity and duration of the pain.

Avoid I.M. injections because drug absorption is unpredictable and the ensuing muscle damage will increase creatine kinase and serum lactate dehydrogenase levels.
• Monitor vital signs when new cardiac medications are added to the drug regimen.
• Assess and document pulmonary artery pressure, pulmonary artery wedge pressure, cardiac output, and systemic vascular resistance, as prescribed, if a pulmonary artery catheter is in place.
• Administer oxygen, as prescribed.
• Administer a stool softener as prescribed, and discourage the use of Valsalva's maneuver.
• Provide an atmosphere that is conducive to rest.
• If chest pain occurs, obtain an ECG reading and blood pressure and pulmonary artery catheter measurements; compare these findings to baseline values. Administer I.V. nitroglycerin, as prescribed.
• Assess for crackles, cough, tachypnea, and edema, which may indicate impending left ventricular failure.
• If an intra-aortic balloon pump is in place, frequently monitor for clinical effectiveness (indicated by increased cardiac output, increased cardiac index, improved ECG changes, and stable blood pressure), ECG changes, and altered vital signs. Also monitor the circulation of lower extremities for diminished pulses, color changes, and decreased sensation or temperature. Keep the patient's legs straight and the head of the bed elevated at no more than 30 degrees. Notify the physician immediately if blood appears in the oversheath of the balloon catheter.

Coronary artery revascularization

On the basis of the patient's symptoms and response to medical treatment, the physician may perform other invasive procedures, such as percutaneous transluminal coronary angioplasty, coronary atherectomy, or coronary artery bypass graft. (For additional information on these procedures, see the entry on "Angina.")

The following nursing interventions should be incorporated into the plan of care:

- Prepare the patient and family for the procedure according to institutional policy.
- Provide appropriate information and offer emotional support.

Prognosis

Current technological advances and improved treatment methods have decreased the MI mortality rate to approximately 25%. As noted, most deaths occur in the first hour after the onset of signs and symptoms; almost half of all MI victims delay seeking help when symptoms first occur. Other factors that can affect a patient's chances for recovery from an MI include:

- the infarction size and location
- complications following the MI
- preexisting illnesses, such as cardiovascular conditions, a previous MI, respiratory disorders, or diabetes mellitus
- age over 80.

Discharge planning

Discharge planning should begin once the patient's cardiovascular status has been stabilized. The following steps should be incorporated into the plan of care to ensure an uneventful discharge:

- Evaluate the patient's support system. Initiate a social services consultation if needed.
- Review the expected recovery period and post-MI activity restrictions with the patient and family. Provide information or initiate a consultation for a cardiac rehabilitation exercise program.
- Provide guidelines for resuming sexual activity.
- Review postdischarge medications, including their actions, dosages, and possible side effects.
- Review what to do if additional signs and symptoms of cardiac problems appear. Instruct the family on how to activate their local emergency medical service.
- Encourage the family to enroll in a cardiopulmonary resuscitation certification class.

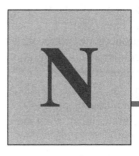

Near drowning

Near drowning, survival for more than 24 hours after submersion in a fluid, can occur from exposure to either salt water or fresh water. In either case, if death ensues after this 24-hour period, usually as a result of pulmonary edema, the incident is considered secondary drowning. Most drowning incidents occur in fresh water. The highest rates of drowning are among preschoolers (commonly as a result of bathtub or swimming pool accidents) and young men between ages 15 and 24 (in most cases, as a result of risk-taking behaviors and alcohol consumption during water activities).

Pathophysiology

Submersion in fluid typically results in initial panic, struggling, and breath holding. This may be followed by swallowing large quantities of water, vomiting, and aspiration. After loss of consciousness, fluid passively enters the lungs. Hypoxemia, the primary pathological process in drowning, may result from severe laryngospasm or aspiration. With laryngospasm, aspiration is prevented and the period of hypoxemia is limited to the time of immersion and inadequate ventilation. With aspiration, the hypoxemia continues even after ventilation is established.

Several factors must be considered when describing the pathophysiological events that occur in a near drowning. These include aspiration, type of water, water temperature, and presence of contaminants. Aspiration of any fluid (fresh water, salt water, or vomitus) causes an inflammatory response in the alveolar capillary membrane that leads to an outpouring of protein-rich exudate. This causes an osmotic gradient, drawing more fluid into the alveoli and resulting in pulmonary edema.

Freshwater near drowning

The hypotonicity of fresh water injures the type II pneumocytes, which, at least temporarily, do not produce surfactant. This alters the alveolar surface tension and leads to focal areas of atelectasis. Perfusion of these atelectatic areas increases intrapulmonary shunting and hypoxic pulmonary vasoconstriction. Loss of surfactant and disruption of alveolar cells can cause pulmonary capillaries to leak, leading to pulmonary edema. Systemic hypoxemia causes reflex pulmonary arterial vasoconstriction, myocardial depression, and an alteration of pulmonary capillary permeability. Therefore, freshwater aspiration results in decreased compliance, increased intrapulmonary shunting, pulmonary hypertension, and ventilation-perfusion mismatch.

Saltwater near drowning

The hypertonicity of salt water causes a temporary osmotic pressure gradient, pulling water and protein-rich plasma into the alveoli and diluting surfactant. The result is alveolar flooding and often diffuse pulmonary edema. The perfusion of fluid-filled alveoli causes a ventilation-perfusion mismatch. Regional hypoxia promotes pulmonary vasoconstriction with increased pulmonary vascular pressures, increased ventilation-perfusion mismatch, decreased lung compliance, and decreased functional residual capacity.

Outcome and length of recovery are not determined by the type or temperature of the fluid, but by the length and severity of hypoxemia. However, aspiration of sea water has a graver prognosis than aspiration of fresh water. Saltwater aspiration causes a greater decrease in arterial oxygen content and results in less improvement in partial oxygen pressure with ventilation. Submersion in salt water, rivers, and lakes has a lower survival rate because of the difficulty in finding the victim, resulting in longer periods of hypoxemia.

Near drowning consequences

Aspiration of contaminants may occur in either freshwater or saltwater near drowning. The victim may aspirate chlorine, mud, algae, weeds, and other foreign material. Saltwater aspiration is considered more dangerous because salt water contains more types of disease-causing bacteria. These contaminants may lead to obstruction, aspiration pneumonia, and pulmonary fibrosis. Aspiration of gastric contents often occurs and contributes to aspiration pneumonia.

A protective effect may be seen in cold water submersion (exposure to temperatures 21° C). Rapid body cooling results in cardiac arrest and decreased tissue oxygen demand. The protective effect is most pronounced in children and may be due to the large ratio of body surface area to mass. Because water rapidly conducts heat away from the body, even persons who drown in warm water may suffer from hypothermia. (See *Physiologic changes in near drowning,* page 448, for the pathways involved.)

All of the consequences of near drowning, with the exception of aspiration pneumonia, are the result of hypoxemia and acidosis:
• Respiratory acidosis results from alveolar hypoventilation, which may be complicated by gastric distention and upper-airway obstruction.
• Metabolic acidosis results from hypoxemia and lactic acid production during the struggle before the victim loses consciousness.
• Cardiac arrest may result from prolonged hypoxemia and acidosis. Circulating catecholamines, released during struggling in the initial drowning phase, increase

Physiologic changes in near drowning

This diagram shows the primary cellular alterations that occur during near drowning. Separate pathways are shown for saltwater and freshwater incidents. Hypothermia presents a separate pathway that may preserve neurologic function by decreasing metabolic rate. All pathways lead to diffuse pulmonary edema.

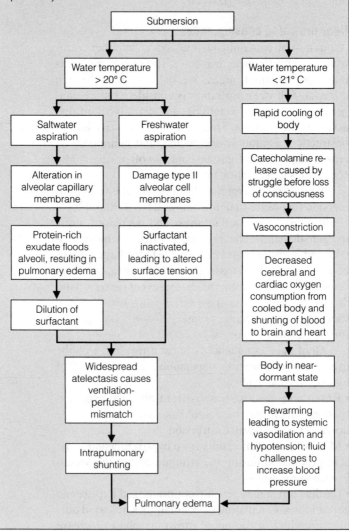

the workload of the hypoxic heart, resulting in an increased oxygen supply-demand deficit, enhancing the possibility of cardiac arrest. After successful resuscitation, supraventricular tachycardias are the most common arrhythmias.

• Anoxic brain damage may occur if the hypoxemia and decreased cardiac output are prolonged. Cerebral hypoxia results in loss of the blood-brain barrier and cerebral edema. Loss of the blood-brain barrier may lead to pathologic bacteria invading cerebral tissue, resulting in abscesses that may not be apparent for several months.

• Renal failure may occur several days after the event because of hypoxia, decreased perfusion, and hemolysis. Acute tubular necrosis secondary to hypoperfusion and hypoxia is the most common form of acute renal failure after a near drowning incident.

• Disseminated intravascular coagulation, which rarely occurs, is thought to be secondary to acidosis, hypotension, and hypoxemia.

• Electrolyte imbalances are rare because of the small amount of fluid aspirated. Acidosis may cause a falsely elevated serum potassium level. When a large amount of salt water is aspirated, hypermagnesemia may occur. The aspirated fluid, which contains levels of magnesium higher than serum plasma, will be absorbed into the circulation and elevate magnesium levels.

• Ischemia and necrosis of the bowel may result from prolonged periods of hypoxemia and hypotension secondary to shunting of blood to more vital areas.

• Pneumonia may result from aspiration of fresh or salt water, or vomitus. Aspiration pneumonia is treated with the appropriate antibiotic after cultures are obtained. Prophylactic antibiotic treatment rarely is given, except in the case of submersion in hot tubs, because of the frequency of *Pseudomonas* species in that environment.

Clinical assessment

Management of near drowning victims requires hospitalization for observation for at least 24 hours for all but the most insignificant submersions. The clinical presentation depends on the degree and duration of the hypoxemia, with victims varying from alert and oriented to those requiring cardiopulmonary support. Frequent focused assessments are conducted on the pulmonary, cardiovascular, and neurologic systems.

History

Several factors affect the prognosis of the near drowning victim and should be obtained during the nursing history:

- length of time submerged
- temperature of the fluid
- associated injuries (especially head and neck)
- aspiration of fluid and the type of fluid aspirated (fresh water versus salt water)
- promptness and aggressiveness of resuscitation.

Physical findings

Any or all of the following may be observed during the physical assessment:

- cough, pleuritic pain; pink, frothy sputum
- tachypnea, or shallow, gasping respirations
- shortness of breath, use of accessory muscles for respiration
- abnormal lung sounds (crackles, rhonchi, wheezes)
- chest pain, arrhythmias (Supraventricular tachycardias are the most common arrhythmias in patients who never have a cardiac arrest and patients resuscitated after a cardiac arrest. Sinus bradycardia, atrial fibrillation, asystole, and ventricular fibrillation may also occur depending upon the degree of hypothermia.)
- hypotension
- cyanosis or pallor
- decreased peripheral tissue perfusion
- decreased level of consciousness (LOC) (Patients may be conscious and alert, unconscious and unresponsive, or at any point in between these extremes.)
- hyporeflexia, seizures, or coma
- vomiting.

Diagnosis

Diagnostic tests help determine the degree of hypoxemia and monitor the success of treatment. The most useful laboratory tests indicate oxygenation status. A list of the diagnostic tests commonly performed can be found in *Confirming near drowning,* page 452.

Treatment and care

Initial treatment of near drowning victims follows established basic life-support measures: ensure airway, breathing, and circulation. The goal is to achieve optimal neurologic function by reversal of hypoxemia and acidosis, promotion of tissue perfusion, and early detection of complications.

Reversing hypoxemia and acidosis

Airway management depends on LOC, patency of airway, presence of secretions, aspiration, and apnea. Oxygen is supplied at the highest level possible until arterial blood gas results are obtained. Victims entering the emergency department with any neurologic dysfunction may need to be intubated to protect the airway and deliver maximum oxygenation. Mechanical ventilation with positive end-expiratory pressure may be required to keep the PaO_2 greater than 60 mm Hg, with a fraction of inspired oxygen of 0.50 or less. According to Fiser (1993), the adult respiratory distress syndrome associated with near drowning, which is not complicated by pneumonia, usually resolves within 3 to 4 days, and mechanical ventilator support can often be terminated at that time. Long-term pulmonary effects are uncommon. The following nursing interventions should be incorporated into the plan of care to reverse hypoxemia and acidosis:

• Maintain the airway with positioning, oral or nasal airways, or endotracheal intubation.
• Administer the prescribed amount of oxygen.
• Maintain prescribed ventilator settings.
• Assess respiratory rate and effort and monitor oxygen saturation of arterial blood via pulse oximetry.

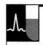

DIAGNOSTIC TESTS

Confirming near drowning

Some of the most common tests used to determine the extent of effects of a near drowning incident are outlined below.

Arterial blood gas (ABG) studies

ABG studies are performed to determine the oxygen status and acid-base balance disturbances caused by a respiratory or metabolic disorder. Hypoxemia and combined respiratory and metabolic acidosis are common in near drowning. Normal values are hydrogen ion concentration (pH), 7.35 to 7.45; $PaCO_2$, 35 to 45 mm Hg; PaO_2, 80 to 100 mm Hg; SaO_2 95%; HCO_3, 24 to 28 mEq/liter; base excess +2 to –2 mEq/liter.

Chest X-rays

Chest radiographs are important in the evaluation of the pulmonary system. They can reveal inflammation, fluid accumulation, excess air accumulation, fractures, and foreign objects. Pulmonary infiltrates indicating pulmonary edema are common findings.

Complete blood cell count

Usually, no change in red blood cell (RBC) values occur in a near drowning victim. However, hemolysis of RBCs is common if the victim aspirates large quantities of fluid, which are rapidly absorbed into circulation. Hypotonic fluid will cause cell enlargement and cell membrane disruption. This will result in decreased tissue oxygenation. Elevated white blood cell (WBC) value secondary to alveolar inflammation is common and not an indicator of infection during the first 24 hours. Decreased WBCs may be observed in the hypothermic near drowning victim. Normal RBC values vary with age and sex: children, 3.9 to 4.2 million/mm^3; adult men, 4.6 to 6.2 million/mm^3; adult women, 4.2 to 5.4 million/mm^3. Normal WBC count ranges from 4.1 to 10.9×10^9/liter.

Potassium

In near drowning victims, hyperkalemia may result from acidosis or hemolysis of RBCs. Normal values in children are 3.4 to 4.7 mEq/liter; in adults, 3.5 to 5.0 mEq/liter.

Coagulation studies

Hypothermia, hypoxemia, or hypotension can initiate the coagulation cascade and cause disseminated intravascular coagulation in which microthrombi are formed throughout the body. This exhausts the coagulation and clot-dissolving factors. Normal values: platelets, 150,000 to 400,000/mm^3; prothrombin time, 12 to 14 seconds; activated partial thromboplastin time, within 5 seconds of the control; fibrinogen degradation products, < 10 µg/ml.

• Monitor for signs of worsening hypoxemia: use of accessory muscles, stridor, nasal flaring, grunting, retractions, restlessness, tachypnea, tachycardia, and cyanosis.
• Monitor serial arterial blood gases for hypoxemia, hypercapnia, and acidosis.

• Monitor serial chest X-rays for changes in pulmonary infiltrates, pneumothorax, and position of endotracheal tube.

• Administer aggressive pulmonary hygiene: positioning, instruction in deep breathing and coughing exercises, suctioning, and postural drainage.

Promoting neurologic perfusion

Aggressive treatment regimens are instituted to control cerebral edema, improve cerebral perfusion pressures, and lower cerebral oxygen demand. These measures to control intracranial pressure (ICP) have included barbiturate comas, paralysis, controlled hyperventilation, hypothermia, diuretic and steroid use, and continuous ICP monitoring. Because these measures have not appreciably improved outcome, a trend is seen toward less dramatic methods to decrease ICP.

The following nursing interventions to promote neurologic perfusion should be incorporated into the plan of care:

• Assess neurologic status each hour for the first 24 hours.

• Promote venous drainage: elevate head 30 degrees, maintain head alignment and neutral head position.

• Observe for signs and symptoms of increased ICP: decreasing LOC, irritability, nausea or vomiting, posturing, altered pupil response, altered motor response, changes in respiratory pattern, disconjugate gaze.

• Observe for impending brain stem herniation: bradycardia, hypertension, widening pulse pressure, alteration in respiratory rate and pattern.

• Provide hyperventilation and osmotic diuresis for increased ICP as prescribed.

• Provide sedation or paralysis as needed to reduce metabolic oxygen consumption.

• Observe for signs and symptoms of the syndrome of inappropriate secretion of antidiuretic hormone or diabetes insipidus: monitor specific gravity every 2 hours, hourly output, and serum and urine osmolality and sodium.

Prevention of complications

The hypoxemia in near drowning affects all body systems. Aggressive treatment often is successful in the return of a spontaneous rhythm and adequate cardiac output. Because of the frequent occurrence of pulmonary edema, patients with continued decreased cardiac output may be monitored with a pulmonary artery catheter to determine fluid resuscitation versus vasopressor therapy. Close monitoring of renal status is required to identify signs of acute tubular necrosis. Cultures of respiratory secretions may be ordered to rule out infection. If necessary, antibiotic therapy may be ordered to combat infection. In addition, measures to rewarm the patient are instituted if required. Removal of wet clothing is the primary method to prevent further heat loss. Core rewarming measures also may be instituted to allow the heart to meet the metabolic demands of the dilating peripheral capillary beds. Such measures include warm I.V. fluids, warm air supply, warm lavage of body cavities, and cardiopulmonary bypass.

The following nursing interventions to prevent, identify, or treat complications should be incorporated into the plan of care:

• Continuously monitor core body temperature.

• Assess heart rate and rhythm and blood pressure every hour.

• Monitor for signs and symptoms of decreased cardiac output and cardiac index: tachycardia, hypotension, decreased peripheral pulses, prolonged capillary refill, color of nailbed or mucous membranes, decreased urine output (monitor hourly), decreased mentation, and absent bowel sounds.

• Continuously monitor ECG for early detection and treatment of arrhythmias.

• Decrease energy expenditure and metabolic demands: provide adequate rest periods, promote a calm environment, and maintain normal temperature.

• Monitor serial electrolytes, glucose, blood urea nitrogen, and creatinine levels to prevent arrhythmias.

• Administer paralytic agents and sedatives to decrease neuromuscular activity and decrease oxygen demands.
• Assess urine for clarity, color, blood, protein, ketones, glucose, hydrogen ion concentration (pH), and specific gravity every 2 to 4 hours.
• Take daily weight.
• Assess respiratory secretions: color, odor, amount, and consistency. Obtain cultures as needed.
• Monitor serial white blood cell count and differential.
• Gradually rewarm the patient (1° C/hour) after sufficient rewarming has occurred to sustain a cardiac output.

Prognosis

The prognosis of the near drowning victim depends on the duration of immersion and degree of cerebral anoxia. The primary cause of death and disability is from cerebral hypoxia. A relative "all or none" effect has been noted, with 85% of victims having little or no neurologic dysfunction and the remaining 15% having profound neurologic dysfunction. Long-term neurologic effects range from vegetative state to impaired verbal skills. Neurologic function at the scene, upon entering the emergency department, and at admission to the intensive care unit is not a reliable indicator of outcome. Neurologic examinations at 24 hours may be the best indicator of good outcome. Comatose near drowning victims who have spontaneous purposeful movements at 24 hours after the event and have normal brain stem functioning have been found to have minimal or no neurological deficit.

Good prognostic signs are listed below:
• return of spontaneous ventilatory efforts in the field with or without cardiopulmonary resuscitation
• cardiopulmonary resuscitation < 10 minutes
• submersion time < 5 minutes
• initial arterial blood gas pH > 7.10
• age over 3 years
• no aspiration.

Discharge planning

Discharge planning should begin once the patient's pulmonary status has stabilized and includes the following:

• Review preventable risk factors. This includes teaching about leaving young children to supervise bathing of toddlers, leaving children unattended around water of any source, the need for fencing around swimming pools, and training in cardiopulmonary resuscitation for parents and swimming pool owners. Adolescents and adults need reinforcement of the dangers of alcohol and water activities.

• Evaluate the support system. Because of the traumatic nature of the near drowning event, the patient may have recurrent nightmares and may require continued support. Parents of child survivors of near drowning may also require additional support because of continued feelings of guilt.

• Review the expected recovery period. The degree of neurologic impairment determines the recovery period, which may vary from a few hours to months or years.

• For a patient returning home after only a 24-hour observation period, review signs and symptoms to consult a health care provider: shortness of breath, increased sputum production, change in sputum color, or changes in LOC or gait. Any of these changes occurring within 2 days after discharge may indicate a delayed complication of the near drowning event.

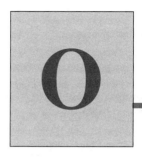

Organ transplantation

Since the first kidney transplant in 1954, the number of organ transplantation procedures has steadily increased and yielded successful results for those with end-stage disease, largely because of better diagnosis and treatment of complications. Many factors have contributed to better graft survival, including refined criteria for recipient and donor selection, development of tissue biopsy as a diagnostic tool, better organ preservation, advances in immunosuppressive therapy, definitive treatment of immunosuppressive complications, and advances in the education of health care personnel caring for transplant patients.

Pathophysiology

Several organs, including the heart, lungs, liver, and kidneys, may undergo transplantation, depending on the patient's physical condition and need (see *Indications for organ transplantation,* pages 458 and 459).

A transplanted organ is considered foreign (nonself) to a normal host recipient. To enable a transplanted organ to survive in a recipient, combinations of therapies have been developed to deceive the normal immune responses. These alterations include masquerading the transplanted organ as self, partially or selectively blinding the immune system so that it does not recognize the transplanted organ

Indications for organ transplantation

The following chart lists potential organ transplantations as well as related diseases and contraindications to transplantation.

Type of Transplantation	Associated Disease	Contraindications to Transplantation
Heart	End-stage heart disease: • Coronary artery disease (ischemic heart disease) • Dilated congestive cardiomyopathy • Valvular heart disease • Congenital heart disease • Life-threatening recurrent arrhythmia	• Active infection • Fixed pulmonary hypertension • Recent pulmonary infection • Insulin-dependent diabetes mellitus • Peripheral vascular disease • Cerebrovascular disease • Chronic pulmonary disease • Cancer
Lung (single or double)	Single: • Idiopathic interstitial pulmonary fibrosis • Sarcoidosis • Primary pulmonary hypertension • Emphysema Double: • Cystic fibrosis • Alpha$_1$-antitrypsin deficiency • Eosinophilic granuloma	• Steroid dependency • Systemic illness • Cardiac insufficiency • Evidence of right ventricular failure • Mechanical ventilator dependence
Heart-lung	• Elevated pulmonary vascular resistance • Eisenmenger's syndrome • Primary pulmonary hypertension	Heart-lung transplantation usually is not chosen because only one patient benefits from the procedure. However, contraindications include: • Systemic disease • Active infection • Irreversible renal or hepatic failure
Liver	• Cholestatic diseases (primary biliary cirrhosis or sclerosing cholangitis, biliary atresia, familial cholestatic syndromes) • Hepatocellular diseases (chronic viral-induced	• Hepatic cancer

Indications for organ transplantation *(continued)*

Type of Transplantation	Associated Disease	Contraindications to Transplantation
Liver *(continued)*	liver disease, chronic drug-induced liver disease, alcoholic liver disease, idiopathic autoimmune liver disease) • Vascular diseases (Budd-Chiari syndrome, veno-occlusive diseases) • Fulminant hepatic failure (viral hepatitis, mushroom poisoning, drug-induced liver disease, metabolic liver diseases)	
Kidney	• End-stage kidney disease in those requiring dialysis	• Severe debilitation • Diabetes without a concurrent pancreas transplant

as foreign, and suppressing the immune response responsible for recognizing nonself.

Once an allograft is recognized as nonself, it can be assaulted or rejected in two ways: cellular rejection or humoral rejection. Cellular rejection is the production of allograft-specific killer T cells. The Class II allograft antigens incite anti-allograft T helper cells to promote the expansion of a donor-specific population of cytotoxic T cells and recruit macrophages into the area of the allograft by releasing various cytokines. The macrophages release interleukin (IL-1), which further fuels the reaction by enhancing T-cell production of IL-2. The cytotoxic T cells then attack allograft antigens and damage the organ.

Humoral rejection, allograft destruction that results from specifically directed antibodies, occurs in two ways. In the first mechanism, a recipient's preformed antibodies (arising from previous blood transfusions or pregnancy) may cross-react with alloantibodies on the endothelium of the new organ. This process causes activation of the complement system and attracts highly destructive neutrophils to the area. It is an example of hyperacute rejection and results in organ death.

In the second mechanism, humoral rejection occurs when allograft-specific antibodies arise after transplantation. These antibodies mediate graft destruction by infiltrating the organ, activating complement, and attracting tissue-destroying neutrophils to the site. Allospecific antibodies also coat allograft cells and make them attractive targets for killer macrophages and lymphocytes. (See *Types of organ transplant rejection,* page 461, for a review.)

Clinical assessment

A thorough understanding of the patient's full medical history, including past surgeries, is necessary during the evaluation process. All potential candidates for transplantation require extensive screening to optimize a donor-recipient match. Generally, pretransplant screening for all transplants should include:

- ABO blood typing
- hepatitis/human immunodeficiency screen
- cytomegalovirus screen
- chemistry and hematology evaluation
- nutritional evaluation
- psychological evaluation.

Because infection is the leading cause of death following transplantation, bacterial infections must be identified and treated aggressively prior to surgery. (For further information about specific screening tests, see *Screening tests for transplantation procedures,* page 462.)

Diagnosis

Patients who require organ transplantation have already undergone a multitude of tests to determine organ function (for more information on end-organ heart disease, lung disease, liver disease, and kidney disease and related diagnostic tests, see the entries on Cardiomyopa-

Types of organ transplant rejection

This chart represents the types of rejections that may occur after organ transplantation as well as the immune system basis for rejection and the potential outcome.

Type of Rejection	Basis for Rejection	Potential Outcome
Hyperacute (white graft rejection) • A rare type of rejection that occurs within minutes to hours after transplantation • May be prevented by screening the potential recipient's blood group and HLA antigens prior to transplantation	• Recipient has preformed cytotoxic antibodies that can react against antigens in the transplanted organ; the antibodies activate the complement system	• Decreased organ perfusion • Ischemic and nonfunctional graft
Acute • Occurs weeks to months after transplantation • Expected to occur 6 to 8 times	• Class I and II HLA antigens in the transplanted organ are recognized as foreign and the recipient activates a cellular immune response • The accumulation of graft-specific cytotoxic T lymphocytes is the chief basis of acute rejection	• Common cause of death or organ loss in the first year • Incidence is reduced over time
Chronic • Occurs months or years after transplantation	• Humoral immune response against the transplanted tissue in which sensitized B cells produce antibodies that activate complement and cause platelet aggregates at the site of the reaction; this leads to accumulation of fibrin on the endothelium and, ultimately, to stenosis and occlusion of the organ vessels	• Gradual deterioration of function of transplanted organ over time • Lack of blood supply to the organ leads to ischemia and eventual necrosis

thy, Hepatic failure, Respiratory failure, and Renal failure).

The major postoperative concern for the organ transplant recipient is the prompt identification of re-

Screening tests for transplantation procedures

Because of the nature of the various transplantation procedures, certain screening tests must be performed preoperatively to optimize the donor-recipient match.

Transplantation Procedure	Screening Tests
Heart transplantation	• Echocardiography • Chest X-ray (to assess lung function and potential complications)
Lung transplantation	• Ventilation/perfusion scan • Pulmonary angiography • Pulmonary function tests • Exercise capacity
Heart-lung transplantation	• Pulmonary function tests • Sizing of donor organs (the donor-recipient chest circumference must be within 3 inches)
Liver transplantation	• Liver function tests • Ultrasound • CT scan and MRI (to evaluate the anatomy of the liver and surrounding structures) • Weight (the donor's weight should not exceed the recipient's by more than 10 kg or the variance in weights should not exceed 20%)
Kidney transplantation	• Dialysis to optimize fluid, electrolyte, and acid-base status • Preoperative monitoring with a pulmonary artery catheter (if patient has preexisting disease) • Culture and cell count of the peritoneal fluid (if patient is managed with peritoneal dialysis)

jection, which is essential to decrease morbidity and mortality. Although organ failure is a diagnostic finding, it is a very late sign. Biopsy is the best method for identifying rejection of solid organs (see *Confirming organ rejection,* page 463).

Treatment and care

The primary medical and nursing goals for postoperative organ transplant patients are to promptly identify

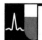

Confirming organ rejection

Several diagnostic procedures are typically performed to help confirm acute organ rejection. Signs and symptoms usually draw attention to the need for diagnostic testing.

Transplanted Organ	Diagnostic Test (Key Finding)	Signs and Symptoms
Heart	• Endomyocardial biopsy • Measurement of hemodynamic pressures (increased pulmonary artery wedge pressure) • Electrocardiogram (arrhythmias) • Echocardiogram • Chest X-ray (infiltrates)	Fatigue, decreased blood pressure, jugular venous distention, S_3 heart sound, fluid retention, tachycardia, peripheral edema, crackles, shortness of breath, decreased urine output, malaise, arrhythmias, cardiogenic shock
Lung	• Endobronchial biopsy • Pulmonary function tests (decreased FEF 25%-75%, decreased FEV_1) • Arterial blood gas levels (increased $PaCO_2$, decreased PaO_2) • Complete blood count (increased WBC count) • Chest X-ray (infiltrates)	Dyspnea, sputum changes, fever, tachycardia, crackles, tachypnea, cough
Liver	• Liver biopsy • Liver function tests, including bilirubin, AST, and ALT (elevated levels)	Malaise, fever, abdominal discomfort (right lower quadrant or flank pain), colorless bile, jaundice, increased PTT, elevated bilirubin, serum transaminase, and alkaline phosphatase levels
Kidney	• Renal biopsy • Elevated BUN and creatinine levels • Elevated fibrin split products	Oliguria, hypertension, graft tenderness, fever

and treat rejection and infection. Common treatments include the use of immunosuppressive agents and infection-control procedures, as outlined below. Also discussed in this section are organ-specific treatment measures for the various types of transplant procedures.

Immunosuppressive therapy

Immunosuppressive medications are used for long- and short-term prevention and treatment of transplant rejection. Immunosuppression may begin before surgery and continue throughout the life of the organ. These therapies are designed to decrease the incidence of acute rejection and are effective in treating acute or chronic rejection (see *Immunosuppressant medications,* pages 466 and 467).

Azathioprine is used as part of triple therapy including azathioprine, cyclosporine, and corticosteroids. Its maximal effect is seen when administered within 24 hours after transplantation, when T cells have been activated and are beginning to produce new DNA. Maintenance dosage is adjusted according to the patient's white blood cell (WBC) count. The dose should be titrated to maintain the WBC count between 4,000 and 5,000 mm^3. If the WBC count drops below 4,000 mm^3, the dose may be lowered or discontinued.

Corticosteroids affect both humoral and cell-mediated immunity. At high doses, corticosteroids interfere with the function of the lymphocytic cell membrane. Thus, lymphocytes are no longer attracted to the graft and those lymphocytes that have already accumulated are rendered ineffective. The side effects of corticosteroids warrant reduction of the dose to every other day or complete or temporary withdrawal. Many of the side effects of steroids can be averted by using the lowest effective antirejection dose.

The introduction of cyclosporine A has improved organ graft survival. Because the agent has little effect on phagocytosis and virtually no bone marrow suppression capability, neutrophils are in good supply and functional, greatly reducing the threat of infection.

Cyclosporine A is beneficial in the prevention of rejection but is not used as a rescue drug. Dosage is adjusted according to kidney function. Intravenous cyclosporine is given until the patient can tolerate oral medications. With the conversion from I.V. to the oral form, there will be an expected decrease in cyclosporine levels related to decreased GI absorption. Blood levels should be monitored to reduce the risk of untoward effects.

Specific nursing interventions for the patient experiencing organ rejection are outlined below.

• Monitor for signs and symptoms of ensuing or worsening graft failure. Notify the physician immediately.

• Administer increased doses of immunosuppressive medications, as prescribed.

• Provide supportive measures for the patient undergoing treatment, such as inotropes or intra-aortic balloon pump for heart recipients, ventilatory support for heart-lung recipients, and dialysis for kidney recipients.

• Monitor for infection, noting the presence of fever or elevated WBC count. Be aware that a sudden decrease in the WBC count can indicate a viral infection and that an increase in bands and a decrease in segmented neutrophils can indicate bacterial infection.

• Monitor kidney and liver function.

• Provide psychosocial support to the patient and family.

Infection control

Infection is one of the most serious and often life-threatening complications of transplantation. The greater the amount of immunosuppression, the greater the potential for infection. The posttransplant patient constantly walks a fine line between acute rejection and infection. Pretransplant conditions that predispose a patient to infection include hepatitis, splenectomy, and diabetes mellitus.

Infections can occur in the immediate postoperative period and are localized at the area of transplantation, such as intra-abdominal sepsis in the liver transplant recipient, pleural and lung infections in the heart and heart-lung transplant recipient, and urinary tract infec-

Immunosuppressant medications

An understanding of dosage, action, and side effects of immunosuppressant drugs is essential to ensure the patient's compliance with therapy.

Drug or Class	Dosage	Side Effects
Azathioprine (Imuran)	I.V.: 2 to 4 mg/kg daily P.O.: 2 to 4 mg/kg daily	• Bone marrow suppression (neutropenia) • GI upset • Hepatotoxicity • Cancer
Corticosteroids (prednisone)	Maintenance dose: 0.2 mg/kg/day P.O. Acute rejection: 1 to 3 mg/kg/day P.O. Tapered dose after rejection episode: 0.5 mg/kg/day	• Short-term effects: glucose intolerance, retention of salt and water, irritability, peptic ulcer disease, increased appetite, insomnia • Long-term effects: cushingoid appearance, osteoporosis, muscle wasting, increased incidence of infection, glaucoma, cataracts, steroid psychosis
Cyclosporine A (Sandimmune)	I.V.: 5 to 6 mg/kg over 2 to 6 hours or continuously over 24 hours P.O.: 10 to 20 mg/kg	• Nephrotoxicity • Hepatotoxicity • Hypertension • Cancer (lymphomas) • Tremors • Headaches • Burning of feet and hands • Hirsutism
Antithymocyte globulin/antilymphocyte globulin	I.V.: 10 to 15 mg/kg over 4 to 6 hours	• Thrombocytopenia, anemia, leukopenia • Serum sickness • Increased risk of infection • Allergic reaction
Muromonab-CD3 (Orthoclone OKT3)	I.V.: 5 mg/day for 10 to 14 days given over 1 minute as a bolus peripherally or centrally	• Hypersensitivity • Aseptic meningitis • Lymphoma • Development of antibodies against drug
Tacrolimus (Prograf)	I.V.: 0.15 mg/kg/day continuous infusion P.O.: 0.15 mg/kg twice daily Maintenance dose: 0.75 mg/kg/day	• Nausea and vomiting • Headache • Hyperglycemia • Insomnia • Renal failure • Hyperkalemia • Tremors and numbness

Nursing Considerations

- Monitor CBC with differential for neutropenia, thrombocytopenia, and anemia.
- Monitor liver enzymes.
- Monitor for signs of infection.
- Observe for jaundice.

- Monitor glucose levels.
- Administer insulin to maintain blood sugar 200 to 250 mg/dl.
- Monitor for signs of infection.
- Take daily weights.
- Monitor hourly intake and output.
- Perform occult stool test for presence of blood.

- Monitor kidney and liver function.
- Take daily weights.
- Monitor hourly intake and output.
- Administer antihypertensive medications, as ordered.
- Mix oral medication with juice or chocolate milk in glass container.
- Be alert to drugs that increase level, including erythromycin, ketoconazole, and diltiazem.
- Be alert to drugs that decrease level, including rifampin, phenytoin, phenobarbital, isoniazid, and carbamazepine.
- Monitor for signs of infection or rejection.

- Administer test dose of 0.1 ml in 1:1,000 dilution prior to full dose.
- Premedicate with Benadryl, Tylenol, or corticosteroids, as ordered.
- Monitor for signs of infection.
- Monitor CBC with differential.

- Monitor temperature, pulse, and blood pressure frequently.
- Assess respiratory status.
- Monitor blood for presence of antibodies.
- Administer Solu-Medrol, Tylenol, or Benadryl, as ordered, to reduce side effects.

- Monitor and maintain drug levels between 0.5 and 1.5 mg/ml.
- Monitor blood glucose levels.
- Monitor serum potassium levels.
- Monitor ECG continuously.
- Record daily weights.
- Monitor hourly intake and output.

tion in the kidney transplant recipient. The most common infections in the postoperative patient include bacterial gram-negative infections; viral infections, including cytomegalovirus (CMV), herpes simplex virus, and varicella zoster virus; fungal infections, such as those caused by *Candida, Aspergillus,* and *Histoplasma* species; and protozoan and parasitic pathogens, which can cause pneumonia in the transplant patient.

Nursing interventions for the patient with infection include the following:

• Monitor for signs of infection, including fever and changes in the WBC count. A sudden decrease in WBC count can indicate a viral infection; an increase in bands and a decrease in segmented neutrophils can also indicate infection.

• Maintain aseptic technique.

• Observe wounds for drainage and edema in the absence of fever.

• Maintain strict handwashing procedures for all persons in contact with the patient.

• Administer antimicrobial agents, as prescribed by the physician.

• Obtain cultures and interpret results; notify the physician.

• Monitor for low-grade fevers; temperatures greater than 99.5° F (37.5° C) may be significant in the transplant patient.

Organ-specific treatment and care

Specific medical treatments and nursing interventions vary depending on the organs transplanted, as discussed below.

Heart transplantation

Patients who have undergone heart transplantation are at increased risk for bleeding and tamponade. Close monitoring of vital signs and chest tube drainage is required to rule out hypovolemia or extreme cardiac failure. Replacement of fluid with crystalloids or colloids may be required.

Initially, the heart often requires inotropic support as a result of primary nonfunction of the heart graft and denervation. Denervation leads to bradycardia and the inability to increase the rate in response to physiologic demand. Because infection is the leading cause of death, prophylactic administration of antimicrobials is important in preventing serious infection.

The following nursing interventions should be incorporated in the plan of care:

- Monitor vital signs and chest tube drainage.
- Replace fluid with crystalloids or colloids.
- Administer inotropic support for hemodynamically significant bradycardia, as ordered.
- Monitor for signs and symptoms of infection.
- Administer prophylactic ganciclovir and trimetho-prim-sulfamethoxazole, as ordered.
- Monitor for signs and symptoms of rejection.
- Prepare for pericardiocentesis for the patient with tamponade.

Lung transplantation

The goals of postoperative treatment in the lung transplant patient include maintenance of adequate pulmonary and cardiac function. Ineffective airway clearance, a common problem during the first 2 to 3 months after transplantation, results from denervation of the transplanted lung, impaired cough, infection, pain, surgery, analgesia, or altered chest wall function. Ineffective gas exchange, another common problem, initially is caused by reperfusion edema in the transplanted lung; it can lead to hypoxemia and the need for increased oxygenation. Later, gas exchange can be hindered by infection or rejection. Also, hypovolemia, myocardial irritability, and depressed myocardial contractility during the immediate postoperative period may lead to hemodynamic instability.

The following nursing interventions should be incorporated in the plan of care:

- Position the patient properly. For single-lung recipients, position with the nonoperative side down; this reduces postsurgical edema and aids in gravitational drainage of the airway. For double-lung recipients, position side to side, 90 degrees each way, every 1 to 2 hours.

• Monitor chest X-rays daily.

• Monitor SaO_2, heart rate, and blood pressure.

• Monitor arterial blood gas levels.

• Monitor chest tube drainage.

• Perform chest physiotherapy every 2 to 4 hours while the patient is awake.

• Perform incentive spirometry after extubation to encourage deep breathing and coughing.

Heart-lung transplantation

The goals of treatment following heart-lung transplantation include maintaining adequate end-organ function and preventing complications, such as pulmonary dysfunction due to reperfusion injury. Monitoring of oxygenation, ventilation parameters, and compliance of new lungs is important. Ventilator management should focus on maintaining normal arterial blood gas levels. Fluid management is imperative to prevent pulmonary edema. Diuretics may assist in decreasing lung water. Chest X-ray should be monitored for appearance of infiltrates.

The major technical problem with heart-lung and lung transplantation is healing of the bronchial anastomosis. This can be complicated by dehiscence and stricture formation. Suctioning is necessary but must be performed carefully to prevent damage to the bronchial anastomosis. Aggressive pulmonary hygiene and early extubation assist in decreasing the risk of infection.

Cardiac and arterial monitoring are important immediately after heart-lung transplantation to assess right-sided and left-sided heart function, monitor blood loss, and determine the need for fluid resuscitation or diuretics, inotropes, or vasodilators. Patients with increased pulmonary pressures and heart dysfunction often have preexisting renal dysfunction. Comparison of posttransplant values with preoperative assessment can help in evaluating therapies.

Fluid management and the need for diuretics are determined by cardiac monitoring. Treatment focuses on careful monitoring of kidney function with serial blood urea nitrogen (BUN) and creatinine levels and of fluid status with hourly intake and output, abdominal girth measurement, and recording of daily weights. Serum levels of nephrotoxic antibiotics and cyclosporine must be closely assessed. Maintaining adequate blood pressure is imperative to reducing the incidence of renal failure.

The following nursing interventions should be incorporated to maintain optimal organ function:
• Assess arterial blood gas levels.
• Monitor intake and output and daily weights.
• Administer diuretics to decrease lung water, if necessary.
• Perform aggressive pulmonary hygiene to decrease incidence of pulmonary infections.
• Monitor for signs and symptoms of fluid overload, including crackles, tachypnea, dyspnea, peripheral edema, jugular venous distention, and hepatomegaly.
• Monitor for signs and symptoms of fluid deficit, including decreased urine output, hypotension, prolonged capillary refill, hypoactive bowel sounds, and pale, cool skin.
• Administer inotropic agents to improve cardiac contractility and maintain the cardiac index, as ordered.
• Monitor serial BUN and creatinine levels.
• Administer nephrotoxic medications carefully.

Liver transplantation

The postoperative plan of care for the liver transplant patient includes close monitoring for acute rejection (which typically occurs within 4 to 10 days), monitoring for signs of infection and bleeding, and evaluating kidney and liver function. The diagnosis of rejection is made by observing for signs and symptoms of liver failure and the results of a liver biopsy. Prior to the liver biopsy, prothrombin time (PT) and partial thrombo-plastin time (PTT) should be assessed and fresh frozen plasma administered, if necessary. Following the biopsy, the patient is placed on the right side and monitored closely for signs of bleeding.

If rejection is suspected, treatment usually includes an intravenous Solu-Medrol bolus. If administration of this steroid is insufficient, OKT3 can be given. Chronic rejection presents as destruction of small intrahepatic bile ducts and cannot be reversed with intensified therapy. Eventually, retransplantation is required for survival. The same criteria used to determine need for the initial transplant are used for retransplantation.

Infection is the primary threat to graft and patient survival. Liver transplant recipients are at higher risk of infection than other solid-organ recipients because the procedure requires five surgical anastomosis sites and multiple invasive catheters. The immunosuppressed patient is at risk for opportunistic infections from such organisms as *Candida albicans, Aspergillus fumigatus, Pneumocystis carinii,* and *Nocardia.*

P. carinii infection typically appears 3 to 6 months after transplantation. Treatment usually consists of Bactrim and pentamidine. *C. albicans* commonly presents in the GI tract and is treated with mycostatin and amphotericin B. CMV infection can be a serious problem, occurring 1 to 4 months after transplantation. The patient with CMV infection typically has a fever and low WBC count. Treatment includes ganciclovir (DHPG) administration and reduction or temporary discontinuation of immunosuppressive agents until the infection is controlled.

The patient with a liver transplant also is at increased risk for bleeding. This is partially due to the large numbers of anastomosis sites and drains and the reduced function of the new liver in the immediate postoperative period, resulting in decreased production of clotting factors.

Several factors predispose the liver transplant patient to acute renal failure. They include hypotension, administration of nephrotoxic antibiotics, administration of cyclosporine, acute severe rejection, acute hepatic failure, and intraoperative or postoperative hypothermia. Treatment focuses on careful monitoring of renal function with serial BUN and creatinine levels and of fluid status with hourly intake and output. Abdominal girths and daily weights should be measured. Serum levels of nephrotoxic antibiotics and cyclosporine must be closely assessed. Maintaining adequate blood pressure is imperative.

Biliary complications occur as a result of biliary anastomosis obstruction, infection, or rupture. If the anastomosis leaks or becomes obstructed, an abscess may form or peritonitis, bacteremia, or cirrhosis can develop. The T-tube should be kept dependent and emptied frequently. Potential T-tube complications include obstruction or dislodgment, leading to infection. This should be suspected if the patient has right upper quadrant pain, nausea, jaundice, vomiting, clay-colored stools, or drainage around the tube. Administration of intravenous prostaglandin may be beneficial.

The following nursing interventions should be incorporated in the plan of care for the liver transplant patient:
• Monitor PT and PTT.
• Assess for signs and symptoms of rejection (elevated AST, ALT, bilirubin).
• Assist with liver biopsy.
• Monitor levels of immunosuppressant drugs.
• Monitor vital signs for signs of infection or hypovolemia.
• Monitor WBC and differential counts, hematocrit and hemoglobin levels, intake and output, and BUN and creatinine levels.
• Obtain serial chest X-rays.
• Obtain serum levels of nephrotoxic antibiotics and cyclosporine.
• Assess function of T-tube.
• Administer prostaglandin, as ordered.

Kidney transplantation

In the first 24 hours after surgery, urine production is the prime concern. A significant decrease in hourly urine output can be one of the earliest signs of dysfunction. If urine output decreases, the nurse should assess the type of renal failure (prerenal, intrarenal, or postrenal). Common causes of postrenal oliguria or anuria include a clot in the bladder obstructing the catheter, obstruction of the transplanted ureter, or a leak at the anastomosis of the ureter to the bladder.

The diagnosis of obstruction can be resolved by ultrasound, which reveals hydronephrosis. A common prerenal cause of oliguria is volume depletion. Adequate hydration with crystalloid solutions to maintain normal central venous pressure is necessary. Intrarenal causes of oliguria include acute tubular necrosis and vascular complications. Acute oliguria can be caused by cyclosporine, which should be administered at the lowest dose possible.

The following nursing interventions should be incorporated in the plan of care:
• Administer fluids, as ordered.
• Monitor hourly intake and output.
• Monitor administration of drugs known to be nephrotoxic (cyclosporine, aminoglycosides).
• Monitor for signs of decreasing renal function (decreased urine output, rising BUN and creatinine levels).

Prognosis

Despite posttransplantation problems, such as rejection, infection, primary graft failure, and consequences of lifelong immunosuppression (hypertension, renal dysfunction, and neurologic sequelae), organ transplantation can restore the quality of life to a patient with an otherwise fatal disease. Heart transplants have a 90% 1-year survival rate. Currently, lung and heart-lung transplants are associated with less favorable outcomes than heart transplants. The 1-year survival rate is 65% to 70%. The 1-year survival for liver transplants is 70%; 5-year survival is 60%.

Discharge planning

The survival of transplant patients depends on their understanding of their illness and treatment regimen and compliance with this regimen. Both the patient and the family must understand prescribed immunosuppressive medications and the signs and symptoms of infection and rejection. Information to be conveyed to the patient and family includes:

• importance of temperature and blood pressure measurements and glucose monitoring
• need to measure daily intake and output and weight
• testing of stool for occult blood
• dietary restrictions (low protein, low sodium)
• testing of urine for blood, protein, or glucose
• medication regimen (name, action, dosages, and side effects of each medication)
• signs and symptoms of rejection, including temperature greater than 100.4° F (38° C), weight gain of 2 to 3 lb in 1 day, increased blood pressure, hyperglycemia, and pain, swelling, or tenderness over the graft site
• need to notify the clinic or physician regarding presence of signs or symptoms of rejection, presence of signs or symptoms of infection, and inability to obtain medications
• importance of regular follow-up visits to the physician or clinic.

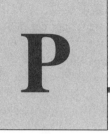

P

Pancreatitis

An acute inflammation of the pancreas caused by premature activation of digestive enzymes, pancreatitis is characterized by severe abdominal pain and persistent nausea and vomiting. About 90% of all cases are attributed to alcohol abuse, gallstone disease, or idiopathic factors. Other causes of pancreatitis are listed in *Major causes of acute pancreatitis,* page 477.

The incidence is 1 per 10,000 in the general population and 1 per 100 in the alcoholic population. The typical male patient is in his 30s to 40s and presents with acute alcoholic pancreatitis. Females have a higher incidence of pancreatitis due to gallstone disease and are generally over age 50. For most patients (85% to 90%), the disease is mild with a rapid recovery within 5 to 7 days. The remaining patients have progressive hemorrhagic pancreatitis and multisystem complications.

Pathophysiology

Acute pancreatitis may occur in one of two forms: edematous (interstitial) pancreatitis, characterized by interstitial edema, polymorphonuclear infiltration, engorgement of capillaries, and dilation of lymphatics; or

Major causes of acute pancreatitis

The most common causes of pancreatitis are alcohol abuse and gallstone disease. Many drugs can cause pancreatitis if they are taken in toxic doses or if they produce drug reactions. Infectious processes also are implicated in pancreatitis.

Drugs
- Corticosteroids
- Nonsteroidal anti-inflammatory drugs
- Rifampin
- Valproic acid
- Thiazide diuretics
- Furosemide
- Estrogens (including birth control pills)
- Procainamide
- Tetracycline
- Sulfonamides

Metabolic conditions
- Alcohol abuse
- Hyperparathyroidism
- Hypertriglyceridemia
- Hypercalcemia
- End-stage renal disease

Infectious processes
- Mumps
- Staphylococcus
- Scarlet fever
- Viral processes
- Infectious mononucleosis

- Viral hepatitis
- Epstein-Barr virus
- Cytomegalovirus

Mechanical
- Biliary disease (gallstones, common bile duct obstruction, biliary sludge)
- Abdominal trauma
- Endoscopic procedures
- Surgical procedures
- Malignancy

Vascular problems
- Ischemia
- Lupus
- Shock states

Other causes
- Ectopic pregnancy
- Ovarian cyst
- Use of total parenteral nutrition
- Hypothermia
- Pregnancy
- Hereditary pancreatitis
- Scorpion venom

necrotizing pancreatitis, characterized by acinar cell death with pancreatic necrosis and hemorrhage.

The inflammation that occurs with both types is caused by premature activation of enzymes, resulting in autodigestion of the gland.

Normally, the acini cells secrete trypsin, chymotrypsin, phospholipase A, elastase, and carboxypeptidase in an inactive form. The mechanism by which these enzymes become prematurely activated is not fully understood. According to one theory, a toxic agent, such as alcohol or a drug, alters the way in which the pancreas secretes enzymes. It is thought that alcohol consumption increases pancreatic secretion and alters the metabolic processes of the acinar cells. It also is believed to promote duct obstruction through precipitation of pancreatic secretory proteins. Another theory speculates that a reflux of duodenal contents containing activated enzymes enters the pancreatic duct, triggering the activation of other enzymes and setting up a cycle of more pancreatic damage.

Regardless of the etiology, the outcome is the same—damage to the pancreatic acinar cells from secretion of prematurely activated enzymes. As these cells are damaged, more enzymes are released, resulting in a destructive cycle. The primary enzyme responsible for cellular damage is believed to be trypsin, which can activate all of the other digestive enzymes.

As activated enzymes cause autodigestion of the pancreas, vasoactive substances are released, causing increased capillary permeability and vasodilation. This leads to massive third-space fluid shifting (as much as 20% to 30% of circulating volume). Up to 12 liters of fluid may collect in the retroperitoneal space and peritoneal cavity.

Clinical assessment

Acute pancreatitis is only one of many causes of abdominal pain. Diagnosis is based on a careful history and physical examination as well as on diagnostic testing.

History

The nurse should ascertain the following during the clinical assessment:
• evaluation of possible causes
• history of pain, including onset, duration, location, intensity, precipitating factors, and relation to meals, anorexia, or food intolerances
• characteristics and frequency of bowel movements
• history of abdominal trauma
• family history of acute pancreatitis (rarely hereditary).

Physical findings

Acute pancreatitis is characterized by severe, persistent, piercing abdominal pain. The characteristic pain is usually midepigastric, although it may be generalized or in the left upper quadrant radiating to the back. It usually begins suddenly after eating a large meal or drinking alcohol. The pain increases with supine positioning and is relieved by assuming the knee-chest position. Pain can be caused by several factors, including:
• extravasation of inflammatory exudate and enzymes into the retroperitoneum
• edema and distention of the pancreatic capsule
• obstruction of the biliary tree.

   Additional findings include:
• weight loss
• nausea and vomiting
• diarrhea; grayish, fatty or bulky, and foul-smelling stool
• orange-red urine (if myoglobin is present)
• low-grade fever (usually under 102° F [38.9° C])
• weakness
• dehydration and hypovolemic shock (associated with hemorrhagic pancreatitis)
• hypotension, tachycardia, increased respiratory rate
• abdominal distention, tenderness, or guarding
• tympany to percussion with dullness over the pancreas
• ascites
• palpable abdominal mass
• hypoactive or absent bowel sounds
• soft abdomen (with severe abdominal pain)
• Turner's sign (ecchymosis of flanks; associated with hemorrhagic pancreatitis)
• Cullen's sign (ecchymosis of periumbilical area; associated with hemorrhagic pancreatitis)
• Halstead's sign (marbled appearance of abdomen; may be found with hemorrhagic pancreatitis)
• jaundice
• Chvostek's sign (elicited by tapping over the side of the face at the level of the eye, leading to twitching of the lip and cheek; indicative of hypocalcemia)

• Trousseau's sign (elicited by applying a blood pressure cuff to the arm and inflating just above systolic pressure—a positive response is evidenced by carpopedal spasm, which occurs within the first 2 minutes; indicative of hypocalcemia).

Diagnosis

Diagnosis of acute pancreatitis is based on the patient's history and clinical assessment and on diagnostic studies. History and assessment can mimic other conditions, such as intestinal ischemia and infarction, bowel obstruction, or ruptured abdominal aortic aneurysm; consequently, laboratory and radiologic studies are important for accurate diagnosis. (See *Diagnostic tests for acute pancreatitis,* page 481, for a summary of commonly ordered tests.)

Other nonspecific laboratory tests may reveal elevated white blood cell (WBC) count due to inflammation, elevated serum glucose due to beta cell damage, elevated liver enzymes, hypokalemia due to vomiting, and hypocalcemia associated with fat necrosis.

Treatment and care

The primary goals for the patient with acute pancreatitis are to achieve fluid and electrolyte homeostasis and to prevent complications. Treatment is aimed at removing the inciting mechanism, limiting the degree of inflammation, and supporting the patient physiologically through treatment of complications.

Fluid volume maintenance

Hypovolemic shock is a common complication of acute pancreatitis and a major cause of death within the first few days after onset. Hypovolemic shock is caused by fluid shifts into the retroperitoneal space and abdominal cavity. The patient attempts to compensate by increasing cardiac output, pulse, and stroke volume. The cardiac output may be insufficient to meet tissue oxygenation demands, resulting in myocardial dysfunction and increased tissue oxygen demands. This may be ev-

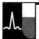

Diagnostic tests for acute pancreatitis

The following tests may help to confirm acute pancreatitis.

Serum amylase
This is the most widely used test in the diagnosis of pancreatitis. Amylase is released as pancreatic cells are destroyed. Serum levels may be elevated 3 to 5 times above normal during the first 24 to 48 hours after onset of symptoms. In mild cases, the level may be normal after 3 to 5 days. In addition, amylase is present in other tissues, so elevated levels may be indicative of other diseases, such as biliary tract disease, acute appendicitis, tumors of the lung or ovary, perforated peptic ulcer, salivary gland dysfunction, pregnancy, pneumonia, chronic alcoholism, or intestinal obstruction. Amylase may not be elevated if serum triglycerides are high. Serum amylase is more specific for pancreatitis if isoamylase also is elevated or if urine amylase is elevated. Normal serum amylase level is 25 to 125 U/liter.

Serum lipase
Lipase is released as pancreatic cells are destroyed. Like serum amylase levels, lipase may be elevated during the first 24 to 48 hours after onset of symptoms and in mild cases and may return to normal after a few days. Prolonged elevation may be suggestive of pancreatic pseudocyst development. Normal serum lipase level is 10 to 150 U/liter.

Serum calcium
Calcium levels are often decreased (under 8 mg/dl) due to intraperitoneal saponification. Trypsin inactivates parathyroid hormone, leading to further hypocalcemia. Normal serum calcium level is 8.4 to 10.2 mg/dl.

Abdominal ultrasound, computed tomography (CT), magnetic resonance imaging (MRI)
Ultrasound is helpful in identifying associated gallstone disease. It also may reveal variations in size and texture of the pancreas relative to edema and fluid collection. It may not provide an adequate view of the pancreas in obese patients or those with abdominal distention. CT scans can detect changes in organ size, abnormalities of pancreatic ducts, peripancreatic fluid collection, and pancreatic necrosis. MRI may assist in detecting pancreatic fluid collection, abscesses, and masses.

Abdominal X-rays
Abdominal X-rays are not specific but may suggest a diagnosis of pancreatitis. Dilatation of the first loop of the jejunum is referred to as "sentinel loop" and is indicative of jejunal ileus. Dilatation of the transverse colon, known as the "colon cut-off" sign, indicates colonic ileus. Ileus is commonly associated with pancreatitis. An elevated hemidiaphragm and pleural effusion may be present secondary to diaphragmatic irritation Peripancreatic gas ("soap bubbles") of a pancreatic abscess are the only findings specific to pancreatitis.

idenced by depression in left ventricular stroke volume and an elevation in pulmonary capillary pressure.

Rapid fluid replacement may be achieved with colloids or Ringer's lactate solution. Hemorrhagic or necrotizing pancreatitis may require packed red blood cells to restore volume. If the patient fails to respond to fluid therapy, pressors (such as dopamine) may be required.

Appropriate nursing interventions are as follows:
• Monitor hemodynamic status. Hemodynamic parameters should be monitored by a pulmonary artery catheter to assess fluid status. Hypovolemia results in decreased renal perfusion and may lead to acute renal failure. Prompt correction of hypovolemia and hypotension is necessary to prevent impairment of renal function. Goals for hemodynamic parameters are as follows: mean arterial pressure > 60 mm Hg; heart rate < 100 beats/minute; pulmonary capillary wedge pressure 11 to 14 mm Hg.
• Assess heart sounds.
• Monitor intake and output.
• Weigh the patient daily.
• Administer fluids, as ordered.
• Assess for fluid overload.
• Administer vasoactive medications to maintain blood pressure, as indicated.
• Monitor daily blood urea nitrogen (BUN) and creatinine levels.

Maintenance of electrolyte balance

Electrolyte imbalances are common in acute pancreatitis due to fluid loss. Potassium replacement is often necessary because of loss from vomiting and nasogastric suctioning. In addition, potassium is abundant in pancreatic juices. An increase in pancreatic juice secretion further lowers serum potassium levels. Hypokalemia is associated with cardiac arrhythmias, muscle weakness, and hypotension.

Hypocalcemia is another common electrolyte abnormality. Serum calcium levels may fall because of intraperitoneal saponification by free fatty acids released during fat necrosis. Fat necrosis can occur within the pancreas as well as at distant sites as a result of lipolytic enzyme release into the bloodstream. Calcium soap formation may result. If excessive calcium is concentrated in the necrotic foci, hypocalcemia may result.

Hypocalcemia also is thought to be related to decreased binding of calcium with proteins in the plasma. Hypomagnesemia may impair parathyroid gland secretion of parathyroid hormone. This in turn may lead to hypocalcemia. Therefore, magnesium levels usually must be corrected before calcium levels can return to normal. If the patient has low albumin levels, calculate the corrected calcium level prior to giving treatment (see *How to calculate a corrected calcium level*, page 484).

Patients with hypocalcemia should be placed on seizure precautions. Calcium replacements should be infused through a central line if possible; infiltration can cause necrosis.

Nursing interventions for the patient receiving electrolyte replacement include:
• Monitor electrolyte levels carefully.
• Monitor for signs of hypokalemia, hyperkalemia, hypocalcemia, hypercalcemia, hypomagnesemia, and hypermagnesemia.
• During calcium replacement, monitor for signs of calcium toxicity, including lethargy, nausea, and shortening of the Q-T interval.
• Prevent infiltration of potassium and calcium preparations.
• Monitor ECG for arrhythmias associated with electrolyte abnormalities.

Maintenance of respiratory function
About 15% of patients with acute pancreatitis develop adult respiratory distress syndrome (ARDS). This is believed to be due, in part, to the release of proteolytic enzymes into the circulation. A significant ventilation and perfusion mismatch often occurs, resulting in further hypoxemia. In addition to ARDS, pleural effusion, atelectasis, and pneumonia may occur, leading to respi-

How to calculate a corrected calcium level

Serum calcium levels in acute pancreatitis can initially be misleading. Albumin may leave the bloodstream and enter the tissues in acute pancreatitis, resulting in decreased serum levels. Hypoalbuminemia may cause the serum calcium level to appear lower than normal.

Serum calcium exists in ionized and nonionized forms. Laboratory results represent a sum of both forms. Ionized calcium is the form necessary for proper functioning of nerves, muscles, and other processes. Nonionized calcium is bound primarily to albumin. There is a 0.8 mg/dl decrease in serum calcium for each 1.0 mg/dl decrease in albumin below 4.0 g/dl. A corrected calcium level takes into account abnormal albumin levels. Normal serum albumin is 3.5 to 5.0 g/dl, and normal serum calcium is 8.4 to 10.2 mg/dl.

Corrected calcium = Total calcium + 0.8(4.0 - albumin)

Example: total calcium = 7.0, albumin = 2.0
7.0 + 0.8(4.0 - 2.0) = 8.6

ratory failure. Hypoxemia may exist when other symptoms are not present. Arterial blood gas (ABG) levels are generally drawn every 8 hours for the first 3 to 5 days to monitor for this complication.

Appropriate interventions include:
• Provide supplemental oxygen.
• Monitor pulse oximetry or $S\bar{v}O_2$ readings.
• Assess for tachypnea and hypoventilation.
• Assess for mental status changes.
• Monitor ABG results.
• Assess breath sounds for crackles, rhonchi, and wheezing every 2 hours.
• Perform pulmonary hygiene measures (encourage coughing, turning, and deep breathing).
• Place the patient in semi-Fowler's position.
• Administer analgesics to prevent shallow respirations, as ordered.
• Monitor for increasing pulmonary inspiratory pressure.

Pancreatic rest
Resting the pancreas is necessary to minimize the autodigestive process. A nasogastric tube set to low inter-

mittent suction is used in patients with ileus or vomiting. This suppresses pancreatic exocrine secretion by preventing the release of secretin from the duodenum. It also decreases nausea, vomiting, and abdominal pain. Other measures used to suppress pancreatic secretion include the use of antispasmodics and anticholinergics. These drugs also reduce ampullary spasm.

A strict NPO (nothing by mouth) status is usually enforced until abdominal pain subsides and serum amylase levels return to normal. Oral intake any sooner may increase abdominal pain by stimulating the autodigestive process. In mild cases of pancreatitis, oral fluids may be started in 3 to 7 days. If prolonged NPO status is anticipated, total parenteral nutrition (TPN) should be initiated. Lipids may or may not be used because they may raise triglyceride levels and increase inflammation. Insulin secretion may be impaired during acute pancreatitis. Hyperglycemia may worsen with TPN administration.

Appropriate nursing interventions are listed below:
• Maintain a nasogastric tube to low intermittent suction.
• Provide frequent oral hygiene.
• Administer medications, as ordered.
• Maintain NPO status, as ordered.
• Administer TPN and lipids, as ordered.
• Monitor for complications of parenteral nutrition, including electrolyte abnormalities.
• Monitor blood glucose levels every 6 hours and treat as necessary.

Pain control

Severe pain in acute pancreatitis is caused by extravasation of enzymes into the retroperitoneum and edema of the pancreatic capsule. Pain increases pancreatic enzyme secretion. Nonopioid analgesics are used for pain control because opiates, such as morphine, can cause spasms of the sphincter of Oddi, which exacerbates pain.

Nursing interventions for pain control include:
• Promote pancreatic rest.
• Administer nonopioid analgesics, as ordered.

• Instruct the patient on relaxation techniques and imagery to assist in pain reduction.

Surgery

Surgery usually is not required unless a pancreatic abscess develops. This complication carries a 100% mortality without surgical intervention. Pancreatic resection has been used as a treatment for acute necrotizing pancreatitis in an attempt to prevent systemic complication.

Appropriate interventions for the postoperative patient include:
• Administer antibiotics, as ordered.
• Monitor for signs of complications (infection, fistulas, gastrointestinal bleeding, intestinal obstruction, and perforation).
• Monitor intake and output.
• Monitor hemodynamic parameters.
• Administer analgesics, as ordered.

Preventing and treating complications

Most patients with mild pancreatitis recover within 5 to 7 days. Early complications include hypotension and organ damage by circulating toxins. The pancreas has the ability to produce vasoactive substances that affect other organs, such as the lungs, heart, and kidneys. Late complications are usually related to problems with the pancreas itself (see *Complications of acute pancreatitis,* page 487).

Clinical trials have shown that long-term (7 days) peritoneal lavage significantly reduces the incidence of pancreatic sepsis and the mortality rate in acute pancreatitis. Pancreatic pseudocysts (collections of pancreatic secretions contained within a fibrous wall) may require invasive intervention. CT-directed percutaneous catheter drainage may assist in the management of this problem.

Broad-spectrum antibiotics are reserved for cases of biliary obstruction, pancreatic abscess, and sepsis.

In addition, in cases of alcoholic pancreatitis, be alert to signs and symptoms of alcohol withdrawal. Benzodiazepines may be used to treat alcohol withdrawal.

Complications of acute pancreatitis

The following complications may occur with acute pancreatitis:

- Pancreatic abscess
- Pancreatic pseudocyst
- Pancreatic phlegmon
- Pancreaticocutaneous fistulas or internal fistulas (to the colon, stomach, bile duct, or small intestine)
- Pulmonary effusions, especially on the left side
- Pulmonary edema
- Atelectasis
- Adult respiratory distress syndrome
- Disseminated intravascular coagulation
- Anemia
- Metabolic acidosis
- Hypocalcemia
- Hypokalemia
- Hyperglycemia
- Myocardial depression
- Hypovolemic shock
- Sepsis
- Peritonitis
- Cholecystitis
- Paralytic ileus
- Intestinal perforation
- Obstruction of biliary tree
- Fistulas from the pancreas through a tract to outside of the body or internally to the bowel, stomach, or bile duct
- Acute renal failure
- Gastrointestinal bleeding

Prognosis

The overall mortality rate for acute pancreatitis is 10%. However, the mortality rate increases with increased severity and multisystem failure. The Ranson Severity Criteria are widely used prognostic indicators for mortality associated with pancreatitis (see *Ranson Severity Criteria,* page 488).

Discharge planning

Discharge planning should begin as soon as the patient is stabilized. Take into consideration the following:
- Assess the patient's support systems.
- Consult social services.
- Instruct the patient to avoid alcohol, smoking, and stress, which can increase stimulation of the pancreas.
- Provide dietary instructions, including the need to follow a low-fat diet and to avoid crash dieting, binge-eating, caffeine, and spicy foods. Consult the dietitian, as needed.

Ranson Severity Criteria

By using the criteria listed below, clinicians can determine a patient's overall prognosis. Mortality rate is estimated based on the number of presenting signs:

   < 3 signs 1% mortality
   3-4 signs 15% mortality
   5-6 signs 40% mortality
   7 or more 100% mortality

Evaluate on admission or on diagnosis:
• Age > 55 years
• Leukocyte count > 16,000/µl

• Serum glucose > 200 mg/dl
• Serum lactic dehydrogenase > 350 IU/ml
• Serum aspartate aminotransferase > 250 IU/dl

Evaluate during initial 48 hours:
• Fall in hematocrit > 10%
• BUN level rise > 5 mg/dl
• Serum calcium < 8 mg/dl
• Base deficit > 4 mEq/l
• Estimated fluid sequestration > 6 liters
• Arterial PaO_2 < 60 torr

Adapted with permission from: Hudak, C.M. & Gallo, B.M. (1985). "Critical care nursing: A holistic approach." *Hospital Practice* 20(4):69, The McGraw-Hill Companies.

• Tell the patient which signs and symptoms to report to the physician (pancreatic abscesses can develop months after discharge).
• Instruct the patient and family about home medications. Insulin and pancreatic enzymes may be required if pancreatic damage is severe.

Pericarditis

Pericarditis is an inflammation of the pericardium, the double-walled sac that encircles the heart. The pericardium consists of a visceral layer, the serosal inner layer that composes the epicardium, and a parietal layer, the fibrous outer layer. The layers are separated by a thin film of pericardial fluid that reduces friction between them.

   The pericardium has several functions:
• It holds the heart in a fixed position in the mediastinum and minimizes friction between the heart and adjacent structures.
• It prevents sudden dilatation of the cardiac chambers.

• It allows for the development of negative intrapericardial pressure during ventricular systole, thereby facilitating atrial filling.

• It impedes the spread of infection from the pleural cavity to the heart.

Pericarditis can be infectious or noninfectious. Infectious pericarditis of the viral type is probably the culprit behind idiopathic pericarditis. The most common cause of noninfectious pericarditis is a condition that occurs following myocardial infarction (MI) (see *Post-myocardial infarction pericarditis,* page 490).

Other causes of noninfectious pericarditis include:
• uremia
• malignancy
• radiation therapy to the chest
• autoimmune disorders
• drugs
• dissecting thoracic aortic aneurysm.

Pathophysiology

Pericarditis can take one of two forms: acute inflammatory pericarditis or chronic constrictive pericarditis.

Acute pericarditis

Acute pericarditis develops in three inflammatory stages: vasodilatation with transudation of serous fluid into the pericardial space, increased vascular permeability with seepage of serum proteins into the pericardial fluid, and leukocytosis of the pericardial fluid. The immune response is the physiologic basis of the pericardial inflammation. Infectious causes of pericarditis can be eliminated by the immune response (phagocytosis); however, the inflammatory cycle itself releases many substances, including prostaglandin and bradykinin, that produce significant tissue damage and are responsible for most of the symptoms of pericarditis.

Four types of pericarditis can be identified by means of open inspection of the pericardium and the pericardial fluid:

Post-myocardial infarction pericarditis

Pericardial inflammation occurs in approximately 10% to 15% of patients with acute myocardial infarction (MI) and results in acute pericarditis within 48 to 72 hours following infarction. A late form of post-MI pericarditis called Dressler's syndrome occurs in approximately 4% of MI patients and causes symptoms 10 days to 2 months after the infarct. Acute post-MI pericarditis and Dressler's syndrome share the same pathophysiology and clinical course, differing only in the timing of the onset of the symptoms.

The classic clinical findings in post-MI pericarditis include:
• Pericardial pain pattern
• Pericardial friction rub
• Dyspnea
• ECG abnormalities occurring in four stages. The stages evolve over several hours to days and may last for several months:
   STAGE I: Diffuse ST-segment elevation in all leads except lead AVR

STAGE II: Return of ST-segments to baseline and PR-segment depression
STAGE III: Diffuse T-wave inversion
STAGE IV: Normalization of the T-wave

Aside from the clinical examination, the patient will have an elevated erythrocyte sedimentation rate and white blood cell count, which reflect acute inflammation and aid in diagnosis. Treatment is symptom-oriented; nonsteroidal anti-inflammatory drugs are quite effective in relieving pain and inflammation.

Post-MI pericarditis is not life-threatening, and the prognosis is based on the severity of the MI. Dressler's syndrome follows a similar course as acute pericarditis; however, significant pleural effusion with consequent cardiac tamponade is more common.

• Serous pericarditis is an early form of pericarditis characterized by serous exudate.
• Serofibrinous pericarditis, the most common form of pericarditis, is characterized by a cloudy pericardial fluid. Portions of the parietal and visceral pericardium may become inflamed and scar tissue can develop, leading to the development of constrictive pericarditis.
• Purulent pericarditis is characterized by a suppurative pericardial fluid and intensely inflamed pericardial tissues. Bacterial infections are the most common cause of purulent pericarditis.
• Hemorrhagic pericarditis, which is characterized by a grossly bloody pericardial fluid, is commonly caused by tuberculosis, malignancy, or a complication of anticoagulation therapy.

It is possible for the pericardial exudate to accumulate and cause a subsequent increase in the intrapericardial pressure. The result is cardiac compression and tamponade. The physiologic sequelae of tamponade are outlined below.

• Elevation of the intracardiac pressure. Normally, the intrapericardial pressure is several millimeters of mercury lower than the ventricular diastolic pressure. When pericardial fluid accumulates in the closed space, the intrapericardial pressure increases to first equal the ventricular diastolic pressure and then to cause a concomitant rise in both the intrapericardial and ventricular diastolic pressures.

• Progressive limitation of ventricular diastolic filling. The increase in intrapericardial pressure compresses the ventricular chambers during diastole, thus reducing the volume capacity of the ventricle.

• Reduction of stroke volume. Because of the reduced diastolic capacity (preload) of the compressed ventricle, stroke volume is reduced despite normal systolic contraction. Consequently, the systemic blood pressure is reduced.

Systemic venous return is impaired by cardiac tamponade because the ventricular capacity to accept the preload is reduced. The result is the accumulation of fluid and pressure in the systemic venous system, causing congestion and transudation of fluid into the extravascular tissues.

Chronic constrictive pericarditis

Constrictive pericarditis is a fibrotic thickening of the pericardium caused by the progression of an initial incidence of acute serofibrinous pericarditis. Chronic inflammation causes fibrous scarring and thickening of the pericardium with subsequent fusion of the visceral and parietal pericardial layers. Calcium deposition occurs and intensifies the stiffness of the pericardium. The constrictiveness affects the pericardium uniformly over all cardiac chambers.

The main pathophysiologic result of pericardial fibrosis is impairment of diastolic filling. An abnormal pattern of diastolic filling occurs wherein nearly all of the venous return to the heart occurs during early diastole. Because of the noncompliance of the pericardium, normal changes in intrathoracic pressure during respiration do not affect diastolic filling. Therefore, the increased venous filling that normally occurs during inspiration does not occur in the constrictive patient, further decreasing the ventricular filling.

This impaired filling leads to:
• increased systemic venous pressure (which produces venous congestion with exudation of plasma fluids into the interstitial tissues, hepatic engorgement, and other symptoms of right-sided heart failure)
• renal retention of sodium and water (decreased diastolic filling stimulates the renin-angiotensin-aldosterone system, which causes sodium and water retention as a compensatory mechanism; however, the increased fluid volume serves to worsen the venous congestion that already exists)
• decreased stroke volume (because of the decreased preload, the stroke volume also is decreased, resulting in decreased cardiac output and hypotension despite normal systolic function).

Clinical assessment
A thorough history and complete physical examination often clinch the diagnosis of pericarditis and its complications.

History
The nurse should be cognizant of etiologic factors associated with pericarditis while obtaining a patient history. Information should be elicited regarding:
• the character of the pain and its radiation points
• factors that relieve the pain, such as position changes
• recent MI
• recent cardiac surgery

• recent illness, including nonspecific cold and flu-like illnesses
• all medications the patient takes and the duration of therapy with each drug
• cancer history, including treatment with radiation therapy or chemotherapy
• history of renal dysfunction
• history of autoimmune or connective tissue diseases
• history of tuberculosis or positive purified protein derivative skin test.

Physical findings

Clinical signs and symptoms of acute and chronic pericarditis are outlined below.

Acute pericarditis

The signs and symptoms of acute pericarditis can mimic those of acute MI. The nurse should pay particular attention to the patient's pain characteristics. The most commonly reported symptoms of pericarditis include:
• chest pain, usually localized to the retrosternal area, left precordium, neck, and trapezius muscles. The pain can mimic that of an acute MI, angina, or pleurisy and is aggravated by deep inspiration, cough, and supine positioning. It is generally relieved when the patient sits upright and leans forward. Only the distal parietal pericardium has pain fibers; therefore, much of the pain results from inflammation of the diaphragmatic pleura.
• fever
• sudden onset of chest pain that is unrelenting in duration
• nonexertional dyspnea, possibly resulting from the patient's reluctance to take a deep breath becaue of pain
• generalized malaise.
The pericardial friction rub is the most significant physical finding in acute pericarditis. An important feature of the pericardial friction rub is that its quality may change from one examination to the next. When accompanied by the typical pericardial pain pattern described above, the combination is considered diagnostic for acute peri-

ASSESSMENT TIP
Pericardial friction rub

Pericardial friction rubs result when the pericardial layers grate together, producing a scratchy, superficial sound best auscultated at the lower left sternal border. Generally, pericardial friction rubs have the following characteristics:
• They are best auscultated early in the course of pericarditis.
• They are noted intermittently.
• They can be exaggerated by having the patient forcefully expire while leaning forward (Mohammed's sign).
• They disappear within several days after their initial presentation due to accumulation of fluid in the pericardium. Fluid accumulation causes the loss of contact of the pericardial surfaces to each other.

Such friction rubs may have one, two, or three components to the sound. The first component occurs during atrial systole. The second component, which is loudest, occurs during ventricular systole. The third component, the softest component, occurs during ventricular diastole. Two- and three-component pericardial friction rubs are the most common. Occasionally, the third component appears to be absent because it is difficult to auscultate.

carditis (see *Assessment tip: Pericardial friction rub,* page 494).

Chronic constrictive pericarditis
The physical findings of chronic, constrictive pericarditis can mimic those of restrictive cardiomyopathy (see the entry on Cardiomyopathy). Findings commonly reflect systemic venous congestion and include:
• abdominal swelling, postprandial fullness, anorexia, flatulence, and dyspepsia secondary to ascites and passive liver congestion
• dyspnea secondary to pleural effusions and hemidiaphragm elevation
• jugular vein distention
• tachycardia
• tachypnea
• hepatomegaly, hepatic pulsations
• lower-extremity edema
• fatigue
• weight loss.

Diagnosis

The diagnosis of acute pericarditis is based largely on the patient history and physical examination. The 12-lead electrocardiogram typically reflects characteristic changes, including the presence of diffuse ST-segment elevation in about 90% of patients. (See *Differential diagnosis of pericarditis,* pages 496 and 497, for specific tests and studies that help confirm diagnosis.)

Treatment and care

Acute pericarditis is a self-limiting disorder that generally runs its course in 1 to 3 weeks, with or without treatment. Depending on the severity of the disease, patients may be treated in the hospital or on an outpatient basis. Treatment is primarily symptomatic and aims to prevent complications.

Relief of pain and inflammation

Pericardial pain, one of the hallmarks of pericarditis, is a result of inflammation of the bottom portion of the parietal pericardial pleura and the pulmonary pleura transmitted by way of stimulation of the phrenic and intercostal nerves. Relieving the inflammation results in relief of pain.

Appropriate nursing measures include:
• Administer nonsteroidal anti-inflammatory agents (NSAIDs), as ordered. NSAIDs are the mainstay of the treatment of pericarditis. Various agents are available, and the choice should be based on the patient's tolerance, cost of medication, and dosing schedule. Ibuprofen generally is administered every 8 hours. Because of its efficacy and low cost, it is a good choice if the GI effects (nausea, vomiting, anorexia, gastritis) are not severe. Indomethacin is another frequently prescribed NSAID for pericarditis patients.
• Administer steroids, as ordered, if the patient does not respond to NSAIDs or if the pericarditis is severe.
• Administer narcotics, if required. Narcotics are rarely necessary but may provide pain relief for patients with

Differential diagnosis of pericarditis

Because the clinical manifestations of pericarditis can mimic those of acute myocardial infarction (acute pericarditis) or restrictive cardiomyopathy (chronic constrictive pericarditis), a careful analysis of differential findings is imperative. The following chart includes both diagnostic tests and clinical signs that aid in definitive diagnosis.

	Acute Pericarditis	Acute Myocardial Infarction
Diagnostic Tests		
Electrocardiogram	Diffuse ST-elevation; PR-segment depression in all leads except AVR	ST-segments elevated only in the infarct leads
Chest X-ray	Normal	Normal (may be sign of heart failure depending on extent of infarct, including pulmonary vascular congestion, interstitial edema, and cardiomegaly)
Echocardiogram	Normal function; pericardial effusion may be present	Akinesis or abnormal wall motion in infarct region
Cardiac catheterization	Normal	Coronary artery disease; akinesis on ventriculogram
Computed tomography	Normal; pericardial effusion may be identified	Normal
Clinical Findings		
Erythrocyte sedimentation rate (normal 0 to 30 mm/hour)	Elevated	Normal
Heart failure	Absent unless cardiac tamponade present	Absent unless large infarct
Pericardial friction rub	Present	Absent
Chest pain	Positional; worsens with inspiration not exertion; not relieved with nitroglycerin	Exertional; relieved with nitroglycerin; unaffected by respiration or position

Constrictive Pericarditis	Restrictive Cardiomyopathy
Low QRS voltage; atrial fibrillation (one-third of patients)	Frequent ventricular ectopy
Normal or mildly enlarged heart; calcification of the pericardium detected in half of patients	Normal or mildly enlarged heart; signs of congestive failure, including pleural effusions, pulmonary vascular congestion, and pulmonary edema
Thickened pericardium (may be difficult to observe); small ventricular cavities; normal systolic contraction; abrupt, early termination of diastole	Normal systolic function; rigid ventricles; normal ventricular cavity size; impaired diastolic filling
Equalization of CVP, PAD, and wedge pressures; early diastolic filling with abrupt cessation; early right atrial emptying with abrupt cessation	Impaired diastolic filling
Thickened pericardium	Normal pericardium
Normal or elevated	Normal
Signs of right ventricular failure more prominent than left ventricular failure	Signs of left ventricular failure more prominent than right ventricular failure
Absent	Absent
Absent	Absent

severe pericarditis until the anti-inflammatory agents become effective.

• Treat fever with aspirin, cool packs, and alcohol baths.

• Administer oxygen therapy, as needed, for patients with dyspnea.

• Discontinue medications that can cause pericarditis, especially procainamide, hydralazine, and diphenylhydantoin.

Activity limitations and rest

Vigorous physical activity increases the interaction of the inflamed pericardial layers, producing increased inflammation and pain. Rest is necessary to reduce inflammation and pain.

Nursing measures include:

• Provide bed rest or reduction of physical activity as guided by the patient's comfort status.

• Position the patient with the head elevated. Semi-Fowler's or high-Fowler's position may be more comfortable than lying flat.

• Administer a sedative, as needed, to reduce anxiety.

Preventing complications

The most severe complications of acute pericarditis are pericardial effusion, cardiac tamponade, and constrictive pericarditis (see *Complications of acute pericarditis,* pages 499 and 500).

Nursing measures are outlined below.

• Avoid anticoagulants to prevent the development of bloody pericardial effusion.

• Take necessary measures to treat the underlying cause of the pericarditis if it has been isolated and is treatable (such as more intensive dialysis for uremic patients or antimicrobial therapy for tuberculosis patients).

• Monitor for early signs of cardiac tamponade.

• Monitor the effects of diuretic therapy in patients with pericardial effusion, including daily weight, intake and output, and assessment of dyspnea.

Complications of acute pericarditis

Acute pericarditis can lead to pericardial effusion, cardiac tamponade, or chronic constrictive pericarditis, as discussed below.

Pericardial effusion

The inflammatory characteristics of pericarditis often cause an increase in the volume of pericardial fluid. Normally, 15 to 50 ml of fluid is found in the pericardial sac and drained via the thoracic duct. Volumes in excess of 50 ml constitute a pericardial effusion. Many pericardial effusions are asymptomatic and require no treatment. The factors that determine the severity of symptoms associated with pericardial effusion include:
• the volume of fluid
• the rate of fluid accumulation
• the compliance of the pericardium (its ability to handle the volume without increasing the intrapericardial pressure).

The volume of fluid constituting a pericardial effusion can be quantified on echocardiogram. The clinical features of a large pericardial effusion include muffled heart tones, absent or decreased intensity of pericardial friction rub, and dullness to percussion of the posterior left lung (Ewart's sign).

Therapy is directed at treating the underlying cause, if one has been identified and is treatable. Only symptomatic effusions are treated because uncomplicated effusions are reabsorbed and resolve without treatment.

Specific nursing interventions include the following:
• Auscultate heart sounds for early detection of complications.
• Monitor continuous electrocardiogram for arrhythmias.
• Administer diuretics to reduce the size of the effusion, as ordered.
• Assist in pericardiocentesis for drainage and analysis of the fluid.
• Prepare the patient and family for the possibility of surgical subxiphoid drainage of the pericardium with drainage tube placement.

Cardiac tamponade

Cardiac tamponade results when pericardial fluid accumulates under high pressure and produces compression of the cardiac chambers and diastolic collapse of the ventricles. The impairment of ventricular filling causes venous engorgement with signs of right-sided heart failure and hemodynamic instability with severely decreased cardiac output, which causes death if untreated.

Definitive diagnosis is made by echocardiogram, which reveals:
• increase in right ventricular dimension and decrease in left ventricular dimension during inspiration
• abnormal excursion of the anterior mitral valve leaflet during inspiration
• right atrial collapse
• right ventricular diastolic collapse
• left atrial collapse
• increase of tricuspid valve flow and decrease of mitral valve flow during inspiration
• engorgement of the vena cava.

Clinical signs of cardiac tamponade include:
• hemodynamic instability, including hypotension and low cardiac output
• distended neck veins
• equalization of the right atrial pressures and pulmonary artery diastolic or wedge pressures
• sinus tachycardia

(continued)

Complications of acute pericarditis *(continued)*

- pulsus paradoxus
- dyspnea.

Emergency treatment includes the following nursing measures:
- Monitor hemodynamic parameters using a pulmonary artery catheter for early detection (pulmonary artery systolic, diastolic, and right atrial pressures equilibrate in tamponade).
- Administer intravenous volume to maintain hemodynamic stability until definitive therapy is started.
- Obtain an arterial blood gas analysis and continuous oxygen saturation to assess ventilatory compromise.
- Provide emotional support to relieve extreme anxiety.
- Avoid administering inotropic drugs (dopamine). These agents are ineffective and may be harmful in supporting blood pressure because the hemodynamic instability is the result of impaired diastolic filling with adequate systolic function.
- Assist in needle pericardiocentesis or percutaneous placement of pigtail drainage catheters.
- Prepare the patient for surgical subxiphoid drainage if a large effusion recurs.
- Be aware that in rare instances, surgical excision of the pericardium is required for recurrent effusion or tamponade.
- Send pericardial fluid for bacterial, viral, and acid-fast bacilli cultures.

Chronic constrictive pericarditis

Constrictive pericarditis follows acute pericarditis when pericardial fluid forms into fibrous scar tissue that adheres to the pericardial layers. The fibrotic pericardium allows for normal systolic contraction, but diastolic filling is impaired because of the inability of the heart to fully dilate with the increased volume. Signs of right-sided heart failure occur during the early stages of constrictive pericarditis, followed by a reduction of stroke volume with signs of left-sided heart failure in later stages.

Definitive diagnosis is made by evidence of a thickened pericardium on CT or MRI scans or in the cardiac catheterization laboratory. Constrictive pericarditis is associated with several classic physical findings, including:
- Kussmaul's sign, an increase in systemic venous pressure during inspiration (this can be observed by assessing the jugular neck veins during the respiratory cycle)
- presence of a diastolic knock, a third heart sound that represents filling of the noncompliant ventricle
- narrow pulse pressure due to the diastolic impairment and normal systolic function
- findings of right-sided failure more severe than left-sided failure
- lessening of dyspnea (may be reported by patient).

Constrictive pericarditis is a progressive and debilitating disease. The only effective treatment of constrictive pericarditis is surgical excision of the pericardium. Although pericardiectomy carries a 12% surgical mortality, most survivors experience symptomatic improvement. The procedure is reserved for patients who continue to have clinical deterioration despite diuretic and diet therapy. Symptomatic management of the heart failure with aggressive diuretic therapy and a low-sodium diet is often necessary before and shortly after surgery.

• Assist the physician in performing pericardiocentesis for drainage and analysis of pericardial fluid.
• Maintain patency of drainage tubes in patients who undergo surgical drainage of a pericardial effusion.
• Administer adequate intravenous volume to patients with cardiac tamponade to maintain stable hemodynamics until definitive treatment can be administered.
• Instruct the patient that pericardectomy may be performed for recurrent effusions or tamponade in those with chronic constrictive pericarditis.

Prognosis

Uncomplicated pericarditis is a self-limiting disease; however, treatment is mandated for symptomatic relief and to observe for and prevent complications. When pericardial effusion progresses to cardiac tamponade, death is imminent unless immediate interventions are implemented. Long-term prognosis depends on the cause of the pericarditis or effusion; however, idiopathic pericarditis has an excellent prognosis.

Discharge planning

Discharge planning centers around teaching the patient to observe for complications of the disease or its treatment. Considerations include:
• instructions about daily weights and the need to report any change of over 2 lb within 1 week
• teaching to always take NSAIDs with food and to report any significant gastrointestinal upset that occurs with the medication
• for those receiving steroids, instructions to observe for signs and symptoms of infection
• instructions regarding signs of hypokalemia and over-diuresis (for patients discharged on diuretics)
• need to immediately report recurrence of symptoms, especially pericardial pain or dyspnea
• instructions on limiting fluid intake and eating a no-added-salt diet until pericardiectomy is performed (for those with chronic constrictive pericarditis).

Peripheral vascular disease

Peripheral vascular disease (PVD) is characterized by a narrowing of the peripheral vasculature and changes in the normal blood clotting mechanism, which lead to tissue ischemia and necrosis. PVD can be acute or chronic and may affect either the arterial or the venous vasculature, primarily involving the lower extremities.

The leading cause of acute PVD is atherosclerosis, which results in clot formation within the arterial vasculature. Other causes include vasospastic conditions (such as Raynaud's disease), inflammatory processes (as in Buerger's disease), and conditions resulting in increased intramuscular compartment pressure (as in compartment syndrome). Chronic PVD is most commonly associated with atherosclerosis and diabetes mellitus.

Acute and chronic arterial PVD affects men and women equally over age 50. Acute PVD involving the venous system occurs in about one-third of those over age 40 who have had recent surgery or acute myocardial infarction (MI). (See *Risk factors for the development of peripheral vascular disease*, page 503, for other predisposing factors.)

Pathophysiology

PVD occurs when either a thrombus forms within a vessel or an embolism lodges within a previously unoccluded vessel. Typically, thrombus formation occurs with venous stasis, hypercoagulability, or injury to the vessel wall. Acute PVD usually follows local vessel trauma or an acute systemic injury that affects the normal circulation. Once a vessel is injured, a thrombus forms from the accumulation of platelets, which aggregate and adhere to the endothelium. Fibrin causes further trapping of white and red blood cells, increasing the thrombus size. This results in a corresponding decrease in mean and pulse pressures within the distal

Risk factors for the development of peripheral vascular disease

The following conditions contribute to the development of peripheral vascular disease to the arterial or venous circulatory system.

Acute arterial occlusion
• Conditions that encourage thrombosis formation:
—sepsis
—low cardiac output states
—hypotension
—aneurysm
—aortic dissection
—bypass grafts
—atherosclerotic PVD
• Conditions that encourage emboli formation:
—atrial fibrillation
—myocardial infarction
—ventricular aneurysms
—aortic or mitral stenosis
—prosthetic valves
—cardiomyopathy
—bacterial endocarditis
—postpartum state
—sepsis or febrile state
—hyperthyroidism
—thoracic aorta trauma
—cardiac catheterization

Acute venous occlusion
• Conditions that encourage thrombosis formation and pulmonary emboli (a potential complication of PVD):
—orthopedic or gynecologic cancer
—abdominal, cardiac, renal, or splenic surgical procedures
—congestive heart failure
—myocardial infarction
—cardiomyopathy
—immobilization from bed rest
—prior development of deep vein thrombosis
—pregnancy
—postpartum cesarean section
—trauma
—estrogen therapy or oral contraceptive use
—age over 50
—varicose veins
—obesity

arteries and a decrease in tissue perfusion and oxygenation, leading to cell hypoxia and necrosis.

In acute PVD caused by an embolism, the wall of the occluded artery usually shows no sign of disease. In such cases, the embolism is thought to originate from the heart, probably as a result of atrial fibrillation, MI, or valvular disease; it then migrates and lodges within a vessel. Because collateral circulation is not commonly present in those with PVD caused by an embolism, limb hypoxia and muscle necrosis may appear within 2 to 3 hours after vessel occlusion. If left undiagnosed and treated, the limb may become paralyzed, with muscle and joint stiffness indicative of rigor mortis. This signifies irreversible damage and the need for amputation to prevent a total body reaction to the byproducts of muscle destruction and systemic sepsis.

In chronic PVD caused by atherosclerosis, the vessels have been lined with plaque, leading to vessel occlusion. In those with diabetes mellitus, the vessels have undergone epithelial lining changes. This, coupled with alterations in normal platelet and clotting factor functions, causes platelets to adhere to vessel walls, thereby narrowing the vessel lumen and reducing blood flow to the extremity. Over time, this mechanism produces vessel occlusion; however, lower-extremity blood flow is usually sustained by collateral circulation.

Clinical assessment
The clinical findings associated with PVD depend on the presence or absence of collateral circulation and whether the episode is caused by thrombosis or embolism. Based on the patient's past medical history and current symptoms, the nurse can plan care appropriate for the acute episode.

History
When assessing the history, the nurse should obtain the following information:
• history of cardiac problems
• history of atherosclerosis, diabetes mellitus, or deep vein thrombosis
• history of pain (usually described as a tightening or pressure or a sharp cramp in the calves or buttocks during ambulation that quickly disappears with rest; indicative of intermittent claudication)
• recent surgical procedures, including cesarean section
• recent prolonged immobilization
• use of estrogen or oral contraceptives
• history of smoking.

Physical findings
Physical findings typically depend on the cause and whether the condition is acute or chronic.

Acute arterial occlusion

The classic signs of acute arterial occlusion include:
• pain resulting from ischemia
• paresthesia of the affected limb caused by reduced blood flow to the peripheral nerves
• loss of position sense when the toes of the affected extremity are extended or flexed
• poikilothermia or reduced temperature of the affected extremity
• paralysis of the affected extremity
• pallor of the affected extremity below the level of the arterial occlusion
• pulselessness of the affected extremity.

Chronic intermittent arterial occlusion

The patient may have any of the following signs:
• intermittent claudication
• pain at rest (usually occurs during sleep and causes the patient to awaken and dangle the legs or walk around)
• coldness of the affected extremity
• hairless, dry, and shiny extremity
• pallor of the extremity when elevated and ruborous when dangling or dependent
• ulcers on the heel, outer ankle area, toes, or dorsum of the foot of the affected extremity (may be painful and typically appear pale gray; toenails may be hypertrophied from chronic reduced arterial blood flow)
• diminished or absent pulses of the affected extremity.

Acute venous occlusion

The patient may have any of the following signs:
• pain of the affected extremity (usually in the region of the thrombosis)
• swelling of the affected extremity below the level of the thrombosis
• redness of the affected extremity around the region of the thrombosis

• palpable cord along the occluded vessel (indicative of vessel engorgement and blockage of normal blood flow)
• positive Homan's sign
• warmth of the affected extremity
• low-grade fever.

Chronic intermittent venous occlusion
Typical findings include:
• lower-extremity ulcers (venous stasis ulcers) usually located on the inner ankle (may be mildly painful, with a pink base and irregular hyperpigmented edges)
• toughened, mottled, or hyperpigmented lower-extremity skin that may be thicker around the ankle
• pain (usually described as an ache or cramp of the affected extremity) that occasionally improves with activity and is relieved with elevation
• presence of pulses over the affected extremity
• edema of the affected extremity at nighttime, particularly in areas of lesions.

Diagnosis
The diagnosis of PVD focuses on determining the cause of the occlusion and preventing further lower-extremity tissue damage. Both noninvasive and invasive tests are used (see *Diagnostic tests for peripheral vascular disease,* pages 507 and 508).

Treatment and care
The successful treatment of PVD depends on the extent of the occlusion, the presence of any underlying health conditions that caused the thrombosis or embolism, and the efforts taken to reduce future occlusive episodes. Depending on the severity of the occlusion, surgery may be indicated.

The initial goals for a patient with PVD are to prevent an existing thrombosis from becoming an embolism, provide pain relief, prevent the formation of a new thrombosis, and restore adequate circulation to the af-

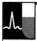

Diagnostic tests for peripheral vascular disease

The following chart reviews the diagnostic tests commonly performed on the patient with peripheral vascular disease.

Diagnostic Test	Vessel Occluded	Findings
Doppler ultrasound	Artery	Helps detect blood flow in the absence of a palpable pulse. Audible flow pattern varies with respiration in normal vessels; no flow pattern heard in occluded vessels.
	Vein	Helps diagnose deep vein thrombosis. Positive findings include no flow pattern change with respiration and no flow pattern heard over a major vein. False-positive results can occur after extremity trauma, edema, inflammation, and arthritis.
Ankle-brachial index	Artery	A ratio of a Doppler-recorded systolic dorsalis pedis or posterior tibial pressure compared with the brachial blood pressure; the value is obtained by dividing the ankle systolic pressure by the brachial systolic pressure. Normal values are between 0.8 and 1.2. A value between 0.4 and 0.8 indicates intermittent arterial occlusion; between 0.0 and 0.4, severe arterial occlusion.
Angiography	Artery	Accurately pinpoints area of occlusion as the inability of the radioactive contrast to advance through an occluded vessel. Identifies presence of collateral circulation and atherosclerotic plaques.
Plethysmography	Vein	This test examines the venous system by recording volume changes in a limb during venous filling and emptying. False-negative results can occur if the patient cannot sustain a position that causes blood to pool in the deep veins of the lower extremities or cannot lie still during the procedure. False-positive results occur when excessive blood pools in the lower extremities, as seen in right ventricular heart failure, vascular compression from abdominal masses, or COPD.

(continued)

Diagnostic tests for peripheral vascular disease *(continued)*

Diagnostic Test	Vessel Occluded	Findings
Venography	Vein	The standard for detecting deep vein thrombosis. Positive findings include filling defects, sharp termination of a column of contrast, and nonfilling of the deep vein system.
Pulmonary arteriography	Pulmonary artery	The only conclusive diagnostic test for pulmonary emboli. Positive findings include identification of an intraluminal filling defect or a sharp cutoff of lobar or segmental vessels.
V/Q scanning	Pulmonary artery	Useful in diagnosing a pulmonary emboli. A mismatch between the ventilation and perfusion scans (adequate ventilation but without gas exchange in the vasculature) suggests the presence of a pulmonary emboli.

fected extremity (see *Key nursing interventions for the patient with peripheral vascular disease,* page 509).

Arterial bypass grafting

In arterial bypass grafting, the patient's own saphenous vein is used to reroute the blood flow around the occluded artery, restoring blood flow to the affected extremity. If the saphenous vein is found to be insufficient to withstand grafting, synthetic materials are used. The most commonly encountered bypasses on the critical care unit are aorto-bifemoral, aorta-iliac, femoral-femoral, and femoral-popliteal.

Nursing management of the patient with a bypass graft includes the following:
• Evaluate the integrity of the bypass graft by assessing the color, temperature, sensation, movement, amount of edema, and peripheral pulses of the extremity every hour for the first 12 hours, then every 4 hours. Also assess the incision site for redness, swelling, and drainage every hour for the first 12 hours, then every 4 hours.

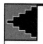

ESSENTIAL ELEMENTS

Key nursing interventions for the patient with peripheral vascular disease

The following chart highlights interventions typically performed for a peripheral vascular disease.

Prevent existing thrombosis from becoming an embolism and restore adequate circulation to affected extremity

Prevent embolic formation	Provide pain relief	Prevent recurrence
• Administer fibrino-lytics, as ordered. • Monitor for bleeding. • Assess for allergic reaction to streptokinase infusion, if applicable. • Keep aminocaproic acid at the bedside as an antagonist to thrombolytic therapy (prevents further plasmin generation and plasmin lysis to control hemorrhage). • Inspect affected extremity every 2 hours. • Position for comfort. • Provide wound care, as prescribed, if ulcers are present. • Monitor for signs of pulmonary emboli. • Apply pressure to venipuncture sites for 15 to 30 minutes. • Assess for bleeding through GI and GU tracts.	• Elevate the foot of bed 6 inches to relieve venous engorgement and associated pain (unless contraindicated). • Apply warm soaks if patient has a venous occlusion. • Administer analgesics, as prescribed.	• Monitor PT/PTT levels. • Adjust medication therapy, as ordered. • Begin oral anticoagulants, as ordered. • Instruct patient on long-term anticoagulant therapy. • Instruct patient on home safety measures, such as avoiding the use of a razor, bumping of legs, and wearing incorrect-fitting shoes. • Teach lifestyle changes to prevent recurrence, including smoking cessation information. • Instruct patient on daily activity and exercise program and weight reduction, if indicated. • Instruct patient on proper foot care.

• Promote circulation by turning and repositioning the patient every 2 hours. Remind the patient to avoid crossing the legs or bending the legs at a severe angle. Add a foot board to the bed to promote optimal circulation.

Embolectomy

During this procedure, the blood clot is removed and the atherosclerotic plaque along the inner arterial wall is stripped. Specific nursing measures are listed below.
• Assess the surgical site for redness, swelling, or drainage.
• Monitor vital signs.
• Assess the skin color, temperature, and peripheral pulses of the affected extremity.
• Encourage movement of the affected extremity.

Percutaneous transluminal angioplasty (PTA, balloon angioplasty)

This invasive, nonsurgical procedure is found to successfully increase the lumen of the affected vessel. During this procedure, a catheter with a distal inflatable balloon ruptures the occlusion and stretches the artery away from the occlusion, resulting in increased blood flow to the extremity.

Nursing care of the patient who has undergone a PTA includes the following:
• Assess the site for signs of reocclusion and bleeding, as evidenced by edema, ecchymosis, or hematoma formation.
• Monitor peripheral pulses every 15 to 30 minutes for 1 hour, then every hour for 4 hours, followed by once every 4 hours.
• Assess for sudden changes in limb color, temperature, muscle cramping, pain, and motor or sensory changes.
• Monitor heparin or other antiembolitic medication therapy; report prothrombin time (PT)/partial thromboplastin time (PTT) values and adjust infusion accordingly.

Prevention and treatment of deep vein thrombosis

The goals for patients with PVD secondary to deep vein thrombosis are to prevent the formation of additional thrombosis, prevent existing thrombosis from becoming an embolism, prevent bleeding complications from anticoagulant therapy, relieve pain, reduce anxiety, and educate the patient to avoid future deep vein thrombosis episodes.

An acute, often fatal complication of deep vein thrombosis is pulmonary embolism. A portion of the clot within the affected vein breaks off, enters the general venous circulation, and lodges within the pulmonary circulation, decreasing pulmonary blood flow. A pulmonary embolism should be suspected if the patient has sudden onset of chest pain with respiration, cough, hemoptysis, diaphoresis, dyspnea, and apprehension. The patient typically has a PO_2 of less than 80 mm Hg because of reduced oxygen reaching the arterial blood and decreased PCO_2 because of hyperventilation.

Nursing interventions for the patient with a deep vein thrombosis include:
• Maintain the patient on bed rest for 5 to 7 days while providing support to respiratory, integumentary, gastrointestinal, and genitourinary systems.
• Elevate the foot of the bed 6 inches while supporting the popliteal area.
• Use lower-extremity elastic stockings or wraps; unwrap and assess pulses and skin every 4 to 8 hours.
• Provide warm soaks to affected area every 4 hours.
• Monitor the effectiveness of analgesic therapy.
• Monitor the effectiveness of I.V. heparin therapy by evaluating the PT/PTT level every 4 hours. Report the PT/PTT levels and adjust the heparin infusion accordingly.

Venous ligation surgery

In the case of an extensive occlusion or multiple recurrences of an occlusion within a vein, venous ligation surgery may be indicated. During this procedure, the great saphenous vein is ligated close to the femoral junction and the occluded veins are stripped through small incisions placed in the groin, above and below the knee, and the ankle.

Nursing management of the patient who has undergone venous ligation surgery includes the following:

• Maintain the patient lying down immediately after surgery, with the affected extremity elevated to promote venous return.

• Assist with ambulation (usually 24 hours after surgery), and instruct the patient to avoid standing still.

Thrombolytic therapy

Medications helpful in treating venous or arterial thrombosis include streptokinase and urokinase. These drugs, which are only administered in a critical care area, can be given through a peripheral vein or an intraarterial catheter. Prior to administration, the nurse must obtain a baseline PT/PTT, thrombin time, platelet count, hematocrit, and white blood cell (WBC) count. In addition, recent streptococcal infection must be identified because this may reduce the effectiveness of the infusion in patients who may be resistant to streptokinase as a result of prior streptococcal infections. (See *Medication therapy for peripheral vascular disease,* pages 513 and 514, for more information.)

Prognosis

The mortality rate for patients with acute arterial occlusion is 25% to 30%, mainly because of the associated cardiac disease. About 5% to 25% of patients who survive the acute episode lose the affected extremity to amputation. The recovery for the patient with acute deep vein thrombosis is good, with most returning to normal activity within 3 to 6 weeks. Of those who develop a pulmonary embolism, the mortality rate is 5% to 8%. The prognosis for chronic venous occlusion depends on the patient's willingness to comply with necessary lifestyle and dietary changes in conjunction with long-term anticoagulant therapy.

MAJOR DRUGS

Medication therapy for peripheral vascular disease

The following chart identifies medications commonly used to treat arterial or venous peripheral vascular disease.

Medication	Dose	Nursing Considerations
Fibrinolytics		
Streptokinase	250,000 IU I.V. load over 30 minutes; 100,000 IU/hour for 24 to 72 hours	• Assess patient's prior exposure to streptococcal infections. • Monitor temperature throughout administration, and administer antipyretics, as ordered (streptokinase is pyrogenic). • Monitor for allergic reaction, and administer antihistamines and/or steroids, as prescribed. • Monitor thrombin time; time of 2 to 5 times the control indicates adequate clot lysis. • Administer from glass container because plastic inactivates medication. • Monitor for signs of hemorrhage.
Urokinase	4,400 IU/kg I.V. load over 10 minutes; 4,400 IU/kg/hour for 72 hours	• Monitor temperature throughout administration, and administer antipyretics, as ordered (urokinase is pyrogenic). • Monitor thrombin time; time of 2 to 5 times the control indicates adequate clot lysis. • Monitor for signs of hemorrhage.
Anticoagulants		
Heparin	5,000 units I.V. load; 20,000 to 30,000 units/day at 0.5 units/kg/minute in 5% dextrose or normal saline solution	• Monitor PTT to 1½ to 2½ times the control in seconds. • If patient scheduled for invasive procedure, discontinue infusion 4 to 6 hours prior to the study, as prescribed. • Monitor for signs of hemorrhage. • Maintain protamine sulfate at the bedside in the event of a hemorrhage; this antagonist neutralizes the effects of heparin.

(continued)

Medication therapy for peripheral vascular disease *(continued)*

Medication	Dose	Nursing Considerations
Anticoagulants *(continued)*		
Heparin *(continued)*		• Monitor peripheral infusion site for signs of tissue necrosis and notify physician. Discontinue the heparin and switch to another anticoagulant, if necessary.
Warfarin sodium	10 to 15 mg/day until prothrombin time therapeutic; 2 to 10 mg/day maintenance	• Administer as prescribed; will be administered along with the heparin infusion because of a slow onset of action. • Monitor prothrombin time to therapeutic range of 2 to 2.5 times the control time. • Monitor for signs of hemorrhage, and instruct patient to contact physician after discharge if any bleeding develops. • Instruct patient to avoid foods rich in vitamin K, a warfarin sodium antagonist.

Discharge planning

Patients recovering from an acute arterial or venous occlusion will require long-term anticoagulant therapy. The nurse should focus on:
• reviewing with the patient the actions, dosage, frequency, and side effects of the prescribed anticoagulant
• the importance of monitoring the effectiveness of the anticoagulant by keeping appointments at the prescribed intervals
• consulting social services about the needs for assistive devices at home, any financial concerns the patient may have, and the patient's support systems.

For patients with PVD affecting arterial circulation, the nurse should focus on:
• patient-teaching measures to promote arterial perfusion, such as maintaining lower extremities in a dependent position, keeping extremities warm, and avoid-

ing the use of vasoconstrictive substances (such as caffeine and cigarettes)
• instructions and information on a daily walking program
• the need to avoid tight, restrictive clothing over the lower extremities
• instructions on inspecting lower extremities daily for ulcers
• instructions on proper foot care
• the importance of an adequate, well-balanced diet to maintain tissue integrity and promote wound healing.

For patients with PVD affecting venous circulation, the nurse should focus on:
• the need to avoid prolonged sitting or standing
• the need to keep lower extremities slightly elevated when sitting
• the need to wear elastic hose or stockings
• avoiding massaging a painful leg area after prolonged sitting or standing
• instructions on when the patient should contact the physician.

Pneumonia

Pneumonia is a parenchymal lung disorder caused by alveolar inflammation and fluid collection in the air spaces that results in a decrease in the ventilation/perfusion ratio. Despite advances in antibiotic therapy and medical technology, pneumonia remains a common and serious illness. It may be characterized as a community- or hospital-acquired (nosocomial) disease.

Community-acquired pneumonia is the sixth leading cause of death in the United States and the leading cause of death from infectious disease. As many as 4 million cases of community-acquired pneumonia are diagnosed each year, and 20% of these patients are hospitalized. The mortality rate for hospitalized patients is estimated at 25%. The most common causative organisms of community-acquired pneumonia are *Strepto-*

coccus pneumoniae (leading cause), *Legionella pneumophila, Staphylococcus aureus,* varicella, *Mycoplasma pneumoniae,* and *Haemophilus influenzae.*

Nosocomial pneumonias account for 18% to 22% of hospital-acquired infections, with the majority of cases occurring in critical care areas. Modes of transmission include direct contact with the hands of hospital personnel, bacterial translocation, and direct contact with contaminated equipment. Gram-negative enteric bacteria, such as *Escherichia coli* and species of *Klebsiella, Enterobacter, Proteus, Pseudomonas,* and *Serratia,* are the most frequently diagnosed microorganisms. The mortality of nosocomial pneumonia is estimated at 50%. Because of its high morbidity and mortality, prevention of nosocomial pneumonia is critical. It is estimated that up to 50% of all nosocomial pneumonias can be prevented.

Pneumonia may also be characterized by its causative organism. The types of pneumonia as classified by causative organisms include bacterial, viral, fungal, and protozoan. Risk factors of bacterial pneumonia include chronic obstructive pulmonary disease, alcoholism, increased age, multiple myeloma, recent influenza, diabetes, immunodeficiency, and mechanical ventilation. Acquired immunodeficiency syndrome (AIDS), lymphomas, organ transplantation, and pregnancy are risk factors of viral pneumonia. AIDS and immunosuppression are risk factors for fungal and protozoal pneumonias. The following factors also are associated with increased risk: stress, malnutrition, dehydration, smoking, bed rest, chronic disease, steroid treatment, and aspiration (see the entry on "Aspiration").

Pathophysiology

The pathophysiology of pneumonia may differ slightly, depending on the causative organism. For a patient to develop pneumonia in the lower respiratory tract, which is normally sterile, a defect in host defenses, a virulent organism, or an overwhelming inoculation must occur.

In general, pathogens may enter the lower respiratory tract by inhalation, aspiration, vascular dissemination, or direct contact with contaminated equipment, such as suction catheters. Once pathogens enter the lower respiratory tract, colonization and infection develop. This infection results in pulmonary inflammation, with or without secretions, a process that produces an area of low ventilation with normal perfusion. This ventilation/perfusion (V/Q) mismatching increases as exudate accumulates in the alveoli and the lungs consolidate.

Occasionally, hypoxic vasoconstriction may decrease blood flow to the affected area. Intrapulmonary shunting with atelectasis and hypoxemia result. Decreased functional reserve capacity (the lung volume at the end of a quiet expiration) and increased work of breathing follow. Ventilation may further decrease as a result of pleural effusions, which further restrict lung expansion. Increased capillary permeability as well as products of inflammation (cells, protein) contribute to the development of pleural effusions in the patient with pneumonia. Tracheobronchial edema and increased secretions increase both airway resistance and the work of breathing. Airway obstruction may also occur as a result of edema or mucus. If untreated, pneumonia may lead to pulmonary fibrosis, necrosis, and loss of functional tissue.

Viral pneumonia, which is generally community-acquired, is a virulent form of pneumonia, as the only cure is support of oxygenation. Cellular changes that occur include inflammation of the alveoli and pulmonary interstices. Severe respiratory distress, cough, chest pain, hypoxemia, and hemoptysis frequently occur. Severe viral pneumonia progresses rapidly (in under 24 hours), presenting as adult respiratory distress syndrome and should be treated in the same manner (see the entry on "Adult Respiratory Distress Syndrome").

Varicella pneumonia is often seen as a complication of severe chickenpox in adults, occurring in 38% of cases. Pregnant women are especially susceptible as a result of their immunosuppression and decreased lung capacity. Pulmonary symptoms begin about 2 days after the original vesicle eruption.

Pneumocystis carinii pneumonia is a complication of AIDS and immunosuppression (generally from organ transplantation). In a normal child or adult, *P. carinii* is not highly virulent, and infection is usually asymptomatic. However, in immunosuppressed patients, it can cause virulent lung disease. Signs and symptoms include fever, shortness of breath, and a nonproductive cough. *P. carinii* often is the first and most common AIDS-indicator opportunistic infection in patients with human immunodeficiency virus.

Clinical assessment

A thorough clinical assessment is essential for all patients in critical care areas. The mere admission to the critical care area places the patient at increased risk for nosocomial pneumonia because of altered defense mechanisms.

History

Information to solicit from the patient or family includes:
• history, character, onset, and duration of cough, fever, chest pain, and sputum production
• amount, color, and consistency of sputum
• treatments initiated at home
• exposure to pulmonary irritants (asbestos, smoking)
• exposure to infection.

Physical findings

For a list of physical findings commonly associated with specific types of pneumonia, see *Clinical findings of pneumonia,* pages 519 and 520. In addition, be aware that immunocompromised patients may not respond with typical immune responses, such as fever, chills, and increased white blood cell (WBC) count. Also, because normal physiologic changes of aging produce decreased vital capacity and decreased residual vol-

Clinical findings of pneumonia

The causative organism, physical findings, medical treatment, and complications related to specific types of pneumonia are included in the chart below.

Causative Organism	Physical Findings	Medical Treatment	Complications
Bacterial pneumonia • *Streptococcus pneumoniae* • *Staphylococcus aureus* • *Haemophilus influenzae* • *Pseudomonas aeruginosa* • *Escherichia coli* • *Klebsiella pneumoniae* • *Legionella pneumophila*	• Pertinent history • Fever and chills • Cough with purulent sputum • Infiltrates and local consolidation on chest X-ray • Leukocytosis • Pleuritic chest pain • Crackles, wheezes • Decreased breath sounds • Decreased P_{O_2} • Egophony and bronchophony over consolidation • Diaphoresis • Hemoptysis	• Depends on presentation and patient history • Broad-spectrum gram-positive and gram-negative antibiotics • Supportive oxygenation • Bronchodilators • Change to pathogen-specific antibiotic after sensitivity testing	• Bacteremia • Meningitis • Endocarditis • Pericarditis • Empyema • Cavity formation • Respiratory failure • Sepsis • ARDS • Death
Viral pneumonia • Cytomegalovirus • Varicella zoster • Herpes simplex	• Pertinent history • Abrupt onset and rapid progression • Dry cough with mucoid or blood-tinged sputum • Tachypnea and dyspnea • Crackles, wheezes • No consolidation • Fever • Decreased P_{O_2}	• Acyclovir • Supportive oxygenation	• Bronchiolitis • Respiratory failure • ARDS • Death
Fungal pneumonia • *Candida albicans* • *Aspergillus fumigatus* • *Cryptococcus*	• Pertinent history • Acute onset • Fever • Chest pain • Dyspnea • Prostration • Weight loss	• Amphotericin B • Supportive oxygenation • Diflucan	• Necrotizing cavity formation • Fibrosis • Emphysema • Respiratory failure • ARDS • Death *(continued)*

Clinical findings of pneumonia *(continued)*

Causative Organism	Physical Findings	Medical Treatment	Complications
Protozoan pneumonia • *Pneumocystis carinii*	• Pertinent history • Sudden or gradual onset • Hypoxemic normocapnic respiratory failure ($PO_2 < 40$) • Dry cough • Dyspnea • Fever • Malaise	• Trimethoprim-sulfamethoxazole • Pentamidine isethionate • Supportive oxygenation	• Pneumothorax • Respiratory failure • ARDS • Death

ume, elderly patients may present with mental confusion, tachycardia, and dyspnea.

Diagnosis

The diagnosis of pneumonia is made on the basis of clinical manifestations, radiology changes, and microbiology data (including arterial blood gas results and WBC counts) (see *Diagnostic tests and findings in pneumonia,* page 521).

Treatment and care

The primary goals of treatment for the patient with pneumonia are to optimize oxygenation and ventilation, promote clearance of secretions, treat the infection, and prevent the spread of infection (see *Key nursing interventions for patients with pneumonia,* page 522).

Complications of pneumonia include respiratory failure, pleural effusions, pulmonary abscess, sepsis, and right ventricular failure. They may lead to chronic ventilator dependence, ARDS, multiple organ dysfunction syndrome, or death. Generally, the complications depend on the causative organism, as well as the patients state of health prior to infection. Prevention of nosocomial pneumonia is a significant contribution of the critical care nurse when caring for the critically ill

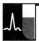

DIAGNOSTIC TESTS
Diagnostic tests and findings in pneumonia

Precise clinical diagnosis of pneumonia is difficult in the absence of a standard diagnostic test. However, one or more clinical findings, including dyspnea, wheezes, fever, and secretions, are present in most patients.

Laboratory tests
Sputum specimen
Gram stains and bacterial cultures to establish the cause of pneumonia have no proven value. Their main value is to exclude certain microorganisms with characteristic smears and cultures. Sputum examination for bacterial infection rules out organisms rather than diagnosing the offending organism.

Sputum culture and sensitivity testing
These tests are helpful for identifying resistance to particular antibiotics.

Complete blood count
This test has marginal value for diagnosing pneumonia, generally indicating only that infection is present, not its location.

Radiology findings
Chest X-ray
Nonspecific pulmonary infiltrates are generally present. Conditions that also cause pulmonary infiltrates on X-ray include atelectasis, pulmonary edema, aspiration, hemorrhage, pleural effusion, and thromboembolism.

Pulmonary tests
Arterial blood gas analysis
Low PaO_2 with a high A-a gradient and pulmonary shunt is often demonstrated. During initial presentation, the $PaCO_2$ is generally low. This increases as the work of breathing increases.

Fiberoptic bronchoscopy
Bronchoalveolar lavage with a protected specimen brush increases the likelihood of obtaining positive cultures, although prior antibiotic treatment will decrease the success of this diagnostic test.

Pulmonary function tests
Decreased vital capacity, decreased functional reserve capacity, and decreased compliance are demonstrated with these tests.

patient (see *Preventing nosocomial pneumonia,* page 523).

Treatment of bacterial infection
Treatment of the infection with antibiotics is indicated. Empirical therapy is an acceptable approach, because it is often impossible to determine the cause of the pneumonia in a timely manner. Sputum culture and sensitivity results may take 48 to 72 hours before a definitive identification of the organism can be made. Often, no

ESSENTIAL ELEMENTS

Key nursing interventions for patients with pneumonia

The following flowchart highlights key interventions that typically are performed when a patient is diagnosed with pneumonia.

Achieve optimal pulmonary status		
Treat infection and prevent cross-infection	**Treat hypoxemia**	**Promote airway clearance**
• Obtain sputum cultures. • Administer antibiotics, as ordered. • Wash hands frequently, especially between patients. • Maintain sterility of artificial airway.	• Administer oxygen, as ordered. • Monitor oxygen saturation and ABG results. • Monitor intrapulmonary shunt. • Provide chemical and physical restraints to assist with ventilation, as necessary. • Ensure that patent airway is maintained.	• Adequately hydrate to thin secretions. • Suction as needed to remove secretions. • Humidify all supplemental oxygen. • Medicate for pain to facilitate turning; incentive spirometry; coughing, deep breathing; and chest physiotherapy. • Avoid cough suppressants if cough is productive.

organisms are defined. In these situations, treatment is based on clinical signs and symptoms.

Empirical therapy consists of selecting the most appropriate antibiotic on the basis of Gram stain results. Antibiotics that offer broad-spectrum coverage against gram-negative or gram-positive organisms should be chosen. Failure of the patient to improve, as indicated by chest X-ray, WBC counts, and amount of sputum produced, indicates a need to reevaluate the therapy. Improvement should be noted within 24 to 48 hours after beginning antibiotics. As culture and sensitivity

Preventing nosocomial pneumonia

The critical care nurse is the most important member of the health care team in preventing nosocomial pneumonia. The following nursing interventions are vital in preventing this complication.

Nursing goal	Interventions
Optimize ventilatory status	• Assess respiratory status every 2 to 4 hours. • Administer analgesics to control pain and to facilitate coughing and deep breathing. • Ensure adequate hydration. • Encourage the use of incentive spirometry. • Assist the mobilization of secretions by performing chest physiotherapy. • Administer humidified oxygen therapy, as ordered. • Turn patient at least every 2 hours. • Consider use of specialty beds.
Prevent respiratory tract contamination	• Use sterile fluids in ventilator humidifiers. • Date fluids when opening and discard after 24 hours. • Discard condensation in reservoir tubing. • Provide sterile suction, as needed, for secretion removal only. • Avoid use of saline flush when suctioning.
Prevent transmission of infection by health care provider	• Wash hands and wear gloves. • Ensure that disposable equipment (hand-held resuscitation bags, ventilator circuits) is replaced per institutional policy. • Ensure that reusable equipment is cleaned per institutional policy during and between patient use. • Monitor critical care unit for infecting organism that may be endemic. • Increase vigilance when special risk factors are present.

results are obtained, the antibiotics can be changed to specifically address the microorganism.

The following nursing interventions should be incorporated into the plan of care:

• Obtain sputum cultures prior to beginning antibiotic therapy, and monitor results.

• Administer antibiotics, as ordered. Monitor for adverse reactions to the antibiotics, including anaphylaxis, hives, rash, and renal and liver failure. In addition, monitor for antibiotic effectiveness.

• Practice good handwashing technique. Because the hands are the most frequent mode of transmission in all nosocomial infections, handwashing and gloving by hospital personnel is vital.

• Maintain sterility of artificial airway at all times.

Treatment of hypoxemia

Critically ill patients with pneumonia frequently require positive-pressure mechanical ventilation to correct the ventilation/perfusion mismatch that occurs. Appropriate nursing interventions are included below:

• Administer humidified oxygen, as ordered.

• Administer bronchodilators, as ordered, to dilate the alveoli to increase oxygenation.

• Maintain oxygen saturation greater than 95%.

• Monitor intrapulmonary shunt. Pulmonary shunting occurs when capillary blood flow is normal, but ventilation is completely lacking as a result of alveoli inflammation and consolidation. Therefore, unoxygenated hemoglobin is returned to the left atrium and mixes with oxygenated blood. In severe pneumonia, the hypoxemia that occurs is a result of this intrapulmonary shunt. Monitor the impact of therapy on the existing ventilation/perfusion mismatch to determine the most effective treatment. With appropriate treatment, the amount of shunt and resulting hypoxemia decreases.

• Monitor for signs of barotrauma secondary to mechanical ventilation.

• Provide anxiolytics and pain medications to decrease anxiety, splinting, and work of breathing to assist with oxygenation, if necessary.

• Apply restraints, if necessary, to prevent airway loss in a mechanically ventilated patient. Always provide anxiolytics or opioids with restraints.

• Ensure maintenance of patent airway.

• Provide frequent rest periods based on oxygen saturation. The patient should not desaturate greater than 4%.

Promote secretion clearance

Clearance of secretions is necessary to ensure an adequate airway and oxygenation and to improve the lungs. Interventions that promote secretion clearance include the following:

• Administer expectorants, as ordered. *Note:* Do not administer cough suppressants.
• Provide adequate systemic hydration.
• Humidify all supplemental oxygen.
• Prevent hypoventilation.
• Hyperoxygenate and suction, as needed; do not lavage. Current research demonstrates that lavaging causes hypoxemia even with hyperoxygenation. In addition, studies indicate that lavaging may actually wash bacteria into the lungs.
• Administer chest physical therapy, including percussion, postural drainage, coughing, and incentive spirometry.
• Turn the patient every 2 hours.
• Consider a specialty bed for secretion mobilization.
• Maintain the head of the bed at 45 degrees.

Prognosis

The prognosis for pneumonia depends on the causative organism, the patient's response to treatment, and the ability to maintain tissue oxygenation. For nosocomial pneumonia, the treatment of choice is prevention, as the mortality rate is 30% to 50% because of concomitant illness and antibiotic-resistant bacteria. In addition, significant changes in pathogens, immunosuppressive diseases, and antimicrobial resistance patterns have increased the virulence of community-acquired and nosocomial pneumonias.

Prevention of community-acquired pneumonia should also be emphasized. Prompt treatment with appropriate antibiotics improves mortality, as untreated pneumonia results in acute respiratory failure and septicemia. Prenatal care should include screening for a history of chickenpox and information regarding varicella pneumonia. Mortality increases with concomitant diseases, such as diabetes, malnutrition, immunosuppression, chronic lung disorders, and increasing patient age.

Discharge planning

Discharge planning for the patient with pneumonia depends on the functional status of the pulmonary system. Generally, patient teaching should focus on:
• prevention of infection
• obtaining extra rest and gradual increasing activity
• proper handwashing techniques
• proper administration of any drugs
• smoking cessation
• proper diet and fluid intake
• coping with any long-term effects, such as decreased lung function.

Ventilator-dependent patients may need long-term placement in an extended-care facility, although many return home after extensive family and patient assessments are completed.

Pneumothorax

Pneumothorax is a condition characterized by the presence of air between the visceral and parietal pleurae that leads to partial or complete lung collapse. As the amount of air increases, the tension also increases, trapping air within the intrapleural space. This causes the lung to further collapse, in some cases impeding venous return to the heart and causing a life-threatening tension pneumothorax.

Pneumothoraces are usually classified by their underlying etiology as either traumatic or spontaneous. A traumatic pneumothorax may be further classified as open (sucking chest wound) or closed (blunt or penetrating trauma). A spontaneous pneumothorax, which is also considered closed, can be further described as primary (idiopathic) or secondary (related to a specific disease). A tension pneumothorax can develop from either a spontaneous or a traumatic pneumothorax.

A spontaneous pneumothorax may occur from unknown causes or from an underlying pulmonary disease, such as chronic obstructive pulmonary disease (COPD) or acquired immunodeficiency syndrome (AIDS). A traumatic pneumothorax occurs when an external blunt force or penetrating injury causes air to enter the negative intrapleural space, as in a chest injury. In such injuries, the intrapleural space may fill with blood, causing a concurrent hemothorax. A massive hemothorax (loss of more than 1,500 ml of blood) can cause hemorrhagic shock and a tension pneumohemothorax.

Most pneumothoraces occur outside the clinical setting. Those that occur in a hospital usually result from complications associated with central line placement, needle thoracentesis, or positive-pressure mechanical ventilation (see *Risk factors for pneumothorax,* page 528).

Pathophysiology

Although the causes of traumatic and spontaneous pneumothorax vary greatly, their pathophysiologic effects are similar.

Traumatic pneumothorax

In most cases, traumatic pneumothorax results from a penetrating or blunt trauma; however, it can result from insertion of a central I.V. line, thoracic surgery, thoracentesis, or pleural or transbronchial biopsy. A penetrating injury from a stab wound, gunshot wound, or impaled object may result in either a traumatic open pneumothorax (sucking chest wound) or a closed pneumothorax or hemothorax. A blunt trauma may result from a car crash, a fall, or a crushing chest injury and cause a closed pneumothorax or hemothorax.

With a traumatic open chest wound, atmospheric air enters the negative-pressure (subatmospheric) pleural cavity from the external chest wound. As air enters the pleural cavity, the pressure becomes positive and the lung collapses on the affected side. This results in

Risk factors for pneumothorax

Spontaneous pneumothorax
• Bleb rupture
• Emphysematous bulla rupture
• AIDS
• Barotrauma from mechanical ventilation
• Necrotizing pneumonia
• Tubercular lesions eroding into pleural space
• Chest tube occlusion or malfunction
• Malignancy
• Rare etiologies:
—cocaine use
—high altitudes
—diving-related injuries
—lymphangial myxomatosis
—ankylosing spondylitis
—menstruation

Traumatic pneumothorax
• Penetrating chest injury (gunshot, knife, foreign object)
• Blunt chest injury (falls, vehicular crashes)
• Chest surgery
• Insertion of a central line
• Needle thoracentesis

substantial decreases in total lung capacity, vital capacity, and lung compliance. The resulting ventilation-perfusion imbalance leads to hypoxia.

A "one-way" valve effect, or sucking chest wound, occurs when air that is sucked through the chest wound into the intrapleural space on inspiration cannot escape on exhalation. This accumulation of air collapses lung tissue and can cause a tension pneumothorax. The defect in the chest wall causes the one-way valve effect. The defect must be occluded during inspiration to prevent air from entering and released during exhalation to allow air to exit the defect. Until the chest wound is surgically repaired, the defect must be temporarily corrected. (See the "Thoracic Trauma" entry.)

Spontaneous pneumothorax

A spontaneous pneumothorax can be caused by multiple chronic diseases that predispose the alveoli and visceral pleura to rupture internally. When this occurs, air moves from the alveoli into the intrapleural space. The negative pressure in the intrapleural space becomes positive, collapsing the lung and resulting in decreased total lung capacity, vital capacity, and lung compliance.

Tension pneumothorax

In a tension pneumothorax, air in the intrapleural space is trapped. The pressure in the intrapleural space is higher than the pressure in the lung and vascular structures and is strong enough to compress the lung tissue, causing tracheal deviation to the opposite side and decreased venous return to the heart. This life-threatening emergency requires immediate lung re-expansion. As the positive pressure is released from the intrapleural space, the lung re-expands and venous return to the heart increases.

Clinical assessment

Depending on the patient's condition on admission, the nurse may have only enough time for a focused cardiopulmonary assessment. If a tension pneumothorax is suspected, the nurse must obtain vital signs, auscultate breath sounds, inspect and palpate the neck and chest, and evaluate for chest pain caused by a collapsed lung. Arterial blood gas values are not used to diagnose a pneumothorax, although they may be used to monitor oxygenation. Oxygen saturation monitoring is quicker, cheaper, noninvasive, and easy to obtain with a pulse oximeter (SaO_2). Oxygenation and physical assessment findings may vary, depending on the degree of lung collapse and the underlying cause.

History

Patients with traumatic and spontaneous pneumothoraces or hemothoraces usually have similar signs and symptoms. Typically, they complain of shortness of breath. They may also complain of sharp pleuritic chest pain that increases with inspiration and coughing. A brief, subjective assessment of the pain is helpful in identifying which lung is collapsed. The nurse should elicit the following information:

• patient's risk factors for pneumothorax (such as a history of pulmonary disease or AIDS)
• history of previous pneumothorax
• history of chest trauma

• location of the chest pain.

Physical findings

It is important to remember that a traumatic or spontaneous pneumothorax may progress to a tension pneumothorax at any time. Signs and symptoms must be evaluated quickly to expedite treatment. Any trauma patient should be inspected for signs of penetration trauma, such as entrance and exit bullet wounds, and open sucking chest wounds.

The patient with a spontaneous pneumothorax (nontension) may have some or all of the following findings:
• decreased or bronchial breath sounds on affected side
• tachypnea, shortness of breath
• tachycardia
• overexpansion or rigidity on affected side
• subcutaneous emphysema, air, crepitus
• decreased vocal fremitus.

The patient with a tension pneumothorax generally presents in acute respiratory distress. Clinical manifestations of impeded venous return include decreased cardiac output, hypotension, compensatory tachycardia, tachypnea, and cardiac arrest. Lung collapse can be caused by air or blood in the intrapleural space. A mediastinal shift and tracheal deviation to the contralateral side may be observed in a tension pneumothorax. Widening of intercostal spaces and diaphragmatic depression are also seen on chest X-ray. The patient typically has several of the following findings:
• neck vein distention (jugular)
• increased central venous pressure
• asymmetrical chest expansion
• tracheal deviation away from affected side
• tachycardia
• hypotension
• pallor or cyanosis
• respiratory arrest
• pulseless electrical activity.

Diagnosis

The diagnosis of spontaneous pneumothorax is based on physical findings and an upright chest X-ray. If a tension pneumothorax is suspected in an unstable patient, immediate treatment is given without taking the time to obtain an X-ray. Chest X-rays are used to diagnose all types of pneumothoraces. In the upright chest film, a pneumothorax is best visualized over the apex. In the supine patient, it is best visualized laterally or at the base of the lung. The X-ray typically shows air in the pleural space, identified by a thin line representing compressed visceral pleura with hyperlucency and an absence of lung marking peripherally.

Treatment and care

A small pneumothorax in an asymptomatic patient may be treated conservatively with close observation only. However, for most patients with moderate or large pneumothoraces, standard treatment includes a pleural chest tube. Symptomatic patients with unstable vital signs and hypotension, including those in cardiopulmonary arrest, require immediate lung re-expansion. Hypotension or cardiopulmonary arrest will not resolve with fluids or emergency medications. Symptoms will resolve when the tension is released from the intrapleural space and cardiac output improves.

Needle thoracentesis or placement of a pleural chest tube may be used to evacuate air in the intrapleural space and re-expand the lung. A "swoosh" sound of air exiting the intrapleural space may be heard when a needle or scalpel enters the intrapleural space and releases the tension.

Emergency lung re-expansion

If a tension pneumothorax is suspected, the nurse must quickly notify the physician, remain with the patient to prepare for lung re-expansion, and ask another nurse to obtain equipment needed for chest tube placement. It is important to remember that a tension pneumothorax

Needle thoracentesis

Needle thoracentesis may be performed in an emergency on an unstable patient to temporarily relieve pleural pressure until a chest tube can be inserted. The patient will probably have unstable vital signs with hypotension, hypoxia, and possibly pulseless electrical activity.

Procedure Steps	Nursing Considerations
• Locate the second intercostal space, midclavicular line. • Prepare the affected side with an antiseptic. • Puncture the parietal pleura with the needle. • Listen for air escape as the needle enters the pleura. • Prepare for chest tube insertion. • Follow with a chest X-ray.	• Place the conscious patient in an upright position. • Monitor continuous pulse oximetry (SaO_2). • Explain the procedure to the patient. • Administer a local anesthetic if the patient is conscious. • Assess patient for relief of symptoms. • Monitor vital signs every 15 minutes until stable.

may lead to cardiopulmonary arrest (see *Needle thoracentesis,* page 532, and *Chest tube insertion,* page 533). A Heimlich valve may be used in a prehospital or triage situation in place of a chest drainage system. This valve is lightweight and easily connected to the distal end of the chest tube. It acts as a one-way valve, allowing air to leave the intrapleural space, and maintains negative intrapleural pressure.

Immediate nursing intervention following emergency lung re-expansion includes the following:

• Obtain an emergency portable chest X-ray, and assess the radiologist's interpretation for chest tube placement and lung re-expansion.

• Assess the patient's comfort level, and take vital signs every 15 minutes for the first hour, once every hour for the next 2 hours, then every 4 hours for 24 hours.

• Assess the amount and color of chest tube drainage every 2 hours for at least 8 hours; mark the drainage level on the side of the drainage unit, using a pen.

• Notify the physician if bloody drainage exceeds 100 ml/hour.

Chest tube insertion

The standard treatment for a pneumothorax is placement of a single pleural chest tube on the affected side.

Important nursing interventions
• Prepare the affected side with an antiseptic.
• Have necessary equipment available at the bedside.
• Explain the procedure to the patient.
• Place the patient in supine position, or the position requested by physician.
• Monitor Sao_2 with continuous pulse oximetry.
• Assist with chest tube insertion.

• If hemothorax is present, be prepared to immediately connect chest tube to drainage system.
• Connect chest tube to chest drainage system.
• Connect the system to suction.
• Secure chest tube with tape or anchoring device.
• Tape connections together.
• Apply dressing or anchoring device.
• Obtain a follow-up chest X-ray.

• Monitor the patient's breath sounds at least every 4 hours.
• Monitor oxygen saturation levels continuously, or spot check as clinically indicated every 2 to 4 hours.

Pulmonary expansion measures

Standard treatment for a patient with a pneumothorax involves placement of a single pleural chest tube on the patient's affected side; the tube is usually left in place for 3 to 5 days. During this time, the nurse must monitor the patient's respiratory status, provide chest tube care, provide comfort measures, encourage mobility, and maintain the chest drainage unit. Chest tubes are removed when the lung is fully expanded (as seen on chest X-ray), drainage from the chest is minimal (25 ml per 8 hours), and the visceral pleural has had time to heal. This usually takes at least 48 hours.

Routine nursing interventions are outlined below:
• Obtain and review radiologist's interpretation of daily chest X-rays.
• Perform a complete cardiopulmonary assessment every 8 to 12 hours if the patient is stable, or more fre-

quently if unstable, documenting findings. If the patient is in ICU, assess every 4 to 8 hours.

• Auscultate breath sounds every 4 hours. To hear breath sounds without interference from the water bubbling in the chest drainage unit, momentarily clamp the wall suction tube to muffle loud bubbling in the water chamber.

• Wash the chest tube insertion site with soap and water and assess it for redness or swelling.

• Assess for the presence of subcutaneous air on affected side of chest.

• Follow institutional procedures regarding the use of dressings for insertion sites.

• Change any dressing placed over the site at least every 48 hours, or as needed.

• Secure the chest tube to the patient with an anchoring device or tape.

• Administer pain medication and nonsteroidal anti-inflammatory drugs (NSAIDs), as prescribed.

• Teach the patient to cough and breathe deeply enough to mobilize secretions and promote lung expansion. Observe return demonstration.

• Help with repositioning at least every 2 hours if the patient is not ambulatory or suffers from impaired mobility.

• Encourage the patient to sit up in a chair whenever possible and to remain ambulatory, if appropriate.

• Stress the importance of keeping the drainage collection chamber below chest level.

• Caution the patient against compressing or kinking the drainage tube.

• Explain to the patient the importance of taking measures to enhance lung re-expansion and promote drainage of air and fluid. Ensure that the patient can verbalize understanding of teaching.

Conservative treatment

Conservative treatment for a spontaneous (nontension) pneumothorax involves close observation, which includes the following:

• Monitor daily chest X-rays.
• Monitor the patient's cardiovascular and pulmonary status to evaluate for changes or deterioration in status.
• Administer NSAIDs, as prescribed.
• Teach the patient to cough and breathe deeply enough to mobilize secretions and to promote lung expansion. Observe return demonstration.
• Encourage the patient to sit up in a chair or ambulate, if appropriate.

Prevention of recurring pneumothoraces

The most successful way to treat recurrent spontaneous pneumothorax is thoracotomy with resection of large cysts or bullae. This procedure prevents recurrence by causing the lung to adhere to the parietal pleura. The patient will have postoperative chest tubes for 3 or 4 days, an incision, and have approximately 5 days of hospitalization.

Thorascopy

Thorascopic treatment is a surgical procedure that is performed by thoracic surgeons and trauma surgeons. Currently, it is extensively used for recurrent pneumothorax and will probably become the standard treatment for spontaneous pneumothorax because it has a 98% success rate. It is effective and reliable in detecting the location, number, and size of bullae. During thorascopy, a thorascope is used to close ruptured bullae, although target bullae must be less than 1 cm in diameter. Larger bullae usually require a resection by thoracotomy. Postoperative care of thorascopy patients is similar to that of patients who have had a thoracotomy, except that the patient has only one pleural chest tube and a small incision.

Pharmacologic intervention

Instillation of intrapleural tetracycline (pleurodesis) is another means of treating recurrent spontaneous pneumothorax. In this instance, the tetracycline serves as a pleural sclerosing agent. Approximately 500 mg of tetracycline, dissolved in 10 ml of isotonic saline solution, is instilled into a chest tube that has been inserted into the intrapleural space. The medication scars the lung tissue sealing and leak. This is a very painful procedure for which a 30% to 100% success rate has been reported. Doxycycline, a tetracycline analog, has also been used as a pleural sclerosing agent. In this procedure, 500 to 1,000 mg of doxycycline, dissolved in 30 ml of isotonic saline solution, is instilled into the chest tube.

The following nursing interventions are done prior to the procedure:

• Discuss the procedure with the patient and explain that there will be pain associated with the instillation of medication. Ensure that the patient can communicate understanding of the procedure.

• Obtain the pleural sclerosing agent from the pharmacy.

• Prepare the agent according to labeled instructions.

• Provide the patient with analgesic pain control.

The physician instills the pleural sclerosing agent; continue nursing care as previously described in maintaining lung expansion.

Prevention of complications

Complications of pneumothorax are infrequent and rarely serious. Most can be prevented or minimized by attentive nursing care (see *Preventing and treating complications associated with pneumothorax,* page 537).

Prognosis

A pneumothorax typically resolves following lung re-expansion. However, the patient's prognosis is related to the underlying disease. AIDS patients have the highest rate of bilateral pneumothorax (34%) and recurrent spontaneous pneumothorax (34%). The mortality rate of spontaneous pneumothorax in this population is also 34%. Patients with subpleural bleb disease or COPD usually have a low rate of bilateral pneumothorax (2%) and recurrent pneumothorax (16%); mortality is about 2%.

Preventing and treating complications associated with pneumothorax

Complication	Means of Prevention or Treatment
Infection of chest tube insertion site	• Cleanse site daily. • Change dressing at least every 48 hours.
Allergic reaction to occlusive tape near tube insertion site	• Secure chest tube with horizontal drain attachment device.
Chest tube that becomes dislodged or falls out	• Anchor chest tube firmly to the chest wall.
Increased size of pneumothorax or hemothorax	• Ensure that chest tube drainage system is not held above level of the heart. • Ensure that suction is maintained.
Large air leak	• Increase level of suction (> 25 cm H_2O). • Perform thoracoscopy.
Tension pneumothorax	• Ensure that chest tube and drainage tubing are not kinked or otherwise obstructed.

Discharge planning

The patient with a recently removed chest tube must be able to verbalize and demonstrate an understanding of the following discharge teaching:

• Clean the insertion site carefully with soap and water; showering is permitted.

• Recognize that fever or drainage may be signs of infection and should be reported to health care provider at once.

• Report to the emergency department if chest pain or shortness of breath recur.

Pulmonary embolism

Pulmonary embolism is the complete or partial obstruction of the pulmonary vasculature by an insoluble substance that compromises pulmonary function and deprives tissue of vital oxygen and nutrients. Blockage may result from thromboembolic fats, migration of tumor cells, amniotic fluid, a foreign object, an infected particle, or fibrin. Diagnosed in over 500,000 patients annually in the United States, pulmonary embolism is responsible for over 50,000 deaths each year.

Pathophysiology

Most pulmonary emboli develop from clots formed distal to the pulmonary vasculature. About 90% of emboli are caused by deep venous thrombosis (DVT), which usually occurs above the knee in the popliteal or iliofemoral veins. Such conditions as lower limb trauma, orthopedic surgery, and peripheral vascular surgery increase the risk of venous thrombosis and embolism.

Other conditions associated with DVT development include immobility or obesity that results in venous stasis, chronic venous disease (as in those with a history of I.V. drug abuse, thromboembolism, phlebitis, or vascular insufficiency), sepsis, burns, heart failure, sickle cell disease, polycythemia, diabetes mellitus, increased blood coagulability (as in cancer or use of high-estrogen oral contraceptives), and pregnancy or postpartum status. Hypercoaguable states leading to increased clot formation are also associated with systemic lupus erythematosus and antithrombin III deficiency, especially when the endothelial lining of the blood vessel has been damaged, making it more susceptible to intravascular clotting and thrombus development.

Pulmonary emboli sometimes result in critical care settings from the introduction of air, fat, infected material, or amniotic fluid into the vascular system. Air emboli may occur secondary to catheter placement. Fat emboli, which may occur following fractures of long bones, hip surgery, or major trauma, do not cause the same type of complete obstruction that occurs with emboli from DVTs. Rather than causing complete occlusion of a larger pulmonary vessel, such emboli cause partial or temporary occlusion of many smaller capillaries as the fat breaks into smaller and smaller particles. Eventually, the fat particles are broken down by lipases. The fatty acid products of lipid digestion injure the pulmonary vasculature, producing toxic vasculitis. This causes capillary leakage and edema within the affected segment, precipitating the development of adult respiratory distress syndrome.

When infected materials cause the obstruction, the source is likely to be from pelvic inflammation, an infected venous catheter or right heart valve, or phlebitis. The resulting disruption is severe, with fever, hemodynamic compromise, and multiple pulmonary sites that can develop into abscesses as the embolus resolves. Amniotic fluid emboli may occur during either spontaneous delivery or cesarean section; massive obstruction leads to shock or death. The thromboplastic nature of the amniotic fluid triggers thrombosis in the pulmonary vasculature and elsewhere.

The physiologic disruption that occurs with pulmonary embolism depends on the source and form of the vascular disruption (see *Pathophysiology of pulmonary embolism,* page 540). The extent of the compromise resulting from the embolism is related to the patient's underlying health status. Typically, over 50% of the pulmonary vasculature must be obstructed to cause significant pulmonary hemodynamic compromise; however, even a small embolus can cause major damage in patients with preexisting pulmonary or cardiac disease (left ventricular failure, mitral stenosis, chronic obstructive lung disease, pulmonary congestion). Such patients are at increased risk for pulmonary infarction. The infarcted area may become necrotic and infected and may develop into an abscess.

Clinical assessment
Recognizing the clinical signs and symptoms of pulmonary embolism can be difficult, but prompt diagnosis and initiation of corrective therapies are essential.

Pathophysiology of pulmonary embolism

The following sequence describes the physiology behind a thrombotic pulmonary embolism.

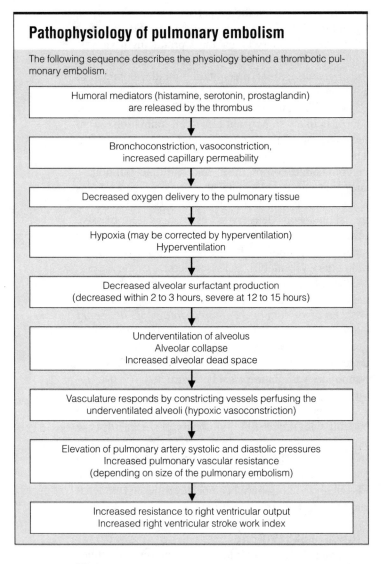

Humoral mediators (histamine, serotonin, prostaglandin) are released by the thrombus

↓

Bronchoconstriction, vasoconstriction, increased capillary permeability

↓

Decreased oxygen delivery to the pulmonary tissue

↓

Hypoxia (may be corrected by hyperventilation) Hyperventilation

↓

Decreased alveolar surfactant production (decreased within 2 to 3 hours, severe at 12 to 15 hours)

↓

Underventilation of alveolus Alveolar collapse Increased alveolar dead space

↓

Vasculature responds by constricting vessels perfusing the underventilated alveoli (hypoxic vasoconstriction)

↓

Elevation of pulmonary artery systolic and diastolic pressures Increased pulmonary vascular resistance (depending on size of the pulmonary embolism)

↓

Increased resistance to right ventricular output Increased right ventricular stroke work index

History

The nurse should obtain information regarding the patient's risk factors for pulmonary embolism, including:

• personal and family history of pulmonary emboli
• recent immobilization

- use of birth control pills
- history of DVT or peripheral vascular disease
- recent surgery, especially involving the hip or long bones
- history of cancer, systemic lupus erythematosus, co-agulation disorders
- recent trauma
- recent ambulation after prolonged immobilization
- intravenous drug use (increased risk of septic emboli).

Physical findings

Recent clinical trials have shown that the symptoms most closely linked with confirmed pulmonary embolism include dyspnea, pleuritic chest pain, tachypnea, and cough. Patients may also present with hemoptysis, calf pain, syncope, nonpleuritic chest pain, and palpitations. Unfortunately, these symptoms are easily attributed to other diseases, such as congestive heart failure, pneumonia, pneumothorax, pulmonary edema, myocardial or pulmonary infarction, and exacerbation of chronic obstructive pulmonary disease. Clinical assessment should include both physical and laboratory-based assessments.

Findings may include:
- sudden onset of mild to severe shortness of breath
- hemoptysis (associated with pulmonary infarction)
- 12-lead ECG findings (right axis deviation or right bundle branch block, prominent P waves, and ST elevations occurring diffusely across precordial leads)
- tachycardia, atrial arrhythmias
- split S_2 on inhalation and exhalation (indicates increased pulmonary resistance and right ventricular overload)
- jugular venous distention, hepatomegaly, peripheral edema that accompanies right ventricular failure from an extensive embolism
- crackles, cough, tachypnea, and wheezes over affected area

• signs of shock (decreased blood pressure, increased heart rate, cool and clammy extremities, cyanosis, and diaphoresis)
• petechiae over axilla and chest (fat embolus)
• change in level of consciousness (syncope)
• agitation, restlessness, anxiety, nausea, and vomiting
• auscultation of pleural friction rub (usually seen with infarction)
• pleuritic chest pain on inspiration
• murmur associated with turbulent flow through the partially obstructed pulmonary artery
• pleural effusion (found in about half of the cases as dullness on percussion) confirmed by chest X-ray
• phlebitis, varicosities, and decreased peripheral circulation.

Diagnosis

The most important part of the diagnostic process is the early recognition of signs and symptoms of pulmonary embolism, which will lead to early testing and more diagnostically conclusive findings. A complaint of radiating chest pain is unlikely to be the result of pulmonary embolism. If chest pain worsens with exhalation and stops when the patient holds the breath, it is likely to be pleuritic; chest pain associated with myocardial infarction is constant. (For a full presentation of diagnostic tests for pulmonary embolism, see *Diagnostic tests for pulmonary embolism,* pages 543 and 544.)

Treatment and care

Caring for a patient with pulmonary embolism centers on stabilizing whatever hemodynamic and respiratory functions have been debilitated by the disease and administering appropriate medications (see *Key nursing interventions for patients with pulmonary embolism,* page 545). This requires maintaining ventilation, circulation, and oxygenation. Supportive ventilation consists of supplemental oxygen and adequate ventilatory excursion.

This process may be as basic as providing oxygen via a nasal cannula or face mask (in some cases, a non-

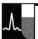

Diagnostic tests for pulmonary embolism

The following tests may be ordered to confirm a diagnosis of pulmonary embolism.

Electrocardiogram (ECG)

ECGs tend to be sensitive but unspecific, unless the patient has had such a severe embolism that right-sided heart failure (cor pulmonale) is occurring; then the ECG will show p-pulmonale, right axis deviation, right bundle branch block, or a classic $S_1Q_3T_3$ pattern. Sinus tachycardia, ST-T wave changes are nonspecific in most cases. More significant findings may be found in the patient with preexisting cardiac compromise.

Arterial blood gas (ABG) analysis

The hyperventilating patient presents with respiratory alkalosis. An increased alveolar-arterial oxygen gradient is indicative of the perfusion abnormality. Hypoxemia may be hidden by the patient's hyperventilation. Normal values do not rule out pulmonary embolism.

Enzymatic evaluation

Lactic dehydrogenase, serum glutamic oxaloacetic transaminase, and bilirubin may be measured to rule out other causes of symptoms, such as myocardial infarction.

Vital signs, blood pressure

Assess for tachycardia, tachypnea, and temperature increase. Decreased blood pressure occurs with massive embolism, which causes an increase in right-sided heart pressure and right ventricular (RV) dilation. The RV dilation causes a shift of the septum into the left ventricle and decreased filling, contractility, and cardiac output.

Chest X-ray

Many patients do not show changes on the chest X-ray. Changes that are present may be nonspecific, such as consolidation. An elevated hemidiaphragm, small pleural effusion, atelectasis, and cutoff of a prominent pulmonary artery are consistent with pulmonary embolism. Segmental oligemia (avascular-appearing lung segment) and Hampton's hump (wedge-shaped pleural-based peripheral consolidation) are associated with pulmonary infarction. A rapidly resolving infiltrate indicates a parenchymal hemorrhage, while one which resolves slowly and has a bloody pleural effusion indicates pulmonary infarction. An infiltrate that resolves but forms multiple spheroid nodules is associated with septic emboli. If the abnormalities on chest X-ray are much greater than found with the perfusion scan, the problem is probably parenchymal in origin rather than a pulmonary embolism.

Ventilation-perfusion scan

Pulmonary emboli classically cause abnormalities in perfusion while ventilation remains normal. Matched defects, with corresponding infiltrates on chest X-rays, can indicate pneumonia or pulmonary infarction. Defects seen on the perfusion scan but not on the ventilation scan are called mismatches and indicate possible sites of pulmonary embolism. Results are given in terms of the likelihood that pulmonary emboli exist: low probability, ~10% to 20% chance; intermediate probability, ~30% to 50%

(continued)

Diagnostic tests for pulmonary embolism *(continued)*

chance; high probability, ~80% to 90% chance.

Angiography
Used for those with intermediate or indeterminate scan with strong clinical symptoms, patients with contraindications for anticoagulation therapy, or those who may require inferior vena cava filter placement. An invasive procedure, it requires direct, rapid injection of radiopaque materials by way of cardiac catheterization into the main pulmonary artery or its branches. It provides a visual image of the pulmonary vessels and intraluminal filling defects and "cut off" of blood flow. Repeated injections directed toward the different lung zones with multiple images and magnification provide the best diagnostic examination. Con-traindications for the procedure include dye allergies, recent myocardial infarction, and ventricular irritability. Use of a compressible peripheral site for catheter insertion may be indicated if the patient is likely to need thrombolytic therapy.

Venous Doppler studies
Used to evaluate presence or absence of deep venous thromboses, usually between the inguinal ligament and popliteal trifurcation. Transmitted waves of sound are sent and returned to a probe. The operator evaluates vessels for flow characteristics indicative of thrombosis, occlusion, narrowing, and compressability of vessels. Studies can now be augmented with color to show direction and speed of flow.

---

rebreather-rebreather mask, which can provide almost 100% oxygen). Keeping the patient upright or in semi-Fowler's position facilitates diaphragmatic excursion, as does the use of pain medication. Good pain management will help promote adequate ventilatory effort but may suppress the respiratory drive. If the patient requires intubation to maintain satisfactory saturations and blood gas level, tidal volume, and respiratory rate will need to be monitored. Whenever possible, decrease the oxygen consumption associated with activities of daily living, and minimize physical activity when oxygen levels are precarious. The mainstay of pulmonary embolism treatment, however, is removal of the offending agent.

Restoring and maintaining perfusion
The goals of anticoagulant therapy are to prevent further clot development and to allow the natural lysing system of the body to dissolve the existing clot. Heparin, the

ESSENTIAL ELEMENTS

Key nursing interventions for patients with pulmonary embolism

The following flowchart highlights key interventions that typically are performed when a patient is diagnosed with pulmonary embolism.

Stabilize the patient		
Stabilize respiratory system	**Stabilize hemodynamic parameters**	**Administer medication, as ordered**
• Monitor for compromise: —oxygen saturation < 90% to 93% —PaO_2 < 110 mm Hg —shortness of breath —dyspnea, tachypnea —increased tidal volume and minute volume —crackles, wheezes. • Administer supplemental oxygen with a nasal cannula, mask, or endotracheal tube. • Support ventilation: —semi- or high-Fowler's position —coughing and deep breathing —pain medication to offset splinting of respirations —mechanical ventilation. • Monitor hemoglobin and hematocrit; supplement as needed.	• Monitor for mental confusion, dizziness, syncope, blood pressure changes, heart rate changes, and changes in central venous pressure, pulmonary capillary wedge pressure, and urine output. • Reestablish hemodynamic stability: —administer positive inotropic agents and vasoconstricting agents —administer normal saline solution, dextran, and blood products. • Monitor hemodynamic parameters. • Monitor for tolerance of infusions and pressor agents, checking breath sounds, peripheral pulses and perfusion, heart rate.	• Administer anticoagulants (heparin or warfarin sodium), as prescribed. —monitor for bleeding —monitor PPT (heparin therapy), PT, INR (warfarin therapy). • Administer thrombolytics (streptokinase, urokinase, tPA), as ordered. —monitor for bleeding —monitor for severe allergic reaction to streptokinase —monitor fibrinogen degradation products, thrombin time, PPT, and platelet count. • Administer pain medications (morphine, midazolam, fentanyl), as prescribed. —prepare patient for long-term therapy and immobility. • Monitor neurologic function.

agent most commonly used, blocks platelet/thrombin interactions on the embolus, thereby inhibiting normal hemostatic mechanisms designed to help maintain the clot. It is also thought to prevent the further release of serotonin, which causes bronchoconstriction and hypotension. High-dose heparin therapy is initiated with a intravenous loading dose of 2,000 to 5,000 units, followed by 800 to 1,200 units per hour I.V. (alternative route and dosing recommendations are listed in *Drugs used in pulmonary embolism*, pages 547 and 548).

Nursing care of the patient receiving anticoagulant therapy includes the following:

• Maintain bed rest for the early portion of heparin therapy to prevent bleeding and decrease the risk of loosening fragile venous thrombi.

• Monitor for bleeding in urine, stool, gums, and skin.

• Administer stool softeners to prevent straining and bleeding.

• Administer antacids to decrease acidity and potential gastric bleeding.

• Keep in mind that the therapeutic goal of heparin therapy is to obtain a partial thromboplastin time (PTT) between 1.5 and 2.5 times control and to maintain it for 7 to 10 days.

• Monitor PTT levels every 12 hours. Full anticoagulation, as measured by the PTT, should be obtained within 48 hours.

• Monitor coagulation levels and prepare for reversal if invasive procedures are scheduled.

Although the use of heparin may be contraindicated in patients with active bleeding or a known bleeding coagulopathy, most patients may start heparin therapy before the clinical diagnosis is confirmed by diagnostic examinations. Heparin-induced thrombocytopenia, a potential side effect, may develop 1 to 20 days after therapy is initiated. Warfarin sodium, an oral anticoagulant that interferes with the synthesis of important clotting factors, is often used for this purpose. Because it takes approximately 3 to 5 days for warfarin sodium to bring the prothrombin time (PT) within the desired

Drugs used in pulmonary embolism

The following table provides information about anticoagulants and thrombolytics, the two classes of drugs that play a key role in the treatment of patients with pulmonary embolism. This table can be used to individualize
patient care when administering thrombolytic therapy.

Drug	Dosage	Side Effects	Reversal Agents
Anticoagulants			
Heparin		• Bleeding • Thrombocyto- penia	• Protamine sulfate
Continuous intravenous	1,000 units/hour		
Intermittent continuous	5,000 units every 4 hours, or 7,500 units every 6 hours		
Subcutaneous	5,000 units every 4 hours, or 10,000 units every 8 hours, or 20,000 units every 12 hours		
Warfarin sodium	5 to 10 mg/day (sufficient to pro- long the PT to 1.5 to 2.5 times control); adjust- ed to maintain therapeutic range, which is affected by liver function and underlying coagulopathies	• Bleeding • Diarrhea • Crosses placen- ta and may injure developing fetus • Rare: warfarin skin necrosis (mi- crovascular throm- bus development 3 to 10 days after starting therapy) • Multiple drug interactions	• Vitamin K
Thrombolytics			
Streptokinase	250,000 IU over 30 minutes, followed by 100,000 IU/hour for 24 hours	• Bleeding • Anaphylactic reaction • Hypotension with rapid infusions	• Aminocaproic acid topically or systemically • FFP and cryo- precipitate *(continued)*

Drugs used in pulmonary embolism *(continued)*

Drug	Dosage	Side Effects	Reversal Agents
Thrombolytics *(continued)*			
Urokinase	4,400 IU/kg loading dose over 10 minutes, then 4,400 IU/kg/hour for 12 hours	• Bleeding	• Aminocaproic acid topically or systemically • FFP and cryo-precipitate
Tissue plasminogen activator	No loading dose; 50 mg/hour over 2 hours	• Bleeding and hematomas, especially at sites of vascular access	• No direct reversal agent

therapeutic range of 1.5 to 2.5 times control, administration is started before the cessation of heparin therapy. Because PT testing can be variable, monitoring of the International Normalized Ration (INR) is increasing. The therapeutic range is 2.0 to 3.0 (which corresponds to a PT value of 1.3 to 1.5 times control).

Thrombolytic therapy is indicated for massive pulmonary embolism, severe hemodynamic compromise that is unresponsive to volume repletion, severe pulmonary hypertension, and patients who are not candidates for surgery. Typically, absolute contraindications to using thrombolytic agents include patients who have had a cerebral vascular accident within the last 2 months or have active internal bleeding. Major contraindications include surgery within the past 10 to 14 days, obstetrical delivery, gastrointestinal bleeding, serious trauma, recent CPR, or hypertension greater than 200 mm Hg systolic/100 to 120 mm Hg diastolic. Careful consideration must be given to the use of thrombolytic therapy in patients with minor trauma, in those at high risk of a left-sided heart thrombus, in patients with bacterial endocarditis or coagulation defects, and in those who are over age 75, pregnant, or suffering from diabetic hemorrhagic retinopathy.

Streptokinase is produced from group C beta-hemolytic streptococci and activates a fibrinolytic precursor that promotes clot dissolution. A patient who has received the drug previously or who has recently had a streptococcal infection will have antibodies to the agent, increasing resistance to the drug and putting the patient at risk for a major allergic reaction. Streptokinase should be started within 7 days after development of an embolism; its maximum effect occurs within 24 hours of administration and can continue for 24 hours after completion of the drug administration.

Urokinase, another thrombolytic, is most effective when started within 5 days of the onset of symptoms since it works best on newly formed clots. It is not associated with the allergic reactions seen with streptokinase. Tissue plasminogen activator is an agent designed to bind to the fibrin in the clot and convert the plasminogen into plasmin, which then initiates clot lysis at the site. Following the completion of thrombolytic therapy, anticoagulant therapy must be initiated to prevent further clot development.

Nursing care for the patient receiving thrombolytic therapy includes the precautions initiated for patients receiving anticoagulant therapy (listed above), as well as the following:

• Maintain strict bed rest during drug infusion and for 24 hours after completion (streptokinase therapy).

• Monitor coagulation panel.

• Take necessary safety precautions, such as avoiding venipunctures and keeping side rails up.

• Evaluate all venipuncture sites for bleeding.

• Maintain pressure on the site for at least 10 minutes after discontinuation of a catheter, followed by reevaluation of the site every 15 minutes for an hour and then once per hour.

• Monitor for signs and symptoms of cerebral bleeding.

• Perform a neurologic assessment every 8 to 12 hours. Notify the physician of any neurologic changes.

Some patients are not candidates for anticoagulation therapy, and in others, the therapy may not be effective. In these cases, surgery may be the only available option. Pulmonary embolectomy, in which the embolus is located by pulmonary angiogram then removed surgically, places the patient at high risk and therefore is not done unless all other management options have been exhausted. Embolectomies are performed when there is severe hemodynamic compromise that is unresponsive to supportive measures. A surgical team skilled in the use of cardiopulmonary bypass equipment must be available.

Hemodynamic support

When there is enough embolic disturbance of the pulmonary vasculature, the result is increased pressure against right ventricular outflow and decreased flow back to the left side of the heart. The decreased preload diminishes cardiac output and blood pressure. Supportive measures must be enacted to correct the imbalance if ischemia, infarction, and multisystem compromise are to be avoided. Measures are designed to correct these by increasing circulating volume and strengthening the quality of cardiac contraction.

Nursing measures are included below:
• Monitor central venous pressure (CVP) and pulmonary capillary wedge pressure (PCWP), blood pressure, heart rate, skin turgor, and intake and output.
• Ensure I.V. access. Solutions of normal saline and dextran (which has anticoagulant properties) are used to maintain CVP between 2 and 8 mm $H_2O/2$ to 6 mm Hg and PCWP between 4 and 12 mm Hg.
• Monitor hemodynamic values. Acceptable hemodynamic values should be established by correlating the cardiac output, stroke volume, and blood pressure with the clinical presentation.

In the patient who shows signs of pulmonary edema, congestive heart failure, intolerance of increased circulating volume, inability to keep fluid within the vascular space, or no response to fluid administration, fluid resuscitation may be balanced by use of inotropic and vasoactive agents. Nursing interventions should include the following:

• Evaluate for increased pulmonary vascular resistance and right-sided heart failure, which may result from pressor use and fluid resuscitation.

• Monitor clinical response to interventions by noting kidney function (quality/quantity of urine output, blood urea nitrogen, creatinine, and potassium levels), mentation ability (mental confusion, syncope, dizziness, convulsions, seizures), cardiac perfusion (ischemic changes, angina), peripheral perfusion (hypotension, cyanosis, decreased quality or absence of peripheral pulses) and pulmonary function (chest X-rays, auscultation for crackles, consolidation, atelectasis; chest expansion, respiratory rate, tidal volumes, arterial blood gas levels, saturations, patient comfort).

Preventing recurrence

Patients will need to continue anticoagulant therapy for 3 to 6 months after trauma or surgery; if the patient is at high risk for development of DVT secondary to the primary disease, duration of therapy may be indefinite. Patients who have had extensive DVTs or large pulmonary emboli identified at the initiation of anticoagulant and thrombolytic therapy require prolonged treatment. Regardless of the length of therapy, continued surveillance of PT is indicated. Should a patient with a history of DVTs or pulmonary embolism be readmitted, low-dose heparin therapy may be instituted as a prophylactic measure, especially if prolonged immobility is expected.

Interruption of the inferior vena cava to prevent further embolization may be achieved by various techniques, such as ligation or clipping of the inferior vena cava. Commonly, interruption is achieved by the implantation of an inferior vena caval "umbrella" to filter out clots. It has been used to decrease the risk of re-embolization, especially in patients who are not candidates for anticoagulant therapy. It is also used for patients who have septic emboli originating from the lower extremities, or for those who have had multiple embolisms and are unlikely to handle the hemodynamic effects of another embolic event. The device can be placed percutaneously through the femoral or internal jugular vessels and requires only local anesthesia.

The average patient will still require some level of anticoagulant therapy to decrease filter clotting and to prevent development of thromboses at the site of vascular interruption and endothelial irritation. Inferior vena cava ligation is appropriate for some patients. The patient with multiple septic pulmonary emboli from septic pelvic thrombophlebitis may die unless ligation of the cava and left ovarian vein is performed. If ligation or clipping is required, patients must be able to tolerate the acute obstruction of venous flow; over time, collateral circulation will develop to bypass the ligation. The filters, which do not obstruct caval flow, are less problematic for most patients. If they should thrombose and clot in the future, however, collateral circulation must be developed to return flow from the lower torso and extremities.

Appropriate nursing interventions are listed below:
• Administer fresh frozen plasma, platelets, cryoprecipitate, and red blood cells, as required, to achieve level of hemostasis prior to surgery or filter placement.
• Evaluate femoral and internal jugular cannulation sites for bleeding and hematoma formation.
• Maintain cardiac output sufficient for the patient's cardiovascular status (venous return will be decreased following ligation/clipping).
• Evaluate for development of increasing pedal edema or lower-extremity edema secondary to obstruction of flow.
• Monitor peripheral pulses for signs of obstruction or insufficient perfusion.

Prognosis

The sooner therapy is started, the better the prognosis. Progressive clinical resolution with partial or complete resolution of the perfusion defects occurs over several weeks in most cases. If the defect remains after approximately 3 months, it is likely to be permanent. Unfortunately, if the patient has had multiple silent emboli before diagnosis, pulmonary hypertension may already exist, leaving the patient more susceptible to compromise with repeated embolic episodes. Pulmonary infarction is uncommon but has the potential to be the source of long-term pulmonary compromise. The extent of compromise is determined by the size of the infarcted area, whether or not it becomes necrotic and infected and develops into an abscess. As part of the healing process, fibrotic and scarred pulmonary tissue develops.

Discharge planning

Discharging the patient postembolization requires consistent and repeated education, which should include:
• review of the medication regimen
• signs and symptoms of pulmonary compromise and circulatory compromise, including development of or increasing pedal edema, which must be reported to the health care provider immediately
• signs and symptoms of gastrointestinal bleeding, including pain, discomfort, bloating, blood in the stool, diarrhea, vomiting, and light-headedness, which require prompt medical attention
• use of an identification card or a medical alert bracelet/necklace if on long-term anticoagulant therapy
• rehabilitation services consultation, if necessary.

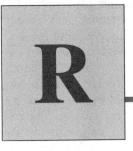

Renal failure

Acute renal failure (ARF) is a rapid deterioration of kidney function that results in a reduced or absent urine output and the subsequent accumulation of metabolic wastes, fluid, and electrolytes. If left untreated, ARF can lead to parenchymal damage, progressing to chronic renal failure or death.

Although ARF can occur at any age, it most often affects previously healthy individuals who have recently sustained a life-threatening trauma or who have ingested or been exposed to a nephrotoxic agent.

ARF is most commonly seen in the immediate postoperative phase of patient care but manifestations of this condition begin during the operative phase.

During surgery, patients are exposed to or physiologically develop conditions that predispose them to ARF. Operative situations that support the development of ARF include hypovolemia and hypotension and the administration of nephrotoxic agents, including general anesthesia. Surgical procedures in which ARF is more likely to occur include cardiopulmonary bypass, abdominal aortic procedures, and major biliary tree surgery. Elderly patients undergoing long surgical procedures, surgical patients with preexisting renal disease, and major trauma patients are also prone to developing ARF.

ARF can develop insidiously, making this disease difficult to detect. If the urine output remains constant with the only change being a decrease in volume, the only signs of developing ARF may be steadily rising serum blood urea nitrogen (BUN), creatinine, and potassium levels.

Pathophysiology

ARF is commonly classified as prerenal, intrarenal (intrinsic), or postrenal, depending on its underlying cause (see *Causes of acute renal failure*, page 556).

Prerenal ARF

Prerenal ARF results from any condition outside of the kidney that causes impaired blood flow to the renal vasculature and subsequently decreases glomerular perfusion, leading to oliguria. The nephrons remain normal, and normal renal function can be resumed if the underlying cause is diagnosed and treated promptly.

Postrenal ARF

Postrenal ARF is caused by a mechanical obstruction of urine outflow backing urine up into the renal pelvis. Normal renal function can be restored if the obstruction is removed.

Intrarenal ARF

Intrarenal ARF may result from any condition that directly damages the renal parenchyma and leads to nephron malfunctioning (such as infection, glomerulonephritis, or sclerosis caused by hypertension or diabetes mellitus). Acute tubular necrosis (ATN), the most common intrarenal condition, is responsible for 75% to 90% of all ARF cases; it is sometimes used interchangeably for the term ARF.

In ATN, the epithelial layer of the nephrons within the tubular portions of the kidney are damaged, leading to changes in urine concentration, waste filtration, and acid-base, electrolyte, and water balance. ATN typically develops after nephrotoxic injury or a prolonged re-

Causes of acute renal failure

The causes and conditions that predispose a patient to acute renal failure (ARF) are included below.

Prerenal ARF
• Hypovolemia (as seen in hemorrhage, shock, burn, and prolonged diarrhea and vomiting)
• Decreased cardiac output (from myocardial infarction, cardiac arrhythmias, congestive heart failure, cardiac tamponade, or open heart surgery)
• Increased intravascular blood pooling (as seen in septic shock or anaphylaxis)
• Renal vascular obstruction secondary to embolic phenomena, renal artery thrombosis, or bilateral renal vein thrombosis
• Obstetrical complications

Intrarenal ARF
• Exposure to nephrotoxic agents
• Infection from gram-negative bacteria leading to sepsis
• Pancreatitis or peritonitis
• Hemolytic blood transfusion reaction

• Rhabdomyolysis with myoglobinuria (as seen in trauma, severe exertion, or seizures or after the ingestion of heroin, barbiturates, intravenous amphetamines, or succinylcholine)
• Glomerular diseases (such as systemic lupus erythematosus, serum sickness, or post-streptococcal glomerulonephritis)
• Ischemic causes (such as toxemia of pregnancy and malignant hypertension)

Postrenal ARF
• Renal calculi
• Benign prostatic hypertrophy
• Bladder and pelvic neoplasms
• Renal papillary necrosis
• Uric acid or sulfonamide crystals in renal collection ducts
• Back, pelvis, or perineal trauma resulting in bladder rupture
• Ureteral strictures
• Spinal cord disease

nal ischemic episode that causes a decrease in renal perfusion, parenchymal damage, or obstruction, such as surgery or use of certain medications (see *Medications that cause or aggravate acute renal failure*, page 557). ATN may result from the release of hemoglobin from hemolyzed red blood cells or myoglobin from necrotic muscle tissue. Both hemoglobin and myoglobin block the renal tubules, causing renal vasoconstriction. Nephrotoxic chemicals can crystallize within the renal tubules, causing further obstruction.

Several theories attempt to explain the pathologic processes involved in the development of ATN and subsequent ARF: renal vasoconstriction, cellular edema,

Medications that cause or aggravate acute renal failure

Certain medications cause or aggravate acute renal failure (ARF).

Medications that can cause ARF include:
- Contrast media
- Diuretics (especially furosemide)
- Heavy metals (such as gold, lead, and mercury)
- Ibuprofen
- Organic or chemical solvents (such as carbon tetrachloride and ethylene glycol)

Medications that can aggravate ARF include:
- Amiloride
- Any medication containing magnesium tetracycline
- Aspirin
- Cisplatin
- Lithium carbonate
- Nitrofurantoin
- Nonsteroidal anti-inflammatory agents
- Phenylbutazone
- Spironolactone

decreased glomerular capillary permeability, intratubular obstruction, and leakage of glomerular filtrate.

In renal vasoconstriction, renin is released in response to ischemia. Renin activates the angiotensin-aldosterone system, leading to the constriction of peripheral and renal afferent arterioles. In conjunction with the decreased blood flow, there is a corresponding decrease in glomerular capillary pressure, glomerular filtration rate (GFR), and tubular dysfunction. Ultimately, renal vasoconstriction will cause oliguria.

Cellular edema, which results from ischemia that leads to cell anoxia and endothelial cell necrosis, raises tissue pressures above the capillary flow pressure. This inadequate blood flow further decreases the GFR and subsequently decreases the formation of urine.

Decreased glomerular capillary permeability results when ischemia alters the glomerular epithelial cells and subsequently changes the capillary permeability of the glomeruli. An altered capillary permeability reduces the GFR, leading to a reduction in tubular blood flow and, ultimately, tubular dysfunction.

Intratubular obstruction results when tubules become damaged and interstitial edema and the accumulation of necrotic epithelial cells within the tubules ensue. The accumulating necrotic cells obstruct the tubules, leading to a lowered GFR and increased intratubular pressure. Damaged tubular membranes permit the filtrate to leak back into the plasma, further decreasing intratubular fluid flow. This leads to a decrease in urine production with concurrent retention of electrolytes, water, and waste.

Physiologic changes

Depending on the classification of ARF, the patient might exhibit a variety of signs and symptoms. A patient with prerenal failure is usually hypovolemic and subsequently has a reduced urine output. In a patient with postrenal failure, the reduction of urine output is not caused by parenchymal disease.

In intrarenal failure caused by ATN, renal failure advances through four phases: onset, oliguria/anuria, diuresis, and recovery.

• The onset phase, which lasts from a few hours to days, is the period between the initial assault to the nephrons and the time when cell damage occurs. If treatment is initiated during this phase, permanent kidney damage can be reversed or reduced.

• The oliguria/anuria phase usually lasts 1 to 2 weeks. If the ATN is caused by ischemic changes, oliguria will be present. Nonoliguria will result in ATN as a result of toxic exposure. During this phase, glomerulofiltration is significantly reduced, leading to increased serum BUN and creatinine levels. In addition, electrolyte abnormalities, such as hyperkalemia, hyperphosphatemia, and hypocalcemia, develop as well as metabolic acidosis.

• The diuresis phase, which also lasts from 1 to 2 weeks, is characterized by an increase in glomerulofiltration and subsequent increase in urine output. Patients can have 2 to 4 liters of urine output per day, leading to sodium and water losses through the urine and volume depletion.

• During the recovery phase, which lasts 6 months to 1 year, renal function slowly begins to improve. Glomerulofiltration slowly recovers to 70% to 80% of normal.

Clinical assessment

Because ARF typically progresses through four phases, the nurse's ability to detect which phase of failure the patient is experiencing will directly influence when the appropriate medical therapy is instituted.

History

The onset phase of ARF may occur prior to hospitalization or during a current stay. When determining the presence and phase of ARF, the nurse should obtain the following information:

• history of chronic illness, such as hypertension or diabetes mellitus
• recent infections, particularly those caused by streptococcal bacteria
• recent episode of hypotension precipitated by major surgery or bleeding
• exposure to nephrotoxic or chemical agents
• recent blood transfusions
• recent urinary tract disorder
• toxemia of pregnancy or abortion
• recent severe muscle damage
• burn trauma.

Physical findings

The signs and symptoms in which the patient presents depend on the phase of the illness, the extent of azotemia, and the degree of metabolic acidosis. Clinical findings, broken down according to the phase of failure, include:

Onset phase
• minor reduction in normal daily urine output
• mild lethargy.

Oliguria/anuria phase
• urine output reduced to a daily total of 400 ml or less

- listlessness, confusion, or altered level of consciousness from electrolyte imbalances or uremia
- ECG changes including tall T waves, depressed ST segments, prolonged PR intervals, loss of P wave, wide QRS complexes, arrhythmias, or cardiac arrest due to decreased potassium excretion
- S_3 or S_4 gallop
- pericardial friction rub, pulsus paradoxus, fever, chest pain, and associated ECG changes including ST segment elevation, depressed PR interval, and low QRS voltage due to pericarditis as a result of pericardial membrane inflammation from uremic toxins
- crackles upon auscultation from fluid overload
- pulmonary edema, shortness of breath due to fluid volume overload or uremic toxins
- onset of productive cough with pink-tinged sputum due to fluid volume overload
- jugular vein distention due to fluid overload
- periorbital, peripheral, or sacral edema due to fluid overload
- capillary fragility evidenced by easy bruising
- metabolic acidosis exhibited by Kussmaul's respirations, hyperkalemia, and mental changes
- behavioral changes, fatigue, and pallor due to uremia
- anorexia, nausea, vomiting, diarrhea, constipation, halitosis, or GI bleeding due to uremia
- stomatitis due to uremic toxins
- uremic frost; pale, yellow, dry, and itchy skin
- muscle soreness or tenderness due to uremic toxins
- tremors due to uremic toxins or electrolyte imbalances
- memory impairment due to uremic toxins
- ascites due to fluid overload.

Diuresis phase
- urine output of 3 to 5 liters over 24 hours
- lethargy and muscle weakness due to reduced serum potassium level
- decreased blood pressure due to fluid volume depletion

• dry mucous membranes, flushed skin, and poor skin turgor due to fluid volume depletion.

Recovery phase
• urine output from 1,500 to 1,800 ml/24 hours
• stabilization of serum potassium, bicarbonate, BUN, and creatinine levels
• stabilization of cardiac rhythm and rate and a reduction in aberrant heart sounds and tracing abnormalities
• reduction in lethargy and shortness of breath
• reduction in adventitious lung sounds.

Diagnosis
Tests used to diagnose and evaluate treatment for ARF include serum and urine analyses and selected diagnostic procedures to visualize the renal parenchymal and vascular system (see *Diagnostic tests for acute renal failure,* pages 562 to 564).

Treatment and care
Treatment for the ARF patient is focused on correcting the cause of the failure, promoting regeneration of the remaining renal functioning, and preventing complications. For prerenal failure, treatment includes replacing lost fluids and stimulating urine output with the use of diuretics. Postrenal failure treatment is centered on identifying the cause of the obstruction of urinary flow, eliminating it, and supplementing with fluids and electrolytes, as necessary. Intrarenal failure is treated by clearing out extra fluids, electrolytes, and toxins from the general circulation through the use of dialysis while managing the patient's status with medications, fluid restriction, and dietary changes.

Dialysis is the treatment of choice when the patient is experiencing fluid excess, uncontrolled hyperkalemia or acidosis, progressing uremia, significant alterations in central nervous system functioning, and pericarditis. The choice of dialysis will depend on any underlying medical conditions and the acuity of the current failure episode.

(Text continues on page 564.)

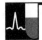

Diagnostic tests for acute renal failure

The following tests are used in the diagnosis and treatment of acute renal failure.

Electrolyte studies
Used to evaluate sodium, potassium, and bicarbonate levels. Positive findings include sodium > 147 mEq/liter (normal 135 to 145 mEq/liter); potassium > 6 mEq/liter (normal 3.5 to 5 mEq/liter); bicarbonate < 15 mEq/dl (normal 15 to 25 mEq/dl).

Blood urea nitrogen
Used to evaluate protein metabolism and the presence of uremia. Level > 20 mg/dl (normal 9 to 20 mg/dl) indicates deteriorating renal function.

Serum creatinine
Precise indicator of renal functioning as creatinine builds up in the blood when renal function is impaired. Level > 1.5 mg/dl (normal 0.7 to 1.5 mg/dl) indicates deteriorating renal function.

Serum phosphorous
Used to evaluate the kidney's ability to excrete phosphorous. Level > 4.5 mg/dl (normal 3 to 4.5 mg/dl) indicates decreased ability of the kidneys to excrete phosphate, leading to phosphate deposits in the skin and soft tissues.

Serum magnesium
Used to evaluate if magnesium is building up in the blood because magnesium clearance is hindered with renal compromise. Level > 2.5 mEq/liter (normal 1.5 to 2.5 mEq/liter) indicates hypermagnesemia and medications with magnesium are to be avoided.

Serum calcium
Used to evaluate the absorption and use of dietary calcium and the conversion of vitamin D. Level < 8.5 mg/dl (normal 8.5 to 10.5 mg/dl) indicates calcium precipitation out of tissues; if secondary hyperparathyroidism present, calcium level > 10.5 mg/dl.

Complete blood count
Evaluates hydration, lysis of red blood cells, and presence of infection. Hemoglobin < 10g/dl (normal 13 to 18 g/dl males, 12 to 16 g/dl females) and hematocrit < 30% (normal 45% to 52% males, 37% to 48% females) means lysis of red blood cell or hemodilution; white blood cell count over 11,000/μ (normal 4,500 to 11,000/μ) indicates infective process.

Prothrombin time (PT)/Partial thromboplastin time (PTT)
Evaluates amount of damage to the platelets because of uremic toxins. Levels > 2 seconds of the control for PT (normal is < 2 seconds from control) and > 37seconds for PTT (normal is 25 to 37 seconds) indicate prolonged bleeding and hindered clotting ability.

Arterial blood gas analysis
Evaluates degree and progression of metabolic acidosis seen in the acute renal failure patient. Bicarbonate level < 22 mEq/liter (normal is 22 to 34 mEq/liter) and blood pH < 7.35 (normal is between 7.36 to 7.44) indicates metabolic acidosis.

Diagnostic tests for acute renal failure *(continued)*

Urinalysis
Used to evaluate the chemical composition of urine. Findings indicative of acute renal failure include sediment consisting of epithelial cells, cellular debris, and tubular casts; with intrarenal disease, protein and red blood cell casts will also be seen; with prerenal disease, the sediment will be normal.

Creatinine clearance test
Believed to be most accurate determination of GFR, the accuracy will depend on a complete 24-hour urine collection. Levels < 50 ml/minute (normal is 95 to 125 ml/minute) seen in intrarenal disease; prerenal disease level varies according amount of time that has elapsed with reduced renal perfusion; postrenal disease levels should be within the normal range.

Urine sodium
Used to evaluate ability of the kidneys to excrete excess sodium. Level < 80 mEq/day (normal is 80 to 180 mEq/day) seen in prerenal and postrenal disease; intrarenal disease levels in the high normal range to over 180 mEq/day indicate damaged nephrons and inability to reabsorb sodium.

Urine specific gravity
Measures density of urine compared to distilled water; evaluates the kidney's ability to concentrate or dilute urine. Normal level is 1.010 to 1.015; prerenal disease level > 1.015; intrarenal and post renal disease approximately 1.010.

Magnetic resonance imaging
Identifies masses; distinguishes cysts from hemorrhages. Increased areas of density indicative of lesions, malformation of tissue, vessels, or tubules, and necrosis.

Computed tomography scan
Identifies masses, hemorrhage, calcifications, or necrosis of renal tissue. Increased areas of density indicative of hemorrhage; white areas indicative of renal calculi.

Ultrasound
Identifies renal structures and the presence of fluid accumulation or obstruction. Determines location and cause of obstruction in postrenal disease.

Intravenous pyelogram
Used to visualize kidney and associated structures. Obstruction seen in postrenal disease; used cautiously in intrarenal disease because contrast medium can exacerbate condition.

Retrograde pyelogram
Used to visualize urinary system Useful in postrenal disease because it visualizes clots, strictures, and stones within the kidneys and urinary system; uses an iodine-based contrast material to reduce exacerbation of intrarenal disease.

Angiogram
Used to visualize renal blood flow. Useful in the diagnosis of stenosis, tumors, clots, cysts, infarctions, and trauma to the kidneys; used cautiously in intrarenal disease because contrast medium may exacerbate condition.

Kidney-ureter-bladder X-ray
Used to visualize overall position, size, and structures of kidneys, ureters, and bladder. Enlarged kidney
(continued)

Diagnostic tests for acute renal failure *(continued)*

may indicate calculi, hydronephrosis, cysts, or tumors; enlarged areas of ureters may indicate calculi.

Biopsy
Directly analyzes the kidney tissue. Although it is the definitive test for

diagnosing the disease within the kidney, it is usually the last resort because of the postprocedural risks of bleeding, hematoma formation, and infection.

Hemodialysis, the separation of excess electrolytes, fluids, and toxins from the blood, works by circulating the blood outside of the body. Through osmosis and diffusion, extra fluid, electrolytes, and toxins are removed from the blood prior to returning to the patient's general circulation. This type of dialysis can only be performed by accessing the patient's vascular system.

Peritoneal dialysis may be indicated if the patient has diabetes mellitus or a history of poor vascular status. This type of dialysis involves introducing dialysate into the patient's abdominal cavity. The dialysate mixture bathes the peritoneum and through the processes of osmosis, diffusion, and active transport, excess fluids, electrolytes, and toxins enter the dialysate. The dialysate is then drained from the abdominal cavity. (For care of the patient receiving hemodialysis or peritoneal dialysis, see *Nursing interventions for patients undergoing hemodialysis and peritoneal dialysis*, pages 566 and 567.)

Newer methods of dialysis fall under the category of continuous renal replacement therapy (CRRT). CRRT is a continuous therapy in which the patient's whole blood is circulated through a hemofilter. The hydrostatic pressure exerted by the patient's mean arterial pressure sets the rate of blood flow through the filter. Currently, there are three forms of CRRT: slow continuous ultrafiltration, continuous arteriovenous hemofiltration, and continuous arteriovenous hemodialysis.

Overall nursing care for the ARF patient is focused on managing fluid and electrolyte balance; identifying, preventing, and treating infections; maintaining adequate respiratory status; supporting nutritional status; and preventing complications and future episodes of failure.

Complications from ARF arise from infections or a worsening of the failure. Most deaths related to ARF are attributed to a secondary infection that develops following recent surgery or a traumatic injury. Pericarditis occurs in up to 18% of patients. Treatment includes administering steroids or nonsteroidal anti-inflammatory agents and may include pericardiocentesis or pericardiectomy if cardiac function becomes significantly compromised.

If normal renal function does not resume, chronic renal failure may be imminent. As the primary complication of ARF, chronic renal failure cannot be reversed and the patient will be dependent on dialysis for the remainder of life.

Prerenal failure

For the patient diagnosed with prerenal failure in the beginning phase, care focuses on the following nursing interventions:

• Replace lost fluid volume. Provide intravenous solutions between 1,500 ml/day for fluid deficits totaling 5% of body weight and 3,000 ml/day for fluid deficits greater than 5% of body weight.

• Reverse or prevent onset of oliguria. Administer diuretics (furosemide or ethacrynic acid), as ordered, to stimulate urine output once the patient is adequately hydrated. Also administer mannitol or low-dose dopamine, as ordered, to increase renal perfusion.

Intrarenal failure

Patients with intrarenal failure respond to the following nursing interventions:

• Identify the cause. Report findings from laboratory data indicating toxic serum values. Discontinue medications that cause nephrotoxicity.

• Prepare the patient for peritoneal dialysis or hemodialysis.

Nursing interventions for patients undergoing hemodialysis and peritoneal dialysis

The following chart provides nursing interventions appropriate for the patient receiving hemodialysis or peritoneal dialysis to treat acute renal failure.

Dialysis Type	Description
Hemodialysis	Circulating blood is filtered through an external device and circulated back into the patient's general blood flow to remove extra fluid, electrolytes, and toxins.
Peritoneal dialysis	Dialysate is introduced through an implanted catheter into the patient's abdominal cavity to remove fluid, electrolytes, and toxins from the bloodstream; indicated for patients with poor arteriovenous access sites

• Support circulating blood volume by providing packed red blood cells and monitoring for transfusion reaction.
• Support nutritional status by providing a high-carbohydrate diet appropriate for the patient's electrolyte status, such as low sodium for the patient with water retention or high sodium for the patient with water loss, by parenteral, enteral, or oral route.

Nursing Interventions

• Assess weight, blood pressure, heart and lung sounds, temperature, access site, and skin condition before the dialysis procedure to serve as a baseline and to evaluate the patient's ability to physiologically tolerate the procedure.
• Monitor vital signs every 30 to 60 minutes during the procedure.
• Monitor for signs of intolerance to the procedure, including nausea, vomiting, confusion, restlessness, headache, muscle cramping, twitching, jerking, or seizures.
• Monitor the vascular access site after dialysis for bleeding or hematoma formation, evidence of clotting, skin discoloration, and signs of infection. Document and report these signs to the physician.
• Avoid blood sampling and taking the blood pressure if the extremity was used for vascular access.

• Assess weight, blood pressure, heart and lung sounds, temperature, and catheter site before infusion of the dialysate.
• Ensure that the dialysate is warmed to body temperature to maintain the blood temperature and maintain the ability of the solutes in the dialysate to diffuse.
• Elevate the head of the bed to decrease pressure on the diaphragm and to aid in breathing if the patient will tolerate it.
• Monitor the patient for abdominal pain, cramping, or lower back pain during the procedure because the introduction of dialysate into the abdominal cavity causes increased intra-abdominal pressure and concurrent pressure to the lower back.
• Monitor for signs of peritonitis, including cloudy dialysate, abdominal pain, rebound tenderness, nausea, vomiting, and fever.
• Instruct the patient about the need for adequate protein and amino acid intake because both are removed during the procedure; estimated intake of protein should be 1.2 to 1.5 grams per kilogram of body weight per day.
• If the patient is diabetic, monitor glucose levels and administer insulin, as prescribed.
• Monitor vital signs during outflow phase to avoid potential hypotension or overhydration.

• Provide pharmacologic support. Administer antihypertensives, as ordered, according to blood pressure; aluminum hydroxide and calcium carbonate antacids to control hyperphosphatemia; sodium bicarbonate for metabolic acidosis; Kayexalate (oral or per rectum) for hyperkalemia.
• Provide water-soluble vitamin supplements post-dialysis because the dialysate filters out water soluble vitamins.

• Support immunosuppressed state by monitoring temperature, white blood cell count, and peripheral and central venous access sites for signs of infection. Provide oral hygiene every 2 hours, turn and reposition every 2 hours, and encourage the patient to deep breathe and cough every 2 hours to prevent pooling of secretions in the lungs. Evaluate need for indwelling urinary catheter as urinary catheters can serve as a cause for infection.

• Support integumentary status by providing skin lubricants or oral antihistamines, as ordered, for pruritus.

• Monitor serum calcium and parathyroid hormone levels because of a decreased excretion of phosphate and synthesis of vitamin D due to the renal failure.

• Support GI status by monitoring for frequency and quality of bowel movements and providing stool softeners or enemas, as ordered, to prevent constipation commonly seen with phosphate antacids.

Postrenal failure

Care of the patient with postrenal failure includes the following interventions:

• Relieve the cause or obstruction.

• Monitor urinary catheter or stent, if present. Stent may be placed in a ureter to optimize the flow of urine from the kidney to the bladder.

• Prepare the patient for surgery (lithotripsy or prostatic resection) if renal calculi or prostatic hypertrophy are found to be the cause of failure.

• Support fluid and electrolyte status by administering replacement fluids, as ordered, and monitoring and replacing serum electrolytes, as indicated.

Prognosis

ARF carries a 30% to 60% mortality rate, depending on the underlying cause. If the cause is from nephrotoxic agents, obstruction, or glomerulonephritis, the mortality rate is lower. The higher mortality rates occur when the failure is caused by surgery or trauma.

Discharge planning

Discharge plans for a patient recovering from ARF should include discussions and instructions on methods to prevent future episodes of failure, indications of fluid volume and electrolyte changes, care of the peritoneal or hemodialysis site, medications review, diet review, and the need for future long-term medical follow-up.

Specific instructions should cover:
• causes of ARF and methods to prevent it
• medication regimen, including the name, dosage, purpose, frequency, precautions, and possible side effects
• prescribed dietary plan, including which foods to avoid, such as bananas, citrus fruits, fruit juices, nuts, tea, and coffee (they are high in potassium). A dietitian can be consulted to provide the most accurate information and ways to aid for an adequate intake.
• indicators of altered fluid or electrolyte status, such as changes in urine output, changes in weight, level of responsiveness, onset of cough, or shortness of breath
• care of the peritoneal dialysis or hemodialysis site, stressing universal precautions and site assessment
• need for social services to assist with outpatient dialysis and financial issues
• need for home nursing care for evaluation once the patient is discharged.

Renal trauma

A serious injury to the kidney that can lead to hemorrhage and loss of functioning renal tissue, renal trauma is rarely seen as an individual injury. Because the thoracic rib cage and heavily muscled back area serve as added protection to the renal tissue and vasculature, direct trauma to the kidneys is usually caused when the patient sustains either a blunt or penetrating trauma to the abdomen, back, or flank area.

Most incidents of renal trauma occur in males under age 30. The incidence of blunt renal trauma is greater and closely associated with motor vehicle accidents, sports injuries, and accidental falls. Blunt trauma can also occur as a result of direct kidney compression by the twelfth rib squeezing the kidney into the lumbar spine. Penetrating renal injuries are usually caused by shotgun and stab wounds, but fractured ribs can also cause kidney lacerations. Approximately 85% of all cases of renal trauma are caused by blunt force, whereas 15% are the direct result of penetrating injuries.

Renal trauma is considered a medical emergency because hemorrhage and permanent kidney damage can directly result. Often overlooked as a site of injury, the kidneys should be thoroughly evaluated for involvement when traumatic injuries to the colon, liver, pancreas, and spleen are present.

Pathophysiology

In the case of blunt trauma, a direct blow or other force is directly applied to the kidney. The renal capsule surrounding the kidney cannot protect the tissue from injury. Even though the resulting contusion or intrarenal hemorrhage is confined within the renal parenchyma, it interferes with normal glomerular functioning.

Additionally, blunt renal trauma can result in either a ruptured or fractured kidney. A ruptured kidney causes hemorrhage between the capsular wall and the renal parenchyma, whereas a fractured kidney results in hemorrhage throughout the entire renal tissue. Either case represents a surgical emergency (see *Types of renal trauma,* page 571).

Penetrating renal injuries can cause either minor or major lacerations to the kidney tissue. With a minor laceration, the tissue ruptures, creating a subcapsular hemorrhage, altering renal function. Major lacerations cause rupturing into the renal pelvis, hemorrhage, extravasation of urine, and impaired function.

Injuries to the renal pedicle can cause impaired vascular flow to the renal tissue or a complete dislocation of the kidney from the pedicle. There may or may not be an associated intrarenal hemorrhage. Impaired blood flow to the renal tissue causes ischemic changes within

Types of renal trauma

The following chart identifies types of kidney injuries, along with their defining characteristics and expected outcome.

Type of Injury	Defining Characteristics	Expected Outcome
Minor trauma		
• Renal contusion • Shallow lacerations • Subscapular hematoma 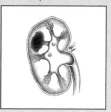	• Renal parenchyma is bruised; superficial lacerations of renal cortex without rupture of renal capsule • Flank tenderness • Hematuria	Usually a full recovery without loss of normal renal function
Major trauma		
• Major lacerations 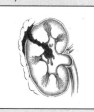	• Major lacerations throughout cortex and medulla; laceration continues through to renal capsule • Flank pain • Hematuria • Hypotension	Nephrectomy may be necessary in 10% of the cases
Critical trauma		
• Fractured kidney • Renal pedicle injury 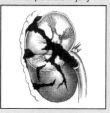	• Trauma to the renal vasculature resulting in a shattered kidney and renal pedicle injury • Rapidly expanding flank mass • Severe blood loss • Shock	• Immediate surgical intervention necessary • Kidney can be saved in 10% to 30% of cases

Source: Swearingen, P. L. & Keen, J. H. (1991). *Manual of Critical Care*. Mosby: St. Louis; pg. 194.

the renal parenchymal cells, creating changes in glomerular filtration and sodium reabsorption. Additionally, urea, creatinine, and other body wastes are unable to filter through the glomerular membrane, creating a buildup of these substances within the circulating blood. Total kidney destruction can occur within 2 hours after kidney dislocation.

Clinical assessment
Trauma sustained to the kidneys is an emergency necessitating immediate surgical intervention for patient survival. The nurse is in the pivotal position to assess the extent of renal injury and support remaining renal tissue function.

History
The patient with renal trauma, depending upon the level of responsiveness, will complain of flank soreness or back tenderness. In addition, the patient should be asked about recent activity that could have caused:
• a blow to the flank region, such as a sporting activity
• penetrating injury to the flank region, such as involvement in a motor vehicle accident.
• severe pressure to the abdominal region.

Physical findings
Often thought of as the universal sign of kidney trauma, gross hematuria is present in only about 50% of diagnosed cases, whereas microscopic hematuria is present in about 80% of diagnosed cases. However, gross hematuria is often present in minor renal trauma. Other, more predictable signs and symptoms of renal trauma include:
• abdominal or flank pain, back tenderness
• intermittent pain associated with the passing of clots through the urine
• confusion, fatigue, restlessness
• dizziness
• nausea, vomiting
• abrasions over the flank or abdominal region
• hypotension, tachycardia

• pallor, diaphoresis
• hematoma over the flank or lower rib region
• obvious wounds
• abdominal distention
• reduced or absent bowel sounds
• Grey Turner's sign (bruising over the flank and lower back region)
• pain upon palpation of the flank region
• evidence of an expanding abdominal or flank mass
• fever.

Diagnosis

The extent of injury to the renal tissue and subsequent viability of the organ can be evaluated through the use of a variety of radiologic tests. Those most frequently used to assess the extent of renal trauma are listed in *Diagnostic tests for renal trauma,* page 574.

Treatment and care

The primary goals of treatment for the patient with renal trauma are to evaluate the extent of renal tissue damage, support optimal circulating blood flow, reverse shock, and maintain remaining renal tissue functioning.

Evaluating extent of renal tissue damage

Patients found to have a renal laceration will either be treated medically, which includes bed rest, observation, and monitoring of hematuria, or receive surgical intervention to repair the laceration.

Specific nursing interventions for the patient with a renal contusion and treated medically include the following:
• Monitor the degree of hematuria, if present.
• Monitor for changes in urine output; report changes that indicate early signs of renal failure, such as a sudden increase or decrease in urine output and alterations in specific gravity value.
• Evaluate serum blood urea nitrogen (BUN), creatinine, and electrolyte levels as well as complete blood

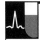

Diagnostic tests for renal trauma

This chart identifies common tests used in the diagnosis of renal trauma.

Kidney-ureter-bladder X-ray

Assists in identifying the location and gross appearance of the kidneys, ureters, and bladder. Displacement or alteration in kidney structure may indicate laceration or contusion.

CT scan and MRI

Identify location, extent, and degree of renal tissue injury; aid in diagnosis of laceration vs. rupture. Able to differentiate between superficial lacerations or major injuries. Increased areas of density indicative of hemorrhage.

Intravenous pyelogram

Used to visualize kidney and associated structures. In combination with the CT scan, this test provides the most accurate information on the extent of injuries. Outlines the collection system and establishes the presence and function of both kidneys. Contrast medium is used for visualization; however, it must be used cautiously because it can cause renal parenchymal damage.

Renal arteriogram

Used to definitively diagnose the quality of renal arterial blood flow and the status of organ circulation. This test is indicated if the IVP fails to fully define the extent of injury, if the entire kidney cannot be visualized, or if CT scanning equipment is unavailable. Outlines the renal vessels, integrity of blood flow, and existence of hematomas; interruption in progression of contrast medium indicates pedicle injury. Contrast medium is used for visualization and should be used cau-

tiously because it can cause renal parenchymal damage.

Electrolyte studies

Used to evaluate sodium, potassium, and bicarbonate levels. Sodium > 147 mEq/liter (normal 135 to 145 mEq/liter), potassium > 6 mEq/liter (normal 3.5 to 5 mEq/liter), and bicarbonate < 15 mEq/dl (normal 15 to 25 mEq/dl) indicate inability of kidneys to regulate hydrogen ion secretion or regulate excess electrolyte excretion, which may lead to fluid overload or an oliguria/anuria phase of acute renal failure.

Blood urea nitrogen

Used to evaluate protein metabolism and the presence of uremia. Level > 20 mg/dl (normal 9 to 20 mg/dl) indicates deteriorating renal function.

Serum creatinine

Precise indicator of renal functioning as creatinine builds up in the blood when renal function is impaired. Level > 1.5 mg/dl (normal 0.7 to 1.5 mg/dl) indicates deteriorating renal function.

Complete blood count

Evaluates hydration, lysis of red blood cells, and presence of infection. Hemoglobin < 10 g/dl (normal 13 to 18 g/dl for males, 12 to 16 g/dl for females) and hematocrit < 30% (normal 45% to 52% for males, 37% to 48% for females) indicates lysis of red blood cells or hemodilution; white blood cell count > 11,000/μl (normal 4,500 to 11,000/μl) indicates infection.

count (CBC) for signs of deteriorating renal functioning; report values as indicated.

If the patient requires surgical intervention to repair the laceration, postoperative nursing care is as follows:
• Monitor urine output and reporting changes that indicate signs of renal failure.
• Monitor cardiac rhythm and rate, and administer antiarrhythmics, if indicated, to treat electrolyte abnormalities secondary to altered renal functioning.
• Monitor central venous pressure (CVP) for signs of fluid overload, and prepare to administer diuretics, as ordered.
• Monitor serum BUN, creatinine, and electrolyte levels as well as CBC; provide electrolyte supplements as ordered; administer packed red blood cells as ordered.
• Maintain patency of nephrostomy tube by supporting efforts to prevent tube dislodgment; evaluating the site for redness, exudate, and leakage of urine or blood; documenting nephrostomy tube output separately from indwelling urinary catheter output; avoiding kinking the tube; and maintaining a sterile closed system.

Patients who have sustained a renal fracture or pedicle injury will undergo immediate surgery. If the fracture can be repaired, care of the patient will mimic that of the renal laceration. Should the kidney be unsalvageable, the patient will need to have a nephrectomy.

Nursing care for the patient undergoing a nephrectomy includes the following:
• Monitor urine output, and report sudden increases or decreases in volume.
• Monitor cardiac rhythm and rate, and monitor and treat electrolyte imbalances secondary to altered renal function.
• Monitor CVP for signs of fluid overload, and prepare to treat, as ordered.
• Monitor peripheral blood pressure, and report increasing values.
• Monitor serum electrolyte, BUN, creatinine, and CBC levels, and administer electrolyte supplements and blood replacement products, as ordered.

Optimizing circulating blood flow

Optimal blood flow is necessary to prevent further renal and cellular damage. Nursing interventions to achieve this goal include:

• Assess for poor skin turgor, dry mucous membranes, thirst, hypotension, tachycardia, and decreasing CVP.

• Assess for signs of bleeding; monitor hemoglobin and hematocrit as well as urine drainage from nephrostomy tube for increasing blood-tinged output.

• Monitor urine output every hour; report output less than 30 ml/hour.

• Monitor and report changes in vomiting, diarrhea, wound drainage, or sudden diuresis.

Reversing shock

Depending on the extent of injury, the patient may experience hypovolemic shock. Appropriate nursing measures are listed below:

• Provide continuous cardiac monitoring.

• Assess for arrhythmias and treat as prescribed.

• Provide ongoing monitoring of blood pressure every 15 minutes.

• Evaluate cardiac rate; report tachycardia and treat with fluids or volume expanders.

• Provide ongoing assessment of level of consciousness.

Maintaining renal tissue function

Depending on the extent of renal injury and subsequent damage, the patient may experience alterations in normal renal regulatory mechanisms. Nursing care to ensure optimal renal tissue functioning includes the following measures:

• Monitor urine output every hour; report output less than 30 ml/hour.

• Monitor for signs and symptoms of fluid overload, including crackles, jugular vein distention, tachycardia, pericardial friction rub, gallop, increasing blood pressure, increasing CVP, shortness of breath, and increasing peripheral edema.

• Monitor fluid intake, and restrict as ordered.
• Monitor serum electrolyte, BUN, and creatinine levels; intervene as ordered.
• Monitor arterial blood gas levels for indications of metabolic acidosis.
• Prepare for hemodialysis, if indicated.

Preventing and treating complications

Common complications associated with renal trauma include renal hypertension, renal artery scarring and fibrosis (which can cause systemic hypertension), and the development of renal failure. However, the leading complication of renal trauma is infection related to the patient's immunosuppressed state associated with the traumatic incident or surgical procedure.

Nursing interventions for the patient with a post-traumatic or surgical infection include:
• Monitor temperature every 2 hours; report elevations of 1° to 2° C.
• Monitor white blood cell count. Report levels greater than 11,000/µl.
• Monitor the surgical wound site for signs of infection; culture drainage.
• Culture urine and nephrostomy drainage; begin antibiotic therapy, as ordered.
• Evaluate peripheral and central venous access sites for signs of infection; use universal precautions.
• Turn and reposition the patient every 2 hours.
• Assist the patient with deep breathing and coughing technique every 2 hours.

Prognosis

With correct, timely diagnosis of the extent of injury and immediate surgical intervention, if indicated, the prognosis for the renal trauma patient is good. Long-term effects of the incident, however, may be a challenge, particularly if the patient has had a nephrectomy or needs long-term dialysis for survival.

Discharge planning

When preparing the patient for discharge, the nurse should provide the following information:

• need to restrict physical activity until permitted by the physician

• need to schedule follow-up appointments for ongoing evaluation of blood pressure, renal function, and serum blood values

• review of all prescribed medications, including the purpose, dosage, and possible side effects

• review of signs and symptoms of altered renal status, including changes in urine output and color

• consultation with social services, especially if the patient is to undergo outpatient hemodialysis or is being discharged with a nephrostomy tube or has had a nephrectomy

• need to reduce high-risk behavior, such as participating in gang activities, if that was the cause of the trauma. If the trauma was sustained during recreation, alternative avenues must be offered to the patient. If the event occurred during employment, such as in law enforcement professions, alternatives might be more limiting. Social services would be in the best position to help the patient make such life-altering decisions and to aid in the reinforcement of nursing's efforts to alter behaviors that could cause additional trauma in the future.

Patients who have had a nephrectomy need to be particularly careful of their lifestyle and choice of employment. Discharge instructions for the patient postnephrectomy should include:

• signs and symptoms of kidney infection: dull flank pain, elevated temperature, cloudy or blood-tinged urine, and nausea or vomiting.

• review of follow-up appointments with the physician for ongoing evaluation of blood pressure, renal function, and serum blood values.

Respiratory failure

Respiratory failure is a general medical condition characterized by the inability of the respiratory system to supply sufficient oxygen for sustaining life or to eliminate carbon dioxide from the bloodstream. Acute respiratory failure, a serious and sometimes fatal condition, occurs when the PaO_2 level falls below 50 mm Hg or the $PaCO_2$ level exceeds 50 mm Hg. If respiratory failure is left undiagnosed and untreated, the ongoing lack of oxygen and continuing carbon dioxide buildup eventually lead to hypoxia and cellular death.

Rarely diagnosed alone, acute respiratory failure commonly develops from some underlying condition that results in increased work of breathing, decreased respiratory drive, or dysfunction of the chest wall and lung parenchyma. Additionally, acute respiratory failure is often misdiagnosed because the major indicator, a change in level of responsiveness, is mistakenly seen as a precursor to congestive heart failure, cerebrovascular accident, or pneumonia. (Specific causative factors are listed in *Common causes of acute respiratory failure,* page 580.) Because of the insidious onset of hypoxia, the diagnosis of acute respiratory failure may be delayed. Consequently, early recognition of signs and symptoms is essential for patient survival.

Acute respiratory failure can be classified as Type I or Type II. In Type I failure, also termed hypoxemic normocapnic respiratory failure, the patient has a low PaO_2 and a normal $PaCO_2$. With Type II failure, or hypoxemic hypercapnic respiratory failure, the PaO_2 is also low, but the $PaCO_2$ is elevated.

Pathophysiology

In acute respiratory failure, alveolar ventilation and pulmonary vascular perfusion are impaired. A reduction in the arterial blood oxygen tension below 50 mm Hg and an increase in $PaCO_2$ greater than 50 mm Hg causes an alteration in the amount of oxygen-carrying

Common causes of acute respiratory failure

Acute respiratory failure may be precipitated by any of the following causes:

Decreased respiratory drive
• Brain disorders, including brain trauma, tumor, and stroke
• Drug-induced states (from use of barbiturates, narcotics, sedatives, or tranquilizers)
• Obesity
• Sleep apnea syndrome

Dysfunction of chest wall
• Use of anesthetic-blocking agents
• Cervical spinal cord injury
• Kyphoscoliosis
• Use of neuromuscular-blocking agents
• Neuromuscular disorders (such as amyotrophic lateral sclerosis, Guillain-Barré syndrome, muscular dystrophy, or polio)

Dysfunction of lung parenchyma
• Adult respiratory distress syndrome
• Inhalation of toxic chemicals, gases, or smoke
• Interstitial lung diseases
• Near-drowning
• Pneumonia
• Pulmonary contusion
• Pulmonary edema
• Smoking

Other factors
• Abdominal distention related to intestinal obstruction
• Ascites
• Carbon monoxide inhalation
• Upper airway obstruction (such as from a foreign body or tumor)

hemoglobin to body tissues. Hypoxia results from the inadequate oxygenation of hemoglobin within the pulmonary capillaries.

Respiratory system mechanisms that cause acute respiratory failure include alveolar hypoventilation, ventilation-perfusion mismatch, diffusion abnormalities, and shunting. Type I failure is the result of ventilation-perfusion mismatch and shunting. A patient who develops alveolar hypoventilation in addition to the ventilation-perfusion mismatch and shunting has Type II respiratory failure.

Alveolar hypoventilation

The reduction in available oxygen reaching the alveolar level causes a buildup of carbon dioxide, resulting in hypoventilation. The alveolar hypoventilation manifests as an alteration in minute ventilation—either a decrease in minute ventilation with normal dead-space ventilation (seen in patients with normal lungs whose respiratory status is impaired by drugs or neuromuscular diseases) or a normal or increased minute ventilation with an increase in dead-space ventilation (seen in patients with pneumonia or chronic obstructive pulmonary disease [COPD]). The amount of dead-space ventilation depends on the underlying medical condition.

Ventilation-perfusion mismatch

For efficient gas exchange to occur, the ventilation-perfusion relationship must be equal: the amount of lung oxygenation must match the amount of blood perfusion to any given area. Mismatching occurs when blood flows to an underventilated area or when areas with a reduced or absent blood flow become ventilated.

Diffusion abnormalities

A diffusion abnormality exists when the equilibrium between the alveolar oxygen pressure and the pulmonary capillary pressure is interrupted. Diffusion can be interrupted when the amount of time red blood cells (RBCs) are in contact with the capillary membrane is reduced, pulmonary capillary blood flow is reduced, or the capillary membrane is thickened, hindering effective RBC oxygenation.

Shunting

Shunting occurs when blood enters the arterial blood circulation before passing through ventilated lung areas. Typically, such shunting occurs in a right-to-left pattern: large volumes of blood pass from the right side of the heart directly into the left side of the heart, entering the general circulation without being adequately ventilated. Viewed as an extreme ventilation-perfusion disturbance, shunting occurs when blood perfuses large areas of nonventilated or underventilated alveoli (as in consolidated pneumonia) or when blood bypasses the alveoli (as in pulmonary embolism). Anatomical causes of shunting include an arterial or septal defect or patent ductus arteriosus.

Clinical assessment

Adequately diagnosing acute respiratory failure depends on early recognition of signs and symptoms and prompt initiation of therapy to reverse the hypoxic state, improve blood oxygen levels, and reduce carbon dioxide blood levels. The nurse's ongoing respiratory assessment is key to early diagnosis and treatment.

History

The patient with acute respiratory failure probably will be hospitalized with an underlying medical condition. Information necessary for a timely diagnosis include:
• reason for the current hospitalization (if appropriate)
• history of smoking
• history of nonprescribed drug use
• preexisting health conditions, such as COPD, asthma, chronic bronchitis, emphysema, myasthenia gravis, multiple sclerosis, or muscular dystrophy
• recent thoracoabdominal surgery.

Physical findings

Clinical signs and symptoms of acute respiratory failure vary with the underlying medical condition. Early signs of pending acute respiratory failure include:
• anxiety or restlessness, fatigue
• cool, dry skin
• headache
• productive or nonproductive cough
• wheezing or shortness of breath
• increased blood pressure
• tachycardia or onset of cardiac arrhythmias.
    Patients who are in the intermediate stages of acute respiratory failure will present with:
• confusion and lethargy
• tachypnea
• hypotension (secondary to vasodilation)
• ongoing cardiac arrhythmias.
    Late signs and symptoms of acute respiratory failure include:
• cyanosis

- diaphoresis
- coma
- respiratory arrest.

Physical assessment findings of acute respiratory failure may include:
- use of accessory respiratory muscles
- asymmetrical chest movement
- intercostal muscle retraction
- tactile fremitus, crepitus, and deviated trachea
- absent or diminished breath sounds
- crackles, rhonchi, wheezes, pleural friction rub, inspiratory stridor, bronchial or bronchovesicular sounds in abnormal location
- peripheral edema (extremities, periorbital, or sacral)
- jugular vein distention
- cyanosis
- reduction in level of responsiveness
- irregular heart rate and rhythm.

Diagnosis

Early diagnosis and appropriate medical intervention is crucial to patient survival. Diagnostic tests useful in the detecting acute respiratory failure include arterial blood gas (ABG) studies, cardiac output and mixed venous blood gas measurement, pulse oximetry, chest X-ray, blood and sputum cultures, bronchoscopy, and lung biopsy (see *Diagnostic tests for acute respiratory failure,* page 584, for more information).

Treatment and care

The treatment goals for the patient in acute respiratory failure are to correct the underlying cause of failure and restore oxygen-carbon dioxide gas exchange to maintain normal physiologic functioning. Medical management involves protecting the airway and establishing ventilation, with endotracheal intubation and mechanical ventilation if necessary; correcting the hypoxemia and the underlying cause; correcting the abnormal pH level; and monitoring for and treating complications.

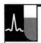

Diagnostic tests for acute respiratory failure

The following diagnostic tests and procedures are used for the diagnosis and treatment of acute respiratory failure.

Arterial blood gas analysis

The most specific diagnostic test available to determine acute respiratory failure and predict future responses to treatment; values expected in the acute respiratory failure patient include $PaO_2 \leq 60$ mm Hg, $PaCO_2 \geq 45$ mm Hg, and pH < 7.35.

Cardiac output and mixed venous blood gas measurement

Normal PO_2 of mixed venous blood is 35 to 40 mm Hg with an average oxygen saturation of 75% (between 60% and 80%); in acute respiratory failure, a $P\bar{v}O_2$ of 60 mm Hg indicates oxygen is not being extracted from the red blood cells; a $P\bar{v}O_2$ of < 35 mm Hg indicates an increased use of oxygen by the tissues.

Pulse oximetry

Electronically measures the optical density of light absorbed by the arterial blood; accuracy depends on the amount of tissue perfusion to the skin. This diagnostic test has limitations: the indicator is accurate within two digits when the arterial oxygen saturation level is between 70% and 100%. Marked changes in the PaO_2 level can occur despite minimal changes seen in the pulse oximeter value; the meter cannot differentiate between oxyhemoglobin and carboxyhemoglobin and might incorrectly interpret the hemoglobin as saturated. Should be used in conjunction with other tests to adequately assess the oxygenation status.

Chest X-ray

A shift in the mediastinum could indicate either atelectasis or pneumothorax; shifts also are seen in pleural effusion and tumors. Findings might include an elevated hemidiaphragm (associated with pneumonia), flattening of the diaphragm (indicates increased air in the lungs as in COPD or pleural effusion), blunting of the costophrenic angle (occurs with pleural effusion, atelectasis, or pneumothorax), evidence of a pleural space (indicates pneumothorax or pleural effusion), increased density of lung tissue (indicates fluid in the lungs or a collapsed lung), and increased radiolucency of the lung tissue (indicates increased air in the lungs as seen in COPD).

Sputum culture

Examined for volume, physical properties, mucopurulence, and color. If a bacterial infection is suspected, a Gram stain followed by a culture and sensitivity is performed. Based on findings, antibiotic medications might be indicated.

Bronchoscopy

Used diagnostically or therapeutically. Diagnostically, bronchoscopy is indicated for patients experiencing hemoptysis and pneumonia. Therapeutically, bronchoscopy is used to remove foreign body aspirates, to treat atelectasis, and to resect benign growths from the airway. Chest X-ray must be performed prior to the procedure in addition to a PT/PTT and ABG analysis. Hypoxic patients will need supplemental oxygen during the procedure. Complications include laryngospasm, epistaxis, fever, pulmonary infiltrates, bronchospasm, and pneumothorax.

Nursing care is focused on promoting effective airway clearance and gas exchange, monitoring and documenting indicators of altered tissue perfusion, monitoring and promoting effective breathing patterns, preventing complications caused by immobility, reducing anxiety, and promoting comfort (see *Key nursing interventions for patients with acute respiratory failure,* page 586).

Mechanical ventilation

Mechanical ventilation is used to restore alveolar ventilation, restore blood pH to normal limits, and decrease the effort of breathing. Intubation at an early stage can prevent further airway collapse and subsequent tissue injury. Mechanical ventilation is continued until the underlying medical condition is diagnosed, treatment is instituted, and the patient is able to resume independent respirations.

Specific nursing interventions are outlined below:
• Adjust the mechanical ventilator according to ABG levels and patient position.
• Assess the mechanical ventilator for proper functioning and settings. Set alarms and free circuitry of any condensed water.
• Monitor for signs that the patient's independent respirations are out of sync with the ventilator's cycle (dysynchrony). This condition is detrimental to gas exchange and causes an increase in airway pressures.
• Encourage the patient to relax to synchronize respirations with the ventilatory cycle. Explain how the ventilator alarms serve as an alert for any accidental disconnections.
• Reassure the patient that ventilatory support may be a temporary measure until normal respiratory functioning is restored.
• Monitor humidification of mechanical ventilator.
• Prepare the patient for weaning from the ventilator by explaining the process and offering reassurance; placing the patient in a sitting or semirecumbent position to facilitate diaphragmatic breathing; suctioning if neces-

ESSENTIAL ELEMENTS

Key nursing interventions for the patient with acute respiratory failure

The following chart highlights interventions typically performed with a patient in acute respiratory failure.

> **Restore oxygen-carbon dioxide gas exchange to maintain normal physiologic functioning**

Promote effective gas exchange	Ensure effective airway clearance	Maximize nutritional status
• Monitor and adjust ventilator according to ABG levels and patient response. • Auscultate breath sounds and over artificial airway. • Report diminished lung sounds and any air leaks over the artificial airway. • Administer prescribed analgesics or sedatives, as ordered. • Monitor patient's tolerance to the weaning process; evaluate ABG levels, lung sounds, and use of accessory muscles during weaning episodes.	• Perform chest physiotherapy every 2 hours as tolerated. • Perform nasotracheal suction, as tolerated. • Report changes in secretions. • Monitor ventilator temperature between 89.6° and 96.8° F (32° and 36° C). • Provide IVF 2 to 3 liters/24 hours, as ordered. • Monitor and report signs of complications or infection. • Practice universal precautions. • Provide oral hygiene every 4 to 8 hours. • Administer antibiotics, as ordered. • Monitor patient's tolerance of mechanical ventilation. • Provide tracheostomy care at least every 4 hours.	• Provide total parenteral nutrition, as ordered; evaluate tolerance. • Administer enteral feedings, as prescribed. • Consult dietitian. • Monitor gastric tube placement. • Aspirate residuals prior to next feeding. • Keep head of bed elevated more than 30 degrees, as tolerated, during feedings to prevent aspiration of tube feeding. • Keep trach cuff inflated during feedings.

sary prior to weaning; and assessing the patient's heart rate, cardiac rhythm, blood pressure, respiratory rate, ABG levels, and level of consciousness.

Correcting hypoxemia
In the correction of hypoxemia, oxygen therapy, chest physiotherapy, and pharmacotherapy will be used. Medications helpful to improve ABG levels include antibiotics, bronchodilators, and steroids. Nursing interventions for correcting hypoxemia include the following:
• Observe, document, and report changes in the patient's condition that indicate an increase in respiratory distress.
• Monitor respiratory rate and rhythm. Report rates less than 11 or greater than 24 per minute.
• Instruct the patient in deep-breathing techniques, if patient is capable of performing them; provide positive reinforcement of efforts.
• Use postural drainage to facilitate clearance of secretions that might pool in the different lung segments.
• If only one lung is affected, position the patient with healthy lung down or in a dependent position to facilitate perfusion and decrease ventilation-perfusion mismatching.
• If both lungs are affected, position the patient with the right lung down (as tolerated) because the right lung has more surface area to combat the effects of ventilation-perfusion mismatch. Reposition the patient every 2 hours.
• Keep a manual resuscitator at the bedside in the event that the patient begins to fight the ventilator or the ventilator malfunctions.

Correction of underlying cause
Successful treatment of acute respiratory failure includes managing the underlying cause. For example, if ventilation-perfusion mismatch is the problem, perfusion must be reestablished; if the cause is secondary to pulmonary embolism, thrombolytic therapy is indicated; if low perfusion is due to low cardiac output, im-

proving the cardiac output is necessary; and if excessive medication and central nervous system depression is the problem, medications must be adjusted to decrease the depression. Specific nursing measures include the following:

• Continuously monitor cardiac rate and rhythm. Report arrhythmias, and begin corrective action as ordered.

• Monitor intake and output.

• Monitor for jugular vein distention and for peripheral or sacral edema.

• Consult a dietitian to determine the patient's caloric requirements.

• Provide parenteral nutrition, as ordered; advance to enteral nutrition as the patient's condition warrants. Implement measures to prevent aspiration.

Correcting the blood pH

Correcting acidosis (blood pH < 7.25) is achieved by administering sodium bicarbonate I.V. Alkalosis, blood pH > 7.45, can be managed by using a rebreathing oxygen face mask or increasing the dead space with the use of mechanical ventilation. Nursing measures include:

• Monitor ABG levels for changes in PaO_2, $PaCO_2$, and pH.

• Report dropping PaO_2.

Monitoring for and treating complications

The major complications seen in acute respiratory failure are caused by mechanical ventilation or a further deterioration of the patient's respiratory status. Common complications caused by mechanical ventilation include barotrauma, fluid imbalances, gastrointestinal disturbances, hypotension, increased intracranial pressure, and tension pneumothorax (see *Complications of mechanical ventilation*, pages 590 and 591).

Nursing interventions include:

• Monitor for and report signs of infection (temperature greater than 100.4° [F38° C], pulse greater than 100 beats/minute, change in odor of sputum).

- Practice frequent handwashing; use protective equipment while suctioning and working with ventilator.
- Use aseptic technique when suctioning.
- Change ventilator circuitry a minimum of every 24 hours.
- Culture sputum or wound drainage; begin antibiotic therapy, as ordered.

Should the patient's respiratory status continue to deteriorate, adult respiratory distress syndrome (ARDS) might occur. Often equated with acute respiratory failure, ARDS is characterized by sudden and progressive pulmonary edema, worsening dyspnea, hypoxemia unresponsive to oxygen therapy, reduced lung compliance, and diffuse pulmonary infiltrates.

ARDS typically presents in patients with normal lungs who have suffered some respiratory system assault, as in lung contusion, fat embolism, aspiration, or massive smoke inhalation. Indirect causes of ARDS include sepsis, shock, multisystem trauma, disseminated intravascular coagulation, pancreatitis, uremia, drug overdose, anaphylaxis, prolonged cardiac bypass surgery, massive blood transfusions, pregnancy-induced hypertension, increased intracranial pressure, and radiation therapy.

Prognosis

The outcome for a patient with acute respiratory failure depends on the diagnosis and treatment of the underlying condition, attaining optimal oxygen-carbon dioxide gas exchange, and preventing complications. If the underlying disease necessitates prolonged bed rest and immobility, additional efforts should be undertaken to prevent complications associated with immobility, ventilator dependency, and infection. In the event of ARDS, the prognosis is poor. The current mortality rate of this disorder stands at 50% to 70%, not because of the progressive respiratory failure, but because of concurrent multiple organ systems failure and recurring infections. The mortality rate of ARDS secondary to sepsis is between 60% and 90%.

(Text continues on page 592.)

Complications of mechanical ventilation

The following chart identifies common complications associated with mechanical ventilation.

Complication	Cause
Barotrauma	Deterioration in respiratory status that occurs when an increase in intrathoracic pressure damages major vessels or organs within the thorax and causes subsequent damage to abdominal structures, leading to a decrease in venous return and cardiac output; pneumothorax can occur.
Fluid imbalances	Increased pressure on baroreceptors in the aorta causes an increased production of antidiuretic hormone and fluid retention.
GI problems	Stress from the respiratory failure can cause a physiologic reaction that leads to the development of peptic ulcers and possible hemorrhage. Also can result from gastric dilatation caused by increased volumes of air swallowed in the presence of an artificial airway.
Hypotension	May develop as a result of decreased venous return secondary to increased intrathoracic pressure; seen transiently when a patient is first placed on mechanical ventilation.
Increased intracranial pressure	Physiologic response to a worsening respiratory status; occurs as a result of decreased venous return with venous blood pooling in the cerebral vasculature.
Tension pneumothorax	Occurs when pressurized air enters the thoracic cavity as a result of positive pressure ventilation.

Treatment	Nursing Indications
If pneumothorax is suspected, immediately disconnect ventilator and ventilate patient manually with 100% oxygen. Chest tube placement is imminent.	• Perform ongoing monitoring of respiratory rate, breath sounds, and cardiac output. • Report changes indicative of pneumothorax, such as tracheal deviation and worsening ABG values.
Diuretic therapy usually is indicated.	• Assess orbital, sacral, and lower extremities for signs of edema. • Auscultate breath sounds for increased crackles. • Monitor effectiveness of diuretic therapy, as prescribed.
Begin antacids, cimetidine, or ranitidine to reduce ulcer formation. Place nasogastric tube and use intermittent suctioning to decompress abdomen and reduce pressure on the diaphragm.	• Monitor GI aspirate for occult blood; administer hydrogen ion agonists, as prescribed. • Monitor NG tube for correct placement; secure suction apparatus, if ordered. • Auscultate bowel sounds every 4 hours.
Temporarily reduce PEEP to below 20 mm Hg.	• Monitor heart rate, blood pressure, and cardiac output every hour. • Alert physician to signs of worsening hypotension.
Immediate efforts to reduce pressure may include administering cerebral diuretics (mannitol) and increasing the head of the bed to at least a 30-degree angle.	• Monitor for signs of altered level of consciousness every hour; report changes in responsiveness, including increased lethargy, change in arousability, and response to pain or pressure. • Administer cerebral diuretics, if prescribed.
Emergency chest tube placement	• Secure chest tube apparatus, ensuring no leaks or breaks in the system. • Monitor blood pressure, respiratory rate, heart rate, and cardiac output every hour. • Auscultate breath sounds every hour. • Monitor ABG values every hour.

Discharge planning

Depending on the treatment success of the underlying condition, discharge instructions should include information concerning:

• underlying disease and prescribed medication therapy
• smoking cessation
• techniques to promote lung drainage, such as frequent position changes and sitting in a semirecumbent position
• deep-breathing and coughing techniques, including breathing in through the nose and exhaling through the mouth several times prior to initiating coughing
• the need to avoid nonprescription medications (barbiturates, sedatives, cocaine, heroin, and alcohol) that can lead to accidental overdose
• techniques to reduce stress and anxiety.

In the case of ventilator dependency, discharge planning will include:

• consultation with social services to plan the transfer of the patient to a long-term care facility equipped to care for the ventilator patient and to evaluate the patient's and family's financial status
• consultation with a speech therapist
• instructions on the care of a gastric or duodenal feeding tube if one is present
• instructions on the signs and symptoms of postoperative infection, tube patency, intolerance to feedings, fluid balance, and other indicators of an adequate nutritional status.

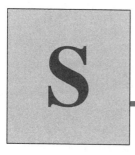

S

Seizures

Seizure result from the spontaneous, excessive, and synchronous discharge by thousands of cerebral neurons. A seizure disorder is a chronic condition of recurrent seizures. Although the terms seizure disorder and epilepsy are synonymous, the former is preferred because of the negative connotation associated with epilepsy. About 2 to 4 million Americans are affected by recurrent seizures.

Pathophysiology

Seizures are symptoms of an underlying structural or functional brain disorder and are primary or secondary in nature. Primary seizures are idiopathic, resulting from a disturbance in the function of cortical neurons. They may result from genetic factors; over 140 genetic syndromes are associated with seizures. Primary seizures also have been linked to a lower threshold for seizure activity. Individuals with a lowered seizure threshold experience seizures in response to relatively benign stimuli, including flickering lights, being startled, certain odors, lack of sleep, emotional stress, alcohol consumption, febrile illness, and hyperventilation.

Secondary seizures result from an insult to the cerebral tissue. An important and sometimes undetected cause of cortical trauma occurs in utero or at birth. Seizures resulting from perinatal trauma may not manifest for years. Secondary seizures that occur later in life commonly result from trauma (especially head injury), exposure to or withdrawal from toxic substances, neoplasms, central nervous system (CNS) infections, cerebrovascular disorders, or metabolic derangements.

Head trauma, especially from motor vehicle accidents, is a leading cause of seizures. About 50% of patients with a penetrating head wound and 5% of those with a closed head injury experience post-traumatic seizures. The interval between the head injury and the development of seizures varies. The frequency of post-traumatic seizures also is highly variable; while some head-injured patients experience only a few seizures, others have many. Over time, however, post-traumatic seizures typically decrease in frequency.

Toxic substances, including alcohol, sedatives, tranquilizers, and antihistamines, can cause seizures, particularly when they are abruptly discontinued. Brain tumors often manifest with seizures. The sudden onset of seizures after age 20 may indicate a neoplasm. Partial seizures, in particular, are produced by a number of lesions, including benign hamartomas, meningiomas, and malignant neoplasms.

CNS infections also can cause seizures. Generalized seizures may result from meningitis and encephalitis; partial seizures, from brain abscesses. Seizures also may occur after severe disruption of the cerebrovasculature, such as occurs with a high-grade subarachnoid or intracerebral hemorrhage. Metabolic disorders, including anoxia, severe hypoglycemia, alkalosis, hyponatremia, and hypo- or hyperosmolality, also cause seizures.

Cellular pathophysiology

Although the pathophysiology of seizures is quite complex and incompletely understood, a number of cellular mechanisms are known to be involved. Researchers postulate that groups of spontaneously discharging (depolarizing) neurons could have at least three defects: alterations in synaptic and neurotransmitter functions, changes in membrane receptors, and altered glial cell function.

The normal function of neuronal membranes is facilitated by a balance of excitatory and inhibitory mechanisms. Neurons within a seizure focus may be adversely affected by either a deficiency of inhibitory neurotransmitters or an excess of excitatory transmitters. Either situation could result in synchronous and spontaneous firing of cells within the seizure focus.

The excitatory neurotransmitter glutamate exerts its effects by binding to specialized receptors within the neuronal cell membrane. Receptor binding by excitatory neurotransmitters triggers the neuron to fire (depolarize). When inhibitory neurotransmitters, such as glycine and gamma-aminobutyric acid (GABA), bind to their receptors, the effect on the cell membrane is hyperpolarization, which makes the neuron less likely to fire (depolarize). Thus, an excess of glutamate or a deficiency of glycine or GABA could result in spontaneous and excessive depolarizations.

Alterations in the membrane receptors at which excitatory and inhibitory neurotransmitters bind also could result in spontaneous depolarization. The function of these receptors is to gate (control) the influx and exit of ions. In normal neurons, membrane depolarization results when glutamate binds to its receptors and opens sodium and calcium channels. As a result, depolarization occurs as sodium and calcium enter the cell. At the same time, potassium channels open to allow potassium to exit so that repolarization of the cell can take place.

When GABA binds to its membrane receptors, chloride channels open, allowing the influx of chloride ions into the cell. The effect this has upon the cell membrane is hyperpolarization, making the membrane less capable of depolarization. A potential mechanism leading to spontaneous neuronal depolarization, then, is decreased potassium or chloride channel activity or increased sodium or calcium channel activity.

Abnormalities in the function of glial cells also could result in spontaneous depolarization. One of the functions of glial cells is to scavenge potassium as it exits the cell during depolarization. Defective glial cell function can prevent the removal of extracellular potassium. As a result, repolarization might be delayed or lessened, which could result in the continuous depolarization of neighboring neurons.

Seizure classification

Seizures commonly are classified according to their focus or origin and presenting symptoms (see *Classification of seizures,* page 597).

Partial seizures arise from a discrete area of cortical tissue, involve only a part of the brain, and result in symptoms in part of the body; they may be further classified as simple (if consciousness is maintained) or complex (if consciousness is impaired). In complex partial seizures, the most common type of seizures among adults, the irritable focus is located in either the temporal or the frontal lobe. Partial seizures arise locally, but may secondarily generalize to involve other parts of the brain.

Generalized seizures involve the entire cortex and subcortical structures and always are accompanied by a diminution in consciousness. Idiopathic generalized seizures arising in adulthood are rare. More commonly, the onset of generalized seizures in the adult is the result of an infection, vascular abnormality, or neoplasm. The sudden onset of a generalized seizure disorder in later life is an ominous sign deserving careful scrutiny.

The reason why some seizures spread to involve the entire cortex and others remain localized is unknown. However, the phenomenon of recruitment may be involved. Recruitment is the process by which many other neurons, most of them normal, are entrained in the process of spontaneous depolarization. Additionally, generalization is thought to involve the engagement of

Classification of seizures

In an effort to categorize seizures, a number of classification systems have been developed. Of these, the most widely used is the International Classification of Epileptic Seizures, which was initially developed in 1964 and revised in 1981.

I. Partial (focal) seizures (beginning locally)
   A. Simple partial (consciousness maintained)
      1. Motor involving the arm, leg or both (including Jacksonian)
      2. Somatosensory or special sensory (visual, auditory, olfactory, gustatory)
      3. Autonomic (tachycardia, tachypnea, flushing)
      4. Psychic (deja vu, feelings of fear)
   B. Complex partial (impaired consciousness)
   Includes cognitive, affective, psychosensory, and psychomotor symptomatology with automatisms
   C. Partial seizures (simple or complex) with secondary generalization

II. Generalized seizures (bilaterally symmetrical and without local onset)
   A. Tonic or clonic or tonic-clonic (grand mal) seizures

   B. Absence (petit mal)
      1. Simple (loss of consciousness only)
      2. Complex (with brief tonic, clonic, or autonomic movements)
   C. Lennox-Gastaut syndrome
   D. Juvenile myoclonic epilepsy (short, abrupt contractions of arms, legs, torso)
   E. Infantile spasms (West syndrome)
   F. Atonic (astatic, akinetic) seizures (abrupt loss of muscle tone)

III. Unilateral or predominantly unilateral seizures (tonic, clonic, or tonic-clonic, with or without impaired consciousness)

IV. Unclassified (because of inadequate or incomplete data)

V. Status epilepticus (a seizure or series of sequential seizures lasting more than 30 minutes without recovery between episodes)

Adapted from the Commission on Classification and Terminology of the International League Against Epilepsy, "Proposal for Revised Clinical and Electroencephalographic Classification of Epileptic Seizures," *Epilepsia* 22:489-501, 1981. Used with permission of Ravin Press, Ltd., New York.

subcortical structures (thalamus and substantia nigra) into the seizure process. Once these areas are mustered, their diffuse projections to the cortex provide a mechanism for seizure spread to areas distant to the original focus.

Status epilepticus (SE) can occur with both partial and generalized seizures, is more common in the extremes of age, and constitutes a medical emergency. Most patients with SE do not have a history of a seizure disorder; rather, SE is a manifestation of an acute event, such as severe metabolic encephalopathy, anoxia, sepsis, electrolyte disorders, acute stroke, and CNS infections.

Clinical assessment

The physical assessment may be entirely normal between seizures, therefore eliciting a thorough description of the seizure activity is of utmost importance.

History

When obtaining the history, the nurse should realize that the patient may not be able to recall the events surrounding the seizure. Consequently, obtaining information from those who witnessed the seizure is crucial.

The following information should be elicited:
• onset, frequency, and duration of the seizure
• nature of the seizure (including symptoms before, during, and after, as well as body parts involved, and any alterations in consciousness)
• precipitating or triggering events (such as alcohol withdrawal and self-discontinuation of antiseizure medication)
• history of family or childhood seizures, head injury, hypoxia, or CNS infection
• presence of other disorders (such as intracranial neoplasm, uremia, stroke, or hypoglycemia)
• dependence on or withdrawal from drugs.

Physical findings

The manifestations of seizures include motor, sensory, autonomic, or psychic phenomena. Altered level of consciousness is a prominent feature of many, but not all seizures. Seizure activity occurs in three phases: preictal, interictal, and postictal.

Preictal manifestations occur prior to the seizure and consist of a prodrome or an aura. A prodrome is a symptom or symptoms that occur hours or days before the actual seizure activity. The prodromal phase is characterized by disturbances in affect or behavior and by headaches, depression, and gastrointestinal (GI) distress. An aura is an unusual sensation occurring immediately before the seizure. The most common aural manifestations include visual, auditory, gustatory, or somatosensory phenomena. Typical visual auras consists of bright spots or zigzag lines. Auditory auras may be in the form of voices or music and gustatory auras include the sensation of unpleasant tastes. Somatosensory auras often take the form of unilateral or bilateral numbness or tingling of the face or extremities. Some researchers believe that auras are simple partial seizures.

Interictal activity is the actual motor, sensory, autonomic, and psychic behavior manifested as a result of the discharging cortex. Automatisms (unusual interictal movements that are purposeful, yet inappropriate) are especially characteristic of partial complex seizures and include lip-smacking, chewing, facial grimacing, swallowing, and picking or rubbing movements.

Postictal symptoms occur after a seizure and consist of depressed level of consciousness, confusion, and sleepiness following a generalized seizure, or weakness or paralysis of the parts involved in a partial seizure.

The specific manifestations of a seizure depend on the location of the irritable (seizure) focus within the brain, the number of neurons involved, and whether the seizure remains localized or spreads throughout the cortex. (For specific signs, symptoms, and physical assessment findings of each type of seizure, see *Clinical manifestations of seizures,* pages 600 and 601.)

Diagnosis

The diagnosis of a seizure disorder is made on the basis of clinical manifestations and EEG findings. Other tests that may be used to evaluate the nature of the seizure disorder are listed in *Confirming a seizure,* pages 602 and 603.

Clinical manifestations of seizures

The manifestations of seizures depend on the location of the seizure focus, the number of neurons involved, and whether the seizure remains localized or generalized.

Partial Seizures	
Focal motor	Originate from an irritative focus on the motor cortex of the frontal lobe. Motor activity usually is clonic in nature and most commonly involves the face, arm, hands, and leg. Focal motor seizures usually begin slowly, involve repetitive jerking of the part involved, increase in intensity over about 15 seconds, and taper off or cease abruptly.
Jacksonian	A specific type of focal motor seizure in which seizure activity spreads in an orderly manner (Jacksonian march) to adjacent areas on the motor cortex. For example, seizure activity may begin in the fingers of one hand and then progresses sequentially to involve the arm, face, and lower extremity on the same side.
Focal sensory (somatosensory or special sensory)	Originate from an irritative focus within the sensory strip of the parietal lobe. Manifestations depend on the function of the cortex involved and include visual or auditory hallucinations; flashing or zigzag lights; odd tastes or smells; or numbness, tingling, burning, or crawling sensations.
Complex partial	Most commonly originate in the temporal lobe, producing an alteration in consciousness as well as cognitive, affective, psychosensory, and psychomotor symptoms. Automatisms and amnesia are characteristic of these seizures which last from 1 to 4 minutes and leave the individual in a post-seizure confusional state.
Generalized Seizures	
Tonic/clonic (grand mal)	Usually begin with an abrupt loss of consciousness followed by generalized tonic contraction (tensing) of the muscles lasting 15 to 60 seconds. During the tonic phase, the patient is apneic and may be incontinent. The clonic phase is characterized by rapid, rhythmic muscle contractions, hyperventilation, excessive salivation, tachycardia, and hypertension. The clonic phase lasts 2 to 5 minutes and is followed by a postictal confusional state.

Clinical manifestations of seizures *(continued)*

Generalized Seizures *(continued)*

Absence (petit mal)	Characterized by an abrupt cessation of activity and consciousness, without loss of posture. The most common manifestation is a blank stare, but minor motor symptoms such as twitching of the eyes or mouth also may be present. These seizures, which affect children between 4 and 12, usually last less than 30 seconds.
Myoclonic	Affect both adults and children and are characterized by sudden, brief, uncontrollable jerking of one or more extremities or of the entire body. Momentary loss of consciousness and postictal confusion also occur.
Atonic (akinetic, drop attack)	Characterized by a sudden and brief loss muscle tone, posture, and consciousness. Atonic seizures usually appear before puberty and are associated with mental retardation and other types of seizures.

Treatment and care

The treatment of seizures includes medical and surgical modalities. Nursing care focuses on monitoring the patient's neurologic status and preventing or treating complications (see *Key nursing interventions for patients with seizures,* page 604).

Up to 80% of patients with medically intractable seizures have complex partial seizures; the remaining 20% experience either generalized seizures or a mixture of seizure types. To be considered for surgery, a patient must meet the following criteria:

• history of intractable seizures for at least 2 years, despite aggressive medical management
• presence of seizures that interfere significantly with daily life or livelihood
• good enough health to tolerate the procedure
• high motivation, psychological preparedness, and adequate support (depression occurs in 50% of patients even if the surgery is a success).

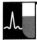

DIAGNOSTIC TESTS

Confirming a seizure

The diagnosis of seizures or a seizure disorder is based on clinical manifestations and electroencephalographic evidence. Other tests used to aid in the diagnosis are presented below.

Standard electroencephalogram (EEG) and video EEG

An EEG provides a recording of the electrical activity of the brain. When an irritable cortical focus fires, it is reflected in the EEG as a series of periodic spike discharges, which increase progressively in amplitude and frequency. Among seizure patients, interictal EEG often shows isolated spikes even though clinical manifestations are absent. Video EEG monitoring is a technique used to simultaneously record EEG and clinical features of seizure activity. This technique reveals movements immediately before the seizure, which may provide clues to the location of the irritable focus.

Telemetry radiotelemetry

This is accomplished using a small 16-channel EEG built into a box that can be worn on the head. This modality allows the patient to resume normal activities while seizure activity is being monitored.

Magnetic resonance imaging (MRI)

MRI is twice as effective as computed tomography for picking up atrophy and subtle lesions such as tumors or an arteriovenous malformation.

Laboratory studies

Because seizures may result from metabolic disorders, a full laboratory analysis may be helpful in identifying the cause. Common tests include complete blood count, blood chemistries, such as glucose and electrolytes, blood urea nitrogen and creatinine, liver profile, toxic screens, and cerebrospinal fluid (CSF) analysis.

Skull X-rays

Skull X-rays demonstrate structural deficits and are used to rule out intracranial lesions, such as fractures, masses, tumors, atrophy, and intracranial calcification.

Computed tomography (CT)

CT is useful for visualizing gray and white matter and CSF. CT can identify tumors 1 or 2 cm in size and is superior to MRI for imaging blood and calcification.

Brain mapping

Brain mapping involves the placement of subdural electrodes or a grid for cortical mapping of the epileptogenic focus and to determine the landmarks for surgical resection prior to seizure surgery. The placement of subdural electrodes also allows for the localization of motor, sensory, or speech areas.

Wada test

As part of a presurgical evaluation, the Wada test is performed to determine the location of the speech center. To perform the test, a catheter is placed in the carotid artery (on the same side of the seizure focus) and amobarbital is injected into the artery. The amytal produces a temporary contralateral hemiparesis, mimicking the effects of surgery on that hemisphere. The goal of the Wada test is to identify the dominant speech center. Accordingly,

---

Confirming a seizure *(continued)*

while the patient is in the hepatetic state, speech, comprehension, and memory are tested.

Positron emission tomography (PET)
PET provides a three-dimensional view of the structure of the brain, as well as allowing for the noninvasive

evaluation of the metabolic activity of the brain. A PET scan will demonstrate cerebral hypermetabolism during a seizure and hypometabolism between seizures. Currently, PET scanning is available at very few locations.

Different types of surgery are available, depending on the type of seizures experienced. However, the vast majority of surgeries are for the treatment of partial seizures.

Status epilepticus, a medical emergency, requires immediate intervention, as outlined in *Emergency treatment for status epilepticus,* page 605.

Pharmacologic measures

Antiseizure medications are the mainstay of medical treatment. Currently, several classes of antiseizure drugs are available, including several new agents. The class of drug chosen depends on the type of seizure the patient experiences (for a listing of these drugs, see *Antiseizure medications,* pages 606 to 609).

When initiating therapy, a single medication is selected on the basis of its efficacy and safety profile. The lowest effective dose is administered to minimize adverse effects. The dose may be gradually increased until the target dose is reached and a therapeutic drug level is attained. Approximately 60% to 70% of patients achieve complete seizure control by using this approach. About 30%, however, will require polytherapy. Among those patients, 30% continue to experience seizures despite the addition of complementary acting antiseizure medications. For some of these patients, surgical intervention may be beneficial.

ESSENTIAL ELEMENTS

Key nursing interventions for patients with seizures

The following flowchart highlights key interventions for caring for patients with seizures.

```
                  Achieve optimal neurologic status
```

Prevent seizure activity.	Protect the patient from injury during a seizure.	Prevent complications.
• To prevent seizure activity: —administer antiseizure medications, as ordered —obtain and monitor antiseizure medication drug levels, as ordered, and report abnormal levels —avoid exposing the patient to precipitating events —monitor laboratory values carefully and report abnormal values promptly —if the patient is unable to take medications by mouth, ensure that parenteral antiseizure medications are administered.	• Remain calm and stay with the patient. • Provide as much privacy as possible. • Make sure side rails are up and padded. • Never force anything into the patient's mouth. • Have an oral airway and suction at hand for the postictal phase. • Guide the patient's arms and legs if possible (do not restrain).	• Position the patient side-lying when the seizure is over to prevent aspiration. • If the SaO_2 is low, provide oxygen. • Allow for rest following the seizure • Carefully document the details of the seizure, including the type of movements, parts involved, duration; whether the patient was incontinent; and whether the patient lost consciousness or suffered postictal confusion or weakness.

Surgery for partial seizures

The goal of surgery for complex partial seizures is to remove as much of the epileptogenic focus as possible, without compromising vital tissues. Surgical candidates are those with a unilateral focus that is caused by an identifiable lesion that is clearly localized to one part

Emergency treatment for status epilepticus

The following protocol is representative of the general treatment provided for patients with status epilepticus.

Within first 5 minutes
- Assess cardiorespiratory function.
- Obtain history.
- Perform physical examination.
- Obtain laboratory specimens (electrolytes, blood urea nitrogen, glucose, antiseizure and other drug levels, metabolic screen).
- Administer oxygen.

Within 6 to 9 minutes
- Begin I.V. of 0.9% NaCl
- Administer 100 mg thiamine, followed by 50 ml 50% glucose I.V.
- Administer lorazepam 0.1 mg/kg I.V. at a rate no faster than 2 mg/minute.

Within 10 to 30 minutes
- If seizures continue, give phenytoin 20 mg/kg I.V., no faster than 50 mg/minute. Always administer in saline solution, using the port closest to the patient. Monitor blood pressure and ECG during the infusion.

- Provide an additional 5 mg/kg (up to two times) for continued seizures (total maximum dose is 30 mg/kg).
- If necessary, provide a second dose of lorazepam; respiratory support may be required.

Within 31 to 60 minutes
- If the patient is still experiencing a seizure, intubate and give phenobarbital 20 mg/kg I.V. at a rate no faster than 100 mg/minute.
- Monitor carefully for cardiovascular depression.

After 60 minutes
- If seizures have not abated, place the patient in a barbiturate coma using pentobarbital 2 to 5 mg/kg I.V. slowly followed by a continuous infusion of 0.5 to 2 mg/kg/hour.
- Continuously monitor EEG for a burst suppression pattern, and slow the infusion rate every 2 to 4 hours to see if seizures have stopped.

of the brain. Providing that the seizure focus is not located in a vital area, lesionectomy or lobectomy (partial or total, usually involving the temporal lobe) may be performed.

About 75% of those treated by either lesionectomy or lobectomy are completely cured of their seizure disorder. An additional 20% experience a reduction in the frequency and number of seizures, as well as a decreased need for antiseizure medications. Prior to seizure surgery, candidates undergo an extensive evaluation to localize the seizure foci.

(Text continues on page 608.)

MAJOR DRUGS

Antiseizure medications

About 75% of patients achieve good seizure control with antiseizure medications, the most common of which are included in the chart below.

Drug	Usage and Characteristics
Traditional drugs	
Barbiturates (phenobarbital, pentobarbital) Dosage: 2 to 3 mg/kg for prophylaxis; 10 to 20 mg/kg for status epilepticus Therapeutic range: 10 to 40 mg/ml	• Principally used in treating pediatric generalized seizures • May be used as a second line for treating generalized or complex partial seizures in adults • Half-life of 96 hours • Moderately protein-bound; increases the metabolism of coumadin, cortisol, and phenytoin
Desoxybarbiturates (primidone) Dosage: 10 to 15 mg/kg	• May be used for generalized tonic-clonic and complex partial seizures • Half-life of 12 hours • Variable protein binding
Hydantoins (phenytoin) Dosage: 4 to 7 mg/kg for prophylaxis; 15 to 20 mg/kg for status epilepticus Therapeutic range: 10 to 20 mg/ml	• Drug of choice for primary generalized seizures • Also used for complex partial seizures • Half-life of 24 hours • Highly protein-bound • May reduce the levels of other medications, such as valproic acid
Iminostilbenes (carbamazepine) Dosage: 4 to 20 mg/kg beginning with a low dose and titrating upward	• Drug of choice for partial complex seizures • Also used for generalized tonic-clonic and simple partial seizures • Half-life of 12 to 18 hours • Moderately protein-bound
Benzodiazepines (diazepam, lorazepam, clonazepam) Dosage: • diazepam: 0.2 to 0.5 mg/kg I.V. • lorazepam: 0.05 to 0.1 mg/kg I.V. • clonazepam: 0.5 to 1 mg daily	• Diazepam and lorazepam are first-line drugs of choice for status epilepticus • Lorazepam is associated with less hypotension and respiratory depress than diazepam • Clonazepam is used for absence and myoclonic seizures • Half-life of 10 to 15 minutes for diazepam and lorazepam; about 20 hours for clonazepam

Probable Mechanism of Action	Adverse Effects
• In routine doses, phenobarbital enhances GABA receptor activity, increasing CNS inhibition by reducing repetitive firing of neurons • In large doses pheno- and pentobarbital block certain Ca^{++} channels, which makes them valuable for treating status epilepticus	• Sedation, slowness, fatigue, and ataxia, because of effects on normal neurons • Large doses cause cardiovascular depression secondary to calcium channel blocking and anesthesia
• Reduces repetitive firing but does not affect GABA inhibition	• Similar to those of barbiturates
• Limits repetitive firing of neurons by inactivating sodium channels • At high concentrations, also limits calcium channel activity	• Rashes, lymphadenopathy, bone marrow suppression, autoimmune syndromes, gingival hyperplasia, hirsutism, osteomalacia • Dose dependent toxic effects include nystagmus (15 to 20 mg/ml), ataxia (20 to 30 mg/ml), stupor (40 mg/ml)
• Action is similar to that of phenytoin by limiting repetitive firing, probably by acting on sodium channels	• Liver function abnormalities and bone marrow suppression • Toxic effects include vertigo, "spaciness," drowsiness, nausea, and diplopia
• Binds to the GABA chloride channel to increase frequency of channel opening, thereby increasing neuronal inhibition • May also block repetitive firing	• Sedation at high doses is related to long elimination half-lives of these drugs

(continued)

Antiseizure medications *(continued)*

Drug	Usage and Characteristics
Traditional drugs *(continued)*	
Fatty acids (valproic acid) Dosage: 20 to 60 mg/kg	• Drug of choice for mixed seizure disorders and absence seizures • Also helpful for myoclonic and tonic-clonic seizures • Half-life of 12 to 18 hours • Highly protein-bound • Can increase phenobarbital levels and decrease phenytoin levels
Newer drugs	
Gabapentin (Neurontin) Dosage: 1,200 to 2,400 mg daily	• Used as an add-on therapy for adults with partial and secondary generalized seizures • Half-life of 5 to 6 hours • Produces no significant interactions with other drugs
Lamotrigine (Lamictal) Dosage: 300 to 700 mg daily	• Used as an add-on in adults with partial and secondary generalized seizures • Half-life of 24 hours • Interacts with other anticonvulsants, increasing the half-life of some and decreasing the half-life of others
Felbamate (Felbatol) Dosage: 3,600 to 4,800 mg daily	• Used as monotherapy in adults with partial and secondary generalized seizures • Half-life of 20 to 24 hours • Inhibits metabolism of most other antiseizure medications

Generalized seizure surgery

Surgical procedures performed include hemispherec-tomies and corpus callosumotomies. The goal of these surgeries is to prevent the spread of the seizure from one hemisphere to the other. The corpus callosum is an important route of seizure generalization and resecting it does not cure, but palliates, severe generalized sei-

Probable Mechanism of Action	Adverse Effects
• Increases GABA levels by inhibiting GABA degradative enzymes • Also limits sustained repetitive firing of neurons	• Tremor, weight gain, sedation, alopecia, and hepatic toxicity
• Mechanism of antiseizure activity is unknown at this time	• Somnolence, fatigue, dizziness, weight gain, ataxia, headache, nausea, and diplopia
• Probably exerts its effects by inhibiting the release of excitatory amino acids, especially glutamate	• Diplopia, drowsiness
• Blocks action of glutamate • Inactivates sodium channels and inhibits glutamate release	• Headache, weight loss, anorexia, insomnia, and irritability • Has been associated with severe bone marrow depression (typically during the first 6 months of therapy) and has resulted in the death of several patients. Patients who opt to continue taking this drug should be monitored carefully, especially during the first 6 months of therapy.

zures and injuries from atonic seizures. Most patients experience little functional deficit when the callosum is interrupted.

Hemispherectomy is a radical form of seizure surgery reserved for patients with intractable generalized seizures. Candidates for hemispherectomy are those with a preexisting hemiplegia and hemianopsia. In these individuals, severe neurological deficits already are present and surgical intervention may provide the only mechanism available for adequate seizure control. Recent modification of the procedure, in which only the cortex and not deeper structures are removed, has resulted in a cure or substantial improvement for most patients.

Complications of seizure surgery

Potential complications include bleeding, infection, and neurologic deficits. Patients with resections in the dominant hemisphere may experience temporary speech and language deficits as a result of postoperative edema. Individuals undergoing temporal lobectomy may experience visual disturbances. Following complete corpus callosotomy, some patients may experience a phenomenon known as disconnection syndrome (language and perception deficits resulting from severing the connections between the two cerebral hemispheres). When blindfolded, these patients can identify an object placed in the right hand but not the left hand.

Prognosis

The prognosis for patients with seizures is continually improving. Recently, several new antiseizure drugs have been added and several other promising agents are in clinical trial. Additionally, refinements in seizure surgery have provided hope for many individuals with intractable seizures.

Discharge planning

In addition to educational needs, the patient and family may require psychological, emotional, and social support. For many individuals, the psychosocial implications of living with a seizure disorder are more incapacitating than the seizures themselves. Patients with poorly controlled seizures may not be able to operate machinery (including a car), work at their desired occupation, or succeed in furthering their education.

Many experience interpersonal difficulties. For many of these individuals, quality of life is poor.

The nurse should offer referrals to various social services to help the patient and family cope with this complex disorder. Patients also should be provided with information about the Epilepsy Foundation of America, which supports both patients and families on a broad range of topics and concerns.

Shock

A clinical syndrome reflective of the body's attempt to adapt to an injury and preserve its vital functions, shock is characterized by ineffective tissue perfusion that causes an imbalance in the supply and demand of oxygen and nutrients to the cells. Although shock can be caused by various factors, the ensuing ineffective tissue perfusion produces a common chain of biochemical events at the cellular level. This alteration in cellular metabolism decreases the effective circulating volume and impairs cardiac output. Ultimately, end-organ damage and death can occur rapidly if general supportive measures and pharmacologic therapy are not instituted promptly.

Shock may be categorized as cardiogenic, hypovolemic, or septic, depending on the cause and course of the decreased perfusion. Cardiogenic shock, which results from decreased cardiovascular function, occurs when the heart is unable to maintain a cardiac output (CO) sufficient to meet the metabolic needs of major organ systems. This is the most severe form of heart failure and is associated with a mortality rate of 80% to 100%.

Hypovolemic shock, which results with a loss of 20% to 25% of circulating blood volume, is the most common type of shock. Usually the result of a traumatic injury that causes some external or concealed hemorrhage, hypovolemic shock also may result from sequestration of fluid within the abdominal viscera, soft tissue, or peritoneal cavity.

Septic shock occurs when an infectious organism or its by-products trigger a host response that compromises cardiovascular function, systemic perfusion, and oxygen delivery and use at the cellular level.

Pathophysiology

Shock progresses through four discrete phases marked by characteristic cellular changes (see *Stages of shock at the cellular level,* pages 613 and 614). The major pathophysiologic responses of the different types of shock are discussed below.

Cardiogenic shock

Cardiogenic shock is characterized by a maldistribution of blood flow with inadequate transport of oxygen at the microcirculatory and cellular level due to ineffective cardiac pumping (see *Causes of shock,* page 615, for common etiologies). This type of shock interferes with tissue perfusion, oxygen transport, and synthesis of adenosine triphosphate (ATP). The patient has sustained systemic arterial hypotension and inadequate tissue perfusion of the kidneys, brain, heart, GI system, and skin. Initially, the body compensates by maintaining blood pressure and marginal perfusion to nonvital organs. However, as the cardiac function continues to deteriorate, the patient progresses into decompensated shock, a stage characterized by profound hypotension that activates ischemic mediators, which stimulate the complement cascade. Later, the patient develops bradycardia and arrhythmias.

Hypovolemic shock

The severity of hypovolemic shock depends not only on the volume deficit but also on the patient's age and preexisting health status. The rate at which the volume has been lost is a critical factor in the compensatory response. Loss of volume over an extended period, regardless of age, is better tolerated than a rapid loss.

Initially, the patient may maintain mean arterial pressure and remain compensated; however, with con-

Stages of shock at the cellular level

The following chart summarizes the changes that occur during different shock stages.

Stage	Cellular Changes
Initial	• Cell membrane becomes damaged and myocardial depressant factor is released from ischemic cells • Complement is activated • Calcium stores are altered; influx of calcium increases when reperfusion occurs • Arachidonic acid metabolism occurs • Coagulation cascade is activated • Cellular death occurs if altered perfusion is not corrected
Compensatory	• Body attempts to maintain cardiac output and blood pressure through increased heart rate and peripheral vasoconstriction • Arteriolar vasoconstriction results in redirection of blood flow from the periphery to the central circulation (heart and brain) • Reduced diameter of vessels increases velocity of flow and decreases blood viscosity as it reaches the ischemic vascular beds, permitting more efficient microcirculatory flow, thereby improving oxygen delivery and reducing tissue acidosis • Cardiac output is supported by tachycardia and fluid shifts from the interstitium that occurred earlier in shock • Secretion of aldosterone and vasopressin increases renal retention of salt and water to assist in maintaining circulating blood volume • Epinephrine, cortisol, and glucagon increase the extracellular concentration of glucose and make energy stores available for cellular metabolism • Fat mobilization increases and serum insulin levels decrease • Autoregulation to the kidney is maintained as long as the mean arterial pressure is between 70 and 160 mm Hg • Autoregulation of the brain's blood supply keeps the flow constant as long as arterial pressure does not drop below 60 mm Hg
Progressive	• Failure of compensatory mechanisms with continued deterioration of tissue perfusion and organ function occurs —decreased cardiac output and vasoconstriction lead to decreased blood flow to the brain, resulting in altered consciousness —decreased blood flow to kidneys causes a further decrease in glomerular filtration rate —blood flow shunts away from GI system, resulting in a decrease in GI mobility and hypoactive bowel sounds —decreased flow to the liver results in decreased function of *(continued)*

Stages of shock at the cellular level *(continued)*

Stage	Cellular Changes
Progressive *(continued)*	the Kupffer cells (causing increased susceptibility to infection), increased aldosterone secretion, and increased ammonia secretion (causing decreased cerebral function) —pancreatic ischemia causes release of myocardial depressant factor, which decreases cardiac contractility —sympathetic nervous system stimulation leads to decreased pulmonary capillary blood flow, resulting in increases in physiologic dead space and decreases in gas exchange • Continued hypoperfusion leads to an inflammatory response that results in release of chemically active substances, or mediators —mediators cause vasoconstriction and endothelial damage associated with increased pulmonary capillary permeability, resulting in interstitial and intra-alveolar edema and increased intrapulmonary shunting. —reduced pulmonary perfusion combined with mediator release results in capillary and alveolar cellular injury, leading to acute respiratory distress syndrome • Increases in sympathetic nervous system stimulation and heart rate lead to decreased blood flow to the coronary arteries, resulting in decreased supply to the myocardium, increased afterload and heart rate, angina, and possibly myocardial infarction
Refractory (irreversible)	• Profound cell dysfunction and multiple organ failure occur; patient is refractory to conventional therapy and undergoes a vicious cycle of cardiac failure, acidosis, blood dyscrasia, and cerebral ischemia —acidosis further decreases blood flow to the cells, resulting in more severe acidosis —severe acidosis leads to cell aggregation of platelets and red blood cells; this produces a fibrin clot that predisposes the patient to disseminated intravascular coagulation —decreased blood flow to brain results in cerebral ischemia, which stimulates the vasomotor center of the medulla —stimulation by the sympathetic nervous system causes cerebral vasoconstriction and further cerebral ischemia • If cycle continues, medullary infarction can occur, resulting in loss of vasomotor function (decrease in heart rate and vasodilation) and brain death, leading to cardiac or respiratory arrest

Causes of shock

The following conditions are considered common causes of cardiogenic, hemorrhagic, and septic shock.

Cardiogenic shock
- Acute myocardial infarction
- Tachyarrhythmias
- Ruptured septum
- Ruptured papillary muscle
- Left ventricular aneurysm
- Severe aortic stenosis
- Anemia
- Sepsis
- Hyperthyroidism
- Multiple arteriovenous fistulae

Hypovolemic shock
- Frank hemorrhage
- Bleeding at fracture site
- GI bleeding
- Hemothorax
- Retroperitoneal bleeding
- Soft-tissue trauma (swelling)
- Sepsis
- Peritonitis
- Ascites
- Intestinal obstruction
- Burn injuries
- Vomiting and diarrhea
- Diuretic therapy
- Excessive sweating

- Diabetes mellitus and insipidus
- Fistulas

Septic shock
- Granulocytopenia
- Diabetes mellitus
- Liver disease
- Neoplasms
- Neonatal status
- Age over 65
- Alcoholism
- Renal failure
- Pregnancy
- Malnutrition
- Autoimmune disorders
- Immunosuppressive therapy
- Pneumonia
- Urinary tract infection
- Cholecystitis
- Peritonitis
- Abscess
- Indwelling urinary or vascular catheterization
- Instrumentation of urinary tract
- Extensive major abdominal or pelvic surgery

tinued or massive volume loss, decompensation ensues, resulting in a decrease in mean arterial pressure. Because of the loss in intravascular volume, venous return to the head and ventricular filling volumes are reduced and ventricular performance falls below normal. The body compensates by an increase in systemic vascular resistance (SVR), which results in maintaining arterial pressure and shunting of blood centrally to maintain perfusion pressure and flow to the brain and the myocardium. The decreased capillary hydrostatic pressure and unchanged colloid osmotic pressure favors fluid movement from the tissue to the intravascular space to restore plasma volume.

Decompensated shock usually accompanies an acute intravascular volume loss greater than 30% of total blood volume. Falling systolic pressure represents a level of shock at which compensatory mechanisms are exhausted. If aggressive fluid replacement is not initiated rapidly, death will ensue.

Septic shock

The distinguishing features of septic shock include an excess of endogenous mediators, peripheral vascular failure, decreased myocardial function, and disturbances in oxygen supply and consumption.

Endogenous mediators, such as cytokines, are chemicals released by immunocompetent cells in response to activation by microbial products; they may be responsible for some of the deleterious effects of sepsis. These include cytokines tumor necrosis factor (TNF) and interleukin-1, which have been shown to cause severe hypotension, fever, chills, nausea, and muscle pain. High doses lead to multiple organ failure and death from shock.

An increase in serum beta-endorphins, protein catabolism, lipolysis, and resting energy expenditure also occur after release of TNF. TNF and interleukin-1 stimulate the release of various eicosanoids, including platelet activating factor. Eicosanoids are physiologically active substances derived from arachidonic acid. The arachidonic acid metabolites cause an intravascular inflammatory response that targets endothelial cells, disrupts capillary integrity, and alters microcirculation. This causes capillary leakage and precapillary shunting, as well as a direct myocardial depressant effect.

Oxygen metabolites are produced when oxygen is incompletely reduced to water. These radical intermediates are extremely toxic because of their effects on lipid bilayers, intracellular enzymes, structural proteins, nucleic acids, and carbohydrates. Phagocytes normally generate oxygen radicals to assist in killing ingested material. Antioxidants protect surrounding tissue if these compounds leak from the phagocytes. Ischemia, followed by reperfusion, has been shown to accelerate the production of toxic oxygen metabolites independent of the activity of inflammatory cells. This ischemia-reperfusion syndrome may lead to extensive destruction of surrounding tissue.

In early septic shock, vasodilation results in vascular shunting while the precapillary arterioles vasoconstrict, leading to significant shunting of blood to the peripheral organs. This shunting of blood leads to acidosis, which perpetuates low systemic vascular resistance and refractory hypotension. Decreased myocardial function usually occurs despite the initial increase in cardiac output. The increase in cardiac output results from an increased heart rate and decreased resistance to ejection.

During the course of sepsis, cells convert from pyruvate oxidation to lactate production in response to shunting of oxygenated blood. As the oxygen supply falls below a critical level, demand exceeds supply, consumption decreases, and lactic acidosis may develop secondary to anaerobic metabolism.

Clinical assessment

The patient with suspected shock requires a quick but thorough clinical assessment to reduce organ dysfunction. Once the patient is stabilized, the source of the symptoms must be identified.

History

Identifying the type of shock is essential to ensure correct treatment. A thorough review of predisposing factors along with the clinical presentation will assist in differentiating the type of shock. Remember, cardiac failure is an end-stage consequence of all forms of shock (see *Assessing and diagnosing shock,* pages 618 and 619).

Generally, cardiogenic shock should be suspected in any patient with known cardiac disease who sudden-

(*Text continues on page 620.*)

Assessing and diagnosing shock

Common assessment findings and helpful diagnostic criteria for the different stages of each type of shock are presented in the chart below.

Type of Shock	Common Assessment Findings	Diagnostic Criteria
Cardiogenic	**Compensated stage** • Cool, pale, clammy skin • Anxiety, restlessness • Tachycardia, tachypnea • Hypoactive bowel sounds **Decompensated stage** • Cold, mottled, or cyanotic skin • Tachycardia, tachypnea, then bradypnea • Absent bowel sounds • Decorticate or decerebrate posturing	**Laboratory values** • Cardiac enzymes to evaluate for acute myocardial infarction • Hyperglycemia with release of epinephrine as a response to physiologic stress • Increased blood urea level as blood flow to the kidneys is decreased **Hemodynamic values** • Systolic blood pressure decreased with narrow pulse pressure • Cardiac index < 2.1/minute/m^2 • Pulmonary artery wedge pressure > 20 mm Hg • Systemic vascular resistance > 1,800 dynes/second/cm^{-5} **Other diagnostic tests** • ECG for diagnosis of myocardial ischemia • Chest X-ray to diagnose for pulmonary edema (enlarged heart with pulmonary clouding) • Ventriculography to evaluate ejection fraction (ejection fraction will be decreased in cardiogenic shock) • Echocardiography to identify pericardial tamponade, valvular defects, and ventricular function
Hypovolemic	**Compensated stage** • Pale, clammy skin • Thready peripheral pulses • Tachycardia, tachypnea • Anxiety, restlessness • Decreased urine output • Narrowing pulse pressure	**Laboratory values** • Hemoglobin changes depending on the cause of hypovolemia, the duration of fluid loss, and replenishment of fluids • Increased lactic acid with anaerobic metabolism • Increased urine specific gravity

Assessing and diagnosing shock *(continued)*

Type of Shock	Common Assessment Findings	Diagnostic Criteria
Hypovo-lemic *(continued)*	• Collapse of cutaneous veins • Collapsed jugular veins • Dilated pupils • Hypoactive bowel sounds Decompensated stage • Cold, mottled, or cyanotic skin • Decorticate or decere-brate posturing • Tachycardia • Tachypnea, then bradypnea • Absent bowel sounds	Hemodynamic values • Central venous pressure < normal range of 2 to 8 mm Hg • Pulmonary artery wedge pressure < normal range of 4 to 12 mm Hg • Cardiac output variable but eventually below normal Other diagnostic tests • X-rays • Gastroscopy • Aspiration of gastric contents to test for occult blood
Septic	Early (compensated-hyperdynamic) stage • Tachycardia, widened pulse pressure, bounding pulse • Tachypnea (respiratory alkalosis) • Decreased level of consciousness • Thrombocytopenia • Warm, flushed pink skin • Hypotension • Fever or hypothermia • Agitation Late (decompensated-hypodynamic) stage • Cold, mottled skin, weak pulses • Tachycardia, hypotension • Obtunded or coma • Tachypnea and hypoxemia Late stage • Decreased cardiac output • Severe hypotension • Anuria • Severe mixed acidosis	Laboratory values • Leukocytosis • Thrombocytopenia • Elevated serum lactate levels • Increased urine specific gravity • Increased urine osmolality • Decreased urine sodium Hemodynamic values • Increased cardiac output, low systemic vascular resistance (early stages) • Decreased cardiac output, increased systemic vascular resistance (late stages) Other diagnostic tests • Positive blood cultures

ly worsens. Common complications in acute myocardial infarction can lead to cardiogenic shock. Manifestations of hypovolemic shock vary according to the patient's age, general health, extent of volume loss, and the time over which such losses have occurred.

Septic shock typically occurs in a series of stages. Early septic shock (hyperdynamic or compensated shock) is characterized by hyperdynamic cardiovascular function, peripheral vasodilation, systemic edema, and relative hypovolemia. In later hyperdynamic shock, the patient begins to decompensate and presents with hypotension, metabolic acidosis, increased capillary permeability producing systemic and pulmonary edema, hypoxemia, and progressive tachypnea, resulting in increased effort in breathing. These factors indicate the development of multisystem dysfunction. During the final stage of septic shock (often called the cardiogenic stage), the patient shows severe and progressive left ventricular dysfunction contributing to a fall in cardiac output, cold extremities, hypotension, and severe mixed acidosis. The patient who reaches this final stage of septic shock has a poor prognosis.

Diagnosis

Diagnosis of shock at the cellular level is somewhat difficult because there are no clinical signs and symptoms. Diagnosis must rely on laboratory tests and indicators of cellular perfusion, as listed in *Indicators of cellular shock,* page 621. (For other possible diagnostic criteria, see *Assessing and diagnosing shock*, pages 618 and 619.)

Treatment and care

Medical and nursing management of shock depends on the patient's clinical status and the type of shock, as discussed below.

Cellular shock

Treatment goals for shock at the cellular level include restoring oxygen delivery and extraction, restoring tis-

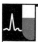

DIAGNOSTIC TESTS

Indicators of cellular shock

The following chart provides information on normal and abnormal laboratory findings that can help diagnose cellular shock.

Lactate levels
Correlate with the extent of tissue perfusion; when oxygen levels are deficient, pyruvate converts to lactate. Normal lactate values are 0.93 to 1.65 mmol/liter. Arterial levels of 4 to 5 mEq/liter may be a more accurate measurement of decreased cellular perfusion.

Anion gap
Measurement of cellular perfusion. An increase in unmeasured anions, lactate, the anion gap rises. Normal anion gap is 5 to 12 mEq/liter. Abnormal findings include levels 20 mEq/liter or higher.

Blood glucose levels
Reflects mobilization of glycogen from the liver by increased catechol-

amines and decreased production and secretion of insulin from a hypoperfused pancreas. Hypoglycemia often is seen just before death. Normal blood glucose is 85 to 125 mg/dl. Levels of 250 to 300 mg/dl are found with cellular shock.

Oxygen extraction ratio (O_2ER)
Fraction of available oxygen that is extracted and consumed by the tissues. Normal ratio is 0.24 to 0.28. Abnormal level is > 0.35. High values indicate increased oxygen consumption or decreased oxygen delivery, or both. Oxygen extraction ratio is a good predictor of survival in the earlier stages of shock.

sue perfusion with optimization of pH, stabilizing lysosomal membranes, and providing substrate for energy production. Restoration of oxygen delivery and extraction usually is accomplished by increasing oxygenation, increasing cardiac output, and normalizing the hemoglobin level. Administration of nitroprusside or phentolamine will help to restore tissue perfusion. Nutritional support with supplemental glucose, free fatty acids, and protein, in combination with administration of insulin, will provide substrate for energy production in the cell.

Insulin administration is needed only if blood glucose levels exceed 200 mg/dl. Bicarbonate should be given to the patient with a pH that cannot be corrected by increased ventilation, or when the bicarbonate level is 12 mEq/liter or less. The early administration of large doses of corticosteroids has been found to stabilize lysosomal membranes in some forms of shock.

Nursing interventions during the treatment of cellular shock include:

• early detection of shock by clinical assessment and patient history

• collaboration with the physician to provide quality patient care

• rapid implementation of therapeutic modalities and reevaluation of the patient.

Cardiogenic shock

The goal of therapy in cardiogenic shock is to enhance cardiac output. This is accomplished by optimizing preload, decreasing afterload, increasing contractility, and optimizing the heart rate. The most common cause of cardiogenic shock is acute myocardial infarction. Therefore, reducing the infarct size also is important (see *Key nursing interventions for patients with cardiogenic shock,* page 623).

Hypovolemic shock

The goals of treatment in hypovolemic shock include ensuring adequate ventilation and oxygenation, identifying and stopping the source of fluid loss, and restoring intravascular volume. The patient in severe hypovolemic shock may be nonresponsive, making airway management a priority.

Often, management of hypovolemic shock requires aggressive fluid replacement, which may lead to overhydration and congestive heart failure, further compromising ventilation and perfusion. A search must be made for sources of blood and fluid loss. Potential sources include GI bleeding, accelerated fluid loss through fistulas, disconnection of intravenous access lines with retrograde bleeding, and disruption of vascular suture lines. When external bleeding is present, direct pressure over the site should be applied until definitive surgical control can be secured.

ESSENTIAL ELEMENTS

Key nursing interventions for patients with cardiogenic shock

The following flowchart highlights typical goals and interventions for the patient in cardiogenic shock.

> **Enhance cardiac output by optimizing preload, decreasing afterload, increasing contractility, and optimizing heart rate**

Improve cardiac output.	Minimize infarct size.
• Monitor hemodynamic parameters (pulmonary artery wedge pressure [PAWP], cardiac index, systemic vascular resistance, left and right ventricular stroke work index). • Assess for signs and symptoms indicative of myocardial ischemia, extension, infarction (chest pain, dyspnea, ECG changes). • Monitor vital signs. • Provide continuous ECG monitoring for arrhythmias and changes consistent with myocardial infarction. • Administer inotropic agents (dobutamine, dopamine). • Administer afterload reducer (nitroprusside). • Administer amrinone and milrinone to increase contractility and decrease preload and afterload. • Administer fluid if low to bring the PAWP up to 15 to 20 mm Hg.	• Administer oxygen as ordered. • Continuously monitor ECG for arrhythmias. • Institute measures to increase oxygen supply and decrease demand. • Assess for chest pain and anxiety. • Administer medication (MSO_4) to relieve pain and anxiety. —administer thrombolytics early in treatment as prescribed —assess for complications of thrombolytic therapy (bleeding, hypotension) —evaluate for the success of therapy (pain will subside, the ST-segment will return to normal, and reperfusion arrhythmias will occur). • Administer nitroglycerin as prescribed to dilate the coronary arteries and increase oxygen supply to the myocardium. • Administer beta-blockers and calcium channel blockers as prescribed to decrease oxygen demand and for their antiarrhythmic activity.

The type of fluid lost generally determines the fluid used for replacement. Solutions that are isotonic with human plasma and have sodium as their principal osmotically active particle should be used for resuscitation. Lactated Ringer's solution has a nearly identical electrolyte concentration as plasma and is often the initial solution of choice. The added lactate is easily metabolized to bicarbonate in the liver, except in the very ill patient.

When isotonic crystalloids are used for resuscitation, administration of approximately three to four times the vascular deficit is required to account for the distribution between the intra- and extravascular spaces. This occurs within 30 minutes after the fluid is given. Within 2 hours, however, less than 20% of the infused fluid remains within the intravascular space. Excessive administration of crystalloids is associated with generalized edema. Recent studies suggest that fluid resuscitation, especially with crystalloids, is contraindicated. It is believed that the excessive fluid produces a dilutional reduction in formed elements (red blood cells, platelets), increasing the tendency to bleed and decreasing the oxygen-carrying capacity, resulting in reduced cellular oxygenation.

Crystalloid-blood component therapy or blood component therapy alone is recommended for volume losses greater than 1,500 ml. Colloids are only partially permeable to the passage through the vessels, tending to remain in the intravascular space for longer periods than crystalloids. Smaller quantities of colloids are required to restore circulating volume. They are significantly more expensive than crystalloids. Albumin is the most commonly used colloid and is available as a 5% or 25% solution. The use of albumin can result in fluid overload.

Hetastarch, an effective volume expander with effects lasting from 3 to 25 hours, may be used up to 1 liter per day. It causes decreased platelet count and prolongation of the partial thromboplastin time due to antifactor VIII effect. The use of desmopressin (DDAVP) corrects the mild coagulopathy associated with hetastarch via a reversal in the decline in Factor VIII.

For the patient without complications, sophisticated monitoring is not required and management of fluids can be accomplished by following blood pressure, heart rate, urine output and by balancing intake and output. The patient with complications usually benefits from invasive monitoring. A fluid challenge that results in increased CO and left ventricular stroke work index (LVSWI) without a significant increase in pulmonary artery wedge pressure (PAWP) indicates that further fluid administration may be beneficial.

A patient with an elevated PAWP that increases abruptly after a fluid challenge without an increase in CO or LVSWI should be given inotropes instead of additional fluids to improve CO. Dopamine is the inotrope most frequently used to increase blood pressure and cardiac output in patients who have already been adequately fluid resuscitated.

The following nursing interventions should be incorporated into the plan of care for the patient with hypovolemic shock:

• Monitor arterial blood gas levels every 2 hours and as needed until stable.

• Observe for hypoxemia, hypercapnia, and acidemia.

• Check respirations every 30 minutes to 1 hour.

• Monitor the patient's breath sounds every 2 hours and observe for tachypnea and dyspnea.

• Monitor level of consciousness.

• Maintain a patent airway.

• Administer oxygen as ordered to maintain a PaO_2 of 80 to 100 mm Hg.

• Suction secretions as needed.

• Turn and position the patient every 2 hours.

• Prepare for mechanical ventilation if the patient is unable to oxygenate or ventilate, unresponsive, or apneustic.

• Monitor for hypotension, tachycardia, and respiratory changes continuously in the early phases of shock, then every hour.

• Assess and document CVP and PAWP every 1 hour and CO every 2 hours, if available.

• Monitor the patient for altered consciousness.

• Monitor input and output and obtain daily weights.

• Monitor for signs of fluid deficit.

Appropriate selection of empiric antibiotics

Empiric antibiotics generally are given to patients with septic shock until the definitive antibiotic can be ordered based on culture studies. Empiric antibiotics are chosen according to organisms associated with suspected infections.

Antibiotic	Suspected Source of Infection
Ampicillin, aminoglycosides, and clindamycin or imipenem	Proven or suspected pathogens in intra-abdominal infections
Aminoglycosides, expanded-spectrum penicillins	Comprehensive coverage and antibiotic synergism for pneumonias
Vancomycin (given until specific microbial sensitivity data is available)	Suspected soft tissue infections
Combination of antibiotics (must be chosen to cover both gram-negative and gram-positive organisms)	No suspected source of sepsis is evident
Amphotericin B (to reduce fungal superinfection)	Immunocompromised patients who are unresponsive to antibacterial therapy

• Administer volume expanders (crystalloids or colloids) as prescribed.
• Administer vasopressors when adequate fluids have been administered.
• Monitor for signs of fluid overload.
• Monitor for signs and symptoms of complications, including renal failure, bleeding tendencies, decreased myocardial function, and decreased calcium.

Septic shock

Treatment goals for the patient in septic shock include maintaining organ function and identifying and treating of the causative organism. Until the organism has been properly identified by culture reports, empiric antibiotics may be given (see *Appropriate selection of empiric antibiotics,* page 626). Organ function may be maintained with appropriate fluid resuscitation and pharmacological agents, and potential sources of infection, such as surgery for closure of bowel perforation, wound debridement, and drainage of abscesses, should be closely monitored (see *Key nursing interventions for patients with septic shock,* page 628).

Because of the high mortality associated with this disorder, emphasis must be placed on preventing infection. Essential preventive measures include hand washing and meticulous aseptic management of wounds and invasive lines. Dressings also can be a source of infection. Occlusive transparent dressings facilitate visualization of the site but may lead to maceration of tissue, which may increase the incidence of line-related sepsis. The use of silver- or antibiotic-impregnated catheters has reduced the need to change catheters as frequently and decreased the incidence of sepsis.

The GI tract is a portal of entry for many pathological organisms. The use of antacids and histamine blockers have reduced the incidence of stress ulcers; however, an increase in stomach colonization has occurred as a result of elevation of gastric pH. Sucralfate is equally effective against stress ulcers without causing bacterial overgrowth in the stomach. Enteral nutrition is preferred over parenteral nutrition because it will preserve the normal natural flora of the gut.

The following nursing interventions should be incorporated in the plan of care for the patient with septic shock:
• Maintain proper hand washing.
• Maintain aseptic care of wounds and invasive lines.
• Observe for signs of infection at line sites.
• Monitor GI pH.
• Administer sucralfate as prescribed.
• Administer antibiotics to neutralize GI flora as prescribed.

Prognosis
The morbidity and mortality from shock varies with the type of shock encountered, patient's health status prior to

ESSENTIAL ELEMENTS

Key nursing interventions for patients with septic shock

The following flowchart highlights goals and interventions typically utilized in caring for a patient in septic shock

Maintain organ function while identifying and treating causative organism

Maintain organ function with appropriate fluid resuscitation and pharmacological agents.	Identify signs of sepsis and treat causative organism or source of infection.
• Administer blood products in conjunction with altered laboratory findings, as ordered (red blood cells for decreased hemoglobin/hematocrit, fresh frozen plasma for clotting factors, cryoprecipitate for decreased fibrinogen, and platelets). • Administer crystalloids or colloids as ordered. • Monitor for signs of fluid overload (dyspnea, tachypnea, crackles, peripheral edema, jugular venous distension, enlarged liver, peripheral edema, increased pulmonary artery pressures). • Monitor vital signs (heart rate, respirations, blood pressure), before and after drug administration. • Administer inotropic drug (dopamine) as ordered. • Assess for signs of inadequate therapy (increased pulse, increased respirations, mottled skin, hypotension, decreased level of consciousness, decreased urinary output).	• Assess for signs of infection (fever or hypothermia, altered white blood cell count with differential, tachycardia, tachypnea). • Obtain cultures (blood, urine, wound, sputum) as ordered. • Administer empiric antibiotics for suspected organisms, as ordered only after cultures have been obtained. • Monitor culture reports for appropriate antibiotic regimen. • Monitor I.V. sites and wounds for signs of infection. • Assist in preparing patient for surgery. • Monitor vital signs for stability before and after surgery. • Administer pain medications, as ordered. • Monitor intake and output and daily weight.

shock, and the therapeutic modalities chosen. The most important factor in survival is the early detection of the shock state. With early detection and aggressive management morbidity and mortality are greatly reduced.

Discharge planning

Discharge planning should begin once the patient has been stabilized. The following guidelines should be considered to prepare the patient for discharge:
• Evaluate the patient's support systems.
• Initiate a social service consultation if needed.
• Review postdischarge medications, including actions, dosages, and possible side effects.

Spinal cord injury

Any damage to the spinal cord resulting from direct or indirect injury to the vertebrae that causes a change in motor and sensory functioning is considered a spinal cord injury. The spinal cord can be damaged by flexion, extension, distraction, compression, rotation, or shearing forces. A direct injury occurs when the muscles, ligaments, and bony structures between the skin and the spinal cord cannot sufficiently protect the cord from the force of the injury. An indirect injury occurs when the vertebral column is injured, the vertebral body ruptures, and the spinal cord is compressed by disk and bone fragments.

Approximately 10,000 spinal cord injuries are reported annually in the United States; about half result in paraplegia, the other half in quadriplegia. The most common sites for spinal cord injury are C1 and C2, C4 to C6, and T11 to L2. Most injuries occur in males between ages 15 and 25. Trauma resulting from motor vehicle crashes, gunshot or knife wounds, falls, and sporting incidents is the most common cause of these injuries. The incidence of injury increases with the use of illicit drugs and alcohol.

Pathophysiology

The major mechanisms of spinal cord injuries include hyperextension, hyperflexion, and compression (see *Mechanisms of spinal cord injury,* page 630). With hyperextension, the spinal cord is stretched against anteri-

Mechanisms of spinal cord injury

The following diagrams illustrate the major mechanisms that can result in a spinal cord injury to the cervical or lumbar region.

Hyperflexion

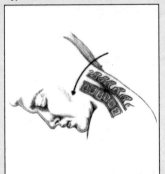

Hyperextension

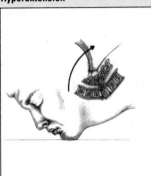

Compression

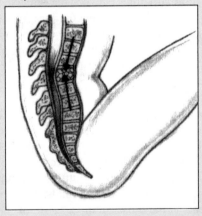

or ligaments leading to cord contusion and posterior vertebral dislocation. This type of injury can occur after falling down a set of stairs. A hyperflexion injury occurs when the spinal cord is stretched against the posterior ligament, also leading to cord contusion but with anterior vertebral dislocation. This type of injury can occur to the cervical spinal cord during a motor vehicle crash. Compression injuries, often caused by falls or jumps, cause vertebral fractures and subsequent cord compression by bone fragments.

When the spinal cord sustains an injury, the central gray area of the cord begins to microhemorrhage. In a matter of a few hours, red blood cells, spinal fluid, and polymorphonuclear leukocytes flood the area, causing vascular stasis and endothelial cell wall damage. The ongoing hemorrhage and accumulating edema contribute to ischemia, leading to cord necrosis both at the level of the injury and below. Cord cells become hypoxic, leading to increased lactic acid and norepinephrine secretion below the level of injury. Norepinephrine causes vasospasm, resulting in ongoing cell hypoxia and furthering necrosis. Because spinal cord cells cannot respond to vasospasm by shunting blood from other sites, the hypoxia-necrosis cycle continues.

Within 4 hours after the initial injury, approximately 40% of the cord's gray matter (at the site and below) will sustain additional necrosis. By 24 hours, this process will progress to the point where the gray matter is entirely consumed by red blood cells and necrotic tissue. Cord edema will extend above and below the site of injury, furthering cord damage and mimicking complete cord transection. Although it is thought that the extent of damage is complete after 48 hours, additional edema that extends beyond the level of injury will not be complete for 72 hours to 1 week following the injury. Prior to this, the full extent of the injury cannot be determined.

The severity of the injury determines the degree of motor and sensory loss. If the injury causes complete transection of the cord, immediate flaccid paralysis and loss of all sensation below the level of the injury occurs. With incomplete cord transection, partial loss of sensory and motor functioning below the level of the injury occurs. About 90% of incomplete lesions can be classified into one of three syndromes: central cord, anterior cord, or Brown-Séquard (see *Incomplete spinal cord injury syndromes,* page 632).

Incomplete spinal cord injury syndromes

Most of the incomplete lesions caused by a spinal cord injury can be categorized according to one of the syndromes listed below.

Syndrome	Characteristics
Central cord	• Most common of the cord syndromes • Caused by sudden hyperextension of the neck • Results in weakness of the arms greater than the legs • About 50% of patients will have return of bowel and bladder control
Anterior cord	• Caused by occlusion of the anterior spinal artery after a flexion injury • Results in abrupt onset of paralysis and loss of pain and temperature sense below the level of the lesion
Brown-Séquard	• Caused by gunshot or knife wound that produces a hemisection of the cord or from fracture of the lateral vertebra • Results in loss of motor function on the side of the injury and hypesthesia on the contralateral side below the lesion

The higher the level of injury, the more serious the effects because of the proximity of the cervical vertebra to the medulla and brain stem. Patients experiencing injuries anywhere within the cervical region will have quadriplegia, whereas those with injuries to the thoracic or lumbar areas will have paraplegia.

In addition to the sequence of events at the site of injury, the entire cord below the level of the injury can fail to function, creating a condition called spinal shock. Spinal shock can last from a few days or weeks to a few months. Initial symptoms include hypotension, bradycardia, warm and dry extremities, and complete loss of motor and sensory functioning below the level of the injury. Once the spinal shock resolves, an active rehabilitation program can be initiated. Signs that spinal shock are resolving include extremity spasticity, hyperreflexia, and reflex bladder and bowel emptying.

Most patients with spinal cord injuries sustain other injuries during the same traumatic event. In addition to

these injuries, the actual spinal cord injury can cause alterations in other body systems. Depending on the level of the lesion, the patient may experience any of the following:
• inability to spontaneously ventilate
• decreased cardiac output, hypotension, and a rapid, irregular heart rate
• aspiration of gastric contents and paralytic ileus
• bladder distention.

Clinical assessment

The clinical findings seen with a spinal cord injury depend on the level and extent of damage to the cord. The nurse must evaluate the extent of dysfunction as it relates to the location of the injury and the type of activity in which the patient participated at the time of injury.

History

When assessing the history, the nurse should elicit the following information:
• activity patient was participating in during the injury
• use of alcohol or illicit drugs
• use of prescribed or over-the-counter medications
• other preexisting medical conditions.

Physical findings

The physical findings associated with a spinal cord injury depend on the level of the lesion (see *Physical findings associated with spinal cord injuries,* page 634). Generally, patients who have sustained a spinal cord injury may present with:
• cuts or bruises over the head, face, neck, or back
• pallor or cyanosis
• pain, tenderness, or muscle spasms along the spinal column
• dyspnea or inability to breath adequately
• cool skin
• absence of perspiration
• bladder distention with possible overflow incontinence

Physical findings associated with spinal cord injuries

Any of the following findings may be noted during the physical examination.

C3 region or above
• Change in level of consciousness or responsiveness secondary to hypoxia from either an associated head injury or an interruption in nervous innervation to the muscles of respiration
• Apnea or inability to cough
• Weak or absent gag reflex
• Bradycardia, hypotension, and postural hypotension
• Flaccid paralysis and parasthesias all four extremities

C4-5 region
• Poor cough, diaphragmatic breathing, hypoventilation
• Some neck movement with normal neck sensation
• Bradycardia, hypotension, and postural hypotension
• Flaccid paralysis and parasthesias all four extremities with sensation present in the shoulders and lateral arm area

C6-8 region
• Bradycardia, hypotension, and postural hypotension
• Sensation in the lateral forearm, the thumb, and the middle finger
• Some motor function of the deltoid and triceps muscles; however, hand muscles remain paralyzed
• Lower-extremity paralysis and parasthesias

T1-3 region
• Normal neck, shoulder, chest, arm, hand, and respiratory function

• Some sensory loss over the medial aspect of the arm and part of the axilla
• Difficulty sitting
• Bradycardia, hypotension, and postural hypotension possible
• Urine retention with overflow incontinence
• Lower extremity paralysis and parasthesias

T4-10 region
• Bradycardia, hypotension, and postural hypotension if the lesion is between the T4-5 area
• Urine retention
• Lower extremity paralysis and parasthesias

T11-12 region
• Urine retention
• Reflex emptying of the bowel
• Difficulty attaining and maintaining an erection
• Lower extremity paralysis and parasthesias

L1-5 region
• Urine retention if the injury is above the L2 level
• difficulty attaining and maintaining an erection
• Varying degrees of lower extremity paralysis and parasthesias

Sacral region
• Anesthesia of the great toe or posterior thigh
• Alterations in bowel and bladder function

• decreased or absent bowel sounds and abdominal distention
• flaccid paralysis and anesthesia below the level of the lesion

• alteration in pain, temperature, pressure, and proprioception below the level of the injury.

Additionally, the patient will experience mild to severe involuntary muscle spasms and twitching. Often misinterpreted as a positive sign by the patient, these spasms do not signal the return of voluntary muscle movement. After a spinal cord injury, the brain no longer controls the spinal cord reflex movements. The section of the spinal cord below the level of the injury begins to function independently, causing reflexive movements. These primitive spinal mechanisms are normally kept inactive with an intact spinal cord.

The presence of hyperactive deep tendon reflexes (DTRs) and a positive Babinski's sign are particularly useful if the diagnosis of a partial or complete cord transection injury has not yet been ascertained. If these reflexes are present, the corticospinal tracts of the spinal cord remain intact, indicating an incomplete lesion has been sustained and the patient has a better prognosis. Hyperreflexic DTRs in the patient who has been areflexic due to spinal shock is a key indicator that the spinal shock is subsiding.

Diagnosis

During the diagnostic phase of spinal cord injury, care should be taken to avoid exacerbating any possible cervical injury by the use of a hard cervical collar. A complete neurologic examination should be performed to include specific diagnostic tests to aid in the diagnosis and extent of spinal cord injury (see *Diagnostic tests for spinal cord injury,* page 636).

Treatment and care

The goals for a patient with a spinal cord injury are to maintain life, prevent further cord damage, support other body systems, control pain, prevent infection, provide emotional support, provide sexual education, and begin the rehabilitative phase when physiologically stable.

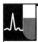

Diagnostic tests for spinal cord injury

The following tests are used to aid in the diagnosis of spinal cord injury.

Spinal X-rays
Both anterior-posterior and lateral X-rays are taken to evaluate for fractures or dislocated vertebra. In addition, the spinal films will detect any cord narrowing (by the location of the vertebral spinous processes) or hematomas.

Computed tomography (CT) and magnetic resonance imaging (MRI)
CT will pinpoint the area of injury and extent of soft tissue damage. An MRI will detect cord edema, necrosis, and evaluate the spinal cord's blood flow pattern and blood vessel integrity.

Myelogram
Although the myelogram has declined in popularity in the diagnosis of spinal cord injury, this test identifies blockages created by bone fragments, dislocations, herniations, or disc protrusions.

Pulmonary fluoroscopy
In the case of a high cervical injury, this diagnostic test will measure the degree of diaphragmatic movement. In injuries above C4, diaphragmatic innervation is interrupted resulting in partial diaphragmatic or paradoxical respiratory movements.

Hemoglobin and hematocrit
A baseline hemoglobin and hematocrit is drawn to evaluate the impact of traumatic injuries on the circulating blood volume. Because abdominal injuries are a frequent occurrence with spinal cord injuries, this blood value aids in ongoing evaluation of continuing hemorrhage within the body.

Urinalysis
Depending upon the level of cord injury, a urinalysis may be beneficial to detect if the kidneys or bladder also were injured during the same episodic event.

Arterial blood gas (ABG) studies
ABG studies are essential when evaluating the effectiveness of ventilation and to support the decision for or against mechanical ventilation. If the PaO_2 is below 60 mm Hg and the $PaCO_2$ is greater than 50 mm Hg, mechanical ventilation is indicated.

Vital capacity
For adequate gas exchange, the spinal cord patient's vital capacity should be greater than or equal to 1 liter.

Oxygen saturation of arterial blood (SaO_2)
Ideally, the SaO_2 should be greater than 90%. Values less than 90% indicate inadequate alveolar ventilation and the need for mechanical ventilation.

Preservation of remaining spinal cord function
Medical and nursing goals to preserve remaining spinal cord function typically focus on maintaining correct spinal alignment, assessing for improvement or deteri-

oration of condition, facilitating progressive mobility, and preventing complications.

Specific nursing interventions are included below:
• Support the spinal column to prevent any exacerbation of injury through the use of skeletal traction or a halo.
• Administer methylprednisolone at a rate of 30 mg/kg I.V. bolus followed by 5.4 mg/kg/hour via continuous I.V. over 23 hours, as prescribed.
• Administer osmotic diuretics (mannitol) to reduce localized edema if systolic blood pressure is high enough to sustain the effect.

Support of other body systems

Nearly all of the body systems are affected by a spinal cord injury. Nursing interventions to support normal physiologic function should include the following:
• Maintain respiratory status by monitoring arterial blood gas studies and pulmonary function tests; evaluate progressive weaning off of mechanical ventilation.
• Maintain cardiovascular status by treating hypotension with vasopressors.
• Decompress the GI tract, and prevent aspiration of gastric contents and paralytic ileus by use of an nasogastric tube.
• Administer antacids, histamine H_2-receptor antagonists, and stool softeners or laxatives as the condition warrants.
• Monitor urine output via an indwelling catheter.

Surgical stabilization

A spinal cord injury may be treated surgically if neurologic deficits continue to worsen, compound vertebral fractures are present, a penetrating wound of the spine has occurred, or bone fragments are in the spinal canal. Procedures undertaken to surgically stabilize a spinal cord injury include decompression laminectomy, closed or open reduction of the fracture, or spinal fusion.

Appropriate nursing interventions include the following:
• Maintain correct spinal alignment through the use of a kinetic therapy bed
• Inspect pins and traction for correct placement; provide pin care with local disinfectant and antimicrobial ointment as prescribed.
• In the event of a halo vest, secure a wrench on the front of the vest to be used for cardiopulmonary resuscitation.

Prevention of complications

Because of changes in mobility and altered body function, the patient is prone to many complications. One major complication that can occur up to 6 years after the initial injury is autonomic dysreflexia (AD), a combination of clinical symptoms that occur simultaneously when areas of the autonomic nervous system are stimulated. Often referred to as a syndrome, AD typically occurs in spinal cord injuries above T7 and is initiated by an overexaggerated response to a noxious stimuli. The most common trigger is a distended bladder, which can be easily treated by immediate straight catheterization, straightening a kinked indwelling catheter, or emptying a collection bag. Examples of other stimuli include bowel distention, pressure ulcers, muscle spasms, pain, accidental pressure on the penis, or uterine contractions.

At the onset of AD, sympathetic responses cause the blood vessels below the level of injury to constrict, resulting in hypertension. In addition, the patient experiences a pounding headache, flushing, diaphoresis, blurred vision, bradycardia, restlessness, and nausea. To prevent seizures or cerebral hemorrhage, AD must be immediately treated by elevating the head of the bed, identifying and removing the source of noxious stimuli, and providing nitrates, nifedipine, or other ganglionic blocking agents (only if the stimulus for the event cannot be found). These medications reduce the blood pressure so that adequate cerebral tissue oxygenation can occur, reducing the likelihood of seizures or cerebral hemorrhage.

Other common complications include the development of deep vein thrombosis (DVTs) and pulmonary emboli, which result because of the venous stasis associated with decreased vasomotor tone and immobility. To prevent the occurrence of DVTs and subsequent pulmonary emboli, the following nursing interventions are appropriate:

• Assess for signs of DVT, including heat and erythema of the calf or thigh, increased calf or thigh circumference, pain or tenderness in the calf or thigh area, positive Homan's sign (pain upon dorsiflexion of the lower extremity; the degree of pain or tenderness depends on the extent and level of the injury).

• Assess for signs of pulmonary emboli, including sudden shortness of breath, pain the chest or shoulder, increased heart rate, decreased blood pressure, pallor, cyanosis, productive cough, blood-tinged sputum, restlessness, and increasing anxiety.

• Turn and reposition the patient every 2 hours.

• Provide passive range-of-motion exercises every 2 hours.

• Instruct the patient to avoid leg crossing or to sit with legs dependent for longer than 30 minutes.

• Apply antiembolitic hose as ordered.

• If ordered, administer low-dose antithrombolytic medication (heparin).

Prognosis

Even though the life expectancy of a patient with a spinal cord injury is estimated to be only 5 years less than that of a person who has not sustained a similar injury, quality of life is a major concern. On average, patients with paraplegia remain in an acute care facility for 15 days, while those with quadriplegia remain hospitalized for 25 days. Once discharged to a rehabilitation facility, the patient's quality of life will be affected by the degree of physical rehabilitation achieved, maintenance of an adequate nutritional status, prevention of infection, efficient bowel and bladder emptying, and the maintenance of an intact integumentary status.

Discharge planning

Planning for discharge from an acute care setting begins upon admission to the critical care area. Efforts are undertaken to prevent further deterioration of mobility while aiding the patient to independently maintain respiratory and cardiovascular functioning.

Specific discharge planning should include:
• consulting a physical therapist to begin evaluating the degree of functional loss, and introducing muscle strengthening exercises
• consulting an occupational therapist to assist with achieving maximum independence in self-care
• consulting social services to begin planning for discharge to a rehabilitation facility
• assessing the patient and family's emotional support system and offering referrals for follow-up counseling on family and sexual concerns
• evaluating the home environment for adaptive equipment or special devices
• beginning a bowel retraining program as soon as the patient is physically able
• Begin a bladder retraining program as soon as the patient is physically able; if arm function is preserved, the patient can be taught to crédé the bladder and practice intermittent self-catheterization.

Syndrome of inappropriate antidiuretic hormone secretion

A condition characterized by water overload, hyponatremia, and hypo-osmolality, syndrome of inappropriate antidiuretic hormone (SIADH) results from excess secretion of antidiuretic hormone (ADH), which leads to an increase in water retention. The severity of signs and symptoms are directly related to the degree of hyponatremia. With rapidly developing hyponatremia coma, convulsions, and even death can occur.

Various diseases and disorders can cause SIADH. Bronchogenic oat cell carcinoma can produce vasopressin and release it independently of normal stimuli. Other cancers known to cause SIADH include cancer of the pancreas, duodenum, prostate, and thymus. Nontumorous lung diseases, including tuberculosis, pneumonia, chronic obstructive pulmonary disease (COPD), asthma, and respiratory failure of any kind also can cause SIADH. The water retention and hyponatremia result from independent synthesis and secretion of vasopressin (ADH) or a change in left atrial filling pressures, resulting in alteration of the stimulus for vasopressin release from the pituitary.

Other causes of SIADH include positive-pressure ventilation, which promotes increased ADH secretion through alteration of the pressure relationships involved in pulmonary volume-sensing mechanisms, and various disorders of the central nervous system (CNS), which can affect the neurohypophysis and increase release of vasopressin, damage the membrane structure of the posterior pituitary (thereby allowing leakage of ADH), or stimulate the sympathetic nervous system as a result of cerebral hypoxia. Such CNS disorders include head trauma with skull fractures, cerebral vascular accident, meningitis, CNS tumors, brain abscess, encephalitis, seizures, and Guillain-Barré syndrome. Certain medications also can alter the secretion of ADH from the pituitary and cause SIADH (see *Drugs that can cause SIADH,* page 642).

Pathophysiology

Vasopressin (ADH) is produced in the supraoptic nucleus of the hypothalamus and transported via the pituitary stalk to the posterior pituitary gland for storage and release. Regulation of ADH release is controlled by several factors. Osmoreceptors in the hypothalamus are sensitive to small changes in osmolality. When stimulated, ADH is secreted and water is reabsorbed via the

Drugs that can cause SIADH

Many drugs are associated with the development of SIADH. The mechanisms of action include increased ADH secretion, increased tubular reabsorption of water, and potentiation of ADH action.

Drugs that increase the secretion of ADH from the pituitary
• Antineoplastic drugs (vincristine, vinblastine)
• General anesthetics
• Barbiturates
• Nicotine
• Morphine

Drugs that increase the tubular reabsorption of water
• Vasopressin
• Oxytocin

Drugs that potentiate ADH action at the distal tubule
• Tricyclic antidepressants
• Nonsteroidal anti-inflammatory agents
• Clofibrate
• Phenothiazines
• Carbamazepine
• Thiazide diuretics
• Chlorpropamide

distal tubule. A decreased blood volume, as reflected by a decrease in the left atrial pressure, also stimulates ADH secretion. These changes in blood volume stimulate baroreceptors in the atria and aortic arch. When plasma volume drops suddenly, as in hemorrhage, increased secretion of ADH helps restore volume.

In congestive heart failure, nephrotic syndrome, and cirrhosis, the effective arterial blood volume is decreased, resulting in a marked increase in ADH levels. In conditions with increased circulating volume, inhibition of ADH release occurs with resulting diuresis (see *ADH release and regulation,* page 643).

Plasma osmolality also affects ADH secretion. When osmoreceptors in the hypothalamus detect increased plasma osmolality, the thirst mechanism promotes increased fluid intake and the posterior pituitary secretes ADH, which promotes fluid retention. Both ADH and the thirst mechanism respond to hyperosmolality by trying to increase extracellular fluid. When increased fluid intake and fluid retention have diluted the extracellular fluid to normal osmolality, ADH secretion falls to a baseline level and thirst disappears.

ADH release and regulation

In response to serum osmolality and reduced circulating volume, the posterior pituitary releases ADH. The circulating ADH alters water permeability at the renal tubule, resulting in increased reabsorption of water. This decreases serum osmolality and increases circulating volume, which through a negative feedback mechanism halts the release of ADH.

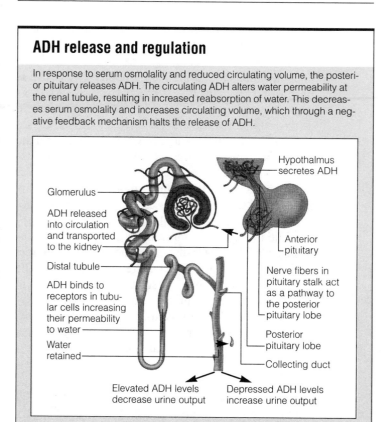

When plasma osmolality is low, the osmoreceptors do not trigger secretions of ADH; consequently, diuresis allows plasma osmolality to rise to normal levels.

ADH acts on the distal tubules and collecting ducts of the kidneys, increasing their permeability to water. This promotes reabsorption of water and reduces urine output. ADH binds to specific receptor sites in the collecting ducts and stimulates production of cyclic adenosine monophosphate (cAMP). This activates the enzyme protein kinase and eventually causes the collecting ducts' epithelium to become more permeable to water. The resulting reabsorption of water reduces volume and leads to concentrated urine.

In SIADH, a breakdown in the normal negative feedback system regulating the release and inhibition of ADH occurs. Circulating vasopressin acts directly on the renal tubules, causing reabsorption of water that is inconsistent with the body's needs. Excessive ADH secretion increases renal tubular permeability, resulting in reabsorption of water into the circulation. This causes water retention and, eventually, water intoxication if the condition remains untreated. The retained water expands the extracellular fluid volume, dropping the serum osmolality. As the serum osmolality decreases, the glomerular filtration rate rises and sodium levels decline, due to increased renal excretion.

Initially, hyponatremia reflects dilution of body fluids by retained water, but subsequently hyponatremia may reflect increased renal excretion of sodium. The increased renal excretion of sodium occurs because, in SIADH, the kidneys are adequately perfused, thereby inhibiting the release of renin-angiotensin-aldosterone. When this cycle is activated, the end result is reabsorption of sodium from the distal tubules.

Clinical assessment

Because the signs and symptoms of SIADH frequently mimic those of other disorders, a careful patient history and physical examination are invaluable for developing nursing goals and planning interventions. The nurse should keep in mind that body weight increases in proportion to retained water. Such water retention usually produces nonspecific signs and symptoms related to the GI tract (abdominal cramps, anorexia, nausea, vomiting) and central nervous system (disorientation, lethargy, confusion, headache, and possible hemiparesis, coma, or seizure).

History

The patient with SIADH usually has an abrupt onset of symptoms that result from increased water retention. If not recognized and treated, these symptoms may progress to water intoxication. During the health history, the

nurse should question the patient regarding a history of disorders leading to SIADH, including:
• oat cell carcinoma or pancreatic tumors
• disorders of the CNS (head injury, cerebrovascular accident [CVA], CNS infections, tumors)
• disorders of pulmonary system.

The nurse also should ask whether the patient has had recent exposure to drugs that cause SIADH, including:
• antineoplastic agents (vincristine, vinblastine)
• chlorpropamide
• tricyclic antidepressants
• general anesthetics or morphine
• nicotine.

Physical findings

Hyponatremia associated with decreased osmolality often is asymptomatic until serum sodium falls below 125 mEq/liter. Subtle neurologic findings, such as decreased ability to concentrate or to perform mental arithmetic, occur. Severe symptoms, such as altered mental status, seizures, nausea, vomiting, stupor, and coma, occur when serum sodium is less than 115 mEq/liter or when hyponatremia develops quickly. Females, children, and elderly patients are more susceptible to hyponatremia because of a lower body water content. (See *Signs and symptoms of hyponatremia,* page 646, for a list of common clinical manifestations.)

The nurse may observe any one or a combination of the following during the physical assessment:
• dyspnea and jugular venous distention
• new onset or worsening of crackles
• restlessness
• hypothermia
• weight gain
• small amounts of very concentrated urine.

Diagnosis

The diagnosis of SIADH usually is made by the finding of inappropriately high urine osmolality with low se-

Signs and symptoms of hyponatremia

The clinical manifestations of SIADH are predominantly due to water retention, hyponatremia, and hypo-osmolality. The severity of the symptoms depends on the degree of hyponatremia and the speed at which symptoms develop.

Mild (130 to 134 mEq/liter)	Moderate (121 to 129 mEq/liter)	Severe (< 120 mEq/liter)
• Headache • Lethargy • Sleepiness • Mental confusion or disorientation • Muscle cramps • Anorexia • Weight gain	• Personality changes • Hostility, irritability • Uncooperativeness • Disorientation • Nausea and vomiting • Diarrhea • Abdominal cramps • Sluggish deep tendon reflexes • Aberrant respirations • Hypothermia • Weakness	• Seizures • Coma • Death

rum osmolality, urine output less than 30 ml/hour, and increased sodium concentration. The urine osmolality may be less than the serum osmolality but still inappropriately high. This is paradoxical because, in a patient with severe hyponatremia, the urine should be maximally diluted (50 mOsm/kg).

Differential diagnosis

Because congestive heart failure, dehydration, hypovolemia, cirrhosis, nephrosis, and renal insufficiency produce a similar clinical syndrome, confirming SIADH requires exclusion of hyponatremia associated with hyperglycemia, hypertriglyceridemia, or hyperproteinemia. It also requires evaluation of fluid volume and of cardiac, hepatic, and renal function. Similarly, hypothyroidism and adrenal insufficiency must also be excluded. Because alterations in thyroid and adrenal function affect fluid balance and ADH secretion, tests to detect hypothyroidism or adrenal insufficiency must be conducted. These disorders must be corrected before SIADH can be confirmed.

Laboratory tests

Serum and urine electrolyte and osmolality abnormalities are the key findings in the diagnosis of SIADH. These abnormalities include:

- decreased serum sodium (< 135 mEq/liter)
- decreased proteins and serum osmolality (< 280 mOsm/liter)
- increased urine sodium (> 30 mEq/liter) and urine osmolality (300 to 500 mOsm/kg)
- increased specific gravity of urine (concentrated)
- increased plasma ADH
- decreased potassium is rare in SIADH
- decreased blood urea nitrogen, creatinine, hematocrit, and albumin.

Other diagnostic findings

The key to identifying SIADH is the relationship between the electrolytes and osmolality of the urine and serum. Other tests to help in diagnosis include X-rays and the water loading test (see *Confirming SIADH,* page 648).

Treatment and care

The cornerstone of therapy in the treatment of SIADH is correction of the underlying cause, restriction of free water, and replacement of sodium in severe cases.

Treatment of underlying cause

Treatment consists of identifying the underlying cause. Surgical resection, radiation, or chemotherapy may alleviate water retention in SIADH caused by cancer. No drugs will successfully inhibit the secretion of ADH from either the pituitary gland or a tumor. When the cause of SIADH is unknown, treatment consists of restricting water intake, giving diuretics to promote water excretion, and giving other drugs that block the action of ADH at the distal tubule and collecting duct, which

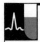

DIAGNOSTIC TESTS
Confirming SIADH

The following diagnostic tests typically are performed to help confirm a diagnosis of SIADH.

X-rays
The most common cause of SIADH is cancer. Carcinomas known to cause SIADH include bronchogenic, pancreatic, duodenal, prostatic, and thymic cancer. These malignant cells synthesize, store, and release biologic ADH. Identification of tumors on X-rays can assist in the diagnosis of SIADH.

Water loading test
The patient is given an oral fluid load (usually 20 ml/kg of body weight) and the urine is collected over the next 5 to 6 hours. To pre-vent any serious side effects from the fluid load, the patient must have a sodium level greater than 125 mEq/liter and must not display any symptoms consistent with hyponatremia prior to administration of the test. Normal individuals will excrete 80% of the fluid load within 5 to 6 hours. Patients with SIADH will excrete less then 50% of the water load given in this period and are unable to dilute their urine. Serial determinations of urine and serum osmolalities after delivery of an exogenous water load also should be conducted.

usually corrects hyponatremia. Medications can be given that reduce ADH secretion (dilantin) or decrease the renal response to ADH (lithium or demeclocycline).

The following nursing interventions should be incorporated into the plan of care:

• Assess the patient frequently for signs of worsening hyponatremia (water overload), including altered level of consciousness, anorexia, vomiting, muscle weakness, and coma.

• Monitor electrolyte levels, serum and urine osmolality, and the results of special diagnostic tests to assist in identifying the underlying cause.

• Monitor hourly intake and output and daily weight.

• Administer thyroid hormone for hypothyroidism.

• Administer glucocorticoids for adrenal insufficiency.

Fluid restriction
Even if the source of ADH secretion cannot be removed or suppressed, water restriction decreases intravascular fluid volume in patients with asymptomatic hyponatre-

mia. The result is decreased renal blood flow and glomerular filtration, which enhances proximal tubular reabsorption of salt and water (and decreases free water generation) and increases aldosterone secretion, enhancing distal tubule sodium reabsorption. However, decreased renal blood flow may predispose the patient to prerenal renal failure.

If the condition is mild to moderate, a fluid restriction of 1,000 to 1,500 ml/24 hours usually is sufficient to increase the serum sodium concentration. Typically, intake should not exceed urine output until serum sodium levels are normal and symptoms subside. Then, fluid intake should equal urine output. Fluid restriction usually is successful in reversing hyponatremia when sodium levels are between 125 and 135 mEq/liter. Normal saline is the fluid of choice in the asymptomatic patient.

The following nursing interventions should be incorporated in the plan of care:
• Monitor intake and output hourly.
• Monitor serum and urine osmolality.
• Administer normal saline, I.V., at a rate not to exceed a total intake of 1,000 to 1,500 ml/24 hours.
• Monitor serum sodium levels every 2 hours. Correct to normal within 24 to 48 hours.

Administration of hypertonic saline solution

Isotonic saline (154 mEq Na/liter) alone may not correct hyponatremia, even though it is hypertonic compared with the patient's plasma. Patients with marked neurologic signs (seizures, coma, focal deficits) or, perhaps, extreme hyponatremia (< 120 mEq/liter) require more aggressive treatment. In those cases, hypertonic (3%) saline should be used (0.1 mg/kg/minute I.V.). Excessive volume or rate of administration of hypertonic saline must be avoided to prevent acute volume overload and pulmonary edema. It is unlikely that the total amount of hypertonic saline will exceed 1,000 ml or a rate of more than 60 to 75 ml/hour.

Free-water diuresis should be induced by giving a loop diuretic concomitantly. This is only a temporary measure to increase the serum sodium; it will prevent the deleterious effects of severe hyponatremia, and the diuresis from the furosemide will help prevent pulmonary edema that might otherwise occur as a result of the fluid overload. A complication of this treatment is hypokalemia, which requires potassium supplements.

Pharmacologic management

Administration of demeclocycline hydrochloride or lithium inhibits the renal effects of ADH. These drugs interfere with the actions of ADH at the distal tubule and collecting duct. Each can be used to limit the effect of ADH on water reabsorption and prevent fluid overload and hyponatremia. The most commonly used drug for this purpose is demeclocycline.

The following nursing interventions should be incorporated in the plan of care:
• Monitor intake and output closely (demeclocycline or lithium can cause an increased output).
• Administer demeclocycline 900 to 1,200 mg/day, I.V. divided every 6 to 8 hours.
• Administer lithium carbonate and monitor for side effects of drugs.

Prevention of complications

Of major concern is the development of central pontine myelinolysis in some patients who have undergone rapid correction of the hyponatremia. This complication of treatment is more likely in female patients or those with alcoholism or malnutrition. Rapid correction (> 1 mEq/liter/hour) may be most appropriate if the hyponatremia is acute, while slower rates of correction (< 0.5 mEq/liter/hour) may be preferred in patients with chronic hyponatremia. Regardless of the initial rate of serum sodium concentration change, the process of correction should initially be to a less dangerous hyponatremic level (serum sodium concentration of approximately

125 mEq/liter), with gradual correction of the patient's serum sodium level to normal thereafter.

Too-rapid correction of chronic hyponatremia also can be deleterious and lead to saline overload. Rapid correction of chronic hyponatremia may result in brain dehydration, cerebral bleeding, demyelination, neurologic injury, or death. Osmotic demyelination syndrome is a delayed complication of rapid reversal of hyponatremia (correction by more than 12 mEq/liter/day). The signs characteristic of hyponatremia improve during correction of the electrolyte disorder, but improvement is followed within 1 to more days by neurologic deterioration (seizures, movement disorders, akinetic mutism, pseudobulbar palsy, quadriparesis, and unresponsiveness). It is suggested that the serum sodium level not be corrected faster than 1 to 2 mEq/liter/hour and that the serum sodium be increased to only 130 mEq/liter. Hypernatremia should be avoided.

The following nursing interventions should be incorporated in the plan of care:

- Administer furosemide as prescribed.
- Administer 3% hypertonic saline solution (60 to 75 ml/hour).
- Monitor sodium levels every 2 hours (increase sodium no faster than 1 mEq/liter/hour to no more than 12 mEq/liter/day).
- Assess for signs of osmotic demyelination syndrome, including seizures, movement disorders, and unresponsiveness.
- Assess for signs of pulmonary edema, including dyspnea, tachycardia, crackles, worsening arterial blood gas levels, and pulmonary shunting.
- Monitor hourly intake and output and daily weight.
- Monitor vital signs hourly.
- Monitor for signs of hypokalemia and replace as needed.

Prognosis

CNS signs of hyponatremia usually improve within 24 to 72 hours after correction of hyponatremia. A small increase in plasma osmolality is sufficient to reduce brain swelling. Continued CNS abnormalities suggest another cause or permanent damage from hyponatremia. After hyponatremia is corrected, careful monitoring of fluid and electrolyte status is required to prevent recurrence.

Discharge planning

Providing patient and family education in chronic disorders of water regulation is imperative. These disorders may be self-limiting or complicate preexisting conditions. The nurse must assume an important role in coordinating maintenance of the patient's fluid status. Early discharge planning with the patient or family may include education in:
• principles of intake and output and daily weights
• drug administration to block or decrease secretion of ADH, such as dilantin, lithium, or demeclocycline
• signs of increased water retention, such as weight gain, peripheral edema, and lethargy.

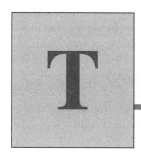

Thoracic trauma

About 50% of all trauma patients suffer some form of thoracic, or chest, trauma. Chest trauma commonly is classified as either penetrating or blunt. With penetrating chest trauma, the injury is inflicted by a foreign object, such as a knife, bullet, knitting needle, pitch fork, or other pointed object, that penetrates the thorax. With blunt chest trauma, injury results from sudden compression or positive pressure inflicted by a direct blow to the organ and surrounding tissue, such as occurs in a motor vehicle accident, a fall, or a crushing injury.

Penetrating chest trauma often is life-threatening, involving isolated injury to the chest and mild pulmonary contusion. If the heart or major vascular structures are penetrated, mortality significantly increases. Penetrating trauma carries an overall mortality of 10%, with an average hospital stay of 3 to 5 days. Urgent thoracotomy is recommended for patients with embedded or impaled objects to facilitate controlled removal of the object and for patients with massive hemothorax.

Pathophysiology

The pathophysiologies of penetrating and blunt chest traumas are very different. Penetrating trauma typically is fairly limited, usually involving isolated organs and lacerated tissues. However, in some cases, extensive tissue damage can occur if a bullet explodes within the chest cavity. Blunt chest trauma can cause extensive injury to the chest wall, lung, pleural space, and great vessels. Injuries resulting from blunt chest trauma include pulmonary contusion, rib fractures, pneumothorax, hemothorax, and rupture of the diaphragm or great vessels.

Penetrating trauma

Tissue damage caused by an impaled object or a foreign body is related to the object size and the depth and velocity of penetration. A penetrating injury inflicted by a bullet has many variables. The extent of injury depends on the range at which the weapon was fired, the type of ammunition, the velocity of the bullet, and the entrance and exit wounds. Factors to consider when assessing the range include the type, caliber, barrel, and length of weapon, the distance at which the weapon was fired, and the powder composition. An intact bullet causes less damage than a bullet that explodes on impact. A bullet that explodes within the chest may break up and scatter fragments, burn tissue, fracture bone, disrupt vascular structures, or cause a bullet embolism.

Blunt trauma

Injury resulting from blunt chest trauma is related to the amount of force, compression, and cavitation. Blunt force that impacts the chest wall at high velocity fractures the ribs and transfers that force to underlying organ and lung tissue. The direct impact of force is transmitted internally, and the energy is dissipated to internal structures. The flexibility or elasticity of the chest wall have a direct effect on the degree of injury.

Because of the noncompliance of the frail elderly, there is more significant injury and mortality, even from minor chest trauma. The first and second ribs take an enormous amount of blunt force to fracture and therefore are associated with significant intrathoracic injuries. Blunt injuries are associated with multisystem organ injuries and carry a higher mortality rate than penetrating injuries.

Traumatic pneumothorax

Several types of traumatic pneumothorax are possible with a traumatic or blunt chest injury: pneumothorax, tension pneumothorax, open (sucking) pneumothorax, hemopneumothorax, hemothorax, massive hemothorax, pneumomediastinum, and chylothorax. The pathophysiology is similar, regardless of the type: the intrapleural space is disrupted, causing air to enter the pleural space and to collapse underlying lung tissue (pneumothorax). If vessels are injured, a hemothorax or a hemopneumothorax will be present.

Injury to the thoracic duct following penetrating trauma causes lymphatic fluid to drain into the pleural space (chylothorax). In a traumatic tension pneumothorax, air in the intrapleural space is higher than the pressure in the lung and vascular structures. This pressure is strong enough to compress the lung tissue, causing tracheal deviation to the opposite side, thereby decreasing venous return to the heart and cardiac output. This results in substantial decreases in total lung capacity, vital capacity, and lung compliance. The resulting ventilation-perfusion imbalance leads to hypoxia (see the "Pneumothorax" entry for further details).

Associated traumatic injuries

When two or more adjacent ribs become fractured at two or more places (segmental fractures), a condition common in elderly patients with blunt chest trauma, a flail chest occurs. The flail segment of ribs is retracted inward during inspiration, causing instability of the chest wall, poor ventilation, and atelectasis. Paradoxical chest wall motion is extremely painful and leads to decreased vital capacity.

Pulmonary contusion occurs with most types of blunt chest trauma. With this injury, the entire lung tissue ruptures, disrupting the alveoli, interstitial membrane, and vascular bed as a result of compression and decompression. Alveolar hemorrhage, edema, and inflammation are present. Large pulmonary contusions cause hypoxia and are associated with an increased risk for adult respiratory distress syndrome (see the "Adult Respiratory Distress Syndrome" entry for more details).

Injuries to the cervical trachea usually result from hyperextension of the neck during a motor vehicle crash or penetrating trauma. Laceration or transection of the trachea occurs at approximately the third tracheal ring. When complete transection occurs, the distal tracheal retracts towards the carina. The recurrent laryngeal nerve surrounding the trachea also may be injured. Tracheobronchial injuries often occur from a crushing or direct blow to the trachea while the glottis is closed. Lacerations of the trachea usually occur near the carina.

Diaphragmatic rupture typically is caused by blunt injury to the abdominal area. The sudden increase in intra-abdominal pressure may rupture the hemidiaphragm, allowing spillage of abdominal contents into the thorax. Lung tissue is compressed and vital capacity is decreased.

Injury to the pericardium, atrium, or ventricles can occur from penetrating or blunt trauma. Bleeding into the pericardial sac can quickly cause cardiac tamponade. Cardiac contusion also can occur from penetrating or blunt trauma to the chest. With this injury, the contused area of the myocardium becomes bruised and may be irritable and hypokinetic; ventricular arrhythmias caused by such ventricular irritability must be treated immediately. Cardiac contusion usually resolves within several days.

Myocardial stunning may occur following an episode of acute ischemia, resulting in acute reversible ventricular dysfunction and decreased cardiac output from decreased ejection fraction and stroke volume. Such stunning may be caused by abnormal energy use, oxygen free radical production, abnormal calcium influx, white cell accumulation in ischemic tissue, or collagen matrix damage; it typically resolves within 24 hours to 2 weeks after the traumatic event.

Intrathoracic bleeding can be caused by injury to the intercostal vessels, pulmonary parenchyma, heart, or great vessels. Most injuries cause a hemothorax and can be managed by pleural chest drainage.

Clinical assessment

A chest trauma assessment typically is performed in the emergency department as part of the primary assessment, usually within 5 minutes after arrival. This assessment focuses on airway, breathing, and circulation and on immobilization of the cervical spine. Life-threatening chest injuries are diagnosed, and immediate intervention is provided to reestablish circulation.

A secondary assessment involves obtaining information on the mechanism of injury and incorporating these findings in a head-to-toe physical assessment. It also involves inspecting and palpating the entire anterior and posterior chest (see *Secondary assessment for chest trauma,* page 658).

If a tension pneumothorax is suspected at any time during the secondary assessment, the nurse must be prepared to assist with placement of a pleural chest tube. The patient history and mechanism of injury alone may indicate the need for a chest tube. A chest X-ray is not necessary to make this diagnosis. The nurse can quickly inspect and palpate the neck and chest, auscultate breath sounds, obtain vital signs, and evaluate for chest pain caused by a collapsed lung.

History

It is important to obtain as much information as possible concerning the mechanism of injury related to the traumatic event. Areas to cover include:
• mechanism of injury
• trauma score at scene
• Glasgow coma scale score
• time from scene to hospital
• prehospital interventions

Secondary assessment for chest trauma

A secondary assessment incorporates determining the mechanism of injury along with a physical assessment to assist with identification of injury.

Inspection
• Respiratory rate, rhythm, depth
• Deviated trachea
• Jugular vein distention
• Use of accessory muscles
• Entrance and exit wounds
• Impaled objects
• Chest wall bruising, lacerations, burns
• Ecchymoses and petechiae

Auscultation
• Breath sounds equal bilateral
• Heart sounds

—diminished: shock or tamponade
—hyperdynamic: normal response

Palpation
• Subcutaneous emphysema
• Fractured ribs or clavicles
• Pain response
• Skin temperature and diaphoresis

Percussion
• Bilateral lung fields
—tympanic: pneumothorax
—dull: hemothorax
• Assess level of diaphragm

• vital signs taken at the scene.

Physical findings

The nurse must rely on the mechanism of injury to assist with assessing for associated injuries and should bear in mind that hypovolemic shock may occur at any time in a patient with chest trauma (see *Clinical findings in chest trauma,* pages 659 to 661).

Diagnosis

Erect or upright chest X-rays remain the gold standard for evaluation of a chest trauma patient. However, such X-rays should be taken only when the patient is stable and has no evidence of cervical involvement. If cervical immobilization must be maintained, a supine chest X-ray usually is taken. However, supine chest X-rays do not always visualize rib fractures, small pneumothoraces, mediastinal width, pulmonary hemorrhage, or cardiac borders. A hemothorax of less than 500 cc does not visualize on chest X-ray.

Computed tomography (CT) of the chest is done to assess suspected organ damage from fractured ribs (liver,

Clinical findings in chest trauma

Correlating the mechanism of injury with clinical findings can expedite the diagnosis and treatment of chest trauma.

Traumatic Injury	Mechanism of Injury	Clinical Findings
Traumatic pneumothorax	• Penetrating or blunt trauma • Air in pleural space	• Dyspnea • Chest pain • Absence of tracheal shift • Breath sounds • Positive chest X-ray • Positive CT scan
Traumatic tension pneumothorax	• Penetrating or blunt trauma • Air in pleural space that becomes trapped and impedes cardiac output	• Dyspnea • Hypoxia • Cyanosis • Displaced trachea • Increased heart rate • Decreased blood pressure • Decreased PaO_2 • Shock, cardiac arrest
Hemothorax	• Blunt or penetrating trauma • Blood in the pleural space	• Dyspnea • Increased heart rate • Increased respiratory rate • Positive chest X-ray
Massive hemothorax	• Blunt or penetrating trauma • Blood in the pleural space • 1,500 ml of blood in pleural space	• Shock • Dullness to percussion • Increased heart rate • Increased respiratory rate • Decreased blood pressure • Treatment based on symptoms
Chylothorax	• Blunt or penetrating trauma • Trauma to left thoracic duct or lymphatics	• Effusion (may not be evident for 2 to 4 weeks) • Left pleural effusion (seen on chest X-ray)
Pneumomediastinum	• Penetrating or blunt trauma • Air in mediastinum	• Dyspnea • Chest pain
Flail chest	• Blunt trauma • Asymmetry of chest wall	• Dyspnea • Hypoxia • Chest wall pain • Crepitus from body fragments • Asynchronous chest expansion *(continued)*

Clinical findings in chest trauma *(continued)*

Traumatic Injury	Mechanism of Injury	Clinical Findings
Sucking chest wall wounds	• Blast wound to chest wall	• Dyspnea • Hypoxia • Chest wall pain • Chest wall defect • Sucking sound audible on inspiration
Pulmonary contusion	• Blunt trauma • Compression or de-compression injury	• Dyspnea • Bloody sputum • Wheezing • Moist crackles • Atelectasis • Shock • Hypoxia
Tracheobronchial injury	• Blunt trauma • Injury to tracheal bronchial tree caused by blunt force	• Dyspnea • Hemoptysis • Difficult intubation • Persistent pneumothorax
Diaphragmatic rupture	• Blunt trauma • Trauma to diaphragm caused by auto deceleration	• Increased respiratory rate • Chest pain • Hypoxemia • Positive chest X-ray findings
Cardiac contusion	• Blunt trauma • Bruising of cardiac muscle from blunt trauma	• Chest discomfort • Increased CPK • Possible normal echocardiogram
Cardiac tamponade	• Penetrating or blunt trauma • Precordial trauma that causes bleeding into pericardial sac and impedes venous return and cardiac output	• Dyspnea • Mid-thoracic pain • Increased heart rate • Increased respiratory rate • Decreased blood pressure, muffled heart tones, neck vein distention (Beck's triad) • Shock • No response to CPR • Increased PAP • Increased CVP • Narrow pulse pressure • Pulses paradox > 15 mm Hg

Clinical findings in chest trauma *(continued)*

Traumatic Injury	Mechanism of Injury	Clinical Findings
Rupture of great vessel	• Blunt trauma • Ruptured aorta (usually caused by external injury from steering wheel or atherosclerosis)	• Dyspnea • Hoarseness • Stridor • Absent femoral pulses • Retrosternal or interscapular pain • Widening mediastinum • Positive aortogram

spleen, kidney), pulmonary contusion, and great-vessel injury. Cardiac ultrasound or transthoracic echocardiography is used to assess pericardial effusion, tamponade, and rupture. Assessment by echocardiogram includes heart structure, valves, papillary muscles, chamber size, ejection fraction, and hypokinesis. Pericardiocentesis also can be done safely using cardiac ultrasound, although trauma surgeons prefer a pericardial window. An electrocardiogram is used to establish the baseline rhythm and to identify areas of ischemia or injury. Initial routine laboratory tests may vary, depending on physician preference or institution standard.

Treatment and care

Most patients with chest trauma have a moderate or large pneumothorax or hemothorax and are treated with a pleural chest tube. Symptomatic patients with unstable vital signs, including those with cardiopulmonary arrest for suspected traumatic tension pneumothorax, require immediate lung reexpansion. Less than 15% of all patients require resuscitative or urgent thoracotomy to repair injuries to the heart, great vessels, pulmonary vasculature, or tracheobronchial tree. Treatments for other specific injuries vary with the type and severity of injury (see *Surgical treatment and nursing interventions of thoracic injuries,* pages 662 to 664).

(Text continues on page 664.)

Surgical treatment and nursing interventions of thoracic injuries

Nursing interventions are identified according to diagnosed or suspected injuries. Surgical treatments also are identified to assist with planning of patient care.

Injury	Surgical Treatment	Nursing Interventions
Traumatic pneumothorax	• Pleural chest tube placement	• Assist with chest tube placement. • Set up chest drainage unit. • Reassess breath sounds for lung reexpansion. • Secure chest tube.
Traumatic tension pneumothorax	• Possible resuscitative thoracotomy (for penetrating trauma with cardiac arrest) • Emergency lung reexpansion	• Assist with lung reexpansion procedure. • Assist with chest tube placement. • Set up chest drainage unit. • Reassess breath sounds for lung reexpansion. • Secure chest tube. • Assess breath sounds.
Hemothorax	• Placement of pleural chest tube with autoinfuser	• Assist with chest tube placement. • Set up chest drainage unit. • Reassess breath sounds for lung reexpansion. • Secure chest tube.
Massive hemothorax	• Urgent thoracotomy (if initial drainage is > 200 ml/hour for 2 hours) • Emergency placement of pleural chest tube with autoinfuser	• Assist with chest tube placement. • Prepare patient for surgery. • Correct hypovolemia with autotransfusion or blood products.
Chylothorax	• Pleural chest tube placement • Thoracotomy: ligation of thoracic duct • Insertion of pleural-peritoneal shunt (rare)	• Assist with chest tube placement. • Set-up chest drainage unit. • Reassess breath sounds for lung reexpansion. • Secure chest tube. • Ensure bowel rest (NPO status) for 2 weeks. • Provide adequate nutrition.

Surgical treatment and nursing interventions of thoracic injuries *(continued)*

Injury	Surgical Treatment	Nursing Interventions
Pneumo-mediastinum	• Repair associated injury • Pleural chest tube placement	• Assist with chest tube placement. • Set up chest drainage unit. • Reassess breath sounds for lung reexpansion. • Secure chest tube.
Flail chest	• Rarely performed	• Provide pulmonary hygiene. • Promote comfort. • Assess for hemothorax and pneumothorax. • Administer analgesics, (consult pain management service). • Monitor intubation and ventilation.
Sucking chest wall wounds	• Pleural chest tube placement • Wound debridement and closure • Myocutaneous flaps for large soft tissue defects	• Assist with chest tube placement. • Cover wound with plastic on three sides, leaving one side to release air on exhalation. • Assess breath sounds. • Prepare patient for operating room and surgery.
Pulmonary contusion	• Urgent thoracoscopy or thoracotomy (for massive intrathoracic hemorrhage)	• Monitor intubation and mechanical ventilation. • Maintain recommended tidal volumes (5 to 7 ml/kg). • Maintain oxygenation and blood pressure during CT scan. • Monitor hemodynamic parameters to maintain adequate cardiac index. • Maintain normal PAWP and CVP levels. • Assess and optimize oxygen delivery.
Tracheobronchial injuries	• Emergency surgical repair of injury	• Establish and monitor airway. • Assess for neck edema, hematoma, and subcutaneous air. • Maintain SpO_2 90%. • Prepare for bronchoscopy and neck CT scan. • Monitor WBC count and chest tube drainage color for mediastinitis. *(continued)*

Surgical treatment and nursing interventions of thoracic injuries *(continued)*

Injury	Surgical Treatment	Nursing Interventions
Diaphragmatic rupture	• Surgical repair • Assess for associated injuries	• Assess breath sounds or bowel sounds in chest cavity. • Prepare patient for operating room and surgery.
Cardiac contusion	• None	• Assess cardiac rhythm. • Treat arrhythmias. • Obtain echocardiogram.
Cardiac tamponade	• Resuscitative thoracotomy (for cardiac arrest) • Pericardial window	• Prepare for pericardiocentesis. • Prepare patient for operating room and surgery. • Assist with echocardiogram, if performed.
Great vessel injury	• Resuscitative thoracotomy • Early diagnosis prior to rupture	• Prepare for transfusion. • Prepare patient for surgery.

Airway stabilization

The decision to intubate a patient usually is based on the patient's clinical presentation during the primary or secondary assessment. The location of injury, tracheal edema, respiratory rate, depth of respirations, oxygen saturation, and level of consciousness play a role in the maintenance of an airway and breathing. If the patient requires mechanical ventilation, arterial blood gas levels are maintained within normal limits by adjusting the oxygen percentage, respiratory rate, tidal volume, and positive end-expiratory pressure.

Appropriate nursing interventions include:
• Maintain gas exchange.
• Minimize oxygen demands.
• Prevent complications.

Emergency lung expansion

Standard treatment involves placement of a single pleural chest tube on the patient's affected side. The chest tube allows air or blood to leave the intrapleural space, allowing the lung to reexpand. Chest tubes usually are required for 3 to 5 days in patients with penetrating trauma.

Nursing interventions to include in the plan of care are listed below:

• After the chest tube is placed, connect the distal end of the tube to the chest drainage system.

• Assess for drainage every hour for 4 hours, then every 2 hours for 24 hours.

• Palpate for subcutaneous air on the affected side.

• Follow institutional guidelines regarding the use of dressing for chest tube insertion site.

• Change any dressing placed over the site at least every 48 hours or more often if it is stained with bloody drainage.

• Secure the chest tube to the patient with an anchoring device or tape.

• To increase patient comfort, administer nonsteroidal anti-inflammatory drugs as prescribed.

• Teach the patient to cough and breathe deeply enough to mobilize secretions and promote lung expansion.

Resuscitative thoracotomy

Resuscitative thoracotomy typically is done for a patient in cardiopulmonary arrest. It is most successful in cases of penetrating trauma in which injuries can be quickly repaired. The nurse's role in resuscitative thoracotomy includes recognition of need and expediting the procedure. It is the nurse's responsibility to provide instruments, prepare a chest drainage system with auto transfusion, prepare infusion of blood, and maintain and record vital signs. Following repair, the patient requires hemodynamic monitoring, frequent vital sign monitoring, continued stabilization, and mechanical ventilation.

Urgent thoracotomy

An urgent thoracotomy is performed in the operating room for patients with stable or unstable vital signs. The patient may have clinical findings of cardiac tamponade, massive hemothorax, or shock from unknown etiology. It usually is done following a positive CT scan or arteriogram. Postoperative nursing interventions include:

• Assess for chest tube drainage every hour for 4 hours, then every 2 hours for 24 hours.
• Palpate for subcutaneous air on the affected side.
• Monitor vital signs and hemodynamic status.
• Assist the patient with turning, coughing, and deep breathing every 2 hours.
• Provide pain management using a pain scale to assess effectiveness of treatment.

Preventing complications

Patients who are elderly or obese and those with multisystem trauma or preexisting cardiac, pulmonary, or renal disease have increased morbidity and mortality; they require careful pulmonary artery monitoring to optimize cardiac output and oxygen availability to the tissues. Aggressive nursing care can prevent the onset of complications (see *Preventing and treating complications associated with chest trauma,* page 667).

Acute lung injury usually occurs within 48 hours after an acute traumatic injury. Tachycardia, tachypnea, and severe hypoxia are present. Chest X-rays reveal diffuse bilateral infiltrates ("white out" of lung fields) as a result of interstitial and alveolar edema. Some evidence suggests that optimizing cardiac output and oxygen delivery and decreasing lactate levels within the first 48 hours after injury reduces the incidence of adult respiratory distress syndrome (ARDS). The presence of sepsis greatly increases the incidence of ARDS and mortality of patients with ARDS. Lateral rotation beds are being used on patients with ARDS to provide constant turning without increasing oxygen consumption.

Preventing and treating complications associated with chest trauma

Pulmonary complications significantly increase mortality in a patient with chest trauma. Aggressive pulmonary care and appropriate ventilator management can help decrease mortality and morbidity.

Complication	Means of Prevention or Treatment
Adult respiratory distress syndrome (ARDS)	• Optimize oxygen delivery to the tissues to decrease incidence of ARDS. • Avoid ventilator-induced lung injury (volutrauma). • Use newer modes of mechanical ventilation, such as pressure support, pressure cycled, inverse ratio, or high-frequency ventilation. • Use a lateral rotation therapy bed to decrease oxygen demand.
Bronchopleura fistula	• Prevent ventilator-induced lung injury.
Ventilatory-induced lung injury	• Maintain peak inspiratory pressure (PIP) < 35 mm Hg to decrease injury to the lung. • Use newer modes of ventilation. • Use tidal volumes of 5 to 7 mg/kg to decrease PIP and thereby decrease volutrauma. • Employ positive end-expiratory pressure to help prevent ARDS and volutrauma.
Pneumonia and at-electasis	• Encourage early mobility (chair and ambulation). • Use a lateral rotation bed for immobile patients. • Employ vigorous pulmonary hygiene. • Be aware that prophylactic antibiotics do not prevent pneumonia.
Infection	• Change soiled or nonocclusive dressings. • Use vigorous wound hygiene and debridement. • Discontinue central lines within 72 hours.
Pulmonary emboli	• Use compression cuffs until patient is ambulating. • Use subcutaneous heparin prophylaxis.

Pneumonia is the most common cause of sepsis in trauma patients. Patients who are immobilized as a result of orthopedic injures requiring traction and extended bed rest are at extreme risk for secretion retention and atelectasis. A pleural chest tube left in longer than 7 days must be cleansed daily or the wound infection rate increases to 60%. Bronchopleural fistula occurs following penetrating trauma to the lung parenchyma and usually heals within 7 days.

Prognosis

The prognosis of patients with chest trauma depends on the mechanism of injury, degree of multisystem involvement, and complications. Sepsis combined with ARDS is associated with the highest morbidity and mortality of greater than 90%. Penetrating chest trauma and blunt chest injury carry a different mortality and morbidity. Blunt chest trauma carries an overall mortality of about 40%; penetrating chest trauma, less than 8%. Injury to the aorta or pulmonary artery frequently leads to immediate death.

Discharge planning

Discharge planning begins at the time of admission and includes an interdisciplinary team approach. A social worker will assist with financial needs, home health, and obtaining adaptive equipment for home use; a dietitian, with nutritional needs and recommendations for nutritional support; a psychiatric clinical nurse specialist, with patient and family coping, managing anxiety, and grieving; and a physical or occupational therapist, with extensive retraining for activities of daily living.

The nurse should ensure that the patient receives adequate information and assistance concerning:
• equipment use (such as the oxygen saturation monitor)
• adjustment to traumatic injury
• infection prevention measures (checking for fever, wound drainage)
• wound or incision care
• pain management
• medications and doses.

Toxic ingestion

Most cases of toxic ingestion reported to poison control centers and treated by health professionals involve overdoses of common prescription or over-the-counter medications. However, other commonly ingested substances that can cause toxicity include street drugs, chemicals in the home or workplace, plants, and foods. Toxicity usually results from ingestion, but other sources of exposure include inhalation, injection, and direct absorption through the skin and mucous membranes.

Clinical symptoms following an accidental or intentional toxic ingestion are influenced by several factors, including the amount of substance ingested, the patient's tolerance to the toxin, the number of toxins ingested, and the time between ingestion and treatment. When more than one toxic substance has been ingested, the effect may be synergistic or antagonistic.

Pathophysiology

Pathological changes produced by toxic ingestion often result from an exaggeration of the toxin's normal therapeutic and side effects. For example, depressed level of consciousness and hypoventilation typically occur after ingestion of sedatives and opiates, while hypotension and arrhythmias occur after ingestion of beta and calcium channel blockers. Some toxins, such as acetaminophen and ethylene glycol, have organ-specific toxic effects that require intensive medical and nursing interventions to prevent complications.

Acetaminophen

Acetaminophen, the active ingredient in many over-the-counter analgesics and antipyretics, is the most commonly reported pharmaceutical ingestion in both adults and children. The drug is rapidly absorbed and metabolized in the liver. Normally, a small amount of acetaminophen (less than 5%) is metabolized to a toxic intermediate metabolite, N-acetyl-para-benzoquinoneimine (NAPQI), which is further metabolized by gluta-thione to nontoxic products.

NAPQI is a powerful oxidizing agent that leads to cell death by bonding to cellular proteins. After an acute single toxic dose (7.5 g in an adult), the glutathi-one is used up and cannot regenerate fast enough to detoxify all of the intermediate metabolite. Conse-quently, the NAPQI builds up, causing liver damage. Evidence of liver damage may not be apparent until 24 to 36 hours after ingestion.

Alcohols

All alcohols, including ethanol, ethylene glycol, meth-anol, and isopropanol, are rapidly absorbed from the GI tract and metabolized by the liver enzyme alcohol de-hydrogenase. Isopropanol and methanol also are easily absorbed through the skin and mucous membranes and can result in toxicity.

Ethanol, the most common alcohol ingested, is a depressant that potentiates the effect of other drugs. Alcohol ingestions complicate treatment and care because they often interact with other medications the patient is receiving (see *Alcohol-drug interactions in trauma patients,* page 671).

Isopropanol, which is found in rubbing alcohol as well as in cleaning and deicing agents, is twice as intox-icating as ethanol. In addition to ingestion, it can be inhaled and absorbed through skin and mucous mem-branes. Isopropanol is metabolized to acetone in the liver by the enzyme alcohol dehydrogenase. Small amounts of isopropanol not metabolized initially by the liver may be excreted back into the GI tract by the salivary glands and then reabsorbed. Isopropanol tends to cause more gastric upset than ethanol, and high doses result in hypotension and hypothermia. Both ethanol and isopropanol can cause respiratory arrest at levels above 400 mg/dl.

Ethylene glycol and methanol are the most toxic alcohols. Ethylene glycol commonly is found in anti-freeze and cleaning solutions; methanol is found in

Alcohol-drug interactions in trauma patients

Many victims of trauma also have ingested alcohol. The following is a list of medications commonly administered to trauma patients that might interact with alcohol. This list also would apply to other intensive care unit patients admitted under the influence of alcohol who receive these medications.

Drug or Therapeutic Class	Interaction with Alcohol
Acetaminophen	Increased risk of liver toxicity
Aspirin	Potentiated disruption of gastric mucosa
Barbiturates	Enhanced CNS depression
Benzodiazepines	Enhanced disruption of psychomotor performance; increased CNS (including respiratory) depression. Benzodiazepines may cause hepatomegaly and hepatotoxicity, but incidence is low.
Beta blockers	Increased elimination and decreased drug effect
Cephalosporins	Flushing, tachycardia, nausea, vomiting
Cimetidine (Tagamet)	Increased alcohol absorption and increased blood alcohol level. These effects do not occur with ranitidine (Zantac).
Disulfiram (Antabuse)	Flushing, headache, chest pain, arrhythmias, cardiovascular collapse, nausea, vomiting
Fentanyl (Sublimaze)	Enhanced CNS depression
Insulin	Unpredictable and varied; often hypoglycemia
Opiates	Enhanced CNS depression
Phenothiazines	Enhanced CNS depression
Phenytoin (Dilantin)	Increased metabolism and increased clearance (particularly during alcohol withdrawal)
Procainamide (Pronestyl)	Increased elimination and decreased blood level
Warfarin (Coumadin)	Excessive anticoagulation

Adapted with permission from Sommers, M. (1994). "Alcohol and trauma: The critical link." *Critical Care Nurse* 14(2):82-92.

windshield washer fluid and solvents. Both are minimally toxic prior to metabolism but, in addition of their inebriating effects, have specific organ toxicity once metabolized. Both alcohols are metabolized in the liver, and blood levels above 20 mg/dl are considered toxic for both.

Metabolism of ethylene glycol produces glycolaldehyde, glycolic acid, glyoxylic acid, and oxalic acid. Symptoms result from the direct effects of these toxins and progress through three stages. Symptoms in stage I (first 12 hours) include altered mental status, seizures, and severe anion-gap metabolic acidosis. Cardiac toxicity occurs in stage II (12 to 36 hours). Stage III, renal failure, the hallmark of ethylene glycol toxicity, occurs at 36 to 48 hours.

Metabolism of methanol produces formaldehyde and formic acid. Folic acid is required for further metabolism to nontoxic products. Symptoms of methanol toxicity appear 12 to 24 hours after ingestion and result primarily from the effects of formic acid. Formic acid damages the optic nerve. Hemorrhages also have been found in a portion of the basal ganglia called the putamen. Symptoms include severe anion-gap metabolic acidosis caused by acid production, hypotension, visual changes that can progress to blindness, coma, and sudden respiratory arrest.

Cocaine

Cocaine blocks the reuptake of norepinephrine, epinephrine, and dopamine, causing excesses at the postsynaptic receptor sites. This leads to central and peripheral adrenergic stimulation and to a generalized vasoconstriction that affects multiple organs. These effects may include hypertension, hyperthermia, tachycardia, excited delirium, and seizures. Hyperthermia can cause rhabdomyolysis and later renal failure. Direct effects on the heart include increased myocardial oxygen consumption, coronary artery spasm, ischemia, myocardial infarction, depressed myocardial contractility, and acute congestive heart failure, sudden death from arrhythmias, and dilated cardiomyopathy. Recent studies also have shown that cocaine increases platelet aggregation and thrombus formation. I.V. drug users also are at risk for endocarditis.

Cyclic antidepressants

Cyclic antidepressants are responsible for almost half of all overdose-related adult admissions to intensive care units and are the leading cause of overdose-related deaths in emergency departments. Cyclic drugs include the older tricyclics, such as amitriptyline and nortriptyline, and such newer agents as the tetracyclic maprotiline hydrochloride (Ludiomil). These drugs are rapidly absorbed from the GI tract, although absorption may be delayed in large overdoses because of anticholinergic side effects. They are metabolized in the liver.

In an overdose, the enzymes responsible for metabolism become saturated and some of the drug and its metabolites are secreted into the bile and gastric fluid and are later reabsorbed. Toxicity results from central and peripheral blockage of norepinephrine reuptake, anticholinergic effects, and quinidine-like effects on the heart. Central nervous system (CNS) effects may include initial agitation followed rapidly by lethargy, coma, and seizures. Anticholinergic effects include tachycardia, mydriasis, dry and flushed skin, hypoactive bowel sounds, and urine retention. Cardiovascular effects include hypotension, arrhythmias, and quinidine-like changes on the ECG with widening of the QRS complex.

Organophosphates and carbamates

Organophosphates and carbamates commonly are found in pesticides and account for 80% of pesticide-related hospital admissions. They are highly lipid-soluble and easily absorbed through skin and mucous membranes. The primary mechanism of toxicity is cholinesterase inhibition. This leads to excess acetylcholine at muscarinic, nicotinic, and CNS receptors. The effects of excessive acetylcholine include excessive salivation and lacrimation, muscle fasciculations and weakness, constricted pupils, decreased level of consciousness, and seizures. Bradycardia usually is present, but tachycardia also has been reported.

Clinical assessment

The clinical assessment of a patient with toxic ingestion must include simultaneous history, assessment of ABCs (airway, breathing, and circulation), and initiation of life support as indicated by physical assessment. Lifesaving initial management may begin before an adequate history is available.

History

An adequate history often is difficult to obtain in the case of toxic ingestion. If the patient is brought to the hospital with a depressed level of consciousness, it may be difficult or impossible to obtain the history from the patient. In such cases, the nurse should try to obtain as much information as possible from others concerning:
• substances ingested and route of exposure
• amount ingested and time since ingestion
• therapy received in the prehospital setting, such as naloxone, ipecac, or activated charcoal, and the results of therapy
• whether ingestion was intentional
• history of alcohol or illicit drug use
• medical conditions that might complicate therapy.

If unidentified tablets or capsules are brought with the patient, the nurse should examine them for imprinted letters and numbers and consult a reference, such as Identadex or Poisindex. The nurse also can contact the regional poison control center, which can provide advice about managing the patient. If the patient has been exposed to toxic substances in the workplace, the nurse should contact the employer's safety officer to obtain information about toxic effects from the material safety data sheet. Another source of information is Chemtrec, a 24-hour hazardous materials hotline (1-800-424-9300).

Physical findings

Assessment begins with the ABCs:

• Look for signs and symptoms specific to the toxin ingested and for signs and symptoms that might help identify an unknown toxin.

• Assess the patient's level of consciousness, pupil size, respirations, and cardiac rate and rhythm.

• Ask about chest pain, especially with cocaine ingestion.

• Assess blood pressure and temperature.

• Note any unusual odors, increased salivation, or flushing of the skin.

• Note the patient's behavior (agitation or hallucinations). Keep in mind that an alert patient, especially one who has ingested a tricyclic antidepressant, may deteriorate rapidly (see *Physical findings associated with common toxins,* pages 676 and 677).

Diagnosis

A diagnosis of toxic ingestion or exposure strongly depends on the history and physical assessment. Toxicological screens are not readily available in all hospitals and, except for specific agents, do not change therapy. (See *Confirming toxic ingestion,* page 678, for specific tests).

Treatment and care

The primary goals of treatment in the care of the patient with a toxic ingestion are to provide life support, administer the appropriate antidote (if available), prevent absorption of the toxin, enhance removal of the absorbed drug, prevent metabolism of the toxin, and prevent complications.

Life-support measures

All patients who present with toxic ingestion should be assumed to have the potential for rapid decompensation until this has been ruled out. Life-support may include the use of oxygen, intubation, mechanical ventilation,

Physical findings associated with common toxins

When a toxin is unknown, signs and symptoms or odors may provide valuable clues to the toxin's identity.

Physical Findings	Common Toxins
CNS depression	Alcohols, carbamates, cyanide, carbon monoxide, opiates, organophosphates, sedatives, tranquilizers, phencyclidine, phenothiazines, phenytoin, salicylates, cyclic antidepressants
Pupil dilation	Amphetamines, cocaine, LSD, anticholinergics, cyclic antidepressants
Pupil constriction	Barbiturates, benzodiazepines, ethanol, isopropanol, opiates (except meperidine), carbamate, organophosphates, PCP, phenothiazines, prazosin
Hallucination	Hallucinogenic amphetamines, PCP, LSD, jimson weed
Bradycardia	Quinidine, beta blockers, calcium channel blockers, carbamates, clonidine, digoxin, organophosphates
Tachycardia	Sympathomimetics (such as beta agonists), amphetamines, cocaine, nicotine, caffeine, theophylline, anticholinergics, cyclic antidepressants
Kussmaul respirations	Salicylates
Hypotension	Vasodilators, cyclic antidepressants, calcium channel blockers, organophosphates
Hypertension	Sympathomimetics, cocaine
Hypothermia	Alcohols, narcotics, phenothiazines, sedatives
Hyperthermia	Amphetamines, anticholinergics, antihistamines, cocaine, phencyclidine, cyclic antidepressants
Seizures	Alcohol, amphetamines, antihistamines, cocaine, heavy metals, lithium, lindane, meperidine (metabolites), mushrooms (Gyromitra), nicotine, organophosphates, phencyclidine, phenothiazines, strychnine, salicylates, theophylline, cyclic antidepressants

Physical Findings	Common Toxins
Physical findings associated with common toxins *(continued)*	
Breath odors	
• Bitter almond	• Cyanide
• Formalin	• Methanol
• Garlic	• Arsenic, organophosphates, phosphorus, selenium, thallium
• Pine fresh	• Pine oil
• Sweet/fruity	• Acetone, ethanol, isopropanol, nail polish remover
• Wintergreen	• Methyl salicylate
• Moth balls	• Camphor, naphthalene, parachlorobenzene

Adapted with permission from Mandl, K., and Lovejoy, F. (1994). "Signs and symptoms associated with common toxins." *Pediatrics in Review* 15(4):151-156.

or I.V. drugs. Specific nursing measures are detailed below:
• Anticipate the need for oxygen, suction, intubation, and mechanical ventilation.
• Anticipate the development of hypertension or hypotension, cardiac arrhythmias, and seizures.
• Place on cardiac monitor; obtain an ECG reading on any patient who has taken a drug that produces known cardiac or acid-base effects.
• Obtain I.V. access; start two large-bore lines with normal saline solution if hypotension is present or anticipated and use a glucose-containing solution, such as dextrose 5% in water (D_5W) if hypoglycemia is anticipated as complication (for example, ethylene glycol, methanol, cocaine, and insulin overdose). Anticipate the need to give a bolus dose of $D_{50}W$ or $D_{10}W$ if hypoglycemia is present.
• Obtain a blood specimen for laboratory studies.
• Prepare to administer vasopressors for severe cyclic drug overdose or vasodilators for cocaine overdose, to increase or decrease blood pressure as appropriate.
• Prepare to assist with cardiac pacing for heart block.
• Administer antiarrhythmic agents for arrhythmias. Beta blockers may be administered to slow the heart rate in cocaine overdoses.

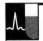

DIAGNOSTIC TESTS
Confirming toxic ingestion

The following diagnostic laboratory and imaging studies may be performed for patients who are believed to have ingested or to have been otherwise exposed to toxic substances.

Glucose test
Used in altered level of consciousness (LOC) and suspected alcohol or salicylate toxicity to rule out hypoglycemia.

Pulse oximetry
Used in altered LOC and respiratory depression to rule out hypoxia; not accurate for testing carbon monoxide toxicity and methemoglobinemia.

Arterial blood gas studies
Used in altered LOC and suspected methanol, paraldehyde, iron, isoniazid, ethylene glycol, salicylate toxicity to rule out hypoxia, hypercapnia, and metabolic acidosis.

ECG
Used in suspected toxicity of cocaine, cyclic antidepressants, and other drugs having cardiovascular effects. Ischemia, arrhythmias, and widened QRS complex are common in cyclic antidepressant toxicity.

Drug screen
Qualitatively used to identify toxin and quantitatively to determine the amount of toxin ingested.

Complete blood count
Ethylene glycol toxicity produces leukocytosis; iron toxicity, potential for bleeding.

Prothrombin time, partial thromboplastin time
Hemopoietic drugs (warfarin, liver toxins) produce potential for bleeding.

Electrolyte levels
High anion gap is associated with methanol, ethylene glycol, paraldehyde, iron, isoniazid, and salicylate toxicity. A low serum ion gap is associated with lithium or bromide toxicity. Serum osmolar gap is associated with acetonitrile, ethanol, ethylene glycol, isopropanol, and methanol toxicity. Hyperkalemia is found with ethylene glycol and methanol toxicity; hypokalemia, with use of loop diuretics and salicylate poisoning. Hypocalcemia is found with ethylene glycol, hydrofluoric acid, and diuretic use.

Hepatic enzyme studies
Elevated levels are produced by Amanita phalloides mushrooms, acetaminophen, chloroform, and other liver toxins.

Urinalysis
Used to test for renal toxins. Ethylene glycol produces calcium oxalate crystals and hematuria; methanol produces a formalin odor; and isopropanol produces ketonuria.

X-rays
Chest X-rays are taken to reveal aspiration caused by a foreign body or gastric contents and to show pulmonary effects of poison. Abdominal X-rays reveal radiopaque toxins, such as heavy metals (iron, lead, mercury), calcium, chloral hydrate, enteric-coated aspirin, and phenothiazines. Also used to identify gastric and intestinal perforation from toxic substances.

Administer antidote

Antidotes are given to halt or reverse the effects of various drugs; however, very few toxins have specific antidotes (see *Common toxins and antidotes,* page 680 and 681). Specific nursing interventions for administering an antidote include the following:

• Anticipate and prepare for potential patient response and complications (for example, seizures or sudden consciousness, agitation, and violence in a previously unconscious patient) prior to administering antidote.

• Administer antidote by the recommended route, dose, and rate. When administering naloxone and flumazenil, watch for signs of withdrawal. Flumazenil may precipitate seizures especially in patients who have ingested cyclic antidepressants or have been on long-term sedation with benzodiazepines.

• Monitor for return of symptoms. Drug may last longer than dose of antidote.

• Monitor for side effects of antidote (for example, alcohol may cause hypoglycemia).

Measures to prevent drug absorption

Various treatments may be used to prevent drugs from being absorbed by the patient's system, including administration of ipecac, gastric lavage, activated charcoal, catharsis, and bowel irrigation. Ipecac, which is used to induce vomiting, should be used only in conscious patients with recent ingestions (usually under 1 hour, although it may be effective up to several hours if an anticholinergic is ingested), those with an intact gag reflex, and those without a potential for rapid change in level of consciousness. Ipecac is contraindicated in patients with caustic ingestion and in those who have ingested petroleum distillates because of the risk of aspiration. Use also is cautioned in digoxin ingestion because of the potential for vagal stimulation and heart block. Appropriate nursing interventions include:

• Place the patient in high-Fowler's position.

• Check the gag reflex prior to administering ipecac.

(Text continues on page 682.)

Common toxins and antidotes

Below is a list of common toxins and their antidotes.

Toxin	Antidote
Acetaminophen	N-acetylcysteine 140 mg/kg followed by 70 mg/kg q 4^0 x 17 doses. Oral only in U.S.; I.V., in Canada and Europe. Enhances conversion of toxic metabolites to nontoxic metabolites.
Ethylene glycol and methanol	Ethanol loading dose 600 to 800 mg/kg oral or I.V. (I.V. route preferred). If oral route, dilute to 50% solution to prevent gastritis. Follow with maintenance dose of 100 to 130 mg/kg/hour to maintain blood level at 100 mg/dl to maintain saturation of alcohol dehydrogenase sites and block metabolism (4-methylpyrazole shown to be effective in experiments).
Co-factors • Ethylene glycol • Methanol	• Thiamine 100 mg I.M. daily and pyridoxine 50 mg I.V. every 6 hours (speeds conversion to nontoxic metabolites). • Folate 1 mg/kg I.V. every 4 hours.
Anticholinergics except cyclic antidepressants	Severe cases only physostigmine (Antilirium) 1 mg slow I.V. push; infusion 2 mg/hour.
Beta blockers	Glucagon 3.5 to 5 mg followed by infusion 1 to 5 mg/hour.
Benzodiazepines	Flumazenil (Romazicon) given I.V. Dose is individualized and titrated to patient effect. Initial dose 0.2 mg over 30 seconds followed by 0.3 mg over next 30 seconds if no response. May be repeated 0.5 mg/minutes over 30-second intervals up to 3 to 5 mg total.
Calcium channel blockers (only if digoxin not co-ingested)	Calcium 10 ml of 10% solution, followed by infusion 20 to 50 mg/hour. Glucagon as for beta blocker.
Ciguatera fish poisoning	Mannitol 1 gm/kg over 30 to 45 minutes.

Common toxins and antidotes *(continued)*

Toxin	Antidote
Cyanide	Lilly Cyanide Kit contains amyl nitrite inhaler and sodium nitrite, used to create methemoglobin, which attracts cyanide away from the respiratory enzyme cytochrome oxidase and sodium thiosulfate used to form nontoxic thiocyanate.
Cyclic antidepressants	Sodium bicarbonate bolus and infusion to maintain pH at 7.5; reverses QRS prolongation and hypotension.
Digoxin, oleander, foxglove	Digoxin immune fab (Digibind); dose based on symptoms and post-distribution serum levels. One vial binds 0.6 mg of digoxin.
Hydrofluoric acid	Calcium gluconate to bind and neutralize free fluoride ion. Administer as topical antidote gel liberally to burns. Calcium gluconate also may be injected intradermally. Administer 10% calcium gluconate slow I.V. push as needed for hypocalcemia (5 to 10 ml). Dose is repeated based on patient response. I.V. magnesium sulfate also may be ordered because it also binds fluoride ion.
Iron	Deferoxamine mesylate 15 mg/kg/hour infusion. Note: Prochlorperazine (Compazine) contraindicated.
Lead	EDTA 50 to 75 mg/day I.V. or I.M. Dimercaprol (BAL) 4 mg/kg q 4^0 I.M. Succimer (Chemet) P.O.
Methemoglobinemia	Methylene blue 1 to 2 mg/kg slow I.V. push.
Opiates (including propoxyphene and dextromethorphan)	Naloxone (Narcan) 2 to 10 mg I.V. repeated as necessary based on patient response; long-acting opiates may require continuous infusion.
Organophosphates	Atropine until mucous membranes become dry (reverses cholinergic effects) pralidoxime 1 g over 45 to 60 minutes (reactivates acetylcholinesterase by breaking its bond with poison, more effective earlier given).
Psychostimulants (cocaine)	Benzodiazepines, labetalol, nitroprusside (to slow heart rate and reverse vasoconstriction).
Salicylates	Alkalinize urine to pH 7.5. Enhances excretion. Isotonic solution given by adding 3 ampules (44 mEq/ampule) to 1 liter D_5W. Monitor for hypokalemia.

• Administer 30 ml of ipecac with 16 ounces of warm water; if vomiting does not occur within 30 minutes, repeat the dose once; if vomiting still does not occur, institute gastric lavage, closely monitoring the patient for decreasing level of consciousness or depressed gag reflex.

Gastric lavage is used in patients with a depressed or potentially depressed level of consciousness because of the increased risk for aspiration of vomitus. Specific nursing measures for gastric lavage are detailed below:

• Initiate necessary airway measures, including intubation with a cuffed endotracheal tube if the patient does not have an intact gag reflex. Have suction available.

• Place the patient in a left-lateral, slightly Trendelenburg position.

• Insert a large-bore (36-F to 40-F) Ewald tube.

• Initiate lavage using tap water by instilling no more than 200 to 300 ml of water at a time. The amount instilled should equal the amount removed. If amounts are unequal, recheck placement of the tube and the patient's position.

• Continue the lavage until at least 5 liters of water have been exchanged and return is clear.

Activated charcoal, which is administered to adsorb the remaining toxin, binds many substances, but does not adsorb alcohols, caustic substances, or small ionic compounds, such as lithium. If a drug is well adsorbed by charcoal, emesis or lavage may be omitted. Nursing interventions for activated charcoal include:

• Administer 1 to 1.5 gm/kg orally only to patients with an intact gag reflex to prevent aspiration. Repeat at a dose of 0.5 to 1 gm/kg every 2 to 6 hours if the patient has ingested sustained-release formulations or drugs that are secreted back into the gut.

• Administer repeat doses only if bowel sounds are present. Constipation and GI obstruction have been reported after multiple doses.

A cathartic may be administered to enhance movement of activated charcoal through the gut. Sorbitol often is added to charcoal. However, if repeated doses of charcoal are administered, only the first dose should contain sorbitol. Repeated doses of sorbitol have resulted in serious electrolyte disturbances.

Prevention of metabolism of absorbed drug
Occasionally, one or more of a drug's metabolites, not the unmetabolized drug, are toxic. Examples include acetaminophen, ethylene glycol, and methanol. In this event, if tests indicate that toxic levels of the drug have been absorbed, then an antidote is given to prevent metabolism of the drug. Drugs also may be given to enhance further metabolism of any toxic metabolites formed to nontoxic compounds. For example, folic acid is necessary for further metabolism of formic acid to nontoxic carbon dioxide and water.

Enhanced removal of absorbed drug
Methods used to enhance removal of absorbed toxins vary according to the toxin. Occasionally, alkalinization (using salicylates) or acidification of the urine is used. Diuretics may be used, especially with drugs that are known to cause renal failure, such as ethylene glycol. In severe toxicity, dialysis is used to remove water-soluble drugs (such as theophylline) that do not bind tightly to plasma proteins and tissues and to correct the severe acid-base disturbances that might occur such as with ethylene glycol, methanol, or salicylate toxicity. Other extracorporeal techniques, such as hemoperfusion with charcoal and exchange transfusion, also are available; their use varies depending on availability and efficacy in removing a particular toxin. Hemoperfusion with charcoal may cause thrombocytopenia.

Nursing measures include those listed below:
• Administer medications to enhance excretion as appropriate.
• Monitor urine output and fluid and electrolyte status.
• Monitor acid base status.
• Facilitate dialysis or hemoperfusion as appropriate.

Prevention of complications

Ongoing assessment is necessary to prevent complications specific to the toxin ingested. For example seizures, hyperthermia, and cardiac complications are common in cocaine ingestions. I.V. drug abusers may develop endocarditis. The following nursing interventions should be incorporated into the plan of care:

• Assess level of consciousness and pupil size.
• Assess respiratory status for signs of pulmonary edema or respiratory failure.
• Monitor the patient's heart rate, pulses, and ECG for changes indicative of arrhythmias.
• Monitor for seizures (if toxin causes seizures).
• Note any blood pressure changes.
• Assess for temperature changes (may be related to toxin or infection).
• Assess electrolyte levels and urine output.
• Monitor patient's response to therapies.

Prognosis

Most cases of toxic ingestion are successfully treated in the emergency department. However, those with significant toxic ingestion or meeting the following criteria may require admission to the critical care unit:

• patients who have ingested drugs with potential cardiac effects (such as cyclic antidepressants, cocaine, ethylene glycol, and methanol)
• patients with altered mental status
• patients with respiratory depression
• patients with significant electrolyte disturbances
• patients with toxic serum levels.

Discharge planning

All intentional toxic ingestions require a psychiatric referral as soon as the patient is stable. Accidental ingestions should be further investigated to determine why the ingestion occurred. Appropriate referrals for home health care, outpatient treatment, rehabilitation, or workplace evaluation may be provided at this time.

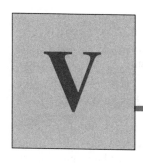

Valvular heart disease

Valvular heart disease, an acquired or congenital condition that commonly strikes the aortic and mitral valves, can result from various causes, including valvular degeneration and acute or chronic obstruction caused by an infection or underlying cardiac disease. Because the most commonly diseased valves are the aortic and mitral valves (tricuspid and pulmonic valvular disease rarely occurs), the following discussion focuses on acquired aortic and mitral valvular disease.

Pathophysiology

The most common cause of all acquired valvular disease is rheumatic fever, which affects the mitral valve in about 40% of all treated cases and the aortic valve in about 25% of cases. Aortic and mitral valvular diseases are characterized primarily by their structural defects and the degree of related stenosis or insufficiency.

Aortic stenosis

Aortic stenosis (AS) is caused by calcification of the cusp fibrosa that eventually results in a nodular deposition on the surface of the valve, within the leaflets, and into the sinuses of Valsalva, impairing forward blood flow through the aortic valve during systole. When the aortic orifice is reduced by 50% or more of normal size (normal aortic valve area is 2 cm^2), left ventricular hypertrophy (LVH) develops. This compensatory mechanism generates enough pressure to force the blood through the narrowed valve, thus creating a pressure gradient between the hypertrophied ventricle and the aorta.

When severe LVH occurs, the left atrium becomes hypertrophied, allowing for ejection into the stiffened ventricle. Left atrial hypertrophy is a late sign of severe aortic stenosis and precedes congestive heart failure. Because AS stenosis causes diastolic dysfunction, stroke volume is compromised, resulting in poor cardiac output and therefore poor peripheral perfusion. Cardiac output is fixed because of the valve obstruction, leading to an inadequate coronary blood supply. When the myocardial oxygen demand increases, such as with exertion, the patient with AS and normal coronary arteries may experience angina.

Aortic insufficiency

Insufficient blood flow through the aorta can result from aortic root dilation (as with aneurysms, Marfan's syndrome, and syphilis) or lesions of the valve leaflets (associated with rheumatic, infectious, or congenital conditions). Any abnormality of aortic valve closure results in regurgitation of blood into the ventricle from the aorta during diastole.

With chronic aortic insufficiency (AI), the left ventricle compensates for the abnormally high diastolic volume by becoming dilated and hypertrophied. The left ventricular (LV) dilation also produces a reservoir for a tremendous amount of regurgitant blood from the aorta and results in elevated systemic systolic pressure (due to the high stroke volume) and decreased systemic diastolic pressure (due to the loss of volume back into the ventricle).

Chronic AI generally is well tolerated for many years because of compensatory mechanisms. However, with acute AI, there is no time for compensatory mechanisms to evolve. Acute AI produces a tremendous increase in LV end-diastolic pressure, which is transmitted to the atrium and pulmonary vasculature. Life-threatening pulmonary edema rapidly results and constitutes a surgical emergency.

Mitral stenosis

Mitral stenosis (MS), a narrowing of the cross-sectional valve area that impedes blood flow from the left atrium into the left ventricle, typically is caused by rheumatic heart disease. It produces the following pathological characteristics:
• short, thick chordae tendineae
• valve leaflet calcification
• thick valve leaflets
• fusion of the valve commissures.

When the mitral cross-sectional area is reduced to cm^2 (normal size is 4 to 6 cm^2), the pressure gradient between the atrium and ventricle becomes high enough to produce left atrial hypertrophy. The left atrial hypertrophy in turn leads to disarray of the conductive tissue through the atrium, which produces atrial fibrillation, and passive pulmonary hypertension, a direct result of the backward pressure transmission. Pulmonary hypertension produces constriction, medial hypertrophy, and intimal fibrosis of the pulmonary arterioles. Although such hypertension relieves the severe pulmonary congestion, it also reduces the available surface area for gas exchange and generates an increase in right heart pressures.

Mitral insufficiency

Insufficient blood flow through the mitrium can result from several causes, including:
• ischemic heart disease with papillary muscle dysfunction (produces acute mitral insufficiency)
• mitral valve prolapse and annular calcification
• endocarditis or rheumatic heart disease
• cardiomyopathy (produces permanent structural myocardial dilatation and damage)

• passive dilatation resulting from left ventricular dilatation (such as occurs with aortic valve disease).

Mitral insufficiency causes regurgitation of blood into the atrium during systole, which reduces stroke volume. Preload (left ventricular diastolic volume) is increased, producing left ventricular dilatation. In cases of chronic insufficiency, two compensatory mechanisms are called into play: left atrial dilatation, which reduces the backward pressure transmission, and left ventricular dilatation, which accommodates the increased preload and activates the Frank-Starling mechanism (see the entry on "Congestive Heart Failure"). Acute mitral insufficiency, however, does not allow for compensatory changes and produces an abrupt increase in left atrial and pulmonary pressures. Consequently, life-threatening pulmonary edema occurs, necessitating emergency surgical replacement.

Clinical assessment

The clinical examination may be the most important tool in the diagnosis of valvular disorders. Differentiating between murmurs and symptoms can lead to the precise diagnosis and allow for streamlined diagnostic testing and accurate evaluation of patient response to treatment.

History

Certain components of the patient history are very useful in determining the medical diagnosis of valvular dysfunction. Inquiries should be made regarding:
• history of acute rheumatic fever or intravenous drug abuse
• presence of dyspnea and its relation to activity
• presence of chest pain, palpitations, or syncope
• medication history
• factors that precipitate or alleviate symptoms
• duration of symptoms.

Physical findings

The physical findings of valvular heart disease vary according to the affected valve and whether it is a stenotic lesion or a regurgitant valve (see *Clinical manifestations in valvular heart disease,* pages 690 and 691, for a breakdown of signs and symptoms and physical findings).

Audible heart sounds probably are the most pertinent physical finding in valvular heart disease (see *Heart sounds in valvular heart disease,* page 692). Murmurs are caused by turbulence resulting from blood flowing:

- in an abnormal direction
- through a narrowed orifice
- through a diseased leaflet that does not open and close normally.

Diagnosis

The diagnosis of valvular heart disease is confirmed by a comprehensive physical examination combined with echocardiographic data (see *Diagnosing valvular heart disease,* page 693). Although a chest X-ray and ECG provide supporting data, echocardiography provides more definitive findings because valvular disease often is multivalvular and clinical signs can either mask or mimic findings associated with any single valvular lesion. Either transthoracic or transesophageal echocardiography can be performed. Transesophageal echocardiography provides a more discrete view of the cardiac valves and can be useful when diagnosis is difficult.

Treatment and care

Treatment for valvular heart disease depends on the severity of the lesion, the state of compensation for the lesion, and the patient's hemodynamic stability and functional status. Generally, treatment is aimed at:

- preventing and alleviating congestive heart failure
- relieving angina and preventing syncope
- halting progression of the disease
- improving dyspneic symptoms

Clinical manifestations in valvular heart disease

The signs and symptoms and physical findings of the major types of valvular heart disease are included below.

Valvular Lesion	Signs and Symptoms	Physical Findings
Aortic stenosis	• Exertional angina • Syncope • Fatigue • Cough • Progressive dyspnea on exertion • Orthopnea • Palpitations • Murmur (in some cases, this is the only physical sign)	• Forceful, sustained apical impulse with displacement downward and to the left • Systolic thrill • Diminished carotid pulse • Prominent A wave on jugular venous pulse or LA waveform • Widened pulse pressure with normal diastolic pressure (in compensated aortic stenosis) • Narrow pulse pressure (in decompensated aortic stenosis)
Aortic insufficiency	• Left-sided heart failure • Angina • Dyspnea at rest • Fatigue • Exertional syncope • Palpitations	• Low diastolic blood pressure • Parasternal lift (visual heave of the chest when pulmonary hypertension is present) • Downward, leftward displacement of apical impulse • Forceful apical impulse • de Musset's sign (nodding head) • Increase in carotid arterial pulse (rises to a single, rapidly collapsing peak [water-hammer pulse] in acute cases) • Widened pulse pressure (in chronic cases)
Mitral stenosis	• Dyspnea • Orthopnea • Paroxysmal nocturnal dyspnea • Pulmonary edema • Hemoptysis • Left-sided heart failure • Hoarseness • Dysphagia	• Signs of congestive heart failure • Atrial fibrillation • Ruddy cheeks (mitral facies)
Mitral insufficiency	• Fatigue • Weakness • Left-sided heart failure	• Atrial fibrillation • Vigorous, sustained apical impulse

Clinical manifestations in valvular heart disease *(continued)*		
Valvular Lesion	**Signs and Symptoms**	**Physical Findings**
Mitral insuffi-ciency *(continued)*	• Dyspnea • Orthopnea • Palpitations	• Downward, leftward displace-ment of the apical impulse • Severe, rapid onset pulmo-nary edema and backward heart failure (in acute cases) • Brisk upstroke followed by a collapsing quality of the carotid pulse • Signs of low forward cardiac output (in chronic cases)

• preventing thromboembolic sequelae
• preventing infectious complications
• prolonging the life span of the patient.

Surgical valve replacement

In many cases, surgical replacement is recommended for patients with valvular heart disease. The prosthetic heart valves currently in use include the mechanical valve, the biological valve, and the human homograft (see *Properties of artificial heart valves,* pages 694 and 695, for characteristics and related nursing considerations).

Nursing considerations for the patient with a prosthetic heart valve include the following:
• Auscultate the valve to listen a prosthetic valve click (a crisp clicking sound that indicates proper closure and the likelihood that no thrombus is present).
• Provide anticoagulation therapy, as prescribed.

Anticoagulation therapy

Anticoagulation is critical in patients with prosthetic heart valves, with the exception of those with aortic homografts. After initial hemostasis is achieved postoperatively, anticoagulation therapy begins with low molecular weight dextran or a heparin infusion. Once stable, the patient is placed on oral warfarin. When the

ASSESSMENT TIP
Heart sounds in valvular heart disease

Auscultating heart murmurs and matching the sound with the specific disorder is a critical part of diagnosing and managing a patient with valvular heart disease. Below is a list of characteristic murmurs and other heart sounds associated with the most common valvular diseases.

Aortic stenosis
• Harsh, systolic, crescendo-decrescendo murmur at the second intercostal space, right sternal border
• Paradoxically split S_2

Aortic insufficiency
• Chronic: High-pitched, blowing diastolic decrescendo murmur at the third or fourth intercostal space, right sternal border
• Acute: Soft murmur, S_3

Mitral stenosis
• Low-pitched, rumbling diastolic murmur at the apex
• Opening snap

Mitral insufficiency
• Chronic: High-pitched, blowing systolic murmur at the apex
• Acute: High-pitched, blowing systolic murmur at the apex with an S_4 and widely split S_2

prothrombin time (PT) has reached therapeutic levels (a PT of 16 to 22 seconds or an international ratio [INR] of 2.5 to 4.0), the low-molecular-weight dextran or heparin can be discontinued.

Patients with biological (porcine or bovine) heart valves usually are on warfarin for 6 weeks to 3 months, only long enough for epithelial tissue to cover the rough edges left by the sutures that hold the valve in place. Patients with mechanical valves or those in chronic atrial fibrillation require lifelong anticoagulation.

Cardiac rehabilitation
Inpatient cardiac rehabilitation is recommended during hospitalization for valve replacement surgery. The cardiac rehabilitation therapist, physical therapist, and nurse should provide instructions regarding the patient's specific rehabilitation prescription. Appropriate nursing interventions include the following:
• Ensure that the patient is free of dyspnea when preforming activities of daily living.
• Ensure that the patient maintains acceptable pulse rate and rhythm and blood pressure during exercise periods.

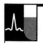

DIAGNOSTIC TESTS

Diagnosing valvular heart disease

Valvular heart disease is diagnosed primarily by echocardiogram in combination with the physical examination. The ECG and chest X-ray provide supplemental information about the severity of the valvular disorder. The normal echocardiogram shows no evidence of valvular dysfunction or abnormalities in the wall thickness.

Disorder	Electrocardiogram	Chest X-ray	Echocardiogram
Aortic stenosis	• Left ventricular hypertrophy	• Left ventricular hypertrophy • Left ventricular enlargement	• Thickened left ventricular wall • High transvalvular gradient • Decreased cross-sectional area
Aortic insufficiency	• Left ventricular hypertrophy	• Enlarged left ventricular silhouette (chronic) • Pulmonary vascular congestion (acute)	• Quantification of the degree of regurgitation • Identification of the structural abnormality
Mitral stenosis	• Atrial fibrillation • Left atria enlargement • Right ventricular hypertrophy (if pulmonary hypertension is present)	• Left atrial enlargement • Pulmonary vascular redistribution • Kerley B lines • Interstitial edema • Prominent pulmonary arteries • Calcification of the mitral valve	• Thickened mitral leaflets • Abnormal fusion of the commissures with restricted separation during diastole • Left atrial enlargement • Possible atrial thrombus • Decreased mitral valve cross-sectional area • High velocity across valve
Mitral insufficiency	• Left ventricular hypertrophy • Atrial fibrillation	• Left atrial enlargement • Left ventricular enlargement • Possible calcification of the mitral annulus	• Identification of the structural abnormality • Vigorous left ventricular contractility • Left ventricular enlargement • Quantification of the degree of regurgitation

Properties of artificial heart valves

Artificial heart valves may be biological (either porcine or bovine), mechanical (usually made of titanium or stainless steel), or human homograft (the newest type). Before implantation, the surgeon must consider certain characteristics of the device, including the hemodynamics produced by the valve, especially the degree of transvalvular gradient (the pressure difference between the chamber above and below the implanted valve). A gradient of zero is considered optimal; the highest gradients are seen with biological valves, the lowest with human homograft valves. Other valve characteristics to consider include the valve's potential for producing thrombi, the durability of the valve, the hemolytic potential of the valve, and the ease of implantation.

Type	Characteristics	Nursing Considerations
Biologic • Porcine • Bovine	• Degeneration and calcification increases after 10 years • Low hemolytic potential; greatest in the aortic position • Porcine type has a limited orifice area and produces restricted flow; results in transvalvular gradients; this type also is associated with low thrombogenicity • Bovine type offers superior hemodynamics over porcine • Implantation of device is similar to that of mechanical type with metal sewing ring attached for ease of implant	• This type requires only short-term anticoagulation, 2 to 3 months of warfarin therapy (warfarin is administered only until epithelial tissue forms over the sutures in the sewing ring). Patients who cannot receive warfarin because of contraindications can receive only 1 tablet of aspirin per day. • Following the initial anticoagulation period, the patient should take 1 aspirin tablet per day. • Biological valves are ideal for older patients whose life expectancy is not longer than that of the valve.
Mechanical • Caged ball • Tilting disk • Bileaflet	• Very durable; should last for life • Hemolytic potential is lowest with bileaflet valve in aortic position • High thrombogenicity; requires lifelong anticoagulation • Caged-ball type is large and obstructs blood flow through the valve and outflow tract • Tilting disc type has minimal obstruction to flow in the open position	• This type is ideal for a young patient because the valve does not degenerate. • Valve is suitable only for patients who can tolerate lifelong anticoagulation. • Assessment of the patient should include auscultation of the heart for the prosthetic valve click.

Properties of artificial heart valves *(continued)*

Type	Characteristics	Nursing Considerations
Mechanical *(continued)*	• Bileaflet type has a large, unobstructed orifice area and unobstructed laminar flow • Implantation is similar to biological valve because of the metal sewing ring	
Homograft (human cadaver valve)	• Durability is uncertain; 10 to 12 years (data pending) • Low hemolytic potential • Low thrombogenicity; no anticoagulation required • Excellent hemodynamics; minimal to zero transvalvular gradient • Difficult to implant because valve is not mounted on sewing ring; only suitable for use in aortic position	• This is the ideal valve for most patients; biggest problem is lack of availability because of a deficiency of donors. • No anticoagulation is required at any time postoperatively. • No immunosuppressants are required because valve tissue is inert and non-immunogenic.

• Assist the patient to gradually increase activity while preventing dyspnea and fatigue.
• Teach the patient how to monitor pulse.
• Instruct the patient to monitor respiratory symptoms and to stop exercising when symptoms reach critical levels.

Prognosis

Prognosis for valvular heart disease varies greatly with the specific lesion. The median survival for patients with aortic stenosis varies with the specific symptoms. Over 75% of symptomatic patients with aortic stenosis who undergo valve replacement have a 10-year survival.

Surgical replacement also dramatically improves the long-term survival in symptomatic patients with aortic insufficiency. Patients with severe or moderately severe chronic aortic insufficiency who do not undergo surgery have the following survival rates:

- 75% survival at 5 years
- 50% survival at 10 years
- death within 4 years after onset of angina
- death within 2 years after onset of heart failure.

Patients with mitral stenosis have a poor survival rate without surgery, about 85% of patients who present with moderate symptoms die within 10 years after initial diagnosis. Those with mitral insufficiency typically have a slow progression of disease; consequently, about 70% survive 15 years without surgery. With mitral valve replacement, about 80% survive over 10 years.

Discharge planning

Discharge planning should include extensive patient teaching about warfarin therapy, including information about:
- dosage instructions, including the need to contact the physician and have a PT taken when a dose is missed
- which foods and drinks can affect the PT; for example, vitamin K-containing foods (green, leafy vegetables) can decrease the PT, and alcohol can increase the PT
- the importance of regularly monitoring the PT
- the need to keep a diary of warfarin levels and doses taken corresponding to the PT
- the possibility of birth defects with warfarin; women receiving warfarin should discontinue therapy during pregnancy and should receive heparin injections through delivery
- warfarin antidotes (parenteral vitamin K is the antidote for warfarin).

Other important instructions for patients with valvular heart disease include:
- education regarding endocarditis prophylaxis; procedures that require prophylactic therapy include dental procedures, invasive GI procedures, invasive genitourinary procedures, and invasive pulmonary procedures
- the need to carry or wear medical identification describing the type of valvular heart disease and the need for anticoagulant therapy.

Appendices

Appendix A

Emergency drugs

This chart summarizes the indications, dosages, routes, and nursing implications for drugs commonly administered for selected emergencies.

Drug	Indications	Dosage and Route	Nursing Implications
adenosine	• Paroxysmal supraventricular tachycardia (PSVT) • Wide-complex tachycardia of unknown origin	*I.V. bolus:* >6 mg rapid followed by 20 ml saline flush; if no response occurs in 1 to 2 minutes, may repeat with 12 mg rapid I.V. bolus and 20 ml saline flush	• Monitor for asystole after bolus, as a brief period may occur. • Monitor for flushing, dyspnea, and chest pain, which should resolve spontaneously in 1 to 2 minutes.
aminophylline	Status asthmaticus	*Loading dose:* 5 to 6 mg/kg I.V. over 20 to 30 minutes (if patient is not on regular oral theophylline therapy) *Maintenance dosage:* 0.4 to 0.7 mg/kg/hour I.V. by continuous infusion	• Use after epinephrine, sympathomimetic aerosol agents, and corticosteroids. • Avoid in patients with supraventricular tachycardia (SVT). • Use cautiously in patients with ischemic heart disease.
atropine	• Symptomatic sinus bradycardia • Asystole • Pulseless electrical activity refractory to epinephrine	*I.V. bolus:* for asystole, 1 mg I.V. push, repeated in 5 minutes if asystole persists; for bradycardia, 0.5 mg I.V. push *Endotracheal:* 1 to 2 mg diluted to a total 10 ml with sterile water or normal saline	• Administer with caution in patients with myocardial ischemia secondary to increased MVO_2. • Monitor for anticholinergic side effects. • Know that denervated transplanted hearts will not respond to atropine and may require pacing.

Emergency drugs *(continued)*

Drug	Indications	Dosage and route	Nursing Implications
bretylium	• Ventricular fibrillation • Pulseless ventricular tachycardia refractory to other therapy	*I.V. bolus:* 250 to 500 mg or 5 mg/kg I.V. push; may double-dose (10 mg/kg) and repeat every 15 to 30 minutes to a maximum dosage of 2.5 g *I.V. infusion:* 1 to 2 mg/minute; add 5 to 10 mg/kg to 50 ml of D_5W	• Know that bretylium may take 2 minutes to reach the central circulation. • Monitor for profound hypotension.
calcium chloride	• Hypocalcemia • Hypokalemia • Calcium channel blocker toxicity	*I.V. bolus:* 500 mg to 1 g I.V. via a central vein, repeat every 10 minutes if necessary	• Monitor ECG. • Monitor for signs of coronary and cerebral artery vasospasm.
diazepam	Status epilepticus	5 to 10 mg I.V. at a rate not to exceed 5 mg/minute; repeated at 10- to 15-minute intervals as needed up to a maximum dosage of 30 mg per seizure episode; repeat regimen in 2 to 4 hours if necessary, but do not exceed total dosage of 100 mg within 24 hours	Observe for respiratory depression.
diltiazem	Control ventricular rate in atrial fibrillation and atrial flutter	*Loading dose:* 0.25 mg/kg over 2 minutes *Maintenance infusion:* 5 to 15 mg/hour titrated to heart rate; doses > 15 mg/hour not recommended	Know that an I.V. infusion lasting longer than 24 hours is not recommended.

Emergency drugs *(continued)*

Drug	Indications	Dosage and Route	Nursing Implications
dobutamine	• Hypotension and low cardiac output • Hypotension with pulmonary congestion and left ventricular dysfunction	*I.V. infusion:* 2.5 to 10 mcg/kg/minute	• Monitor for tachycardia, arrhythmias, fluctuations in blood pressure, and worsening myocardial ischemia. • Administer via an infusion pump to ensure precise flow rates.
dopamine	• Cardiogenic shock • Hypotension in the absence of hypovolemia • Hypotension with symptomatic bradycardia	*I.V. infusion:* 2 to 5 mcg/kg/minute *I.V. infusion:* 5 to 20 mcg/kg/minute; increase the dosage gradually, if needed, in increments of 5 to 10 mcg/kg/minute until the optimum response is achieved	• Monitor for pulmonary congestion even at low dosages. • Monitor for induced or exacerbated SVT. • Add norepinephrine to dopamine dosage if greater than 20 mcg/kg/minute. • Taper dopamine gradually to avoid acute hypotension.
epinephrine	• Ventricular fibrillation and pulseless ventricular tachycardia • Asystole • Refractory pulseless electrical activity • Symptomatic bradycardia	*I.V. bolus:* 1 mg (1 to 10 ml of a 1:10,000 solution) I.V. push, repeated every 3 to 5 minutes until myocardial contractility is restored *Endotracheal:* 1 mg (10 ml of a 1:10,000 solution) followed by 2 to 3 ml of sterile saline solution *I.V. infusion:* 1 to 4 mcg/minute, titrated according to effect	• Do not mix epinephrine with alkaline solutions. • Monitor for effect of increased MVO_2 (myocardial oxygen consumption).

Emergency drugs (continued)

Drug	Indications	Dosage and Route	Nursing Implications
epinephrine (continued)	Status asthmaticus, severe anaphylaxis	Initially, 0.1 to 0.5 mg (0.1 to 0.5 ml of a 1:1,000 solution) S.C. or I.M., repeated at 10- to 15-minute intervals if needed; or 0.1 to 0.25 mg (1 to 2.5 ml of a 1:10,000 solution) I.V. slowly over 5 to 10 minutes, repeated every 5 to 15 minutes as needed or followed by a 1 to 4 mcg/minute I.V. infusion	Do not mix epinephrine with alkaline solutions.
glucagon	Insulin shock	0.5 to 1 mg S.C., I.M., or I.V., repeated once or twice if patient does not awaken within 5 to 20 minutes of the first injection.	• Do not mix the glucagon I.V. solution with solutions containing calcium, potassium, or sodium chloride because precipitation may occur. Glucagon does not precipitate in dextrose solution. • Monitor the patient's blood glucose level before, during, and after glucagon administration.
isoproterenol	Refractory bradyarrhythmia and significant bradycardia in the denervated heart	Dose is 2 to 10 mcg/minute I.V. infusion	• Use a volumetric infusion pump. • Monitor for increased MVO_2. • Monitor for serious arrhythmias.
labetalol	Hypertensive crisis	*I.V. bolus:* 10 to 20 mg I.V. push over 2 minutes, repeated every 10 min-	• Monitor the patient's blood pressure frequently during and after labe-

702

Emergency drugs *(continued)*

Drug	Indications	Dosage and Route	Nursing Implications
labetalol *(continued)*		utes if needed until a total of 300 mg is reached *I.V. infusion:* 2 mg/minute until blood pressure is controlled	talol administration. • Do not mix labetalol with 5% sodium bicarbonate injection because they are incompatible.
lidocaine	• Ventricular tachycardia • Ventricular fibrillation • VPCs especially with myocardial infarct or ischemia	*I.V. bolus:* 1 mg/kg I.V. push, followed by additional 0.5 mg/kg boluses every 8 to 10 minutes, if needed, until a total of 3 mg/kg is reached *I.V. infusion:* after successful resuscitation, 1 to 4 mg/minute	Monitor for signs of CNS toxicity, especially slurred speech and altered level of consciousness.
magnesium sulfate	• Refractory ventricular fibrillation and pulseless ventricular tachycardia • Torsades de pointes • Post-infarct arrhythmias or PSVT • Hypomagnesemia	Administer 1 to 2 g I.V. push over 1 to 2 minutes; for I.V. infusion, 0.5 to 1 g/hour for 24 hours with magnesium deficiency	Monitor for hypotension and asystole. Monitor for signs of hypermagnesemia.
morphine sulfate	• Acute myocardial infarction • Acute cardiogenic pulmonary edema	Administer 1 to 3 mg I.V. push every 5 minutes and titrate for desired hemodynamic response	• Monitor for respiratory depression; use 0.4 to 0.08 mg I.V. naloxone for excessive narcosis. • Hypotension is most common and most severe in volume-depleted patients.

Emergency drugs *(continued)*

Drug	Indications	Dosage and Route	Nursing Implications
naloxone	Opiate drug overdose	0.4 mg I.V., S.C., or I.M., repeated every 2 to 3 minutes for three doses	Dilute naloxone in D_5W or normal saline solution for I.V. administration; use it within 24 hours of mixing or discard it.
nitroglycerin	• Acute myocardial infarction • Angina • Congestive heart failure	0.3 to 0.4 mg tablets S.L. every 5 minutes for a total of 3 tablets; 12.5 to 25 mcg I.V. bolus at initiation of infusion followed by 10 to 20 mcg/ minute; I.V. infusion increments titrated to desired clinical effect	Monitor for hypotension; use hemodynamic monitoring during therapy. • Monitor for ventilation-perfusion mismatch with resultant hypoxia.
nitroprusside	• Hypertensive crisis • Acute left ventricular failure	*I.V. infusion:* 0.5 to 10 mcg/kg/ minute	• Monitor the patient continuously to detect a rapid, profound decrease in blood pressure. • Protect I.V. solution from light by wrapping the I.V. bag in opaque material. • Know that cyanide toxicity can occur after prolonged infusion of high doses. • Administer nitroprusside using an infusion pump. • Reconstitute the drug in D_5W only. • Discard any remaining nitroprusside 24 hours after reconstitution.

Emergency drugs *(continued)*

Drug	Indications	Dosage and Route	Nursing Implications
norepi-nephrine	Hemodynamically significant hypotension refractory to other sympathomimetic amines	*I.V. infusion:* 0.5 to 1 mcg to start and titrate to achieve desired affect; adult dose 2 to 12 mcg/minute	Infuse via a central line and avoid extravasation, which results in tissue ischemia, necrosis, and sloughing. • Monitor blood pressure continuously. • Monitor for affect of Increased MVO_2. • Monitor for arrhythmias.
procainam-ide	• Ventricular fibrillation • Pulseless ventricular tachycardia refractory to other therapy, including bretylium	*I.V. bolus:* 20 to 30 mg/minute until arrhythmia is suppressed, hypotension occurs, QRS complex is >50% baseline value, or a total of 1 g has been administered *I.V. infusion:* 1 to 4 mg/minute	• Decrease the dosage as prescribed for a patient with renal dysfunction. • Monitor the blood concentration levels; continued dosages are based on these levels. • Administer via an infusion pump.
sodium bi-carbonate	Hyperkalemia • Preexisting metabolic acidosis • Tricyclic or phenobarbital overdose • After CPR to buffer "acid wash-out"	*I.V. bolus:* 1 mEq/kg I.V. push; then 0.5 mEq/kg every 10 minutes according to arterial blood gas values	• Base repeated doses on arterial blood pH or laboratory values. • Causes other drugs to precipitate out and become inactive.
verapamil	• PSVT after administration of adenosine • Reentry atrial fibrillation and atrial flutter	2 to 2.5 mg I.V. slow over 2 minutes; if no response occurs, 5 to 10 mg I.V. over 2 minutes every 15 to 30 minutes up to a total of 20 mg	• Do not use in patients with Wolff-Parkinson-White syndrome or left ventricular dysfunction. • Monitor for hypotension.

Appendix B

Common laboratory test values

BLOOD CHEMISTRY
Acid phosphatase
0.5 to 1.9 U/L
Alanine aminotransferase
Men: 10 to 32 U/L
Women: 9 to 24 U/L
Alkaline phosphatase, serum
1.5 to 4 Bodansky units/dl
4 to 13.5 King-Armstrong units/dl
Chemical inhibition method: Men,
90 to 239 U/L; Women < age 45, 76
to 196 U/L; women > age 45, 87 to
250 U/L
Ammonia, plasma
< 50 µg/dl
Amylase, serum
30 to 220 U/L
Anion gap
8-14 mEq/liter
Arterial blood gases
pH: 7.35 to 7.42
PaO2: 75 to 100 mm Hg
PaCO2: 35 to 45 mm Hg
O_2CT: 15% to 23%
O_2Sat: 94% to 100%
HCO_3-: 22 to 26 mEq/liter
Aspartate aminotransferase
8 to 20 U/L
Atrial natriuretic factor, plasma
20-77 pg/ml
Bilirubin, serum
Adult: direct, < 0.5 mg/dl; indirect, ≤
1.1 mg/dl
Blood urea nitrogen
8 to 20 mg/dl
C-reactive protein, serum
Negative
Calcium, serum
4.5 to 5.5 mEq/liter
Atomic absorption: 8.9 to 10.1 mg/dl
Carbon dioxide, total, blood
22 to 34 mEq/liter
Catecholamines, plasma
Supine: epinephrine, 0 to 110 pg/ml;
norepinephrine, 70 to 750 pg/ml; do-
pamine, 0 to 30 pg/ml

Standing: epinephrine, 0 to 140
pg/ml; norepinephrine, 200 to 1,700
pg/ml; dopamine, 0 to 30 pg/ml
Chloride, serum
100 to 108 mEq/liter
Cholesterol, total, serum
0 to 240 mg/dl
CK-BB: None
CK-MB: 0 to 7 IU/liter
CK-MM: 5 to 70 IU/liter
Creatine
Males: 0.2 to 0.6 mg/dl
Females: 0.6 to 1.0 mg/dl
Creatine kinase
Total: Men, 25 to 130 U/L; Women,
10 to 150 U/L
Creatinine, serum
Males: 0.8 to 1.2 mg/dl
Females: 0.6 to 0.9 mg/dl
Free thyroxine, serum
0.8 to 3.3 ng/dl
Free triiodothyronine
0.2 to 0.6 ng/dl
Gamma glutamyl transferase
Males: 8 to 37 U/L
Females: < age 45, 5 to 27 U/L; >
age 45, 6 to 37 U/L
Glucose, plasma, fasting
70 to 100 mg/dl
**Glucose, plasma, 2-hour post-
prandial**
< 145 mg/dl
Hydroxybutyric dehydrogenase
Serum HBD: 114 to 290 U/ml
LD/HBD ratio: 1.2 to 1.6:1
Iron, serum
Men: 70 to 150 µg/dl
Women: 80 to 150 µg/dl
Lactic acid, blood
0.93 to 1.65 mEq/liter
Lactate dehydrogenase
Total: 48 to 115 IU/liter
LD_1: 14% to 26%
LD_2: 29% to 39%
LD_3: 20% to 26%
LD_4: 8% to 16%
LD_5: 6% to 16%

Common laboratory test values *(continued)*

Lipase
< 300 U/L
Lipoproteins, serum
HDL-cholesterol: 29 to 77 mg/dl
LDL-cholesterol: 62 to 185 mg/dl
Magnesium, serum
1.5 to 2.5 mEq/liter
Atomic absorption: 1.7 to 2.1 mg/dl
Phosphates, serum
1.8 to 2.6 mEq/liter
Atomic absorption: 2.5 to 4.5 mg/dl
Potassium, serum
3.8 to 5.5 mEq/liter
Protein, total, serum
6.6 to 7.9 g/dl
Albumin fraction: 3.3 to 4.5 g/dl
Globulin level: alpha$_1$-globulin, 0.1 to 0.4 g/dl; alpha$_2$-globulin, 0.5 to 1 g/dl; beta globulin, 0.7 to 1.2 g/dl; and gamma globulin, 0.5 to 1.6 g/dl
Sodium, serum
135 to 145 mEq/liter
Thyroxine, total, serum
5 to 13.5 µg/dl
Triglycerides, serum
Men: 40 to 160 mg/dl
Women: 35 to 135 mg/dl
Uric acid, serum
Men: 4.3 to 8 mg/dl
Women: 2.3 to 6 mg/dl

HEMATOLOGY
Activated partial thromboplastin time
25 to 36 seconds
Bleeding time
Template: 2 to 8 minutes
Ivy: 1 to 7 minutes
Duke: 1 to 3 minutes
Clot retraction
50%
Erythrocyte sedimentation rate
Males: 0 to 10 mm/hour
Females: 0 to 20 mm/hour
Fibrin split products
Screening assay: < 10 µg/ml
Quantitative assay: < 3 µg/ml
Fibrinogen, plasma
195 to 365 mg/dl
Hematocrit
Men: 42% to 54%

Women: 38% to 46%
Hemoglobin, total
Men: 14 to 18 g/dl
Women: 12 to 16 g/dl
Platelet aggregation
3 to 5 minutes
Platelet count
130,000 to 370,000/mm^3
Platelet survival
50% tagged platelets disappear within 84 to 116 hours
100% disappear within 8 to 10 days
Prothrombin time
10 to 14 seconds
Prothrombin consumption time
20 seconds
Red blood cell count
Men: 4.5 to 6.2 million/ml venous blood
Women: 4.2 to 5.4 million/µl venous blood
Red cell indices
MCV: 84 to 99 fl
MCH: 26 to 32 fl
MCHC: 30 to 36 g/dl
Reticulocyte count
0.5% to 2% of total RBC count
Sickle cell test
Negative
Thrombin time, plasma
10 to 15 seconds
White blood cell count, blood
4,100 to 10,900/µl
White blood cell differential, blood
Neutrophils: 47.6% to 76.8%
Lymphocytes: 16.2% to 43%
Monocytes: 0.6% to 9.6%
Eosinophils: 0.3% to 7.0%
Basophils: 0.3% to 2.0 %
Whole blood clotting time
5 to 15 minutes

URINE CHEMISTRY
Amylase, urine
10 to 80 amylase units/hour
Bence Jones protein, urine
Negative
Bilirubin, urine
Negative

Common laboratory test values *(continued)*

Calcium, urine
Males: < 275 mg/24 hours
Females: < 250 mg/24 hours
Calculi, urine
None
Catecholamines, urine
24-hour specimen: 0 to 135 µg
Random specimen: 0 to 18 µg/dl
Creatinine clearance
Men: 107 to 139 ml/minute
Women: 87 to 107 ml/minute
Creatinine, urine
Men: 1.0 to 1.9 g/24 hours
Women: 0.8 to 1.7 g/24 hours
Glucose, urine
Negative
17-Hydroxycorticosteroids, urine
Men: 4.5 to 12 mg/24 hours
Women: 2.5 to 10 mg/24 hours
17-Ketogenic steroids, urine
Men: 4 to 14 mg/24 hours
Women: 2 to 12 mg/24 hours
Ketones, urine
Negative
17-Ketosteroids, urine
Men: 6 to 21 mg/24 hours
Women: 4 to 17 mg/24 hours
Phenolsulfonphthalein excretion, urine
15 minutes: 25% of dose excreted
30 minutes: 50% to 60% of dose excreted
1 hour: 60% to 79% of dose excreted
2 hours: 70% to 80% of dose excreted
Protein, urine
≤ 150 mg/24 hours
Red blood cells, urine
0 to 3 per high-power field
Sodium, urine
30 to 280 mEq/24 hours
Sodium chloride, urine
5 to 20 g/24 hours
Urea, urine
Maximal clearance: 64 to 99 ml/minute
Uric acid, urine
250 to 750 mg/24 hours
Urinalysis, routine
Color: Straw
Odor: Slightly aromatic

Appearance: Clear
Specific gravity: 1.005 to 1.035
pH: 4.5 to 8.0
Sugars: None
Epithelial cells: Few
Casts: None, except occasional hyaline casts
Crystals: Present
Yeast cells: None
Urine concentration
Specific gravity: 1.025 to 1.032
Osmolality: > 800 mOsm/kg water
Urine dilution
Specific gravity: < 1.003
Osmolality: < 100 mOsm/kg
80% of water excreted in 4 hours
Urobilinogen, urine
Men: 0.3 to 2.1 Ehrlich units/2 hours
Women: 0.1 to 1.1 Ehrlich units/2 hours
Vanillylmandelic acid, urine
0.7 to 6.8 mg/24 hours
White blood cell count, urine
0 to 4 per high-power field

MISCELLANEOUS
Cerebrospinal fluid
Pressure: 50 to 180 mm H_2O
Lupus erythematosus cell preparation
Negative
Esophageal acidity
pH > 5.0
Occult blood, fecal
< 2.5 mg/24 hours
Rheumatoid factor, serum
Negative
Pericardial fluid
Amount: < 50 ml
Appearance: clear, straw-colored
Urobilinogen, fecal
50 to 300 mg/24 hours
VDRL, serum
Negative

708

Appendix C

Therapeutic and toxic drug levels

The following chart presents therapeutic or toxic levels for selected drugs or ingested toxins that are frequently encountered in the hospital setting.

Drug or Ingested Toxin	Adult Therapeutic Range	Toxic Level
acetaminophen	Not applicable	>150 g/ml[*]
digoxin	0.8 to 2 ng/ml	0.2 ng/ml
ethanol and isopropanol	Not applicable	>400 mg/dl (causing respiratory arrest)
ethylene glycol	Not applicable	.20 mg/dl
iron	Not applicable	>20 mg/kg ingested
lidocaine	1.5 to 5 mcg/dl	>5 mcg/ml
lithium[**]	1 to 1.5 mEq/liter for acute mania 0.6 to 1.2 mEq/liter to prevent relapse of bipolar disorder	>2 mEq/liter
methanol	Not applicable	>20 mg/dl >50 mg/dl (causing blindness)
nitroprusside	3 to 10 mcg/kg/minute	> 15 mcg/kg/minute (causing cyanide toxicity
phenobarbital	15 to 40 mcg/ml	> 40 mcg/ml
phenytoin	10 to 20 mcg/ml	> 20 mcg/ml
salicylate	10 to 30 mg/100 ml for arthritis	> 20 mg/100 ml (causing mild toxicity) > 30 mg/100 ml (causing tinnitus)
theophylline	10 to 20 mcg/ml	> 20 mcg/ml

[*] Based on nomogram for acute ingestion and only accurate if time of ingestion is known.
[**] Potential for toxic symptoms in therapeutic range.

Appendix D

Normal hemodynamic variables

Invasive hemodynamic monitoring is widely used in the critical care setting. Various monitoring devices allow health care personnel to diagnose a patient's hemodynamic status and to evaluate the effectiveness of treatments. The chart below lists the normal values for certain hemodynamic parameters.

Hemodynamic variable	Definition	Normal value
Pulmonary artery systolic (PAS) pressure	Peak pressure of the right ventricle	20 to 30 mm Hg
Pulmonary artery diastolic (PAD) pressure	Lowest pressure produced in the pulmonary artery; also an indirect measurement of the left atrial pressure (LAP)	10 to 15 mm Hg
Mean pulmonary artery pressure (PAP)	Average of the systolic and diastolic pulmonary artery pressures; also known as mean pulmonary artery pressure	10 to 20 mm Hg
Pulmonary capillary wedge pressure (PCWP)	Indirect measurement of LAP and left ventricular end diastolic pressure (LVEDP)	4 to 12 mm Hg
Cardiac output (CO)	Volume of blood ejected from the left ventricle per minute	4 to 6 liters/minute
Cardiac index (CI)	Cardiac output per unit time divided by patient's body surface area	2.5 to 4.2 liters/minute/m^2
Systemic vascular resistance (SVR)	Measurement of left ventricular afterload	900 to 1,200 dynes/second/cm^{-5}
Pulmonary vascular resistance (PVR)	Measurement of right ventricular afterload, that is, the total resistance to blood flow in the pulmonary circulation	20 to 120 dynes/second/cm^{-5}

Normal hemodynamic variables *(continued)*

Hemodynamic variable	Definition	Normal value
Mixed venous oxygen saturation ($S\bar{v}O_2$)	Measurement of the balance between oxygen supply (delivery) and oxygen demand (consumption); decreased hemoglobin, decreased oxygen saturation, and decreased cardiac output can cause decreased oxygen supply, whereas conditions that increase the metabolic rate, such as fever or sepsis, can cause an increased rate of oxygen consumption	60% to 80 %

Appendix E

Commonly encountered nursing diagnoses in critical care

This chart links the disease pathologies addressed in the text with the associated nursing diagnoses most commonly encountered in the critical care setting.

	Abdominal trauma	Acquired immunodeficiency syndrome (AIDS)	Adult respiratory distress syndrome (ARDS)	Angina	Aortic aneurysm	Arrhythmias	Aspiration	Asthma	Bowel disorders	Brain tumors	Burns	Cardiac trauma	Cardiomyopathy	Cerebral aneurysm	Cerebrovascular accident (CVA)	Congestive heart failure (CHF)	Diabetes insipidus	Diabetic ketoacidosis	Disseminated intravascular coagulation	Electrolyte imbalances	Encephalopathy	Gastrointestinal hemorrhage	Head trauma	Hepatic failure
Altered urinary elimination									x	x				x	x								x	
Altered nutrition: less than body requirements	x	x	x		x				x		x							x				x	x	x
Altered oral mucous membranes		x	x								x													
Altered tissue perfusion			x	x		x		x			x	x	x	x	x	x		x	x			x		x
Body image disturbance		x							x	x	x					x							x	
Bowel incontinence	x				x				x	x	x				x	x				x		x		x
Bowel constipation											x									x	x		x	
Decreased cardiac output	x			x	x	x		x			x	x	x			x	x		x					
Dysfunctional ventilatory weaning response		x					x	x													x			
Hyperthermia											x			x	x								x	
Hypothermia														x	x							x		
Impaired gas exchange	x		x	x	x		x	x			x		x			x			x					
Impaired physical mobility	x			x	x				x	x	x			x	x	x							x	
Impaired skin integrity	x										x											x		x
Impaired tissue integrity	x										x													
Impaired verbal communication		x								x				x	x								x	
Inability to sustain spontaneous ventilation		x					x	x																
Ineffective airway clearance		x						x																
Ineffective breathing pattern		x						x																x
Ineffective individual coping		x		x					x	x														
Knowledge deficit	x	x	x	x	x											x		x				x		
Pain	x	x		x	x		x		x	x	x	x		x						x	x	x	x	x
Risk for activity intolerance	x	x	x	x	x	x	x	x	x	x	x	x	x	x	x	x	x		x	x	x	x	x	x
Risk for aspiration		x					x	x						x	x								x	
Risk for fluid volume deficit	x								x		x	x					x	x	x	x				x
Risk for fluid volume excess									x				x	x						x	x	x		x
Risk for infection	x	x	x	x			x		x	x	x												x	x
Risk for peripheral neurovascular dysfunction										x		x		x	x					x	x		x	
Risk for suffocation		x					x			x					x									
Sensory/perceptual alterations									x	x	x			x	x							x	x	x
Sleep pattern disturbance		x					x			x	x			x	x							x	x	
Unilateral neglect										x				x	x								x	

Commonly encountered nursing diagnoses in critical care (continued)

	Hyperosmolar hyperglycemic nonketotic syndrome (HHNS)	Hypertensive crisis	Hypoglycemia	Immunosuppression	Myocardial conduction defects	Myocardial infarction	Near drowning	Organ transplantation	Pancreatitis	Pericarditis	Peripheral vascular disease	Pneumonia	Pneumothorax	Pulmonary embolism	Renal failure	Renal trauma	Respiratory failure	Seizures	Shock	Spinal cord injury	Syndrome of inappropriate antidiuretic hormone secretion (SIADH)	Thoracic trauma	Toxic ingestion	Valvular heart disease
Altered urinary elimination							x								x	x			x	x				
Altered nutrition: less than body requirements			x									x	x		x		x		x	x			x	
Altered oral mucous membranes				x											x		x						x	
Altered tissue perfusion		x			x	x	x	x		x	x		x	x	x		x		x	x		x	x	x
Body image disturbance								x			x									x				
Bowel incontinence	x																			x				
Bowel constipation																				x				
Decreased cardiac output		x			x	x		x		x				x					x	x		x		x
Dysfunctional ventilatory weaning response								x				x					x		x					
Hyperthermia												x							x					
Hypothermia							x												x					
Impaired gas exchange	x	x				x	x					x	x	x	x	x	x		x	x		x		
Impaired physical mobility						x	x		x		x	x				x			x	x				
Impaired skin integrity								x			x													
Impaired tissue integrity								x			x													
Impaired verbal communication																				x				
Inability to sustain spontaneous ventilation								x				x					x		x	x		x	x	
Ineffective airway clearance								x				x					x		x					
Ineffective breathing pattern								x				x	x	x			x		x		x	x	x	
Ineffective individual coping				x		x					x				x		x		x		x			x
Knowledge deficit			x			x					x				x		x		x		x		x	x
Pain		x				x			x	x	x		x	x	x	x			x	x		x	x	x
Risk for activity intolerance	x	x	x	x	x	x	x	x	x	x	x	x	x	x	x	x	x		x		x	x	x	x
Risk for aspiration	x							x									x	x	x				x	
Risk for fluid volume deficit	x						x	x				x							x			x	x	x
Risk for fluid volume excess								x							x	x								
Risk for infection	x		x	x			x	x	x	x	x				x	x					x		x	x
Risk for peripheral neurovascular dysfunction								x			x			x					x	x				x
Risk for suffocation								x				x	x	x		x			x				x	x
Sensory/perceptual alterations			x				x											x	x	x			x	
Sleep pattern disturbance								x		x								x	x	x	x		x	
Unilateral neglect																			x	x				

Selected References

Allen, M.A., and Shelton, B.K. "Neutropenia," in Wright, J.E., and Shelton, B.K., eds. *Desk Reference for Critical Care Nursing.* Boston: Jones & Bartlett, 1993.

Alspach, J.G., ed. *AACN Core Curriculum for Critical Care Nursing,* 4th ed. Philadelphia: W.B. Saunders Co., 1991.

Armstrong, Shanna L. "Cerebral Vasospasm: Early Detection and Intervention," *Critical Care Nurse,* 14(4): 33-37, 1994.

Barrett, W.L., et al. "Critical Course of Malignancies in Renal Transplant Recipients," *Cancer,* 72(2):2186-2189, 1993.

Beauchamp, T.L., and Childress, J.F. *Principles of Biomedical Ethics.* New York: Oxford University Press, 1994.

Brown, K.K. "Critical Interventions in Septic Shock," Part 2. *American Journal of Nursing,* 94(10): 21-26, 1994.

Brown, K.K. "Septic Shock: How to Stop the Deadly Cascade," Part 1. *American Journal of Nursing,* 94(9): 20-26, 1994.

Calfee, B. "7 Things You Should Never Chart," *Nursing94,* 24(3): 43, 1994.

Cardona, V.D., et al., eds. *Trauma Nursing: From Resuscitation Through Rehabilitation.* Philadelphia: W.B. Saunders Co., 1994.

Clochesy, J.M., et al., eds. *Critical Care Nursing.* Philadelphia: W.B. Saunders Co., 1993.

Conover, M. "Wellen's Syndrome: Identification of Critical Proximal Left Anterior Descending Stenosis," *Critical Care Nurse,* 10: 30-36, 1990.

Critical Care Skills: A Nurse's Photoguide. Springhouse, Pa.: Springhouse Corporation, 1996.

Currie, Donna L. "Pulmonary Embolism: Diagnosis and Management," *Critical Care Nursing Quarterly,* 13(2): 41-49, Aspen Publishers, 1993.

Dossey, B.M., et al. *Critical Care Nursing,* 3rd ed. Philadelphia: J.B. Lippincott Co., 1992.

Dotson, R.G., et al. "Gastroesophageal Reflux with Nasogastric Tubes: Effect of the Nasogastric Tube Size," *Am J Resp Crit Care Med,* 149(6): 1659-1662, 1994.

Falk, J.L., et al. "Fluid Resuscitation in Traumatic Hemorrhagic Shock," *Critical Care Clinics,* 8(2): 323-340, 1992.

Fan, H., et al. *The Biology of AIDS,* 3rd ed. Boston: Jones and Bartlett Publishers, 1994.

Hudak, C.M., and Gallo, B.M. *Critical Care Nursing: A Holistic Approach.* Philadelphia: J.B. Lippincott Co., 1994.

Jacobs, D.S., et al. *Laboratory Test Handbook.* Cleveland: Lexi-Comp Inc., 1994.

Kay, G.N., and Bubien, R.S. *Clinical Management of Cardiac Arrhythmias.* Gaithersburg, Md.: Aspen Publishers, 1992.

Krause, E. "Radiosurgery: A Nursing Perspective," *Journal of Neuroscience Nursing,* 23(1): 24-28, February 1991.

Lederle, F.A. "Management of Small Abdominal Aortic Aneurysms," *Annals of Internal Medicine,* 113: 731-732, 1990.

Lentz, Steven R. "Disorders of Hemostasis," in Woodley, M., and Whelan, A., eds. *The Washington Manual: Manual of Medical Therapeutics,* 27th ed. Boston: Little, Brown and Co., 1992.

Lewis, S.M. *Medical-Surgical Nursing: Assessment and Management of Clinical Problems,* 3rd ed. St. Louis: Mosby Year Book Inc., 1992.

Lorell, B., and Braunwald, E. "Pericardial Disease," in Braunwald, E., ed. *Heart Disease: A Textbook of Cardiovascular Medicine.* Philadelphia: W.B. Saunders Co., 1988.

Luckman, J., and Sorensen, K. *Medical-Surgical Nursing: A Physiological Approach,* 4th ed. Philadelphia: W.B. Saunders Co., 1993.

Malon, J.F., et al. "Lung Transplantation," *Critical Care Nursing Clinics of North America,* 4(1): 111-129, 1992.

March, Karen. "Retrograde Jugular Catheter: SjO_2 Monitoring," *Journal of Neuroscience Nursing,* 1(26): 48-51, 1994.

McConnell, E.A. "Loosening the Grip of Intestinal Obstruction," *Nursing94,* 3: 34-41, 1994.

Mullan, H., et al. "Risk of Pulmonary Aspiration among Patients Receiving Enteral Nutrition Support," *J Parent Nutr.,* 16(2): 160-164, 1994.

Murrihead, J. "Heart and Heart-Lung Transplantation," *Critical Care Nursing Clinics of North America,* 4(1): 97-109, 1994.

Papadimitriou, L., et al. "Protecting Against the Acid Aspiration Syndrome in Adult Patients Undergoing Emergency Surgery," *Hepato-Gastroenterol,* 39(6): 560-561, 1992.

Paradiso, Catherine. "Liver and Biliary Disorders," in *Lippincott's Review Series: Pathophysiology.* Philadelphia: J.B. Lippincott Co., 1995.

Payne, J.L. "Immune Modification and Complications of Immunosuppression," *Critical Care Nursing Clinics of North America,* 4(1): 43-61, 1992.

Reising, D. "Acute Hypoglycemia: Keeping the Bottom from Falling Out," *Nursing95,* 25(2): 41-48, 1995.

Richard, R.L., and Staley, M.J. *Burn Care and Rehabilitation: Principles and Practice.* Philadelphia: F.A. Davis Co., 1994.

Rippe, J.M., et al. *Intensive Care Medicine,* 2nd ed. Boston: Little, Brown, & Co., 1991.

Ross, A.M., et al. "Prognosticators of Outcome After Major Head Injury in the Elderly," *Journal of Neuroscience Nursing,* 2(24):88-93, 1992.

Schwartz, G.R., et al. *Principles and Practices of Emergency Medicine,* 3rd ed. Philadelphia: Lea & Febiger, 1992.

Shantz, D., and Spitz, M.C. "What You Need to Know About Seizures," *Nursing93,* 11:34-40, 1993.

Sheehy, S.B., and Jimmerson, C.L. *Manual of Clinical Trauma Care: The First Hour,* 2nd ed. St. Louis: Mosby, 1994.

Shlafer, M. *The Nurse, Pharmacology, and Drug Therapy: A Prototype Approach,* 2nd ed. New York: Addison-Wesley, 1992.

Slutsky, A.S. "ACCP Consensus Conference: Mechanical Ventilation," *Respiratory Care,* 38(12): 1389-1413, 1993.

Springhouse Certification Review: Critical Care Nursing. Springhouse, Pa.: Springhouse Corporation, 1996.

Strong, J. "Tuberculous Pericarditis in Transkei," *Clinical Cardiology,* 5: 667, 1984.

Swearingen, P.J., and Keen, J.H. *Manual of Critical Care,* 2nd ed. St. Louis: Mosby, 1991.

Teplitz, L. "Transcatheter Ablation of Tachyarrhythmias: An Overview and Case Studies," *Progress in Cardiovascular Nursing,* 9(3): 16-31, 1994.

Testani-Dufour, L., et al. "Traumatic Brain Injury: A Family Experience," *Journal of Neuroscience Nursing,* 6(24):317-323, 1992.

Thelan, L.A., et al. *Critical Care Nursing: Diagnosis and Management,* 2nd ed. Philadelphia: Mosby, 1994.

Thompson, C. "Managing Acute Pancreatitis," *RN,* 3: 52-56, 1992.

Wait, M., and Estrada, A. "Changing Spectrum of Spontaneous Pneumothorax," *American Journal of Surgery,* 164(5): 528-31, 1992.

Warbinek, E., and Wyness, M.A. "Caring for Patients with Complications after Elective Abdominal Aortic Aneurysm Surgery: A Case Study," *Journal of Vascular Nursing,* 12: 73-79, 1994.

White-Williams, C. "Immunosuppressive Therapy Following Cardiac Transplantation," Critical Care Nursing Quarterly, 16(2): 1-10, 1993.

716

Index

A

Abdominal trauma, 14-24
assessment for, 15, 16t, 17, 18t-19t
cardiac function in, 23
complications of, 21t
diagnosis of, 19, 20t
discharge planning for, 24
fluid and electrolyte balance in, 20-22
infection control in, 22-23
organ injuries associated with, 18t-19t
pathophysiology of, 14-15
prognosis for, 24
respiratory function in, 23
surgery for, 23-24
treatment for, 19-24
Aberrant conduction, 92i
Ablation, 97, 415t
Abscess formation, 21t
Absence seizures, 601t
Accelerated idioventricular rhythm, 88i, 88t-89t
Accelerated junctional rhythm, 86i, 86t-87t
Accessory pathways, 414-416, 422-423
Acetaminophen, toxic ingestion of, 669-670
Acidosis
diabetic ketoacidosis and, 241-242
near drowning and, 451-453
Acoustic neuroma, 135t
Acquired immunodeficiency syndrome (AIDS), 25-36
assessment for, 26-27, 30t
cancer therapy for, 34-35
case definitions for, 28t-29t
diagnosis of, 27, 31t-32t
discharge planning for, 36
drug therapy for, 29-30, 32
immunologic function in, 35-36
infection prevention in, 32-34
pathophysiology of, 25-26

Acquired immunodeficiency syndrome (AIDS) (continued)
prognosis for, 36
treatment for, 29-36
Activated charcoal, 682
Addison's disease, 276
Adhesion, 124i
Adult respiratory distress syndrome (ARDS), 37-51, 667t
assessment for, 39-40, 41t, 46t
complications of, 46t, 50
decreased lung compliance in, 38-39
diagnosis of, 40-41, 42t-43t
discharge planning for, 51
drug therapy for, 48-49
hemodynamic monitoring in, 47-48
hypoxemia in, 39
nutritional support in, 49
pathophysiology of, 37, 38t, 39
prognosis for, 50
pulmonary edema in, 38
stages of, 37, 40, 41t, 42t-43t
treatment for, 41-50
ventilatory management of, 44-47
Advance directives, 11-12
Aging, myocardial conduction defects and, 413
AIDS. See Acquired immunodeficiency syndrome; AIDS dementia complex.
AIDS dementia complex, 291, 295t, 298t, 300t
Alcohol
hepatic failure and, 341, 348t
toxic ingestion of, 670, 671t, 672
Aldosteronism, 276
Allograft, 459
American Nurses Association's Code for Nurses, 12

Aneurysm
aortic, 65-77
cerebral, 188-200
Angina, 51-65
assessment for, 54-55, 56t
complications of, 63
diagnosis of, 56, 57t, 58
discharge planning for, 65
drug therapy for, 60, 61t-62t
ECG changes in, 58i
myocardial oxygen consumption in, 53t
pathophysiology of, 52, 53t, 54t
prognosis for, 63
revascularization for, 60, 62, 64t-65t
severity of, 56t
treatment for, 59-60, 61t-62t, 63, 64t-65t
Wellens' syndrome and, 54t
Angiography, 57t, 128t, 317t
Angioplasty, 64t, 510
Antiarrhythmic drugs, 95t-96t
Anticoagulation therapy, 547t, 691-692
Antidepressants, toxic ingestion of, 673
Antidiuretic hormone (ADH), 227-230, 275, 640-652
Anuria, 558, 559-560
Anxiety, hypertensive crisis and, 378-379
Aortic aneurysm, 65-77
assessment for, 70, 71t
classification of, 66, 67i-68i
complications of, 76t
diagnosis of, 71, 72t
discharge planning for, 77
location of, 68i, 71t
morphology of, 67i
pathophysiology of, 68, 69t
prognosis for, 77
risk factors for, 69t
surgery for, 74-76
treatment for, 72-73, 74i, 75, 76t

Burns *(continued)*
  fluid replacement in, 157t
  pathophysiology of, 148-151
  prognosis for, 161
  severity of, 148t, 152i
  treatment for, 155-156, 157t, 158-159, 160t
  types of, 148t
  wound care for, 160t

C

Calcium, 270t-271t, 484t
Calcium channel blockers, 61t
Cancer. *See* Acquired immuno-deficiency syndrome; Brain tumors; Chemotherapy.
Carbamates, toxic ingestion of, 673-674
Cardiac catheterization, 57t, 181t
Cardiac enzyme studies, 57t
Cardiac output, myocardial conduction defects and, 418-419
Cardiac tamponade, 164i, 499t-500t, 660t, 664t
Cardiac trauma, 162-173
  assessment for, 165-167, 171t-172t
  cardiac function and, 170
  cardiac tamponade and, 164i
  complications of, 171t-172t
  diagnosis of, 167t, 168t
  discharge planning for, 172-173
  hemodynamic support in, 170
  myocardial contusion and, 163i
  pathophysiology of, 162-165
  pericardiocentesis and, 168t
  prognosis for, 172
  respiratory function and, 170
  treatment for, 168, 169i, 170-172
Cardiogenic shock, 611, 612, 615t, 618t, 622, 623i
Cardiomyopathy, 173-188
  assessment for, 176-177, 178t-179t
  classification of, 174i
  diagnosis of, 177, 180t-181t

Cardiomyopathy *(continued)*
  discharge planning for, 187-188
  pathophysiology of, 173, 174i, 175-176
  pericarditis and, 496t-497t
  prognosis for, 187
  treatment for, 177-179, 181, 182i, 183-184, 185i, 186-187
Cerebral aneurysm, 188-200
  assessment for, 191-192
  classification of, 193t
  complications of, 198-200
  diagnosis of, 192, 194t
  discharge planning for, 200
  drug therapy for, 196-197
  fluid therapy for, 196-197
  pathophysiology of, 188-190
  prognosis for, 200
  subarachnoid hemorrhage in, 188, 193t, 194t
  surgery for, 197-198, 199t
  treatment for, 192, 194-198, 199t, 200
  types of, 190t
Cerebral edema, 136
Cerebral perfusion pressure, 336t
Cerebrovascular accident (CVA), 200-213
  assessment for, 203, 204t, 205, 206t, 207
  cerebral circulation and, 202i
  diagnosis of, 207, 210t
  discharge planning for, 212-213
  Glasgow Coma Scale and, 206t
  location of, 208t-209t
  neurologic deficits and, 208t-209t
  pathophysiology of, 201-203
  predisposing factors for, 203t
  prognosis for, 212
  transient ischemic attacks and, 204t
  treatment for, 204t, 208-209, 211-212
Chemotherapy
  acquired immunodeficiency syndrome and, 34-35
  brain tumors and, 145

Chest pain. *See* Angina.
Chest trauma. *See* Thoracic trauma.
Chest tube insertion, 533t
Cholecystitis, 21t
Chylothorax, 659t, 662t
Cirrhosis, 344, 346, 347t
Coagulation factors, 255i-256i
Cocaine, toxic ingestion of, 672-673
Colon, injury to, 19t
Colonoscopy, 128t, 313t
Coma, hepatic, 340t
Computed tomography (CT) scan, 20t, 72t, 143t
Concussion, 326t
Conduction defects. *See* Myocardial conduction defects.
Congenital anomalies, 414
Congestive heart failure (CHF), 213-226
  assessment for, 218-219, 220t
  classification of, 219t
  diagnosis of, 219, 221t-222t
  discharge planning for, 226
  drug therapy for, 220, 222, 223t-224t
  fluid volume management in, 224-225
  Frank-Starling mechanism in, 215, 216i
  pathophysiology of, 213-215, 216i, 217-218
  prognosis for, 226
  treatment for, 220, 222, 223t-224t, 225-226
Contusion, 325t
Coronary arteries, 427i, 443-444
  bypass surgery and, 65t
  stent placement and, 64t
Coronary artery disease. *See* Myocardial infarction.
Coronary ultrasound, 57t
Corticosteroids, 117t-118t
Cranial nerve deficits, 141t-142t
Craniopharyngioma, 136t
Creutzfeldt-Jakob disease, 291
Critical pathways, 3-4
Cyclic antidepressants, toxic ingestion of, 673

i refers to an illustration; t, to a table

---

i refers to an illustration; t, to a table

W-Z